CLINICAL BIOCHEMISTRY
OF
DOMESTIC ANIMALS

Second Edition
VOLUME I

Contributors

J. C. Bartley

D. F. Brobst

Charles E. Cornelius

George T. Dimopoullos

J. J. Kaneko

Mogens G. Simesen

John S. Wilkinson

CLINICAL BIOCHEMISTRY
OF
DOMESTIC ANIMALS

Second Edition
VOLUME I

Edited by

J. J. KANEKO

Department of Clinical Pathology
University of California
Davis, California

and

C. E. CORNELIUS

Department of Physiological Sciences
Kansas State University
Manhattan, Kansas

ACADEMIC PRESS   1970   New York and London

ACADEMIC PRESS, INC.
111 Fifth Avenue, New York, New York 10003

United Kingdom Edition published by
ACADEMIC PRESS, INC. (LONDON) LTD.
Berkeley Square House, London W1X 6BA

LIBRARY OF CONGRESS CATALOG CARD NUMBER: 72-117089

PRINTED IN THE UNITED STATES OF AMERICA

Contents

9. CALCIUM, INORGANIC PHOSPHORUS,
    AND MAGNESIUM METABOLISM IN
    HEALTH AND DISEASE

    Mogens G. Simesen

10. IRON METABOLISM

    J. J. Kaneko

List of Contributors

Numbers in parentheses indicate the pages on which the authors' contributions begin.

J. C. Bartley (53), Bruce Lyon Memorial Research Laboratory, Children's Hospital Medical Center of Northern California, Oakland, California

D. F. Brobst* (231), Department of Veterinary Microbiology, Pathology and Public Health, Purdue University, Lafayette, Indiana

Charles E. Cornelius (161), Department of Physiological Sciences, Kansas State University, Manhattan, Kansas

George T. Dimopoullos (97), Department of Veterinary Science, Agricultural Experiment Station, Louisiana State University, Baton Rouge, Louisiana

J. J. Kaneko (1, 131, 293, 377), Department of Clinical Pathology, University of California, Davis, California

Mogens G. Simesen (313), Department of Special Pathology and Therapeutics, Royal Veterinary and Agricultural University, Copenhagen, Denmark

John S. Wilkinson (247), Department of Veterinary Clinical Pathology, School of Veterinary Science, University of Melbourne, Australia

*Present address: Department of Veterinary Clinical Medicine and Surgery, Washington State University, Pullman, Washington

Preface to the Second Edition

The marked expansion of knowledge in the clinical biochemistry of animals since publication of the first edition of this book seven years ago has necessitated this major revision. In this period, a wealth of new information on clinical biochemical aspects of disease in animals has become available. This has been made possible by the continued rapid advances of modern biochemistry, the increasing awareness of the usefulness of animal models of human disease in biomedical research, and the ever increasing growth of both veterinary and human medicine. In keeping with this expansion of knowledge, this edition is comprised of two volumes. Chapters on the pancreas, thyroid, and pituitary–adrenal systems have been separated and entirely rewritten. Completely new chapters on muscle metabolism, iron metabolism, blood clotting, and gastrointestinal function have been added. All the chapters of the first edition have been revised with pertinent new information, and many have been completely rewritten.

Emphasis continues to be placed on the interpretation of biochemical findings in disease of the domestic animal species. A notable exception is the inclusion of information on subhuman primates in the chapter on liver function. We can already anticipate a marked expansion of biochemical knowledge on primates as well as on laboratory animal species that will be included in subsequent editions.

Keeping pace with the explosive expansion of new biochemical knowledge among a variety of animal species is a formidable task for the veterinary student, his teachers, the veterinary practitioner, the biomedical researcher, and the experimental biologist. It is our hope that this volume, primarily devoted to the interpretation of biochemical findings in diseases of animals, will contribute to the accomplishment of this task.

We are deeply indebted to the contributors for their dedicated efforts and perseverance. Thanks are also due to the users of the first edition whose many helpful suggestions have guided this revision. Finally, we extend our greatest appreciation to our wives, Frances and Bette, and our families who have cheerfully persevered through this second edition.

J. J. Kaneko
June, 1970   **C. E. Cornelius**

Preface to the First Edition

Interest in the clinical biochemistry of animals has increased rapidly in the past decade owing to the expansion and growth of veterinary science as well as the increasing use of domestic animals in comparative medical research. Selected data concerning the changes which occur in the chemical constituents of the blood and tissues can provide for a better understanding of the disease process as well as supply information helpful in differential diagnosis, therapy, and prognostication. This book represents a first attempt to provide the veterinary student, the practitioner of veterinary medicine, and the experimentalist with a specific volume of information concerning the interpretation of biochemical findings in diseases of domestic animals, and it does not purport to be a laboratory manual. Methods, however, are included whenever their understanding is believed to greatly enhance the interpretation of the blood chemical findings. The normal values of the various blood constituents as determined by more recent methods should be of help to all experimental biologists. The information has been gathered from the internationally available scientific literature and, in addition, includes original data obtained in the laboratories of the Department of Clinical Pathology, University of California.

Experience in the clinical laboratory has impressed the editors with the difficulty students and practicing veterinarians encounter in bridging the gap between the fundamental sciences and the practice of clinical animal medicine. It is the hope of the editors that this volume will be of help in the application of some of this highly specialized basic knowledge to animal diseases. The topics included in this volume reflect the diagnostic areas of emphasis presently taught in the second semester of a year course in clinical pathology at the School of Veterinary Medicine of the University of California. The editors welcome suggestions for topics to be added in subsequent editions.

C. E. Cornelius

J. J. Kaneko

March, 1963

Contents of Volume II

1   Carbohydrate Metabolism

J. J. Kaneko

I. INTRODUCTION

The sustenance of animal life is dependent on the availability of chemical energy in the form of foodstuffs. The ultimate source of this energy is the sun, and the transformation of solar energy to chemical energy in a form usable by animals is dependent on the chlorophyll-containing plants. The photosynthetic process leading to the reduction of CO_2 to carbohydrates may be summarized:

$$CO_2 + H_2O \xrightarrow[\text{chlorophyll}]{\text{light}} (CH_2O)_x + O_2 \uparrow$$

The principal carbohydrate synthesized by plants and utilized by animals is starch. The large amounts of indigestible cellulose synthesized by plants are utilized by the herbivorous animals, which depend on the cellulolytic action of the microbial flora in their digestive tracts.

The biochemical mechanisms by which the chemical energy of foodstuffs are made available to the animal are collectively described as metabolism. Thus, the description of the metabolism of a foodstuff encompasses the biochemical events which occur from the moment of ingestion to its final breakdown and excretion. It is convenient to retain the classical division of metabolism into the three major foodstuffs: carbohydrates, lipids, and proteins. The metabolism of the lipids and proteins are discussed in other chapters.

The major function of the ingested carbohydrate is to serve as a source of energy and its storage function is relatively minor. Carbohydrates also function as precursors of essential intermediates for use in synthetic processes. When the metabolic machinery of an animal is disrupted, a disease state prevails, e.g., diabetes. The widespread interest and present status of knowledge concerning metabolism and disease is a direct result of the contributions of modern biochemistry. As a corollary, a knowledge of biochemistry is essential. This chapter is not presented as an exhaustive treatise on the subject of carbohydrate biochemistry, but rather as a basis for the better understanding of the disorders associated with carbohydrate metabolism.

II. DIGESTION

The digestion of carbohydrates in the animal organism begins with the initial contact of these foodstuffs with the enzymes of salivary juice. Starch of plant foods and glycogen of meat are split into their constituent monosaccharides by the action of amylase and maltase. This activity ceases as the food matter passes into the stomach, where the enzymic action is destroyed by the hydrochloric acid. Within the stomach, acid hydrolysis may occur, but the stomach empties too rapidly for complete hydrolysis to take place. Thus, only a small portion of the ingested carbohydrate is acted upon prior to entrance into the small intestine. Here digestion of carbohydrates takes place quickly by action of the carbohydrate-splitting enzymes contained in the copious quantities of pancreatic juice and in the succus entericus. Starch and glycogen are hydrolyzed to glucose by amylase and maltase; lactose to glucose and galactose by lactase; and sucrose to glucose and fructose by sucrase.

These monosaccharide products, glucose, fructose, and galactose, of enzymic hydrolysis of the complex carbohydrates are the principal forms in which absorption occurs.

III. ABSORPTION

The monosaccharides are almost completely absorbed through the mucosa of the small intestine and appear in the portal circulation as the free sugars. Absorption occurs by two methods: (1) simple diffusion and (2) by an as yet inadequately explained active method. Glucose and galactose are absorbed rapidly and by both methods. Fructose is absorbed at about half the rate of glucose with a portion being converted to glucose in the process. Other monosaccharides, e.g., mannose, are absorbed slowly at a rate consistent with a simple diffusion process. A theory which has remained prevalent to explain the active absorption of glucose across the intestinal mucosa is that the carbohydrates are phosphorylated in the mucosal cell. This process assumes that the phosphorylated sugars are transferred across the mucosal cell and then rehydrolyzed, because free glucose appears in the portal circulation.

IV. METABOLISM OF ABSORBED CARBOHYDRATES

A. GENERAL

The carbohydrate absorbed from the intestine is transported to the liver via the portal circulation. Within the liver, there are several general pathways by which the immediate fate of the absorbed carbohydrate is determined. Fructose and galactose first enter the general metabolic scheme through a series of complex reactions to form glucose phosphates (Fig. 1). The enzyme, galactose-1-P uridyl transferase, which catalyzes the reaction:

$$\text{Galactose-1-P} + \text{UDP-glucose} \longrightarrow \text{UDP-galactose} + \text{glucose-1-P}$$

is blocked or deficient in congenital galactosemia of man (Isselbacher, 1959). The glucose phosphates formed may be converted to and stored as glycogen, catabolized to CO_2 and water or, as free glucose, may return to the general circulation. Essentially then, intermediate carbohydrate metabolism of animals evolves about the metabolism of glucose, and the liver becomes the organ of prime importance.

B. STORAGE AS GLYCOGEN

Glycogen is the chief storage form of carbohydrate in the animal organism and is analogous to the storage of starch by plants. It is found primarily in the liver and in muscle, where it occurs at about 3–6% and about 0.5%, respectively (see Table I).

Glycogen is comprised solely of α-D-glucose units linked together through carbon atoms 1 and 4 or 1 and 6. Straight chains of glucose units are formed by the 1–4 links and these are crosslinked by the 1–6 links. The result is a complex ramification

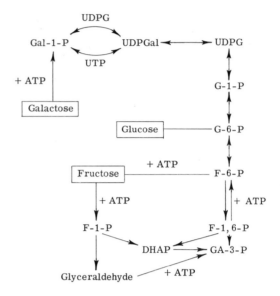

Fig. 1. Pathways for hexose metabolism. ATP = adenosine triphosphate; DHAP = dihydroxy-acetone phosphate; F-1-P = fructose-1-phosphate; F-6-P = fructose-6-phosphate; F-1, 6-P = fructose-1,6-diphosphate; G-1-P = glucose-1-phosphate; G-6-P = glucose-6-phosphate; GA-3-P = gluceral-dehyde-3-phosphate; Gal-1-P = galactose-1-phosphate; UDPG = uridine diphosphate glucose; UDPGal = uridine diphosphate galactose; UTP = uridine triphosphate.

of chains of glucosyl units with branch points at the site of the 1–6 links (Fig. 2). The internal chains of the glycogen molecule have an average length of four glucosyl units. The external chains beyond the last 1–6 link are longer and contain between seven and ten glucose units (Cori, 1954). The molecular weights may range as high as four million and contain upward of 20,000 glucosyl units.

In Table II, the amount of carbohydrate available to meet the theoretical requirements of a hypothetical dog is shown. The amount present is sufficient for about half a day. It is apparent that the needs of the body which must be continually met are satisfied by alternate means and not solely dependent on continuous ingestion of carbohydrates. During and after feeding (postprandial), absorbed hexoses are converted to glucose by the liver and enter the general circulation. Excesses may be stored as glycogen or as fat. During the fasting or postabsorptive state, glucose

TABLE I   LIVER GLYCOGEN OF ANIMALS

Species	Percent glycogen in liver	Reference
Dog	6.1	Lusk (1928)
Sheep	3.8	Roderick et al. (1933)
Cow (lactating)	1.0	Kronfeld et al. (1960)
Cow (nonlactating)	3.0	Kronfeld et al. (1960)
Baby pig	5.2	Morrill (1952)
Baby pig (newborn)	14.8	Swiatek et al. (1968)

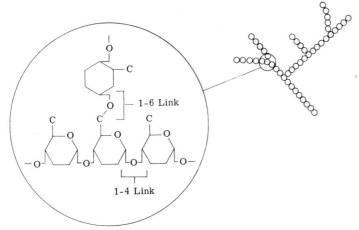

Fig. 2.   Glycogen structure. (Adapted from Cori, 1954.)

is supplied by the conversion of protein (gluconeogenesis) as well as by the breakdown of available glycogen. The continued rapid synthesis and breakdown of glycogen, i.e., turnover, is well illustrated by the finding that the biological half-time of glycogen is about a day.

C. GLYCOGEN METABOLISM

The process by which liver glycogen is formed from the absorbed sugars is known as glycogenesis. On degradation, or glycogenolysis, glucose is released. It had long been assumed that the synthesis and breakdown of glycogen was a direct reversal of the synthetic process. Recently, however, the work of Leloir *et al.* (1959; Leloir and Cardini, 1957) has served to clarify these mechanisms and provides a basis for their discussion as two separate pathways.

1. Glycogenesis

The initial reaction required for the entrance of glucose into the series of metabolic reactions which culminate in the synthesis of glycogen is the phosphorylation

TABLE II   CARBOHYDRATE BALANCE OF A DOG[a]

Muscle glycogen (0.5%)	25	gm
Liver glycogen (6%)	18	gm
Carbohydrate in fluids (100 mg%)	2.2	gm
	45.2	gm

Caloric value (45.2 × 4 kcal/gm) = 181 kcal
Caloric requirement (70 kg$^{3/4}$ = 70 × 5.6) = 392 kcal/day

$$\frac{181}{392} \times 24 \text{ hours} = 11 \text{ hours}$$

[a]Body weight = 10 kg; liver weight = 300 gm; muscle weight = 5 kg; volume of blood and extracellular fluid = 2.2 liters.

of glucose at the C-6 position. Glucose is phosphorylated by adenosine triphosphate (ATP) in liver by an irreversible enzymic reaction which involves the presence of a specific glucokinase:

$$\text{Glucose} + \text{ATP} \xrightarrow[\text{(hexokinase)}]{\text{glucokinase}} \text{glucose-6-P} + \text{ADP} \tag{1}$$

Liver contains both a nonspecific hexokinase and a glucose-specific glucokinase. The high Michaelis constant ($K_m = 10^{-2}$) of the glucokinase which is found only in the liver, indicates a low affinity for glucose. The rate of the phosphorylation reaction catalyzed by glucokinase is therefore controlled by the glucose concentration. The activity of this enzyme is increased by glucose feeding and by insulin and is decreased during fasting and in diabetes. The low Michaelis constant ($K_m = 10^{-5}$) of the nonspecific hexokinase, which is also found in liver, muscle, and in all tissues, indicates a high affinity for glucose and the hexokinase-catalyzed phosphorylation is not controlled by glucose concentration. Activity of this enzyme is not affected by fasting or carbohydrate feeding, diabetes, or insulin treatment.

This unidirectional phosphorylation permits the accumulation of glucose in the liver cells since the phosphorylated sugars do not pass freely in and out of the cell, in contrast to the readily diffusible free sugars. The glucose-6-phosphate (G-6-P) trapped in the cell next undergoes a mutation in which the phosphate grouping is transferred to the C-1 position of the glucose molecule. This reaction is catalyzed by the enzyme phosphoglucomutase and involves glucose-1,6-diphosphate as the intermediate:

$$\text{G-6-P} \longleftrightarrow \text{G-1-P} \tag{2}$$

Glycogen is synthesized from this glucose-1-phosphate (G-1-P) through reactions involving the formation of uridine derivatives. Uridine diphosphoglucose (UDPG) is synthesized by the transfer of glucose from G-1-P to uridine triphosphate (UTP). This reaction is catalyzed by the enzyme UDPG pyrophosphorylase:

$$\text{UTP} + \text{G-1-P} \longrightarrow \text{UDPG} + \text{PP} \tag{3}$$

In the presence of a polysaccharide primer and the enzyme UDPG glycogentransglucosidase (glycogen synthetase), the glucose moiety of UDPG is linked to the polysaccharide by an α-1–4 link:

$$\text{UDPG} + (\text{glucose-1,4})_n \xrightarrow[\text{transglucosidase}]{\text{UDPG glycogen}} (\text{glucose-1,4})_{n+1} + \text{UDP} \tag{4}$$

Through repeated transfers of glucose, the polysaccharide chain is lengthened. When the chain length of the polysaccharide reaches an as yet undetermined critical level (between 7 and 21 glucose units), the brancher enzyme, amylo-1,4–1,6-transglucosidase, transfers the terminal portion from an α-1–4 linkage to an α-1–6 linkage. The newly established 1–6 linkage thus becomes a branch point in the glycogen molecule. Approximately 7% of the glucose units comprising a glycogen molecule are involved in these branch points (Illingworth and Cori, 1952).

2. *Glycogenolysis*

The breakdown of liver glycogen to glucose takes place via a separate pathway. In the presence of inorganic phosphate, the predominant 1–4 linkages of glycogen are successively broken by an active phosphorylase. This reaction cleaves the 1–4 link by the addition of orthophosphate in a manner analogous to a hydrolytic cleavage with water, hence the term "phosphorolysis." Phosphate is added to the C-1 position of one glucose moiety while H^+ is added to the C-4 position of the other. Extensive investigations of Sutherland and co-workers (Rall *et al.*, 1956; Sutherland and Wosilait, 1956) have clarified the influence of glucagon and epinephrine in the phosphorolytic breakdown of glycogen. The phosphorolytic enzyme exists in liver in two forms: an active form designated liver phosphorylase (LP), which contains phosphate, and an inactive form, in which phosphate has been removed, which is designated dephosphophosphorylase (dephospho-LP). The transformations between the active and inactive forms are catalyzed by specific kinase enzymes.

The level of an active form then becomes the resultant of the rates of activation and deactivation. Normally, the level of active form is low, with most of the enzyme in its inactive form. Epinephrine and glucagon shift the equilibrium toward a higher level of LP. The net result is an increase in the phosphorolytic breakdown of glycogen to glucose, a fact reflected in the well-known hyperglycemia observed after injection of these hormones. The mechanism of action of glucagon and epinephrine (also serotonin) is through their stimulation of the liver cell via adenyl cyclase (Robison *et al.*, 1968) to form a special nucleotide, 3',5'-adenosine monophosphate (3',5'-AMP) from ATP (Rall *et al.*, 1957; Rall and Sutherland, 1958). The 3',5'-AMP in turn stimulates the activation of LP.

Cyclic 3',5'-AMP has now been shown to be a key regulating factor in a number of cellular processes in addition to LP activation. It is a requirement for the activation of inactive phosphorylase b to active phosphorylase a in muscle (Anstall, 1968). The actions of other hormones known to be mediated by increasing cyclic 3',5'-AMP include ACTH, LH, TSH, MSH, T_3, and insulin (Robison *et al.*, 1968). From these findings, a general concept of hormone action has evolved in which the hormone is the first messenger and cyclic 3',5'-AMP is the second messenger which is found in the target cell.

The action of glucagon appears to be confined to liver glycogen, whereas epinephrine acts on both liver and muscle glycogen in a similar manner. In liver, glucagon promotes the formation of glucose but the end result with muscle glycogen is different. Since the enzyme glucose-6-phosphatase (G-6-Pase) is absent from muscle, glycogen breakdown here results in the production of pyruvate and lactate rather than glucose.

The continued action of LP on the 1–4 linkages results in the successive formation of G-1-P units until a branch point in the glycogen molecule is reached. The residue is a limit dextrin. The debrancher enzyme, amylo-1,6-glucosidase, then cleaves the 1–6 linkage, releasing free glucose. The remaining 1–4 linked chain of the molecule is again open to attack by LP until another limit dextrin is formed. Thus, by the combined action of LP and the debrancher enzyme, the glycogen molecule is successively reduced to G-1-P and free glucose.

G-1-P is converted to G-6-P by the reversible reaction catalyzed by phosphoglucomutase (Section IV,C,1, reaction 2). The G-6-P is then irreversibly cleaved to free glucose and phosphate by the enzyme G-6-Pase, which is found in liver and kidney. The free glucose formed can, unlike its phosphorylated intermediates, leave the hepatic cell to enter the general circulation, thereby contributing to blood glucose. In muscle tissue, there is no G-6-Pase and muscle glycogen cannot supply glucose directly by glycogenolysis. Muscle glycogen contributes to blood glucose indirectly via the lactic acid cycle (Section IV,D). The series of reactions described are illustrated schematically in Fig. 3.

3. Hormonal Influences on Glycogen Metabolism

The biochemical basis for the glycogenolytic and hyperglycemic action of glucagon and epinephrine is discussed in Section IV,C,2. This effect of epinephrine is the basis for the epinephrine tolerance test commonly employed to assess the availability of liver glycogen for providing blood sugar. Many other hormones are known to have effects upon carbohydrate metabolism, a fact which further indicates that metabolism should be considered an integrated concept.

One of the results of successful insulin therapy is a restoration of the depleted glycogen reserve. The mechanism of insulin action upon carbohydrate metabolism continues to be a subject for debate and is discussed more fully in Section VI.

The early reports from Cori's group (Colowick et al., 1947) formed the basis for a useful concept of integrated hormonal action at the phosphorylation (glucokinase) level. Under this hexokinase theory, which is not generally accepted, the glucokinase reaction is inhibited by the presence of the diabetogenic anterior pituitary factor growth hormone (GH) or somatotropin (STH). Growth hormone has among its effects, enhancement of liver glycogen storage, a sparing of carbohydrate, and enhancement of fat utilization. The inhibition of the glucokinase reaction by GH is relieved by the presence of insulin. The net result is that these two hormones act antagonistically. Under the permeability theory, the result of insulin action appears

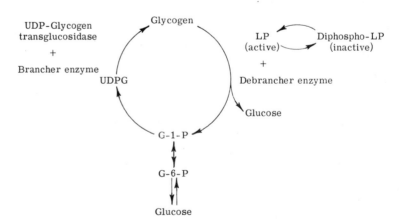

Fig. 3.   Summary of liver glycogen metabolism. In muscle, phosphorylase a is the active form and phosphorylase b is the inactive form. See text for abbreviations.

to be that it promotes glucose entry into the cell. Thus, intracellular glucose would accumulate, and glucose utilization toward glycogen synthesis or oxidation would be favored. This concept is now generally accepted as a major mechanism of insulin action.

Promotion of liver glycogen storage is also one of the effects of the glucocorticoids. This effect may be attributed to their enhancement of the conversion of noncarbohydrate substances, primarily protein, to glucose. Explanations for gluconeogenesis from protein, however, remain inadequate. A possible explanation may lie in the observation by Rosen et al. (1959) that the glucocorticoids have a stimulatory influence upon the glutamic-pyruvic transaminase system. The transaminase systems provide a pathway for entrance of amino acids into the Krebs tricarboxylic acid (TCA) cycle, from which a pathway leading to the formation of glucose is available.

A tendency toward a mild hyperglycemia is present in hyperthyroid states in man. The observed hyperglycemia is probably the result of a number of factors influencing carbohydrate metabolism. Thyroxine is thought to render the liver more sensitive to the action of epinephrine, thus resulting in increased glycogenolysis. Increased glycogenolysis and gluconeogenesis may also be the compensatory result of the increased rate of tissue metabolism. A recent observation by Freedland et al. (1968) that hepatic G-6-Pase activities increased markedly in rats made hyperthyroid is consistent with the viewpoint that hepatic glucose production is increased in hyperthyroid states.

4.   Glycogen in Disease

In disease states, alterations in glycogen are generally observed as decreases. Depletion of liver glycogen stores is seen in diabetes mellitus, bovine ketosis, and ovine pregnancy toxemia. Pathological increases in liver glycogen content are seen in the rare glycogen storage diseases (GSD) of man. Much of the present information concerning the metabolism of glycogen is a direct result of the intensive interest in this disease in the last decade. No clearly established counterpart of these diseases has yet been reported in domestic animals. A von Gierke-like syndrome in the dog, however, has been reported (Bardens, 1966). It will become apparent that the ultimate diagnosis of these conditions depends on biochemical studies of the tissues involved, and procedures for their analysis are available (Illingworth and Cori, 1952). This group of disease entities has been classified into six types on the basis of clinical and biochemical findings (Field, 1966).

Liver glycogen is found in high concentration in classical von Gierke's disease or type 1 according to the Cori classification (Cori, 1954), which leads to a hepatomegaly. The response of the blood sugar to the epinephrine tolerance test is minimal or absent. The liver glycogen in this form of GSD has been shown to have a normal structure, and the defect to lie in a deficiency of the enzyme G-6-Pase. Enzyme deficiencies also account for the abnormal structures of glycogen found in types 3 and 4 of GSD. Glycogen analyses have indicated that in type 3 the debrancher enzyme is deficient. The glucose chains are shorter, and the glycogen molecule has an increased number of branch points. In type 4, with a brancher enzyme deficiency, the chains are longer, and fewer branch points are present. Muscle and liver phosphorylase are absent in types 5 and 6, respectively.

D. Catabolism of Glucose

Carbohydrate in the form of glucose is the principal source of energy for the life processes of the mammalian cell. All cells require a constant supply of this indispensable nutrient, and only relatively small changes may be tolerated without adverse effects on the health of the animal. Glucose is not oxidized directly to CO_2 and H_2O, but rather through a series of stepwise reactions involving phosphorylated intermediates. The chemical energy of glucose is "stored" through the synthesis of "high-energy" phosphate bonds during the course of these reactions and is used in other metabolic reactions.

The subject of carbohydrate metabolism continues to be extensively studied and a voluminous literature is available. The principal pathways of glucose catabolism have been elucidated sufficiently to permit their discussion separately. Emphasis is, however, being placed on the interrelationships of the pathways rather than on the details of the individual reactions. Detailed discussions of the individual reactions involved may be found in the many excellent texts on biochemistry presently available.

1.   Pathways of Glucose-6-Phosphate Metabolism

The fundamental conversion required to initiate the reaction sequences for the oxidation of glucose by the cell is a phosphorylation to form G-6-P. This reaction has been described in Section IV,C,1. The G-6-P formed as a result of the glucokinase (or hexokinase) reaction occupies a central position in glucose metabolism. There are at least five different pathways which may be followed: free glucose; glycogenesis; glycolysis; pentose cycle; and glucuronate pathway.

a. Free Glucose. The simplest pathway is the separate reverse reaction by which G-6-P is cleaved to form free glucose and inorganic phosphate. This reaction is catalyzed by the enzyme G-6-Pase:

$$G\text{-}6\text{-}PO_4 \xrightarrow{\text{G-6-Pase}} glucose + phosphate$$

The energetics are such that this is an essentially irreversible reaction and opposes the previously described unidirectional glucokinase reaction. These two opposing independently catalyzed enzyme reactions offer a site of metabolic control, whereby the activities of the enzymes play a regulatory role. Significant amounts of G-6-Pase are found only in liver and to a lesser extent in the kidney. This is in accord with the well-known function of the liver as the principal source of supply of free glucose for the maintenance of blood glucose concentration.

Muscle tissue, due to the absence of G-6-Pase, cannot contribute glucose to the blood directly from muscle glycogen breakdown. Muscle glycogen does, however, contribute indirectly via a pathway designated the lactic acid or Cori cycle. Lactic acid formed in muscle via muscle glycolysis is transported to the liver, where it is resynthesized to glucose and its precursors as outlined in Fig. 4.

b. Glycogenesis. This pathway for G-6-P leading to the synthesis of glycogen has been discussed in Section IV,C,1.

c. Glycolysis. One of the three oxidative pathways of G-6-P is the classic

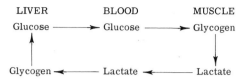

Fig. 4.   Lactic acid cycle. Muscle glycogen indirectly contributes to blood glucose by this pathway.

anaerobic Embden-Meyerhof (E-M) glycolytic pathway. The intermediate steps involved in this pathway of breakdown of G-6-P to three-carbon compounds are summarized in Fig. 5. A mole of ATP is used in the phosphorylation of fructose-6-phosphate (F-6-P) to form fructose-1,6-diphosphate (F-1,6-P). This phosphorylation is essentially an irreversible reaction catalyzed by a specific kinase, phosphofructokinase (PFK). The opposing unidirectional reaction is catalyzed by a specific phosphatase, fructose-1,6-diphosphatase (F-1,6-Pase). The opposing PFK and F-1,6-Pase catalyzed reactions offer a second site of metabolic control regulated by the activities of the two enzymes. It should be noted that, starting from glucose, a total of two high-energy phosphates from ATP have been donated to form a mole of F-1,6-P.

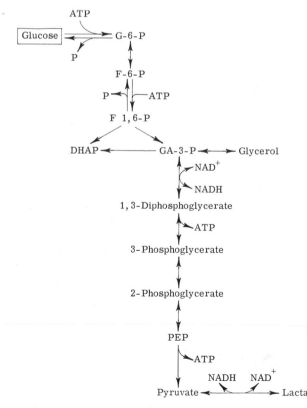

Fig. 5.   The glycolytic or classic E-M pathway. P = phosphate. See text for other abbreviations.

Fructose-1,6-diphosphate is then cleaved to form two 3-carbon compounds as shown in Fig. 5. Next, an oxidative step occurs in the presence of glyceraldehyde-3-phosphate dehydrogenase (GA-3-PD) with oxidized nicotinamide adenine dinucleotide (NAD$^+$), formerly called diphosphopyridine nucleotide (DPN$^+$) as the hydrogen acceptor. During the process, the molecule is phosphorylated. In the succeeding steps, the molecule is dephosphorylated at the points indicated, and a mole of ATP generated at each point.

A third site of control of glycolysis is the unidirectional formation of pyruvate by the pyruvic kinase (PK) reaction which is circumvented by two enzymic reactions. Pyruvic carboxylase (PC) catalyzes the carboxylation of pyruvate to oxalacetate (OAA) and the OAA is converted to phosphoenolpyruvate (PEP) by the enzyme PEP carboxykinase (PEP-CK) (Figs. 5 and 8). Thus, the overall conversion of 1 mole of glucose to 2 moles of pyruvate requires 2 moles of ATP for the initial phosphorylations, and a total of 4 moles of ATP are generated in the subsequent dephosphorylations. This net gain of 2 moles of ATP represents the useful energy of glycolysis.

For repeated functioning of the glycolytic pathway, a supply of NAD$^+$ (DPN$^+$) must be available for use in the oxidative step. In the presence of molecular O_2, reduced NADH (DPNH) is reoxidized via the cytochrome system:

$$H^+ + NADH + \tfrac{1}{2}O_2 \xrightarrow[\text{(system)}]{\text{(cytochrome)}} NAD^+ + H_2O$$

In the absence of O_2, i.e., anaerobiosis, NADH (DPNH) is reoxidized to NAD$^+$ (DPN$^+$) in a reaction catalyzed by lactic dehydrogenase, whereby pyruvic acid is reduced to lactic acid. Thus, by this "coupling" of enzymic reactions, glucose breakdown may continue in periods of anaerobiosis.

d. PENTOSE CYCLE.   This alternate route of G-6-P oxidation has been referred to by a number of terms such as the pentose cycle, direct oxidative pathway, Warburg-Dickens scheme or the hexose monophosphate "shunt." The initial step involves the oxidation of G-6-P at the C-1 position to form 6-phosphogluconic acid as summarized in Fig. 6. The reaction is catalyzed by G-6-P dehydrogenase (G-6-PD), and in this pathway, oxidized NAD phosphate (NADP$^+$), formerly called triphosphopyridine nucleotide (TPN$^+$) serves as the hydrogen acceptor. In the second oxidative step, 6-phosphogluconate (6-PG) is oxidatively decarboxylated by 6-PG dehydrogenase (6-PGD) to yield a pentose phosphate, ribulose-5-phosphate, again in the presence of NADP$^+$ (TPN$^+$). Thus, in the initial reactions, which are essentially irreversible, 2 moles of NADPH (TPNH) are formed. It should be noted that in this pathway only the C-1 carbon atom of the glucose molecule is evolved as CO_2. By contrast, glucose catabolism via the glycolytic scheme results in the loss of both the C-1 and C-6 carbon atoms when pyruvate is oxidatively decarboxylated to form acetyl coenzyme A (Ac-CoA). This phenomenon has been employed in a number of studies in which the relative contributions of the glycolytic and pentose phosphate pathways have been assessed in domestic animals (Black et al., 1957). The subsequent metabolism of the ribulose-5-phosphate formed is also shown in Fig. 6. As a result of the series of transformations, F-6-P and glyceraldehyde-3-phosphate are formed.

For continued functioning of this pathway, a supply of NADP$^+$ (TPN$^+$) must be available to function as a hydrogen acceptor. NADP$^+$ (TPN$^+$) is regenerated from NADPH (TPNH) via the cytochrome system in the presence of O_2, and thus the

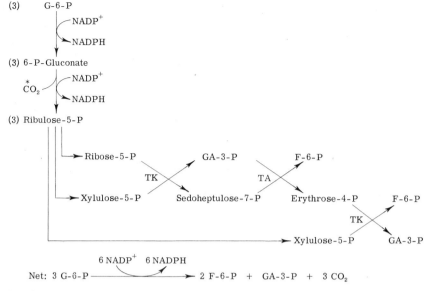

Fig. 6. The pentose cycle or hexose monophosphate shunt pathway. TK = transketolase; TA = transaldolase; C^*O_2 = derived from C-1 of glucose; $NADP^+$ = nicotinamide adenine dinucleotide phosphate.

pentose cycle is an aerobic pathway of glucose oxidation. Reduced NADPH (TPNH) is also required as a hydrogen donor in the synthesis of fatty acids. This has led to the formulation of a hypothesis for a link between carbohydrate metabolism and that of fat (Siperstein and Fagan, 1957). According to this hypothesis, the availability of NADPH (TPNH) generated in the pentose cycle is essential for use in the synthesis of fat. In general, the pentose cycle is a major source of the NADPH (TPNH) required to maintain the reducing environment in synthetic processes using NADPH (TPNH) as cofactor.

    e. GLUCURONATE PATHWAY.   In recent years, another alternate pathway of G-6-P oxidation has been elucidated. This pathway has been termed the uronate pathway, glucuronate pathway, or the C-6 oxidative pathway. This pathway is shown in Fig. 7. Important contributions to its clarification, particularly in relation to L-xylulose

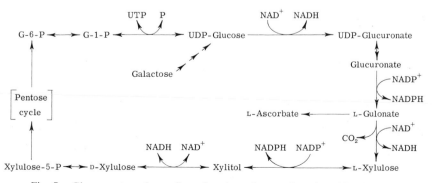

Fig. 7.   Glucuronate pathway. P = phosphate. See text for other abbreviations.

metabolism and ascorbic acid synthesis, may be found in the studies of Touster *et al.* (1957) and Burns and Evans (1956). The initial steps of this pathway involve the formation of UDPG, which, as previously discussed, is also an intermediate in glyco-genesis. Glucose-6-phosphate is first converted to G-1-P, which then reacts with UTP to form UDPG. This product is then oxidized at the C-6 position of the gluscose molecule in contrast to the pentose cycle. This reaction requires NAD^+ (DPN^+) as a cofactor, and the products of the reaction are uridine diphospho-glucuronic acid (UDPGA) and NADH (DPNH). This UDPGA is involved in a number of conjugating reactions in animals, such as bilirubin diglucuronide formation and the synthesis of mucopolysaccharides (chondroitin sulfate) which contain glu-curonic acid.

D-Glucuronic acid is next reduced to L-gulonic acid in the presence of the enzyme gulonic dehydrogenase, and in this reaction NADPH (TPNH) serves as the hydrogen donor. The L-gulonic acid formed may follow a pathway leading to the synthesis of a pentose, L-xylulose, the compound found in the urine in xyloketosuria of man. In this reaction the C-6 carbon of glucose is evolved as CO_2. As shown in Fig. 7, further reactions of L-xylulose lead to the formation of D-xylulose-5-P, and a cyclical pathway including the pentose cycle may occur. L-Gulonic acid may also follow a pathway leading to the synthesis of L-ascorbic acid. For the synthesis of L-ascorbic acid, evidence has been presented (Evans *et al.*, 1959) that D-galactose may be an even better precursor than D-glucose. This pathway is also included in Fig. 7.

2. Terminal Oxidation

The metabolic pathways described thus far have been those followed essentially by carbohydrates alone. Similarly, the breakdown of fats and proteins follow in-dependent pathways leading to the formation of organic acids. Among the organic

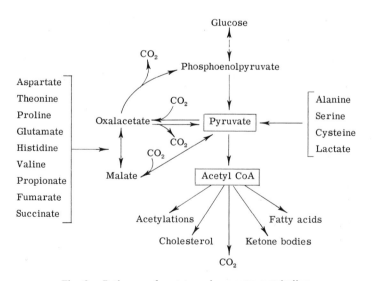

Fig. 8.   Pathways of acetate and pyruvate metabolism.

acids formed are acetate from β-oxidation of fatty acids, and pyruvate, OAA, and α-ketoglutarate from transamination of their corresponding α-amino acids. These intermediate metabolites are indistinguishable in their subsequent interconversions. Thus, the breakdown of the three major dietary constituents converges into a pathway common to all, which then serves as a site for the interconversions between them as well.

a. PYRUVATE METABOLISM.   The pathway for breakdown of glucose to pyruvate has been described in Section IV,D,1. Pyruvate is then oxidatively decarboxylated in a complex enzymic system requiring the presence of lipoic acid, thiamine pyrophosphate, coenzyme A, NAD$^+$ (DPN$^+$), and pyruvic dehydrogenase to form Ac-CoA and NADH (DPNH). Pyruvate may follow a number of pathways as outlined in Fig. 8. The conversion of pyruvate to lactate has already been described in Section IV,D,1. By the mechanism of transamination, pyruvate may be reversibly converted to alanine. The general reaction for transamination may be written

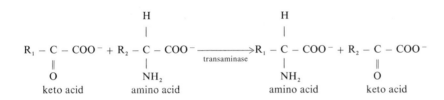

where the amino group of an amino acid is transferred to the α position of an α-keto acid and as a result, the amino acid is converted to its corresponding α-keto acid. This reaction requires the presence of vitamin B_6 as pyridoxal phosphate and is catalyzed by a transaminase specific for the reaction. Measurements of the serum levels of these enzymes have been particularly useful in the assessment of liver and muscle disorders. These are discussed more fully in later chapters.

The energetics of the reaction from PEP to form pyruvic acid are such that this is essentially an irreversible process, as is the breakdown of pyruvate to Ac-CoA. An alternate pathway resulting in an effective reversal of this process has been elucidated. Through a carbon dioxide fixation reaction in the presence of NADP$^+$ (TPN$^+$) -linked malic dehydrogenase, malate is formed from pyruvate. Malate is then oxidized to OAA in the presence of NAD$^+$ (DPN$^+$)-linked malic dehydrogenase. Oxalacetate may also be formed directly from pyruvate by the reaction catalyzed by pyruvate carboxylase. Oxalacetate formed by either route may then be phosphorylated and decarboxylated to form PEP in a reaction catalyzed by PEP-CK. Thus, a pathway which bypasses the direct reversal of the pyruvate to PEP reaction is available for gluconeogenesis from lower intermediates. These pathways for pyruvate metabolism are also outlined in Fig. 8 which includes the dicarboxylic acid cycle.

b. TRICARBOXYLIC ACID CYCLE.   Acetyl CoA formed as a result of the oxidative decarboxylation of pyruvate also has a number of metabolic routes available. This compound occupies a central position in synthetic as well as oxidative pathways as shown in Fig. 8. The oxidative pathway leading to the breakdown of Ac-CoA to CO_2 and H_2O follows a cyclical pathway termed the tricarboxylic acid (TCA) cycle, citric acid cycle, or the Krebs cycle. The major steps involved are shown in Fig. 9.

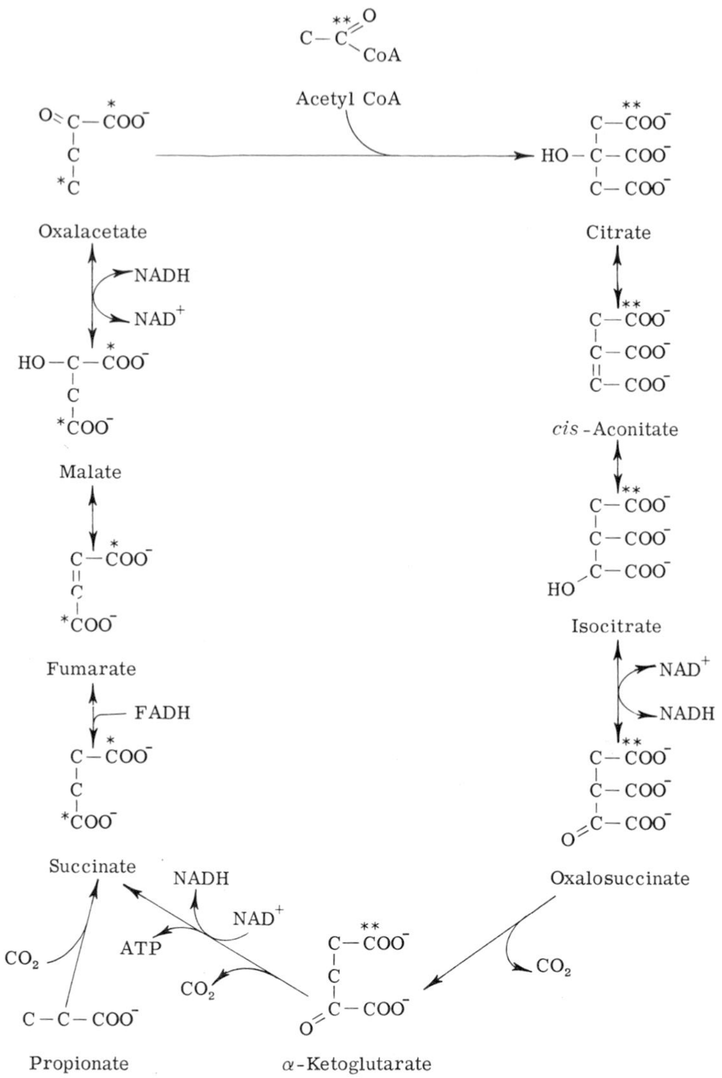

Fig. 9.   Tricarboxylic acid cycle. The pathway for the entry of propionate into the metabolic scheme is also included. The asterisks show the expected distribution of isotopically labeled carbon in a single turn of the cycle starting with acetyl CoA.

In a single turn of the cycle, 2 moles of CO_2 are evolved, and 1 mole of OAA is regenerated. The regenerated OAA may then condense with another mole of Ac-CoA, and the cycle continues. It should be noted that citric acid is a symmetrical molecule which behaves asymmetrically as shown in Fig. 9. The CO_2 is also not derived directly from the portion of the molecule contributed by Ac-CoA. The CO_2 is derived from the portion of the molecule contributed by oxalacetate during each turn of the cycle. In view of the great interest in this cycle, the expected distribution of isotopically labeled carbon atoms in one turn of the cycle is also shown in Fig. 9.

During one turn of the cycle, a randomization of label occurs at the succinate level such that CO_2 derived from the carboxyl group of acetate will be evolved during the next turn of the cycle.

In the process, 3 moles of NAD^+ (DPN^+) and 1 mole of a flavin nucleotide (FAD) are reduced, and 1 mole of ATP generated as noted in Fig. 9. In animal tissues, there is also a $NADP^+$ (TPN^+)-linked isocitric dehydrogenase (ICD), which is cytoplasmic and not associated with the mitochondria as is the NAD^+ (DPN^+)-linked ICD and the other enzymes of the citric acid cycle. The $NADP^+$ (TPN^+)-ICD is among the growing list of clinical serum enzyme determinations used as aids to diagnosis of liver disorder (Cornelius, 1961).

3. Carbon Dioxide Fixation in Animals

According to Fig. 9, the TCA cycle is a repetitive process based on the regeneration of OAA at each turn. Other metabolic paths, however, are also available for intermediates in the cycle. Reversal of the transamination reactions previously described would result in a withdrawal of OAA and α-ketoglutarate (α-KG) from the cycle. By decarboxylation, OAA may form PEP, and malate may form pyruvate and thence other glycolytic intermediates as shown in Fig. 8. Continued losses of these intermediates into other metabolic pathways would theoretically result in a decrease in the rate of operation of the cycle. A number of metabolic pathways are known, whereby the losses of cycle intermediates may be balanced by replacement from other sources and are shown in Fig. 8. The amino acids, aspartic and glutamic, may function as sources of supply as well as for withdrawal. The CO_2-fixation reactions which are the reversal of the reactions previously described

$$PEP + CO_2 \longrightarrow OAA$$
$$Pyruvate + CO_2 \longrightarrow malate$$
$$Pyruvate + CO_2 \longrightarrow OAA$$

may also function as important sources of supply. A fourth CO_2-fixing reaction is known

$$Propionate + CO_2 \longrightarrow succinate$$

which is of especial importance in ruminant metabolism for maintaining the supply of intermediates in the TCA cycle. Propionate is one of the three major fatty acids involved in ruminant metabolism.

4. Energy Relationships in Carbohydrate Metabolism

The energy of carbohydrate breakdown must be converted to high-energy phosphate compounds to be useful to the organism, otherwise it is dissipated as heat. The total available chemical energy in the reaction

$$Glucose \longrightarrow lactate$$

is about 50 kcal/mole or about 7% of the 690 kcal/mole which is available from the total oxidation of glucose to CO_2 and water. In glycolysis, it has been noted that the useful energy is represented by the net gain of 2 moles of ATP, the available energy of each being about 7 kcal. Thus, the efficiency of glycolysis starting from glucose is about 28%.

The major portion of the energy of oxidation is obtained in the further aerobic oxidation of pyruvate to CO_2 and H_2O. In the oxidative or dehydrogenation steps, NADH (DPNH) or NADPH (TPNH) (FAD in the succinate step) is formed. In the presence of molecular O_2, these compounds are reoxidized to NAD^+ (DPN^+) or $NADP^+$ (TPN^+) in the cytochrome system. During the sequence of reactions comprising this system, 3 moles of ATP are formed per mole of NADH (DPNH) or NADH (TPNH) oxidized to NAD^+ (DPN^+) or $NADP^+$ (TPN^+). This phenomenon is known as oxidative phosphorylation. The yield of high-energy phosphate bonds in the form of ATP in the system per atom of oxygen consumed ($\frac{1}{2}O_2$) is conventionally referred to as the P:O ratio, in this case, 3.

In Table III, a balance sheet of the ATP's formed in the various steps are given. The total oxidation of a mole of glucose to CO_2 and water yields about 690 kcal; the net gain of 38 ATP's in the biological scheme represents about 266 kcal or an overall efficiency of 38%.

TABLE III   ATP YIELD IN GLUCOSE OXIDATION

Glucose			
$\downarrow$ ⟵——— ATP (2X)			− 2
F-1,6-P			
⎮ ———→NADH (DPNH) ———→3 ATP (2×)			+ 6
$\downarrow$ ———→ATP (4×)			+ 4
2 Pyruvate			
$\downarrow$ ———→NADH (DPNH) ———→3 ATP (2×)			+ 6
2 Ac-CoA			
⎮ ———→NADH (DPNH) ———→3 ATP (6×)			+18
⎮ ———→ATP (2)			+ 2
$\downarrow$ ———→FADH ———→2 ATP (2×)			+ 4
4CO_2			
Net: Glucose ———→6CO_2			+38 ATP

V. INTERRELATIONSHIPS OF CARBOHYDRATE, LIPID, AND PROTEIN METABOLISM

The mechanism by which the breakdown products of lipids and proteins may enter the common metabolic pathway have been described in previous sections. The principal points at which carbohydrate carbon may be interconverted between amino acids and fatty acids are outlined in Fig. 10. Thus, certain amino acids (glucogenic) can serve as precursors of carbohydrate, and by reversal of the reactions involved, carbohydrates can contribute to the synthesis of amino acids.

The relationship between carbohydrate and lipid metabolism deserves special mention for the carbohydrate economy and the status of glucose oxidation strongly influence lipid metabolism. A brief description of lipid metabolism follows, and greater detail may be found in Chapter 2, on lipid metabolism.

A. Lipid Metabolism

Recent advances in the field of fatty acid metabolism have led to the appreciation that the pathways of oxidation and synthesis may be considered separately.

1. Oxidation of Fatty Acids

Fatty acid oxidation begins in the extramitochondrial cytoplasm with the activation of fatty acids to form fatty acyl CoA. The fatty acids are synthesized in the cytoplasm or taken up as FFA. The activated fatty acyl CoA is bound to carnitine for transport across the mitochondrial membrane into the mitochondria where fatty acyl CoA is released for intramitochondrial oxidation (Fritz, 1967).

The classical β-oxidation scheme for the breakdown of fatty acids whereby two carbon units are successively removed is firmly established. This scheme is a repetitive process involving four successive reactions. After the initial activation to form a CoA derivative, there is (1) a dehydrogenation, (2) hydration, and (3) a second dehydrogenation which is followed by (4) a cleavage. The result is the formation of Ac-CoA and a fatty acid shorter by two carbon atoms which may in turn reenter the cycle. In the case of odd-chain fatty acids, propionyl CoA is formed in the final cleavage reaction. It should be noted that the hydrogen acceptors in the oxidative steps are NAD^+ (DPN$^+$) and FAD. The further oxidation of Ac-CoA to CO_2 and water proceeds in the common pathway of the TCA cycle. In the process, 2 moles of CO_2 are evolved per mole of Ac-CoA entering the cycle. Therefore, fatty acids could not theoretically lead to a net synthesis of carbohydrate. Net synthesis of carbohydrate from fatty acids would require the direct conversion of Ac-CoA into some glucose precursor, i.e., pyruvate. The reaction

$$\text{Pyruvate} \longrightarrow \text{Ac-CoA} + CO_2$$

however, is irreversible. Thus, the only route by which fatty acid carbon could theoretically appear in carbohydrate is through the TCA cycle intermediates, and this occurs without a net synthesis.

2. Synthesis of Fatty Acids

It had long been assumed that the pathway for lipogenesis was a direct reversal of the β-oxidation scheme. It is now apparent that the pathway of lipogenesis diverges from that of oxidation. The first point of divergence involves the initial condensation reaction. Carbon dioxide is a requirement, yet there is no evidence of the incorporation of this CO_2 into the fatty acid (Porter et al., 1957; Gibson et al., 1958). This has suggested a pathway involving the initial synthesis of malonyl CoA. Malonyl CoA is condensed with an aldehyde (Brady, 1958) or Ac-CoA (Wakil, 1958), and in subsequent reactions, the original CO_2 moiety is cleaved from the condensation product. This malonyl CoA pathway of extramitochondrial cytoplasmic synthesis of fatty acid has now been well established.

The second point of divergence involves the requirements for NADPH (TPNH) as the hydrogen donor rather than NADH (DPNH) or FADH. NADPH (TPNH) is generated significantly when glucose is oxidized in the pentose phosphate pathway.

NADPH is also high in the extra mitochondrial cytoplasm of tissues such as liver and adipose where pentose cycle activity is high. The availability of this NADPH (TPNH) forms the basis for the hypothesis linking carbohydrate oxidation to lipogenesis (Siperstein, 1959).

3. Synthesis of Cholesterol and Ketone Bodies

Acetyl CoA is also the precursor of cholesterol and the ketone bodies (acetacetate, β-OH-butyrate, acetone). The synthesis of cholesterol proceeds through a complicated series of reactions starting with the stepwise condensation of 3 moles of Ac-CoA to form β-hydroxy-β-methyl glutaryl CoA (HMG-CoA). Details of the metabolic pathway may be found in Chapter 2, on lipid metabolism. As shown in Fig. 10, HMG-CoA is a common intermediate for the synthesis of both cholesterol and ketone bodies which occurs in the liver. In liver, a deacylating enzyme is present which cleaves HMG-CoA to yield Ac-CoA and free acetacetate (AcAc). This is termed the HMG-CoA cycle. This accumulated AcAc may freely diffuse from the cell and enter the general circulation. In order for further oxidations to occur, AcAc must be "reactivated" by condensation with CoA. This is accomplished in extrahepatic tissues (muscle) by the transfer of CoA from succinyl CoA to AcAc.

Current views portray increased ketogenesis as the net result of alterations in metabolic pathways and/or enzymes, which, in turn, favor the accumulation of AcAc-CoA.

According to Krebs (1966) increased ketogenesis is always associated with an increased rate of gluconeogenesis which is in turn associated with increases in the key gluconeogenic enzyme, PEP-CK. The increased rate of gluconeogenesis is considered to deplete OAA. Wieland (1968) also concludes that a depletion of OAA occurs but that it is the result of an increase in the reductive environment of the cell which is required for synthetic purposes, i.e., gluconeogenesis. The increased

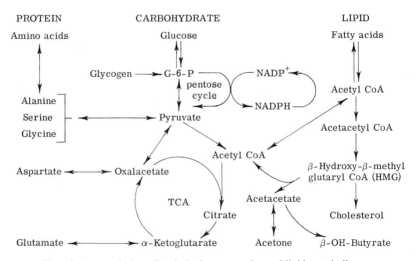

Fig. 10.   Interrelation of carbohydrate, protein, and lipid metabolism.

NADH/NAD ratio is cited as evidence which would promote the conversion of OAA to malate, thereby depleting OAA. By either mechanism, the common area of agreement is the depletion of OAA associated with increased gluconeogenesis which is in turn associated with a deficiency of carbohydrate.

The increased mobilization and utilization of fatty acids is well known under conditions of starvation and diabetes. Under these same conditions, lipogenesis from Ac-CoA is also depressed. The net effect of either or both of these alterations would tend to favor the accumulation of AcAc-CoA and thus ketogenesis. It has also been suggested that an important factor favoring the accumulation of AcAc-CoA is the increase in fatty acid utilization seen in starvation and in the diabetic state (Fritz, 1961). Depression of TCA cycle activity might also be expected to result in AcAc-CoA accumulation due to a decrease in Ac-CoA units traversing the cycle. This depression, particularly as a result of OAA deficiency, appears to have regained support at present (see Section X,D).

B. The Influence of Glucose Oxidation on Lipid Metabolism

In addition to the separation of metabolic pathways, an anatomical separation of lipid metabolism has also been established. The liver is more closely associated with fatty acid oxidation. The major site of lipogenesis in animals is now known to be in the adipose tissue. The rate of fat synthesis by the liverless animal is comparable to that of the intact animal (Masoro et al., 1949) and, in vitro, adipose tissue also converts glucose to fatty acids faster than does liver tissue.

It is well known that, with excessive carbohydrate intake, fat depots in the body increase. Fasting an animal, on the other hand, depresses the respiratory quotient (RQ), an indication that the animal is now utilizing body fat as an energy source. During fasting, unesterified fatty acids in plasma also increase and, when carbohydrate is supplied, they decrease. The presence of glucose has been shown to both stimulate lipogenesis (Hirsch et al., 1954) and have a sparing effect on fatty acid oxidation (Lossow and Chaikoff, 1955). In a condition with relative lack of carbohydrate, e.g., diabetes, where there is an inability to utilize glucose, depression of lipogenesis is a characteristic finding.

These findings provide an indication of the strong influence of the breakdown of glucose on fat metabolism. In the presence of adequate glucose oxidation, the balance of lipid metabolism tends toward lipogenesis from acetate, and this occurs primarily in adipose tissue. In the presence of decreased glucose oxidation, mobilization of depot fat ensues. Mobilized fat in the form of FFA (bound to albumin) is transported to the liver, where the balance is directed toward degradation. In severe diabetic ketosis, the increased mobilization of fat may release triglycerides as well, and a frank lipemia may occur. With increased fat mobilization, AcAc-CoA is generated in excess and may accumulate. The accumulation of AcAc-CoA is also favored by the depression of lipogenesis, which removes one of the possible pathways for metabolism of acetate. The depletion of OAA, the condensing partner for Ac-CoA (Section V,A) also favors the accumulation of AcAc-CoA. The accumulated AcAc-CoA may then follow alternate pathways which are less affected by the relative deficiency of glucose, namely ketogenesis.

VI.   INSULIN AND CARBOHYDRATE METABOLISM

The internal secretions of the anterior pituitary, adrenal cortex and medulla, and the pancreas are closely associated with carbohydrate metabolism. The pituitary and adrenal factors have previously been discussed in Section IV,C together with glucagon. Following the successful extraction of insulin by Banting and Best in 1921, a vast amount of literature has accumulated on its role in carbohydrate metabolism. Although the specific mode(s) of insulin action is still debatable, the contributions to date provide for a clearer understanding of the biochemical events which occur in animals with and without insulin.

A. INSULIN

The elucidation of the structure of insulin by Sanger (1959) has been one of the signal advances of protein biochemistry. Insulin is a relatively small protein comprised of two polypeptide chains designated chain A and chain B, which are linked together by disulfide bridges. Chain A is the shorter and is made up of 21 amino acids residues. The longer chain B is made up of 30 amino acid residues. The molecular weight of this molecule is about 6000, and it is the smallest unit possessing biological activity. Under physiological conditions, it is likely that two molecules are linked together to form a "dimer" or four to form a tetramer. Insulin obtained from various species differs in amino acid composition in chain A or chain B or both of the molecule (Sanger, 1959). The chemistry of insulin has been extensively reviewed (Young, 1963). These structural differences among the various species of animals are not located at a critical site, however, since they do not affect the biological activity. They probably affect their immunological behavior, however.

Insulin is synthesized by the β-cells of the pancreatic islets probably from a single chain precursor called Proinsulin (Steiner and Oyer, 1967; Chance and Ellis, 1969). The granules of the β-cells presumably function in the storage mechanism by providing zinc and protein for the binding of insulin. The amount of insulin stored in the pancreas by various species differs (Marks and Young, 1940). The dog has been found to store about 3.3 units/gm pancreas, which amounts to about 75 units in a 10-kg dog, an amount which, if suddenly released, would be fatal. The release of insulin is normally governed by the level of glucose in the circulating blood.

More recently, it has been shown that the gastrointestinal hormones, secretin (Unger et al., 1967) and pancreozymin (Meade et al., 1967), enhance insulin release by the pancreas. This has been more fully reviewed by Sharkey (1968). This phenomenon may account for differences in the oral vs the iv glucose tolerance which are not explainable by route alone.

Once in the general circulation, insulin is transported to responsive tissues in combination with β-globulin. In the tissues and prior to exertion of its effect, insulin is again bound. All tissues, especially liver and kidney, also are able to inactivate insulin by hydrolysis with the enzyme insulinase. It becomes apparent that a finely balanced system of release, action, and inactivation is available to maintain homeostatic levels of insulin.

B. Mechanism of Insulin Action

It is well established that a principal site of insulin action is in the initial phases of glucose metabolism. This initial site of action has been localized prior to G-6-P in the metabolic events of glucose. In order for extracellular glucose to gain entry into the metabolic pathways, it must first enter the cell and then be phosphorylated. It is now generally accepted that insulin affects glucose entry into the peripheral tissue cells such as muscle (permeability theory). Whether insulin acts on the phosphorylation step continues to be debatable. The earlier hypothesis (Colowick *et al.*, 1947) that insulin acted on the glucokinase system by releasing it from the inhibitory effect of the anterior pituitary (GH or STH) has not received experimental support (Stadie and Haugaard, 1949; Stadie, 1954). The bulk of the current evidence favors the initial entry of glucose into the cell as the principal site of insulin action. Levine *et al.* (1950) obtained evidence that insulin increased the transfer to galactose out of the plasma and into the tissues of nephrectomized eviscerated animals; they postulated that the effect of insulin was to facilitate the transfer of galactose (since galactose is not metabolized in this experimental animal) across the cell membrane. This hypothesis was extended to include glucose. E. J. Ross (1953) obtained direct evidence for the increased transfer of glucose into the aqueous of the rabbit eye by insulin. The mechanism of membrane transfer of glucose has received considerable attention and there is little doubt that insulin increases membrane transport of glucose. This transport step is independent of the phosphorylation step. The reader is referred to reviews by Park *et al.* (1959) and by Randle and Morgan (1962) for further discussion of a postulated transport mechanism. On the other hand, the transport mechanism is also unlikely to be the sole mechanism of insulin action. It does not explain all actions of insulin including many of its effects on liver metabolism since insulin does not affect glucose transport into liver cells.

C. Effects of Insulin

The principal effects of insulin administration to an animal are summarized in Table IV. The most characteristic finding following insulin administration is a hypoglycemia. This occurs regardless of the nutritional state, age, etc., of the animal and is a net result of the increased removal of glucose from the plasma into the tissues. The respiratory quotient (RQ) increases toward unity, indicating that the

TABLE IV   EFFECTS OF INSULIN

Decrease	Increase
Blood glucose	Glucose utilization
Gluconeogenesis	Glycogen deposition in liver and muscle
Ketone bodies	Fat synthesis
Serum phosphate	Protein synthesis
Serum potassium	Food intake
	Respiratory quotient (RQ)

animal is now primarily utilizing carbohydrate. The increased utilization of carbohydrate is a well-established finding. The consequences of this increased utilization of glucose follows a pattern of an increase in those constituents derived from glucose and a decrease in those which are influenced by increased glucose oxidation. The conversion of glucose to glycogen, fat, and protein is enhanced while gluconeogenesis and ketogenesis are inhibited. The decreases in serum phosphate and potassium levels which parallel those of blood glucose are presumably due to their involvement in the phosphorylating mechanisms. As such, they may be considered as reflections of increased glucose utilization, a point, however, which has not been adequately established.

VII. BLOOD GLUCOSE AND ITS REGULATION

A. GENERAL

The dependency of the blood glucose concentration upon a wide variety of factors is apparent, and the concentration at any time is the net result of the rates of entry and of removal of glucose in the circulation. As such, all the factors which exert influence upon entry or removal become of importance in the regulation of blood glucose concentration. Furthermore, when the renal reabsorptive capacity for glucose is exceeded, urinary loss of glucose becomes an additional factor to be considered in the maintenance of the blood glucose concentration. The blood glucose levels at which this occurs vary between species and are listed in Table V.

B. GLUCOSE SUPPLY AND REMOVAL

Glucose may be supplied by intestinal absorption of dietary glucose and production from other dietary carbohydrates such as fructose and galactose, amino acids (gluconeogenesis), or glycogen. The dietary sources of supply are especially variable. The absorptive process itself may vary with the degree of thyroid activity. In the postabsorptive state, the hepatic source is of prime importance in maintenance of the supply of blood glucose. The hormonal influences (epinephrine, glucagon) involved in the release of glucose from glycogen have already been indicated in Section IV,C,2. The influence of the glucocorticoids is probably related to its effect on gluconeogenesis.

TABLE V   RENAL THRESHOLDS FOR GLUCOSE IN DOMESTIC
ANIMALS

Species	mg%	Reference
Dog	175–220	Shannon et al. (1941)
Horse	180–200	Stewart and Holman (1940)
Cow	98–102	Bell and Jones (1945)
Sheep	160–200	McCandless et al. (1948)
Goat	70–130	Cutler (1934)

Removal of glucose is also governed by a variety of factors, almost all of which ultimately relate to the rate of utilization of glucose by the animal. All tissues constantly utilize glucose either for energy purposes or for conversion into other products (glycogen, pentoses, lipids, amino acids). As such, an outflow governed by the rate of utilization occurs at all times. The level of blood glucose itself partially governs the rate of utilization and therefore, in a sense, is autoregulatory. At high levels, the rate of glucose uptake by tissues such as muscle and liver increases, presumably due to a mass action effect. The presence of insulin increases the rate of utilization, whether by increased transfer (muscle) or increased phosphorylation (liver). The action of insulin is opposed, in effect, by the diabetogenic factor of the anterior pituitary, GH.

The liver can thus supply as well as remove glucose and therefore occupies a central position in the regulatory mechanism for blood glucose concentration. The metabolic activities of liver, however, are primarily directed toward supply rather than utilization of glucose. It has been estimated in liver slices that about 25% of glucose is oxidized to lactate or CO_2 and that the remainder goes to glycogen or free glucose (Cahill et al., 1959). Muscle, on the other hand, does not contain G-6-Pase and is therefore primarily a glucose-utilizing tissue.

C. The Role of the Liver

The rate-limiting role of the membrane transfer system in peripheral tissues (muscle) which are sensitive to insulin is now generally accepted. In the liver, however, this mechanism is not rate-limiting because free glucose diffuses freely across the liver cell membrane (Cahill et al., 1958). It has been demonstrated (Soskin et al., 1938; Cahill et al., 1958) that at a glucose level of approximately 150 mg%, the liver ceases to take up or supply glucose to the circulation. This level might then be termed the "steady state" at which those mechanisms of importance in supply and removal are operating at equal rates. Above this level, glucose removal is greater than supply, and the balance is reversed when the blood glucose level is below 150 mg%. This effect may be partially due to a mass action effect but a greater degree of control appears to be exercised by insulin and the rate-limiting enzymic reactions in the liver. Madison (1969) presented evidence that insulin directly decreases liver glucose output and glycogenolysis and increases glucose uptake by the liver. This effect is likely to be secondary to the action of insulin enhancing glucokinase and glycogen synthetase activity.

The sensitivity of the glucokinase reaction to insulin in the intact liver cell, as opposed to cell free systems, is readily demonstrated (Chernick and Chaikoff, 1951). The opposing reaction is catalyzed by G-6-Pase, an enzyme found primarily in the liver. The concentration of hepatic G-6-Pase increases in fasting (Ashmore et al., 1954), a change which would favor the production of glucose by the liver. An even greater increase is found in insulin deficiency, i.e., diabetes, in spite of the hyperglycemia. Increases in the other three key enzymes of gluconeogenesis, F-1,6-Pase, PEP-CK, and PC, are also observed in diabetes (Ashmore and Weber, 1968), although PC may not increase in alloxan diabetes (Krebs, 1966). The increase in activity of G-6-Pase and other gluconeogenic enzymes together with decreased utilization offers an explanation for the excessive production of glucose by the diabetic

liver. The effect of insulin on hepatic glucokinase activity also suggests an anatomical separation for insulin action between muscle and liver. This dual role for
insulin, affecting membrane transport in muscle and glucokinase in liver, has been
suggested by Cahill *et al.* (1959).

The amelioration of diabetes in an experimental animal by hypophysectomy
(Houssay animal) is well established. The pituitary factor, which, in effect, opposes
the action of insulin, is associated with GH. The influence of the glucocorticoids is
probably exerted through their effect upon increasing gluconeogenesis and thereby
the intracellular concentration of G-6-P. An increase also results from the glycogenolytic action of epinephrine and glucagon, and the equilibrium again is shifted
in favor of free glucose production. Therefore, it appears that the factors which influence the two opposing enzyme systems involved or the concentrations of the
reactants, glucose and G-6-P, govern the net inflow or outflow of glucose from the
liver. The hormones which directly or indirectly exert influence upon these reactions
then become a means of control of hepatic glucose uptake or production and therefore influence blood glucose concentration.

D. Glucose Tolerance

The regulatory events which occur in response to changes in blood glucose concentration may be summarized by a description of the consequences of the ingestion
of a test dose of glucose. When administered orally to a normal animal, a typical
change in blood glucose concentration with time is observed as shown in Fig. 11.
During the absorptive phase, phase I, the rate of entry of glucose into the circulation
exceeds that of removal, and the blood glucose concentration rises. As the level
rises, hepatic glucose output is being inhibited, and the secretion of insulin is being
stimulated. This stimulation of insulin secretion is the result of glucose stimulation
per se and also by the insulin-releasing effect of secretin, pancreozymin, gastrin,

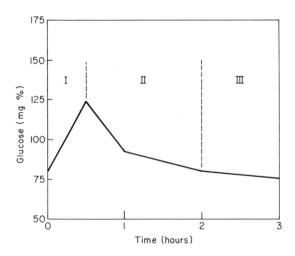

Fig. 11.   Oral glucose tolerance in the dog. I, II, and III are phases of the curve. For discussion,
see text.

and glucagon. In 30–60 minutes, a peak level is reached, after which the blood glucose level begins to fall. During this phase of falling blood glucose, phase II, the rates of removal exceed those of entry, and the regulatory mechanisms directed toward removal of glucose are operating maximally. The increased glucose utilization is enhanced by a decrease in hepatic output of glucose and the blood glucose level falls rapidly. When the glucose level reaches the original level, it continues to fall to a minimal level and then returns to the original level. This hypoglycemic phase (phase III) is considered due to the inertia of the regulatory mechanisms for, in general, the higher the glycemia, the greater the subsequent hypoglycemia.

VIII. METHODOLOGY

A large number of tests have been devised to assess the status of the carbohydrate economy of animals. A selected number will be discussed.

A. Blood Glucose

1. Methods

All blood glucose methods which have been commonly employed are based on the reducing properties of glucose. These methods employ an alkaline copper solution containing cupric (Cu^{2+}) copper which is reduced to the cuprous (Cu^+) form. The reduced copper then reacts with a reagent, phosphomolybdate or arsenomolybdate, to form a color. Another color reaction employs the reduction of ferricyanide to ferrocyanide to form Prussian blue. This is the basis for a micro method (Folin and Malmros, 1929) which employs 0.05 ml of blood. The colored solutions obtained in all these methods are then compared with standard glucose solutions in a colorimeter or photometer.

An important consideration in the use of the reduction methods is that blood contains significant amounts of nonsaccharoid-reducing substances. These include glutathione, ergothionine, creatine, creatinine, and uric acid. These substances must be excluded by the method in order to obtain a measure of the circulating blood glucose. The classical clinical method of Folin and Wu (1920) is the least specific and generally gives values 20–30% higher than other available methods. The Nelson (1944) modification of the Somogyi method largely avoids measurement of these nonsaccharoid-reducing substances by deproteinization of the blood sample with barium and zinc solutions. For this reason, the results have often been referred to as "true" glucose values. Details of this method may be found in a number of clinical laboratory manuals and texts (Hawk et al., 1954). This method has been widely used and, unless specified, all values given in this chapter refer to "true" glucose values obtained by it.

Another important consideration in the use of the Nelson-Somogyi method, particularly with ruminant bloods, is its lack of sensitivity at low concentration of blood glucose. Below 40 mg%, this method underestimates glucose (Campbell and Kronfeld, 1961) up to 20% as compared to the glucose oxidase method. The glucose oxidase method is an even more specific method for blood glucose which employs the enzymes glucose oxidase and peroxidase, and a dye. Glucose oxidase catalyzes the conversion of glucose in the filtrate to gluconic acid:

$$\text{Glucose} \xrightarrow{\text{glucose oxidase}} \text{gluconic acid} + H_2O_2$$

The hydrogen peroxide formed in the reaction, in the presence of peroxidase, oxidizes a dye to form a colored product. This same principle is employed in the glucose-specific paper strips in common use for the estimation of urine glucose. The glucose oxidase method is now the method of choice for blood glucose and is readily available commercially for clinical laboratory use.

However accurate a method for blood glucose may be, it cannot compensate for loss of glucose in the improperly handled blood sample. Glucose breakdown, i.e., glycolysis, takes place very rapidly, about 10% per hour loss, at room temperature and is even more rapid if the sample is contaminated by microorganisms. For these reasons, glucose in the blood sample must be protected from glycolysis if immediate preparation of the filtrate is impractical. This may best be accomplished by the use of sodium fluoride (10 mg/ml blood), thymol (1 mg/ml blood) and by refrigeration. The sodium fluoride will act both as an anticoagulant and a glucose preservative. Sodium fluoride may also be added to the blood sample vial containing an anticoagulant.

2. Blood Glucose Levels in Animals

The normal ranges for blood glucose as reported by a number of authors are given in Table VI. From the preceding sections, it is apparent that a standard procedure for sampling must be employed to minimize variations in blood glucose, especially those due to diet. This is accomplished in the nonruminant and in the young ruminant by a standard 24-hour fast prior to sampling. This is not necessary in the older ruminant for it has been shown that carbohydrate given orally elicits no blood glucose response (Bell and Jones, 1945).

B. Tolerance Tests

1. Glucose Tolerance Tests (GTT)

Tolerance in its original usage referred to the amount of glucose which could be ingested by an animal without producing a glucosuria, hence, tolerance for glucose. Since in the normal animal the absence of a glycosuria indicates only a limited rise in blood glucose such that the renal threshold is not exceeded, glucose tolerance now refers to the blood glucose level following its administration. Accordingly, an animal with an increased glucose tolerance is one which shows a limited rise in blood glucose while the animal with a decreased tolerance shows an excessive rise.

It is important to ascertain the nature of the animal's diet, especially in the dog, prior to performance of this test. A diabetic type of glucose tolerance curve is obtained when dogs are placed on a diet of horse meat alone for 1 week (Hill and Chaikoff, 1956). These dietary variations should be obviated by placing the dog on a high carbohydrate diet (100–200 gm/day) for 3–5 days prior to performance of the

TABLE VI   BLOOD GLUCOSE IN DOMESTIC ANIMALS [a,b]

Horse	Cow	Sheep	Goat	Pig	Dog	Cat	Reference
(3) 60–100	(3) 35–55	(3) 35–60	(3) 45–60	(3) 65–95	(3) 55–90	(3) 60–100	Kaneko (1963)
(4) 54–95							Stewart and Holman (1940)
(3) 66–100							Alexander (1955)
	(1,3) 47–63	(1,3) 42–76					Campbell and Kronfeld (1961)
	(1,5) 39–52	(1,5) 35–74					Campbell and Kronfeld (1961)
		(3) 25–50					Reid (1950a)
			(3) 35–72				Houchin et al. (1939)
			(3) 24–65				Cutler (1934)
				(2,6) 65–95			Eveleth and Eveleth (1935)
				(3,8) 76–149			Sampson et al. (1942)
					(6) 80–120		Baer et al. (1957)
					(4) 70–100	(4) 77–118	Bloom (1957)
					(3) 70–86	(7) 66–80	Bodo et al. (1937)

[a]Whole blood unless otherwise specified.
[b]Numbers in parentheses refer to the following:
(1) plasma; (2) serum; (3) Somogyi method; (4) Folin-Wu method; (5) Somogyi filtrate–glucose oxidase; (6) tungstate filtrate-Benedict's method; (7) Folin micro method; (8) baby pigs, 12–48 hours old.

test. The tolerance curve may also be affected by the status of the intestinal absorptive process, i.e., inflammation, increased motility, thyroxine. The variations due to absorption and the excitement often attending intubation (if used) may be largely avoided by use of the intravenous route of administration.

a. ORAL GLUCOSE TOLERANCE TEST.   In Section VII,D, the blood glucose curve following the oral administration of a test dose of glucose was described. The oral GTT is ineffective in the ruminant animal because the ingested carbohydrate is almost totally fermented by the rumen microflora. This method has been used in dogs by feeding of a test meal consisting of 4 gm glucose/kg body weight mixed with a few grams of horse meat. A fasting blood sample is taken, the test meal given and blood samples taken at 30-minute intervals for 3 hours. The glucose tolerance curves in dogs receiving either glucose or galactose together with meat in their daily diet exhibited normal curves as described in Section VII,D. The maximum level, 120–140 mg%, was reached at 1 hour and returned to the fasting level, 65–95 mg%, in 2–3 hours. The oral GTT may be simplified to the taking of a single

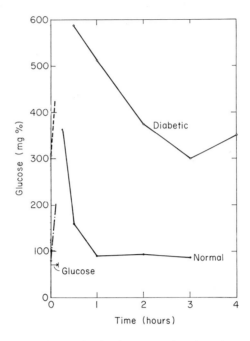

Fig. 12.   Intravenous glucose tolerance in the dog. Note that there is no ascending portion of the curve since there is no absorptive phase.

sample at 2 hours after giving the glucose, i.e., 2-hour postprandial glucose. A normal blood glucose level at 2 hours postprandially indicates that diabetes is unlikely. A persistent hyperglycemia at this time is indicative of a diabetic curve and should be confirmed with the complete GTT.

b. INTRAVENOUS GLUCOSE TOLERANCE TEST. After a standard 24-hour fast (except the adult ruminant which need not be fasted), 0.5 gm glucose/kg body weight is injected intravenously as a 50% solution. In small animals, the glucose solution is injected over a period of 3–5 minutes and in larger animals, at the rate of about 20 cm³/min. A blood sample for glucose analysis is taken before injection and at 30-minute intervals from the start of injection for 3 hours.

A glucose tolerance curve obtained by this method is illustrated in Fig. 12. Since the alimentary tract has been bypassed, phase I or the absorptive phase has, in effect, been eliminated from the resulting curve. Phase II and phase III are similar to those described for the oral GTT. It should be remembered in the use of this test that, in effect, the curve has been shifted to the left, and glucose returns to normal earlier than in the oral test. The peak occurs at the end of injection and has less significance than in the oral method. The height of the peak will vary with the rate of injection and the amount of glucose injected. The amount and rate of injection may vary considerably (between 0.5 gm/kg and 2 gm/kg) but the most significant finding in the curve is the return to normal in 60–90 minutes.

A quantitative measure of the rate of glucose utilization can also be obtained from the half-time ($T_{\frac{1}{2}}$) for clearance of the injected dose of glucose during the first hour after injection if blood samples are taken at 15-minute intervals. By this method the turnover rate of blood glucose in a spontaneously diabetic cow was determined to be one-fifth that of normal cows (Kaneko and Rhode, 1964) and the values were comparable to those obtained by more sophisticated ^{14}C-labeled glucose techniques (Kaneko *et al.*, 1965).

A further modification of the GTT may at times be more applicable. From inspection of the intravenous tolerance curve of the normal animal, the blood glucose returns to its original level in about $1\frac{1}{4}$ hours while the diabetic curve has not yet returned. On this basis, the test may be simplified, at the sacrifice of some accuracy, to the withdrawal of a single blood sample at $1\frac{1}{4}$ hours after glucose injection and comparing it to the fasting blood glucose level. Hyperglycemia persisting at this time is indicative of a diabetic curve.

The GTT is of greatest value in the diagnosis of diabetes, particularly those with a mild hyperglycemia and with no or intermittent glucosuria. Decreased tolerance is also observed, though less consistently in hyperthyroidism, hyperadrenalism, hyperpituitarism, and in severe liver disease. An increased tolerance is observed in hypofunction of the thyroids, adrenals, pituitary, and in hyperinsulinism.

2. Insulin Tolerance Test

The blood sugar response of a normal animal after the administration of a test dose of insulin exhibits a characteristic response as shown in Fig. 13. After obtaining a fasting blood sample, 0.1 unit of crystalline zinc insulin/kg body weight is injected intramuscularly or subcutaneously, and blood samples are taken at $\frac{1}{2}$-hourly intervals for 3 hours. The test measures (*1*) the sensitivity of the blood glucose level to a test dose of insulin and (*2*) the response of the animal to insulin-induced hypoglycemia. Normally, the blood glucose level falls to 50% of its fasting level in 20–30 minutes and returns to its fasting level in $1\frac{1}{2}$–2 hours. Two types of abnormal responses are seen. If the blood glucose level does not fall to the 50% level or requires longer than 30 minutes to reach the maximum hypoglycemic level, the

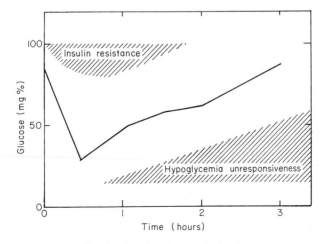

Fig. 13.   Insulin tolerance in the dog.

response is described as "insulin-insensitive" or "insulin-resistant." Insulin resistance is found, though inconsistently, in hyperfunction of the pituitary and adrenals.

If the hypoglycemia is prolonged and fails to return to the fasting level in 2 hours, the response is described as "hypoglycemia unresponsiveness." This type of response may be observed in hyperinsulinism, hypopituitarism, and hypoadrenalism and is most often employed in suspected cases of the latter two conditions. In carrying out this test, since hypoglycemia is being induced, a glucose solution should be readily available for injection.

3. Epinephrine Tolerance

The response of the blood glucose level which follows the injection of epinephrine is characteristic. The blood glucose level rises to a maximum of 50% above the fasting level in 40–60 minutes and returns to the original level in $1\frac{1}{2}$–2 hours. The test is performed by obtaining a fasting blood sample, injecting 1 ml of 1:1000 epinephrine-HCl (in the dog) intramuscularly, and obtaining blood samples at $\frac{1}{2}$-hourly intervals for 3 hours.

The characteristic increase in blood glucose has been used as an index of the availability of liver glycogen for the production of blood glucose. On the basis of a lowered response to epinephrine, J. C. Shaw (1943) concluded that liver glycogen in bovine ketosis was depleted, a finding later confirmed by direct measurement of glycogen in biopsy samples (Kronfeld et al., 1960; Ford and Boyd, 1960). A lowered glycemic response is also a characteristic response in the classic von Gierke's type of GSD of man.

4. Leucine-Induced Hypoglycemia

The oral administration of L-leucine induces a marked and persistent hypoglycemia in hyperinsulinism due to pancreatic islet cell tumors. The hypoglycemia is associated with a rise in plasma insulin (Yalow and Berson, 1960) as a result of its release by tumorous islet cells. The test is performed by the oral administration (stomach tube) of 150 mg L-leucine/kg body weight as an aqueous suspension to the fasting dog. A fasting blood glucose sample is taken before administration and at $\frac{1}{2}$-hourly intervals for 6 hours. A hypoglycemic effect is seen quickly at $\frac{1}{2}$–1 hour and may persist for as long as 6 hours in hyperinsulinism. The normal dog exhibits no hypoglycemic effect.

5. Tolbutamide Test

The intravenous administration of tolbutamide, an oral hypoglycemic agent, results in the release of insulin from the pancreas and is utilized as a test of the available insulin in the pancreas. The blood glucose curve during the test parallels the insulin tolerance test. This test has not received wide application in animals.

IX.   DISORDERS OF CARBOHYDRATE METABOLISM

From the preceding sections, it is evident that alterations in blood glucose levels may occur in a variety of disease states and are of particular importance in the endocrine disorders. Normal blood glucose levels are the result of a finely balanced system of hormonal interaction affecting the mechanisms of supply and removal. When imbalance occurs, a new equilibrium is established. Whether this equilibrium is clinically evident as a persistent hypoglycemia or hyperglycemia depends on the total interaction of the hormonal influences on carbohydrate metabolism. Further discussions concerning the disorders of the pituitary, adrenals, and the thyroids may be found in the chapters on endocrine function. The following sections discuss the conditions in which the principal manifestations are closely related to derangements in carbohydrate metabolism.

A. DIABETES MELLITUS

Although diabetes mellitus has been reported in horses, cattle, sheep, and pigs, it is most frequently found in dogs and cats. Estimates of the incidence of diabetes range as high as 1:152 for dogs (Krook *et al.*, 1960) and 1:800 for cats (Meier, 1960). The literature of diabetes mellitus in animals has been extensively reviewed by Wilkinson (1957, 1958). The clinical aspects have been described by Schlotthauer and Millar (1951). The classic and still the most detailed study of diabetes in the dog and cat was published by Hjarre (1927).

In dogs, the disease occurs most frequently at 8 years of age (Wilkinson, 1957). It has been diagnosed more often in females and frequently in association with obesity (Krook *et al.*, 1960). In contrast, male cats appear to be more commonly affected than females. Little is known of the genetic aspects of diabetes in animals as compared to man, in which the hereditary predisposition is well known. Diabetes has, however, been reported in the female offspring of a diabetic bitch (Roberts, 1954). The recent finding of hereditary diabetes in a laboratory animal, the Chinese hamster (Meier and Yerganian, 1959), should have important consequences in the study of the nature of the disease. Contributory factors to the onset of the disease most often mentioned are pancreatitis, obesity, infection, stress, and estrum (Wilkinson, 1960).

Recently, autoimmunity has been investigated as a possible cause of diabetes mellitus. An immune response is suggested because lymphocytic infiltration is frequently associated with immune processes and lymphocytic infiltration is found in spontaneous diabetes of cattle (Kaneko and Rhode, 1964) and man. It is also observed in cattle (Le Compte *et al.*, 1966) and/or rabbits (Grodsky *et al.*, 1966) immunized with bovine insulin.

The high estimates of the incidence of the disease provide an indication of its importance as a clinical consideration. Furthermore, the similarities of the clinical picture of diabetes with other wasting diseases showing polyuria and polydipsia attest to the importance of laboratory examinations in the early and accurate diagnosis of diabetes. In no other disease is an understanding of the metabolic alterations so important in diagnosis and proper treatment.

The fundamental defect in diabetes mellitus is a real or relative lack of insulin resulting in an inability to utilize glucose. The lack of insulin has been demonstrated in the spontaneously diabetic cow by the failure of a large test load of glucose to elicit a serum insulin response (Kaneko and Rhode, 1964). In the absence of insulin, the inability of the diabetic cow to utilize glucose is clearly shown in its inability to convert glucose-^{14}C to $^{14}CO_2$. This inability was corrected by insulin (Kaneko et al., 1965). The inability of the animal to utilize glucose is reflected in the clinical signs of diabetes, loss of weight, polyuria, polydypsia, and, in the advanced stages, acidosis.

1. Hyperglycemia

The finding of a fasting hyperglycemia is one of the most important diagnostic criteria of diabetes mellitus. As previously stated, the homeostatic level of blood glucose is maintained in the normal animal as a result of an equilibrium established between glucose supply and removal. The endocrine balance is particularly important in establishing this equilibrium. The effect of insulin tends to lower blood glucose, whereas the opposing effects of the anterior pituitary and adrenal cortical factors tend to raise it. In the diabetic animal, with a real or relative lack of insulin, the equilibrium is shifted to a higher level of blood glucose. This new equilibrium level is a result of the interaction of all the factors of importance in maintaining blood glucose levels. Peripheral glucose utilization is lowered, hepatic glucose production is increased due to alterations in enzymic balance with increases in the gluconeogenic enzymes, and gluconeogenesis is favored by the unopposed action of the pituitary and adrenocortical factors.

In the diabetic animal, the hyperglycemia itself tends to compensate in part for the decrease in peripheral utilization. This occurs partially as a mass action effect and results in an inflow of glucose into the tissues. Thus, the diabetic animal continues to utilize glucose in the absence of insulin but only at the expense of increased glucose production and hyperglycemia. As the deficiency of insulin progressively becomes more severe, the equilibrium level of blood glucose is established at higher and higher levels and equilibrium may never be established. Blood glucose values in canine diabetes have been reported as high as 1250 mg% (Wilkinson, 1960). Whenever the renal threshold for glucose is exceeded, the diabetic animal is also faced with excessive loss of glucose for which further compensation must be made.

2. Glucose Tolerance

The GTT is of particular value in those cases of diabetes in which the fasting blood sugar level is only moderately elevated. It is also helpful in moderately severe cases where there is some doubt as to the diagnosis. In no case should this test be applied to a severely diabetic animal.

The blood glucose curve characteristically shows a decreased tolerance for glucose (Fig. 12) and reflects the inability of the animal to dispose of a test dose of glucose. It has long been held that the diabetic curve is a reflection of the inability of pancreas to provide additional insulin in response to the glucose load. More recent postulates delegate a primary role to the homeostatic mechanisms of the liver.

The former is encompassed in the nonutilization theory of diabetes, whereas the latter is expressed in the theory of overproduction of glucose by the liver. Though not yet clearly established, it would seem likely that both mechanisms play a part. The decreased peripheral utilization of glucose in insulin lack is well known, as well as the fact that the diabetic liver continues to provide glucose in the presence of a hyperglycemia. The GTT is, in effect, added to the burden of an existing oversupply of glucose. Since the steady-state level at which the liver ceases to supply or remove glucose is elevated, the liver continues to supply glucose, which may then delay the return of the tolerance curve to its original level. In spite of the debatability of the mechanisms involved for explaining the decreased tolerance curve, this test remains a well-established and valuable test in the diagnosis of diabetes.

3. Ketonemia and Lipemia

As the utilization of glucose progressively decreases in the diabetic animal, the utilization of fatty acids for energy purposes progressively increases. The supply of fatty acids for hepatic utilization is obtained by mobilization from the body fat depots. Mobilization progressively increases as insulin deficiency becomes more severe and as the relative excess of the adrenal and pituitary factors increases. In severe diabetic states, excessive mobilization may result in the appearance of neutral fat in the circulation, and frank lipemia may occur. In severe lipemia, this may be observed visually in whole blood by a milky-white cast and as a white layer above the plasma column in the centrifuged hematocrit tube.

Concurrently with increased utilization of fatty acids, a progressive decrease in hepatic fatty acid synthesis occurs. This lipogenic block is a well-established feature of the diabetic liver. The net effect of the alterations in fatty acid metabolism is the production of Ac-CoA units in excess of the liver's capacity for their further metabolism. Fatty acyl CoA resulting from fat mobilization is also a marked inhibitor of citrate synthase which would remove another route for disposal of Ac-CoA. The accumulated Ac-CoA units are then diverted into alternate pathways, as described in Section V,B, and result in the excessive production of ketone bodies and cholesterol. The capacity of the peripheral tissues to utilize ketone bodies as important sources of energy is unimpaired in the diabetic animal, and these mechanisms are operating maximally. Ketosis thus occurs when the production of ketone bodies exceeds the capacity of the peripheral (muscle) tissues for their utilization. In the acidotic state, cholesterolemias as high as 700 mg% have likewise been observed in clinical diabetes of the dog as compared to the normal range between 125 and 250 mg%. It has been pointed out that net gluconeogenesis from fatty acid does not occur and that the precursors for gluconeogenesis are primarily the proteins. The relative excess of adrenal and pituitary factors in the diabetic animal also serves to stimulate protein catabolism and gluconeogenesis. The reduced cofactors which provide the reductive environment which is required for gluconeogenesis can be provided by the increased production of reduced cofactors as a result of increased fatty acid oxidation (Renold and Cahill, 1966). This increase in the reductive environment has been proposed (Wieland, 1968) as the underlying mechanisms which drains OAA to gluconeogenesis, thereby leading to ketosis.

4. Electrolyte Balance and Acidosis

A mild glycosuria of the order of a few grams of glucose loss per day does not in itself directly precipitate the acidotic state, for a degree of compensation may occur. With continued and severe loss of glucose, all the attending phenomena in attempts to compensate are exaggerated. Liver glycogen stores are depleted, and replacement supplies of glucose are obtained by increased protein breakdown and gluconeogenesis. The oxidation of fatty acids is accelerated and, with it, the accumulation of AcAc, β-OH-butyrate, and acetone in the plasma. The vapor pressure of acetone (bp 56.6°C) is high at body temperature and thus this volatile compound is often detected in the breath of the severely ketotic animal. The other two ketone bodies, being acidic, combine with fixed base in the plasma and thereby reduce the alkali reserve. The plasma bicarbonate (normal range = 18–24 mEq/liter) and the serum sodium (normal range = 137–149 mEq/liter) are below normal. In hyperketonemia, large amounts of ketones are wasted in the urine, together with losses of water and base. The acidic ketones are largely buffered by ammonia synthesized from glutamine in the renal tubules. However, the excessive amounts are ultimately buffered with fixed base, sodium, and potassium, and are lost in the urine. Even without ketonuria, the loss of electrolytes in the polyuria of diabetes may be considerable. Thus, the acidosis of the diabetic is a primary alkali deficit fundamentally related to the ketonemia and to the loss of base in the urine.

The passage of excess glucose provokes an osmotic diuresis leading the loss of water, thirst, and dehydration. The progressively severe loss of water and electrolytes and the accompanying dehydration and acidosis may lead to collapse and coma. This is of particular importance in diabetics which have progressed to the state of renal impairment. Not all the extracellular sodium deficit is due to urinary loss, however, for as increasing amounts of potassium leave the intracellular compartment in the acidotic state, sodium enters the cells. As the dehydration progresses, extracellular potassium concentration may actually be within normal limits due to the decrease in size of the extracellular fluid compartment. This is an important consideration in the fluid and electrolyte replacement therapy of diabetic acidosis, for without the addition of potassium, the rapid expansion of the extracellular fluid compartment may result in hypokalemia. Further discussion of this acidosis and its treatment may be found in Volume II, Chapter 2, on electrolytes and fluid balance.

5. Urinalysis

Considering that the renal threshold for glucose in the dog is about 200 mg % the detection of even trace amounts of glucose in the urine is an important finding and would warrant further investigation. In a total of 56 cases which were tentatively diagnosed as diabetes mellitus on the basis of glycosuria alone, the diagnosis was later confirmed in all (Wilkinson, 1960). Therefore, glycosuria, in any case, should be considered presumptive evidence of diabetes. Renal diabetes, although always a consideration, would seem to be an extremely rare occurrence. The fluctuations in blood glucose levels following feeding have been discussed in Section VII,D and should be considered in the interpretation of the results of urine glucose determinations. Transient glycosurias may occur for $1-1\frac{1}{2}$ hours after a heavy carbohydrate meal, but a 2-hour postprandial glycosuria, or a fasting glycosuria, is a strong indication of diabetes.

An elevated urinary specific gravity has often been considered a good index of the degree of glycosuria and, hence, of diabetes. Specific gravity is a measure of the concentration of solids in the urine. These are principally the cations (sodium, potassium, and ammonium) and their anions (phosphate, sulfate, bicarbonate, and chloride) and urea. The observed specific gravity of urine is the result of the additive effect of the contributions of each (Price *et al.*, 1940). Albumin in urine increases the specific gravity 0.003 units for each gm/100 ml, whereas glucose increases it by 0.004 units for each gm/100 ml. Even though the presence of glucose does increase the specific gravity linearly, a 4$^+$ reaction (2.5 mg% glucose) would increase the specific gravity only 0.010 unit. Therefore, while specific gravity is a valuable measure of renal function, it is of little value with respect to the glycosuria of diabetes, except, of course, in extreme glycosurias. Conversely, by subtracting the contribution of albumin and glucose from the observed specific gravity, a more accurate measure of the renal function in diabetes may be obtained.

Proteinuria is a common sign of renal disease and is often observed in diabetes in dogs (Wilkinson, 1957). There is doubt whether this is associated with chronic nephritis so common in dogs or whether it is due to a renal failure as an aftermath of diabetes. A degree of renal arteriosclerosis is common in diabetic dogs (Meier, 1960), but this lesion may not be exactly comparable to the Kimmelstiel-Wilson lesion seen in man. In advanced cases, this lesion is manifested by proteinuria and uremia.

The ketone bodies are low renal threshold substances (Schwab and Lotspeich, 1954) and their appearance in the urine is an early sign of developing ketonemia. It is not, however, necessarily diagnostic of diabetes, for ketonuria may be observed in starvation and is often absent in the mild diabetic. Ketonuria of varying degrees is, however, common in the more advanced diabetic state. Ketonuria is also a valuable sign of developing acidosis and useful for prognostication. Urinary pH is of little value in detecting acidosis, for only in extreme cases does the pH vary beyond normal limits.

6. Summary

The alterations in blood plasma which have been described are briefly summarized in Fig. 14. In the diabetic state, the uptake of glucose by muscle and adipose tissues is depressed. In these tissues, protein and lipid breakdown are enhanced, and increased amounts of their constituent amino acids and fatty acids are released to the circulation and carried to the liver. Increased hepatic urea production results from the metabolism of the amino acids. Increases in the key gluconeogenic enzymes of the liver, G-6-Pase, F-1,6-Pase, PEP-CK, and PC directs G-6-P metabolism toward increased release of free glucose. At the same time, lipogenesis is suppressed, which, together with the increased mobilization of fatty acids, promotes the accumulation of Ac-CoA and ketosis ensues.

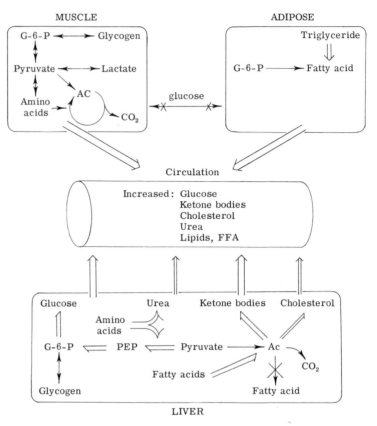

Fig. 14. Summary of metabolic alterations in tissues of major importance in the diabetic animal. Increased flow in the metabolic pathways are noted by larger arrows.

B. Hyperinsulinism

Following the discovery of insulin, a clinical state showing marked similarities to insulin overdosage was recognized as a disease entity in man and termed hyperinsulinism. It is now well established that the disease is due to a persistent hyperactivity of the pancreas, usually as a result of insulin-secreting islet cell tumors. In the now classic case of Wilder *et al.* (1927), excess insulin was extracted from metastatic foci in liver as well as from the pancreatic tumor. The counterpart of this disease in dogs has been reported by Slye and Wells (1935), Hansen (1949), and Cello and Kennedy (1957).

The disease as seen in dogs is characterized by a persistent hypoglycemia in association with periods of weakness, apathy, fainting, and during hypoglycemic crisis, convulsions and coma. A history relating the attacks to periods after fasting or exercise provides a clinical basis for further investigations. Establishment of the diagnosis depends upon the finding of a significant hypoglycemia (below 50 mg%) at the time of occurrence of symptoms and the symptoms are relieved by the administration of glucose. In mild cases, the fasting level may be normal, in which case, diagnostic hypoglycemia may often be provoked in the dog by sequentially (1) placing on a low carbohydrate diet (meat only) for 1 week, then (2) placing on a 24-hour fast, and then (3) moderate exercising. Blood glucose levels are determined at the end of each step, and if hypoglycemia is evident at any step, the provocation should be terminated.

The GTT, as performed in the conventional manner, is of little value in hyperinsulinism. The shape of the tolerance curve is markedly influenced by the previous carbohydrate intake of the dog (Hill and Chaikoff, 1956). A high carbohydrate diet favors a low peak, and conversely, a low carbohydrate diet shows a high peak in the tolerance curve. Diabetic (high) peaks are not unusual in states of hyperinsulin (disease or therapy). This has been interpreted by Somogyi (1959a,b) as due to a transitory excess of insulin antagonists, the hormones of the anterior pituitary, adrenal cortex, and epinephrine, which is provoked by the hypoglycemia and likened to "adrenalin diabetes."

The glucose tolerance curve is usually characteristic, however, if (1) the animal is placed on a high carbohydrate diet for 3–4 days, (2) the intravenous test is used, and most important, (3) blood sampling is continued for 6–8 hours. A prolongation of the hypoglycemic phase (phase III, Fig. 12) is the most significant portion of the curve. A curve of this type has been observed in the dog in which the hypoglycemic phase persisted for 7 hours (Cello and Kennedy, 1957).

An animal with a tendency toward persistent hypoglycemia is likely to show an abnormal response to the insulin tolerance test. The tolerance curve usually shows a minimal drop in blood glucose and remains below the original level for a prolonged length of time. Therefore, the curve shows "insulin resistance" and "hypoglycemia unresponsiveness." Use of this test, however, is not without risk, and if used, glucose solution for intravenous administration should be at hand.

More recently, the hypoglycemia which follows oral administration of leucine in children (Cochrane et al., 1956) has been employed in studies of patients with islet cell tumors (Flanagan et al., 1961). Marked hypoglycemia occurred within 30–60 minutes after L-leucine administration. It has also been shown that leucine-induced hypoglycemia is associated with a rise in plasma insulin levels (Yalow and Berson, 1960). In the patients with islet cell tumors, leucine sensitivity disappeared after removal of the tumor, a finding which would indicate that the tumorous islet cells alone were being stimulated in these cases. This test is routinely employed in our laboratories in hypoglycemic dogs and a description of its successful application in pancreatic islet cell tumors of dogs has been published (Bullock, 1965).

C. HYPOGLYCEMIA OF BABY PIGS

Hypoglycemia of baby pigs was first observed by Graham et al. (1941) and our present knowledge of this condition is largely based upon the work of Sampson and associates (Sampson, 1958). The condition occurs during the first few days of life and is characterized by hypoglycemia (below 40 mg%), apathy, weakness, convulsions, coma, and finally death.

The newborn baby pig is particularly susceptible to hypoglycemia. At birth, the blood glucose level is high (103 mg%) and, unless the pig is fed, drops rapidly to hypoglycemic levels within 24–36 hours. The liver glycogen which is high (14.8%) at birth is almost totally absent at death (Morrill, 1952). In contrast, newborn lambs (Sampson *et al.*, 1955), calves, and foals (Goodwin, 1957) are able to resist starvation hypoglycemia for more than a week. The ability of the baby pig to withstand starvation progressively increases from time of birth, and a 10-day-old pig can be starved up to 3 weeks before symptoms of hypoglycemia occur (Hanawalt and Sampson, 1947).

These findings have recently been confirmed by the studies of Swiatek *et al.* (1968) who concluded that gluconeogenesis was impaired in the newborn pig which was associated with a decrease in plasma FFA. These findings suggest that the gluconeogenic mechanisms of the baby pig are not fully developed at birth and are stimulated or induced by the initial feeding. A study of the hepatic gluconeogenic enzymes and their induceability by feeding would be of great value in understanding the mechanism of baby pig hypoglycemia.

The association of the condition with complete or partial starvation is shown by the findings that the stomachs are empty at necropsy and the syndrome itself is indistinguishable from experimental starvation of the newborn baby pig. Starvation of the newborn pig may occur due to factors relating to the sow (agalactia, metritis, etc.) or to the condition of the baby pig (anemia, infections, etc.), either case resulting in inadequate intake. If feeding is required to induce the hepatic gluconeogenic enzymes in the newborn baby pig, this would explain its inability to withstand starvation as can the newborn lamb or foals.

X.   DISORDERS OF RUMINANTS ASSOCIATED WITH HYPOGLYCEMIA

A. GENERAL

The principal disorders of domestic ruminants in which hypoglycemia is a salient feature are bovine ketosis and ovine pregnancy toxemia. Pregnancy toxemia characteristically is a widespread disease of high mortality occurring in the pregnant ewe just prior to term which is the time when carbohydrate demands are highest, especially in those ewes carrying more than one fetus. Bovine ketosis, on the other hand, occurs in the high-producing dairy cow characteristically during the early stages of lactation, when milk production is generally the highest. Abnormally high levels of the ketone bodies, acetone, AcAc, β-OH-butyrate, and isopropanol appear in blood, urine, and milk. These alterations are accompanied by the clinical symptoms of the disorder: loss of appetite, weight, and milk production, and nervous disturbances.

The energy metabolism of the ruminant is centered about the utilization of the VFA produced by rumen fermentation rather than carbohydrate. The carbohydrate economy of the ruminant is significantly different from that of the nonruminant, and an appreciation of these differences is important to a clearer understanding of the alterations in these metabolic disorders of the ruminant.

B. CARBOHYDRATE BALANCE

1.   *Glucose Requirements*

The heavy demands for glucose in early lactation and in late pregnancy are well known. Kleiber (1959) has calculated that about 60% of the lactating cows' daily

TABLE VII   CARBOHYDRATE BALANCE OF A COW

A. Cow's Daily Glucose Flux[a]

1. *In 12.5 kg milk:*   *Carbohydrate carbon*
   610 gm lactose   257 gm C/day
   462 gm milk fat with 58 gm glycerol   23 gm C/day
   Carbohydrate carbon in milk per day   280 gm C/day
2. *Daily glucose catabolism:*
   Cow produced daily 3288 liters CO_2 = 1762 gm C
   Transfer quotient plasma glucose ——— CO_2 is 0.1
   Thus glucose to CO_2 per day   176 gm C/day
   1 + 2 = Daily flux of glucose   456 gm C/day

$$\frac{180}{72} \times 456 = 1140 \text{ gm glucose/day}$$

B.   Cow's Glucose Sources

Cow secreted daily in urine 34 gm N
This indicates catabolism of 213 gm protein with   110 gm C/day
In urea   14 gm C/day
Maximum available for glucose synthesis from protein   96 gm C/day

Glucose flow in milk and respiration   456 gm C/day
Thus glucose flow from nonprotein sources   360 gm C/day

$\frac{180}{72} \times 360 = 900$ gm glucose daily must have been supplied from nonprotein source

[a]By kind permission of Kleiber (1959).

glucose requirement is for the production of milk. The balance sheet (Table VII) indicates a total daily glucose requirement of 1140 gm of which 700 gm appear in the milk. For sheep in late pregnancy, Kronfeld (1958) calculated from data of others that between one-third and one-half of the daily glucose turnover of 100 gm was utilized by the fetus.

An alternate approach toward assessment of the glucose requirements of an animal is to measure the rate at which glucose enters or leaves the circulation. This is best measured by the use of isotopically labeled glucose. In recent years, reports from Kleiber's laboratory using this technique have given estimates of the daily turnover or requirements for glucose by the lactating cow. Baxter *et al.* (1955), estimated a transfer out of the circulation of about 70 gm/hr or 1680 gm/day in a lactating cow, a figure which they realized may have overestimated the daily glucose turnover. A later report by this group gave an average estimate of 1440 gm/day (60 gm/hr) in four cows. For sheep, similar techniques gave an average turnover of about 144 gm/day in normal pregnant ewes just prior to term (Kronfeld and Simesen, 1961). It would appear that a reasonable estimate of the average daily glucose requirement would be about 50 gm/hr or 1.20 kg/day for a 1000-lb lactating cow and about one-tenth of this or 120 gm/day for the ewe in late pregnancy.

2.   Glucose Sources

The large amounts of indigestible carbohydrates ingested by ruminants are fermented to VFA by the rumen microflora. Little, if any, of the digestible carbohydrates (starch, glucose) in the diet escapes this fermentation. It has previously been emphasized that the oral route is ineffective for the performance of the GTT in the mature ruminant. Thus, glucose absorption by the digestive tract accounts for little of the daily glucose requirement in contrast to the case in nonruminants. It is known, however, that the glucose, which might have escaped rumen fermentation, is readily absorbed (Larsen *et al.*, 1956) as in other species.

A possible source of blood glucose is ruminal lactic acid. Lactic acid is a product of many fermentation reactions, and it is known that blood lactate can be a source of blood glucose via the lactic acid cycle (see Fig. 4). Normally, blood lactate is derived principally from the breakdown of muscle glycogen. It has been demonstrated, however, that sodium lactate placed in the rumen results in increased blood lactate and glucose (Hueter *et al.*, 1956). Thus, some of the glucose requirement may be met from this source but it is likely to be minimal since excesses of lactic acid in the rumen are toxic.

The carbohydrate balance sheet (Table VII) provides an indication of the contribution of protein as a source of carbohydrate for the lactating cow. Since glucose absorption in the ruminant is minimal, the balance sheet also illustrates the importance of an alternate nonprotein source of carbohydrate. These sources are the ruminal VFA. It is now generally recognized that the principle products of rumen fermentation are the VFA, acetic, propionic, and butyric acid, that these acids are absorbed across the rumen wall and are the major source of nutriment for the ruminant. Various authors have used a variety of techniques to arrive at estimates of production and absorption of these acids. These fatty acids are found in approximate proportions of: acetate, 65; propionate, 20; and butyrate, 10. Further details of fatty acid production and absorption by the ruminant may be found in Chapter 2, on lipids.

According to established concepts, carbon from acetic acid, although it appears in carbohydrate (blood glucose, milk lactose) through the mechanism of the TCA cycle (see Fig. 9), cannot theoretically contribute to the net synthesis of carbohydrate. Numerous studies have shown that this is the case and there is extensive evidence that acetate is not a glucogenic compound. The large amounts of acetate provided by rumen fermentation are utilized for energy purposes and for the synthesis of fat. A possible mechanism for the direct incorporation of acetate into a glucose precursor is the so-called glyoxylate pathway (Kornberg and Madsen, 1957), which occurs in plants but has not been demonstrated in animals.

Propionate, on the other hand, is a well-known precursor of carbohydrate (Kleiber *et al.*, 1953; Johnson, 1955; Armstrong and Blaxter, 1957). The pathway leading to a net synthesis of glucose from propionate is available via the reaction

$$\text{Propionate} + CO_2 \longrightarrow \text{succinate}$$

as shown in Fig. 9. According to the scheme, 2 moles of propionate are theoretically required for the synthesis of 1 mole of glucose. A more recent refinement of the pathway for the glucose production from propionate has been proposed by Ballard *et al.* (1968) which separates a mitochondrial pathway from the cytoplasmic. The overall reaction is, however, the same and thus 1 gm of propionate theoretically can provide 1.23 gm of glucose. The amounts of propionate available from rumen fermentation can theoretically supply at least the glucose requirements not accounted for by protein sources.

The contribution of the third major fatty acid from rumen fermentation, butyric acid, in the production of glucose remains controversial. According to the pathway for β-oxidation of fatty acids, butyrate oxidation should lead to acetate production and hence should be a ketogenic substance similar to acetate. There is yet no adequately supported pathway of butyrate oxidation which would bypass the formation of acetate. The labeling patterns of the amino acids of casein after injection of specifically labeled butyrate were consistent with β-oxidation of butyrate (Kleiber et al., 1956). Also, the appearance of radioactive carbon in the respiratory CO_2 after injection of either 1- or 3-labeled butyrate was almost equal, a finding which lends further support to the β-oxidation mechanism (Kleiber, 1959). Nevertheless, butyrate has been shown to have glucogenic properties in lactating cows (Kleiber et al., 1954). A similar glucogenic effect of butyrate in sheep (Potter, 1952) has also been demonstrated. Therefore, while it appears that butyrate is not only ketogenic but glucogenic as well, its significance in the carbohydrate balance of the ruminant remains obscure.

3. Utilization of Glucose

The overall utilization of glucose by the ruminant exhibits some significant differences from that observed in other animals. Reid (1950b), on the basis of carotid-jugular differences in glucose concentration, concluded that glucose was less important as an energy source for the sheep than for the nonruminant and that acetate oxidation plays the more important role in energy metabolism of the ruminant. The oxidation of glucose is also reflected in the excretion of its carbon atoms as respiratory CO_2. Using this technique with radioactive glucose, Baxter et al. (1955) estimated that only about 10% of the respiratory CO_2 arises from glucose oxidation, which is considerably less than the estimates, ranging between 25 and 60% for the rat, dog, and man. The glucose tolerance of the cow (Holmes, 1951) and sheep (Reid, 1952) were reported to be decreased but more recently (Kaneko and Rhode, 1964), the glucose tolerance of the cow was shown to be comparable to that of other animals. The plasma clearance $T_{\frac{1}{2}}$ was 33 minutes which is also similar to that observed in dogs and man.

Black et al. (1957) estimated that about 60% of the glucose oxidized in the mammary gland of the lactating cow occurred via the pentose cycle (see Fig. 6). The same percentage of pentose cycle activity has been observed in rat mammary gland (Abraham et al., 1954). Pentose cycle activity in the mammary gland has also been shown by measurement of the activities of G-6-PD and 6-PGD in the sheep (McLean, 1958) and cow (Raggi et al., 1961). Enzyme activities in sheep gland, however, were not as high as in rat gland. Thus, while the overall utilization of glucose may be lower in ruminants, the pathways, although not necessarily the proportions, by which glucose is catabolized are essentially similar to those of other animals.

The other major pathway for glucose oxidation is the classic E-M pathway and the TCA cycle. The presence of TCA cycle activity in the lactating mammary gland of the cow has been firmly established by Black and Kleiber (1957). Through this mechanism, carbon atoms from acetate, derived from any source, appear in milk products (Fig. 15). Thus, glucose carbon atoms may be given off as CO_2, appear

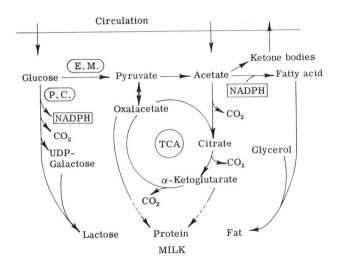

Fig. 15.   Summary of some metabolic pathways in the mammary gland.

in the amino acids of milk protein via transamination of OAA and α-KG or appear in milk fat. The shorter chain fatty acids of butterfat are synthesized from acetate in the mammary gland in contrast to the higher chain acids of butterfat, which are derived from blood lipids. The synthetic pathway for fatty acids in the gland appears to be the same as that in other animal tissues (see Section IX).

The major portion of the glucose uptake by the mammary gland, however, provides for the biosynthesis of milk. The glucose and galactose moieties of lactose are probably derived solely from blood glucose. The rate of lactose synthesis is also constant over a wide range of blood glucose concentrations (20–80 mg/100 ml) (Storry and Rook, 1961), a finding which indicates that lactose synthesis is maximal even under hypoglycemic conditions. The mammary gland, therefore, is a glucose-utilizing tissue, principally for biosynthesis and less for oxidation. The principal metabolic pathways involved are summarized in Fig. 15.

Ruminant nervous tissue, i.e., brain, is similar to that of other animals in being an obligatory glucose-utilizing tissue (McClymont and Setchell, 1956). The gluco-kinase activity of sheep brain, however, is significantly lower than in rat brain (Jarrett and Filsell, 1958; Gallagher and Buttery, 1959). These observations would suggest that, in spite of the glucose requirement, its utilization by this tissue is lower in the ruminant than in other animals. The same authors observed that the glucokinase activity of sheep intestine was similarly low when compared to rat intestine. Ruminant muscle also utilizes less glucose than muscle tissue of other species (Reid, 1950a,b).

Studies of the activities of ruminant liver enzymes, particularly with respect to gluconeogenesis and ketosis, have been conducted. Although highest G-6-Pase activities were found in liver as compared to other organs of sheep at slaughter, they were only about two-thirds of the activities found in rats (Raggi et al., 1960). Hepatic G-6-Pase activities in older calves and lactating cows were slightly higher than G-6-Pase activities of rats and could be reduced by intraduodenal infusions of glucose (Bartley *et al.*, 1966). This is in general agreement with the concept that liver is a glucose-producing tissue and that increased production of glucose by liver is associated with increased G-6-Pase activity. It should be noted, however, that Ford (1961) has observed that hepatic G-6-Pase activities remained relatively constant during early lactation, the period during which a cow's glucose requirement is even higher than during pregnancy (Brody *et al.*, 1948).

Ballard *et al.* (1968) and Baird *et al.* (1968) have recently reported their studies of a number of gluconeogenic enzymes of cow liver. Ballard *et al.* (1968) found that the PEP-CK, a key gluconeogenic enzyme, of cow liver is already very high in comparison to that reported in rat liver (Krebs, 1966). This would further support the concept that the high-producing dairy cow that has been genetically selected for these qualities, is already synthesizing glucose maximally under normal conditions.

To summarize, the ruminant appears to be an animal well adapted to a carbohydrate economy based upon the endogenous synthesis of glucose from non-carbohydrate sources (gluconeogenesis). The enzymic mechanisms for gluconeogenesis are already operating at near maximal levels on the high-producing dairy cow. Glucose oxidation by individual tissues as well as by the intact animal is lower in ruminants than in nonruminants. Although overall oxidation may be different, the pathways by which this oxidation is accomplished are essentially similar to those of other animals (Fig. 15). Considering that the endocrine relationships of ruminants are also qualitatively similar to those of nonruminants, the normally low blood glucose concentration might also be considered to be a reflection of the degree of influence rather than kind. For example, the blood glucose response of the ruminant to insulin (Reid, 1951a,b; Jasper, 1953a,b) as compared to that of the dog shows a slower rate of fall, i.e., insulin resistance.

C. Biochemical Alterations in Body Fluids

1. Hypoglycemia

The occurrence of a significant hypoglycemia in bovine ketosis and in ovine pregnancy toxemia has been repeatedly confirmed. Normal blood glucose levels range between 35 and 55 mg/100 ml for cows and from 35 to 60 mg/100 ml for sheep. The importance placed upon this finding has led to suggestions that a better name for bovine ketosis would be "hypoglycemia." This hypoglycemia has played an important role in ketosis, not only as a rationale for therapy but as a basis for the concept of ketosis and pregnancy toxemia as manifestations of a carbohydrate deficiency which occurs under conditions of excessive and insurmountable demands.

2. Ketone Bodies

Ketosis is defined as a condition with an elevation of ketone bodies in the body fluids and is a characteristic of bovine ketosis and pregnancy toxemia of sheep. The ketone bodies in these animals are the same as those previously mentioned (Section V,A,3), AcAc, β-OH-butyrate, and acetone. A fourth compound, isopropanol, should also be included for the ruminant and interconversions can occur between these ketone bodies (Thin *et al.*, 1959).

a. SITE OF KETONE BODY PRODUCTION. It has been previously mentioned (Section IX,A,3) that increased ketogenesis occurs under conditions which favor the accumulation of acetate. In the nonruminant, the liver is the principal, if not the sole, source of ketone bodies, and they appear in the body fluids when production exceeds the capacity for utilization. In the ruminant, the liver may not be the sole significant source of ketone bodies. It has been demonstrated that rumen epithelium (Pennington, 1952) and mammary gland (Kronfeld and Kleiber, 1959) can also be sources of ketone bodies. The extent of their contribution to the ketone bodies of the body fluids, however, is uncertain although it could be considerable in the ketotic animal.

b. HYPERKETONEMIA. Elevations of ketone bodies in the body fluids may be influenced by a number of conditions which relate to the carbohydrate economy of the ruminant. Starvation is the best-known method of producing ketosis. Some degree of elevation of ketones is also often seen without detrimental effects in association with early lactation, late pregnancy, underfeeding, and with high fat diets. In these states, the continuing demands of the body for carbohydrate are not adequately met.

Elevated blood ketones are a consistent finding in bovine ketosis and pregnancy toxemia, though the degree of ketonemia does not necessarily parallel the severity of the clinical signs. Normally, total blood ketones in sheep or cows is less than 10 mg/100 ml (Thin and Robertson, 1953). Total ketone bodies as acetone may best be determined quantitatively by the salicylaldehyde method or modifications thereof (Adler, 1957; Thin and Robertson, 1952). These methods, however, do not lend themselves for routine use in the office laboratory. The measurement of ketone bodies in the blood has been essentially displaced in clinical practice by the rapid qualitative tests applied to urine and milk. These same rapid tests can be applied to serum diluted 1:1 with water and employed as screening tests for the detection of ketonemia.

c. KETONE BODIES IN URINE AND MILK. The rapid qualitative tests for urinary ketones (see Vol. II, Chapter 11) may also be applied to milk with a slight modification as described by Sampson (1947). The tests containing sodium nitroprusside are widely known as the Ross modification (S. G. Ross, 1931) of Rothera's test.

The results of the qualitative tests on urine and milk are often employed as indices of the degree of ketonemia. The correlation of these tests with blood ketone levels, however, is poor. Adler *et al.* (1957) studied the correlation of these tests on urine and milk with the degree of ketonemia. They employed a modification of the Ross test in which a flake of sodium hydroxide was substituted for the ammonium hydroxide. Statistically, only three divisions for urine and two divisions of color intensity for milk were justifiable. The Ross test applied to urine is very sensitive, and false positives are not uncommon in the urine of normal cows. The test is not as sensitive when applied to milk and a 1+ reaction is of much greater diagnostic significance than the same reaction with urine. For this reason, urine should be diluted 1:10 with water to take advantage of its sensitivity and increase its diagnostic accuracy.

Reagents:	For urine	For milk
Sodium nitroprusside	1 part	2 parts
Ammonium sulfate	99 parts	98 parts

Mix the dry reagents and store in a brown bottle.

Procedure:

For urine: dissolve 1 gm of the dry mixture for urine in 5 ml or urine. Overlay the urine with a 1 ml of concentrated ammonium hydroxide. Note the intensity of the purple color which develops at the interface in 5 minutes according to the scale:

tr = trace purple
1+ = slight purple
2+ = moderate purple
3+ = dark purple

For milk: Repeat the above procedure using 2.5 gm of the dry mixture for milk.

The tests which employ nitroprusside detect acetone and AcAc in the body fluids. These tests are much more sensitive to AcAc than to acetone and, therefore, fresh samples, in which less breakdown of AcAc to acetone has occurred, usually give darker reactions. The presence of Bromsulphalein (BSP) will give a false positive. Gerhardt's test, which uses $FeCl_3$, has also been employed clinically to detect ketone bodies. The $FeCl_3$ tests, however, detect only one ketone body, AcAc, are less sensitive and generally less satisfactory than the nitroprusside tests.

D. RUMINANT KETOSIS

It has been repeatedly mentioned that the finely balanced carbohydrate economy of the ruminants plays an important role in the development of ketosis in cows and sheep. In the cow, large amounts of glucose must be produced by gluconeogenesis to meet the heavy demands for lactose, particularly in early lactation, when the demand is highest. There is also general agreement that, in sheep a failure to meet the obligatory demands for hexoses by the fetus is a precipitating cause of ketosis. The mechanisms whereby imbalances occur and are manifest as ketosis, however, are uncertain and have been the subject of numerous investigations.

The principal concept of a decade ago has been that centered about a slowing of the TCA cycle and a deficiency of its intermediates, namely, OAA (see Fig. 9). According to this hypothesis, the heavy demands of late pregnancy and early lactation for glucose and intermediates for biosynthesis result in a depletion of these intermediates of the TCA cycle with a resulting slowing of the TCA cycle operation. The limiting factor is likely to be the TCA cycle intermediate, OAA, which occupies a central position in the metabolic scheme. Oxalacetate may be withdrawn for amino acid synthesis, for gluconeogenesis, and it is also the condensing partner of Ac-CoA which is required for operation of the TCA cycle. A deficiency of OAA would be expected to lead to a decrease in operation of the TCA cycle and hence a decrease in the oxidation of acetate to CO_2 by this pathway.

This would favor the accumulation of acetate by removing a major pathway for its disposal, and its diversion to ketone body production would be enhanced.

This OAA deficiency theory which had earlier been criticized and rejected (W. V. Shaw and Tapley, 1958; Krebs, 1961) has in recent years been revived and supported (Krebs, 1966; Wieland, 1968; Baird et al., 1968). Only the mechanism by which mitochondrial OAA deficiency occurs has been modified. Under conditions of increased glucose demand (lactation, pregnancy) gluconeogenesis is increased and the major common precursor for glucose, OAA, is excessively drained and is likely to be depleted. Gluconeogenesis is increased either by increase in activity of the gluconeogenic enzymes (Krebs, 1966) or by an increase in the "reducing pressure" (Wieland, 1968) as a result of increased fatty acid oxidation. It has been shown that gluconeogenesis is increased in bovine ketosis as it is in alloxan diabetic rats (Baird et al., 1968). By either mechanism, a deficiency of mitochondrial OAA would be expected to lead to a diversion of Ac-CoA units to ketone body production.

The accumulation of acetate and hence increased ketogenesis would also be favored in conditions where fatty acid oxidation was increased and its synthesis was decreased. It is well known that, in association with decreased glucose utilization, lipid mobilization and oxidation are increased and that fatty acid synthesis is decreased. As previously discussed (Section V), in the presence of decreased glucose oxidation via the pentose cycle, hepatic NADPH (TPNH) generation would be decreased and lipogenesis depressed. This proposal may be modified for the ketotic cow since, even though overall glucose utilization is normal, the pentose cycle activity has been shown to be depressed (Tombropoulos and Kleiber, 1960). As a consequence of decreased NADPH (TPNH) generation in the mammary gland, lipogenesis from acetate would be impaired, again enhancing ketone body production. Recently, this mechanism has been employed to explain the impaired lipogenesis from acetate-^{14}C by the fasting ketotic cow (Simesen et al., 1961). It has been suggested that if a tissue such as mammary gland (Pearce, 1960) or a pathway for glucose oxidation, i.e., the pentose cycle (Tombropoulos and Kleiber, 1960) takes priority for available glucose, the metabolic alterations observed in ketotic cows can be explained. Such a mechanism would consider the mammary gland of the cow as an important site in addition to the liver of the biochemical events which culminate in the development of the ketotic state. The cows' gluconeogenic mechanisms in the liver are likely to be already operating at maximal levels to meet the heavy demands of lactation. This would then suggest an inability of the susceptible cows' enzymic mechanisms to increase to supply sufficient glucose for both lactose production and oxidative purposes during periods of excessive demand. In this respect, it is interesting to note that hepatic G-6-Pase activities of the cow remained constant during the period 60 days before to 60 days after calving (Ford, 1961). Furthermore, Baird et al. (1968) found no differences in gluconeogenic enzyme activity between normal and ketotic cows. Ballard et al. (1968) found that the activity of the key gluconeogenic enzyme, PEP-CK, in cow liver was already very high in comparison to rat liver and did not change. There was also no decrease in OAA in contrast to the report by Baird et al. (1968). Thus, a degree of controversy prevails even while clarification of the biochemical basis of ketosis appears to be nearing.

REFERENCES

Abraham, S., Hirsch, P. F., and Chaikoff, I. L. (1954). *J. Biol. Chem.* **211**, 31.

Adler, J. H. (1957). *Cornell Vet.* **47**, 354.

Adler, J. H., Roberts, S. J., and Steel, R. G. D. (1957). *Cornell Vet.* **47**, 101.

Alexander, F. (1955). *Quart. J. Exptl. Physiol.* **40**, 24.

Anstall, H. B. (1968). *Am. J. Clin. Pathol.* **50**, 3.

Armstrong, D. G., and Blaxter, K. L. (1957). *Brit. J. Nutr.* **11**, 247.

Ashmore, J., and Weber, G. (1968). *In* "Carbohydrate Metabolism and Its Disorders" (F. Dickens, P. J. Randle, and W. J. Whelan, eds.), Vol. 1, p. 336. Academic Press, New York.

Ashmore, J., Hastings, A. B., and Nesbett, F. B. (1954). *Proc. Natl. Acad. Sci. U.S.* **40**, 673.

Baer, J. E., Peck, H. M., and McKinney, S. E. (1957). *Proc. Soc. Exptl. Biol. Med.* **95**, 80.

Baird, G. D., Hibbitt, K. G., Hunter, G. D., Lund, P., Stubbs, M., and Krebs, H. A. (1968). *Biochem. J.* **107**, 683.

Ballard, F. J., Hanson, R. W., Kronfeld, D. S., and Raggi, F. (1968). *J. Nutr.* **95**, 160.

Bardens, J. W., (1966). *Vet. Med.* **61**, 1174.

Bartley, J. C., Freedland, R. A., and Black, A. L. (1966). *Am. J. Vet. Res.* **27**, 1243.

Baxter, C. F., Kleiber, M., and Black, A. L. (1955). *Biochim. Biophys. Acta* **17**, 354.

Bell, F. R., and Jones, E. R. (1945). *J. Comp. Pathol. Therap.* **55**, 117.

Black, A. L., and Kleiber, M. (1957). *Biochim. Biophys. Acta* **23**, 59.

Black, A. L., Kleiber, M., Butterworth, E. M., Brubacher, G. B., and Kaneko, J. J. (1957). *J. Biol. Chem.* **227**, 537.

Bloom, F. (1957). *North Am. Vet.* **38**, 114.

Bodo, R. C., Cotui, F. W., and Benaglia, A. E. (1937). *J. Pharmacol. Exptl. Therap.* **61**, 48.

Brady, R. O. (1958). *Proc. Natl. Acad. Sci. U.S.* **44**, 993.

Brody, S., Worstell, D. M., Ragsdale, A. C., and Kibler, H. H. (1948). *Missouri, Univ., Agr. Expt. Sta., Bull.* **412**, 1.

Bullock, L. (1965). *Calif. Vet.* **19**, 14.

Burns, J. J., and Evans, C. (1956). *J. Biol. Chem.* **223**, 897.

Cahill, G. F., Jr., Ashmore, J., Earle, A. S., and Zottu, S. (1958). *Am. J. Physiol.* **192**, 491.

Cahill, G. F., Jr., Ashmore, J., Renold, A. E., and Hastings, A. B. (1959). *Am. J. Med.* **26**, 264.

Campbell, L. A., and Kronfeld, D. S. (1961). *Am. J. Vet. Res.* **22**, 587.

Cello, R. M., and Kennedy, P. C. (1957). *Cornell Vet.* **47**, 538.

Chance, R. E., and Ellis, R. M. (1969). *Arch. Intern. Med. Symp.* **123**, 229.

Chernick, S. S., and Chaikoff, I. L. (1951). *J. Biol. Chem.* **188**, 389.

Cochrane, W. A., Payne, W. W., Simpkiss, M. J., and Woolf, L. I. (1956). *J. Clin. Invest.* **35**, 411.

Colowick, S. P., Cori, G. T., and Slein, M. W. (1947). *J. Biol. Chem.* **168**, 583.

Cori, G. T. (1954). *Harvey Lectures* **48**, 145.

Cornelius, C. E. (1961). *Cornell Vet.* **51**, 559.

Cutler, J. T. (1934). *J. Biol. Chem.* **106**, 653.

Evans, C., Conney, A. H., Trousof, N., and Burns, J. J. (1959). *Federation Proc.* **18**, 223.

Eveleth, D. F., and Eveleth, M. W. (1935). *J. Biol. Chem.* **111**, 753.

Flanagan, G. C., Schwartz, T. B., and Ryan, W. G. (1961). *J. Clin. Endocrinol. Metab.* **21**, 401.

Field, R. A., (1966). *In* "The Metabolic Basis of Inherited Disease" (J. B. Stanbury, J. B. Wyngaarden, and D. S. Fredrickson, eds.), p. 149. McGraw-Hill, New York.

Folin, O., and Malmros, H. (1929). *J. Biol. Chem.* **83**, 115.

Folin, O., and Wu, H. (1920). *J. Boil. Chem.* **83**, 115.

Ford, E. J. H. (1961). *J. Comp. Pathol. Therap.* **71**, 60.

Ford, E. J. H., and Boyd, J. W. (1960). *Res. Vet. Sci.* **1**, 232.

Freedland, R. A., Murad, S., and Hurvitz, A. I. (1968). *Fed. Proc.* **27**, 1217.

Fritz, I. B. (1961). *Physiol. Rev.* **41**, 52.

Fritz, I. B. (1967). *Perspectives Biol. Med.* **10**, 643.

Gallagher, C. H., and Buttery, S. H. (1959). *Biochem. J.* **72**, 575.

Gibson, D. M., Titchener, E. B., and Wakil, S. J. (1958). *Biochim. Biophys. Acta* **30**, 376.

Goodwin, R. F. W. (1957). *J. Comp. Pathol. Therap.* **67**, 289.

Graham, R., Sampson, J., and Hester, H. R. (1941). *Proc. Soc. Exptl. Biol. Med.* **47**, 338.

Grodsky, G. M., Feldman, R., Toreson, W. E., and Lee, J. C. (1966). *Diabetes* **15**, 579.

Hanawalt, V. M., and Sampson, J. (1947). *Am. J. Vet. Res.* **8**, 235.

Hansen, H. J. (1949). *Nord. Veterinarmed.* **1**, 363.

Hawk, P. B., Oser, B. L., and Summerson, W. H. (1954). "Practical Physiological Chemistry," 13th ed., p. 573. McGraw-Hill New York.

Hill, R., and Chaikoff, I. L. (1956). *Proc. Soc. Exptl. Biol. Med.* **91**, 265.

Hirsch, P. F., Baruch, H., and Chaikoff, I. L. (1954). *J. Biol. Chem.* **210**, 785.

Hjarre, A. (1927). *Arch. Wiss. Prakt. Tierheilk.* **57**, 1.

Holmes, J. R. (1951). *J. Comp. Pathol. Therap.* **61**, 15.

Houchin, O. B., Graham, W. H., Jr., Peterson, V. E., and Turner, C. W. (1939). *J. Dairy Sci.* **22**, 241.

Hueter, F. G., Shaw, J. C., and Doetsch, R. N. (1956). *J. Dairy Sci.* **39**, 1430.

Illingworth, B. A., and Cori, G. T. (1952). *J. Biol. Chem.* **199**, 653.

Isselbacher, C. J. (1959). *Am. J. Med.* **26**, 715.

Jarrett, I. G., and Filsell, O. H. (1958). *Australian J. Exptl. Biol.* **36**, 433.

Jasper, D. E. (1953a). *Am. J. Vet. Res.* **14**, 184.

Jasper, D. E. (1953b). *Am. J. Vet. Res.* **14**, 209.

Johnson, R. B. (1955). *Cornell Vet.* **45**, 273.

Kaneko, J. J. (1963). *In* "Clinical Biochemistry of Domestic Animals" (C. E. Cornelius and J. J. Kaneko, eds.), p. 32. Academic Press, New York.

Kaneko, J. J., and Rhode, E. A. (1964). *J. Am. Vet. Med. Assoc.* **144**, 367.

Kaneko, J. J., Luick, J. R., and Rhode, E. A. (1965). *Cornell Vet.* **56**, 401.

Kleiber, M. (1959). *Proc. 2nd Interam. Symp. Peaceful Appl. Nucl. Energy, Buenos Aires*, p. 161.

Kleiber, M., Black, A. L., Brown, M. A., and Tolbert, B. M. (1953). *J. Biol. Chem.* **203**, 339.

Kleiber, M., Black, A. L., Brown, M. A., Luick, J. R., Baxter, C. F., and Tolbert, B. M. (1954). *J. Biol. Chem.* **210**, 239.

Kleiber, M., Black, A. L., and Brubacher, G. B. (1956). *Abstr. 20th Intern. Physiol. Congr., Brussels*, p. 165.

Kornberg, H. L., and Madsen, N. B. (1957). *Biochim. Biophys. Acta* **24**, 651.

Krebs, H. A. (1961). *Arch. Internal Med.* **107**, 51.

Krebs, H. A. (1966). *Vet. Record* **78**, 187.

Kronfeld, D. S. (1958). *Cornell Vet.* **48**, 394.

Kronfeld, D. S., and Kleiber, M. (1959). *J. Appl. Physiol.* **14**, 1033.

Kronfeld, D. S., and Simesen, M. G. (1961). *Cornell Vet.* **51**, 478.

Kronfeld, D. S., Simesen, M. G., and Dungworth, D. L. (1960). *Res. Vet. Sci.* **1**, 242.

Krook, L., Larsson, S., and Rooney, J. R. (1960). *Am. J. Vet. Res.* **21**, 120.

Larsen, H. J., Stoddard, G. E., Jacobson, N. L., and Allen, R. S. (1956). *J. Animal Sci.* **15**, 473.

Le Compte, P. M., Steinke, J., Soeldner, J. S., and Renold, A. E. (1966). *Diabetes* **15**, 586.

Leloir, L. F., and Cardini, C. E. (1957). *J. Am. Chem. Soc.* **79**, 6340.

Leloir, L. F., Olavarría, J. M., Goldemberg, S. H., and Carminatti, H. (1959). *Arch. Biochem. Biophys.* **81**, 508.

Levine, R., Goldstein, M. S., Huddlestun, B., and Klein, S. P. (1950). *Am. J. Physiol.* **163**, 70.

Lossow, W. J., and Chaikoff, I. L. (1955). *Arch. Biochem. Biophys.* **57**, 23.

Lusk, G. (1928). "The Elements of the Science of Nutrition," 4th ed., p. 321. Saunders, Philadelphia.

McCandless, E. L., Woodward, B. A., and Dye, J. A. (1948). *Am. J. Physiol.* **154**, 94.

McClymont, G. L., and Setchell, B. P.(1956). *Australian J. Biol. Sci.* **9**, 184.

McLean, P. (1958). *Biochim. Biophys. Acta* **30**, 303.

Madison, L. L. (1969). *Arch. Internal Med. Symp.* **123**, 284.

Marks, H. P., and Young, F. G. (1940). *Nature* **146**, 31.

Masoro, E. J., Chaikoff, I. L., and Dauben, W. G. (1949). *J. Biol. Chem.* **179**, 1117.

Meade, R. C., Kneubuhler, H. A., Schulte, W. J., and Barboriak, J. J. (1967). *Diabetes* **16**, 141.

Meier, H. (1960). *Diabetes* **9**, 485.

Meier, H., and Yerganian, G. (1959). *Proc. Soc. Exptl. Biol. Med.* **100**, 810.

Morrill, C. C. (1952). *Am. J. Vet. Res.* **13**, 164.

Nelson, N. (1944). *J. Biol. Chem.* **153**, 375.

Park, C. R. Reinwein, D., Henderson, M. J., Cadenas, E., and Morgan, H. E.(1959). *Am. J. Med.* **26**, 674.

Pearce, P. J. (1960). *Vet. Rev. Annotations* **6**, 53.

Pennington, R. J. (1952). *Biochem. J.* **51**, 251.

Porter, J. W., Wakil, S. J., Tietz, A., Jacob, M. I., and Gibson, D. M. (1957). *Biochim. Biophys. Acta* **25**, 35.

Potter, B. J. (1952). *Nature* **170**, 541.

Price, J. W., Miller, M., and Hayman, J. M., Jr. (1940). *J. Clin. Invest.* **19**, 537.

Raggi, F., Kronfeld, D. S., and Kleiber, M. (1960). *Proc. Soc. Exptl. Biol. Med.* **105**, 485.

Raggi, F., Hansson, E., Simesen, M. G., Kronfeld, D. S., and Luick, J. R. (1961). *Res. Vet. Sci.* **2**, 180.

Rall, T. W., and Sutherland, E. W. (1958). *J. Biol. Chem.* **232**, 1065.

Rall, T. W., Sutherland, E. W., and Wosilait, W. D. (1956). *J. Biol. Chem.* **218**, 483.

Rall, T. W., Sutherland, E. W., and Berthet, J. (1957). *J. Biol. Chem.* **224**, 463.

Randle, P. J., and Morgan, H. E. (1962). *Vitamins Hormones* **20**, 199.

Reid, R. L. (1950a). *Australian J. Agr. Res.* **1**, 182.

Reid, R. L. (1950b). *Australian J. Agr. Res.* **1**, 338.

Reid, R. L. (1951a). *Australian J. Agr. Res.* **2**, 132.

Reid, R. L. (1951b). *Australian J. Agr. Res.* **2**, 146.

Reid, R. L. (1952). *Australian J. Agr. Res.* **3**, 160.

Renold, A. E., and Cahill, G. F., Jr. (1966). *In* "The Metabolic Basis of Inherited Disease" (J. B. Stanbury, J. B. Wyngaarden, and D. S. Fredrickson, eds.), p. 101. McGraw-Hill, New York.

Roberts, I. M. (1954). *J. Am. Vet. Med. Assoc.* **124**, 443.

Robison, A., Butcher, R. W., and Sutherland, E. W. (1968). *Am. Rev. Biochem*, **37**, 149.

Roderick, L. M., Harshfield, G. S., and Merchant, W. R. (1933). *Cornell Vet.* **23**, 348.

Rosen, F., Roberts, N. R., and Nichol, C. A. (1959). *J. Biol. Chem.* **234**, 476.

Ross, E. J. (1953). *Nature* **171**, 125.

Ross, S. G. (1931). *J. Lab. Clin. Med.* **16**, 908.

Sampson, J. (1947). *Illinois, Univ., Agr. Expt. Sta., Bull.* **524**, 405.

Sampson, J. (1958). *In* "Diseases of Swine" (H. W. Dunne, ed.), p. 521. Iowa State Univ. Press, Ames, Iowa.

Sampson, J., Hester, H. R., and Graham, R. (1942). *J. Am. Vet. Med. Assoc.* **100**, 33.

Sampson, J., Taylor, R. B., and Smith, J. C. (1955). *Cornell Vet.* **45**, 10.

Sanger, F. (1959). *Science* **129**, 1340.

Schlotthauer, C. F., and Millar, J. A. S. (1951). *J. Am. Vet. Med. Assoc.* **118**, 31.

Schwab, L., and Lotspeich, W. D. (1954). *Am. J. Physiol.* **176**, 195.

Shannon, J. A., Farber, S., and Troast, L. (1941). *Am. J. Physiol.* **133**, 752.

Sharkey, T. P. (1968). *J. Am. Dietet. Assoc.* **52**, 108.

Shaw, J. C. (1943). *J. Dairy Sci.* **26**, 1079.

Shaw, W. V., and Tapley, D. F. (1958). *Biochim. Biophys. Acta* **30**, 426.

Simesen, M. G., Luick, J. R., Kleiber, M., and Thin, C. (1961). *Acta Vet. Scand.* **2**, 214.

Siperstein, M. D. (1959). *Am. J. Med.* **26**, 685.

Siperstein, M. D., and Fagan, V. M. (1957). *Science* **126**, 1012.

Slye, M., and Wells, H. G. (1935). *A.M.A. Arch. Pathol.* **19**, 537.

Somogyi, M. (1959a). *Am. J. Med.* **26**, 169.

Somogyi, M. (1959b). *Am. J. Med.* **26**, 192.

Soskin, S., Essex, H. E., Herrich, J. F., and Mann, F. C. (1938). *Am. J. Physiol.* **124**, 558.

Stadie, W. C. (1954). *Physiol. Rev.* **34**, 52.

Stadie, W. C., and Haugaard, N. (1949). *J. Biol. Chem.* **177**, 311.

Steiner, D. F., and Oyer, P. E. (1967). *Proc. Natl. Acad. Sci.* **57**, 473.

Stewart, J., and Holman, H. H. (1940). *Vet. Record* **52**, 157.

Storry, J. E., and Rook, J. A. F. (1961). *Biochim. Biophys. Acta* **48**, 610.

Sutherland, E. W., and Wosilait, W. D. (1956). *J. Biol. Chem.* **218**, 459.

Swiatek, K. R., Kipnis, D. M., Mason, G., Chao, K., and Cornblath, M. (1968). *Am. J. Physiol.* **214**, 400.

Thin, C., and Robertson, A. (1952). *Biochem. J.* **51**, 218.

Thin, C., and Robertson, A. (1953). *J. Comp. Pathol. Therap.* **63**, 184.

Thin, C., Paver, H., and Robertson, A. (1959). *J. Comp. Pathol. Therap.* **69**, 45.

Tombropoulos, E. G., and Kleiber, M. (1960). *Biochem. J.* **80**, 414.

Touster, O., Mayberry, R. H., and McCormick, D. B. (1957). *Biochim. Biophys. Acta* **25**, 196.

Unger, R. H., Kelterer, H., Dupré, J., and Ersentraut, A. M. (1967). *J. Clin. Invest.* **46**, 630.

Wakil, S. J. (1958). *J. Am. Chem. Soc.* **80**, 6465.

Wieland, O. (1968). *Advan. Metab. Disorders* **3**, 1.

Wilder, R. M., Allan, F. N., Power, M. H., and Robertson, H. E. (1927). *J. Am. Med. Assoc.* **89**, 348.

Wilkinson, J. S. (1957). *Vet. Rev. Annotations* **3**, 69.

Wilkinson, J. S. (1958). *Vet. Rev. Annotations* **4**, 93.

Wilkinson, J. S. (1960). *Vet. Record* **72**, 548.

Yalow, R. S., and Berson, S. A. (1960). *J. Clin. Invest.* **39**, 1157.

Young, F. G. (1963). *In* "Comparative Endocrinology" (U. S. von Euler and H. Heller, eds.), Vol. 1, p. 371. Academic Press, New York.

2   Lipid Metabolism

J. C. Bartley

I. INTRODUCTION

Of the three basic organic foodstuffs, the chemical nature of common animal and vegetable lipids was known prior to similar basic knowledge of carbohydrates and proteins (Chevreul, 1823). Further studies, however, on the biochemical nature of lipid were inhibited by the lack of techniques for dealing with compounds insoluble in water. Hence, for many years the basic knowledge of lipid biochemistry developed more slowly than that of carbohydrate and protein. This situation no longer exists. The recent development of techniques, such as thin layer and gas–liquid chromatography, specific for the separation of nonpolar compounds has resulted in a rapid accumulation of biochemical data on lipids. Similar rapid increases in our knowledge of the form in which lipid occurs in the plasma occurred since the introduction of the methods for the isolation of lipoproteins by means of ultracentrifugation and gel electrophoresis. The intellectual fallout from these technical advances continues to propel the development of physiological chemistry of lipids at a rapid pace.

Lipids have special importance physiologically as the hydrophobic members of membranes and as the most concentrated source of energy (kcal/gm) of any of the major foodstuffs. Lipids include compounds found in living organisms that are insoluble in water and soluble in so-called fat solvents (diethylether, petroleum ether, chloroform, hot alcohol, benzine, carbon tetrachloride, and acetone) (Deuel, 1951). Such a definition is not all-inclusive; for example, lecithin is insoluble in acetone and yet is considered a lipid.

II. CLASSES OF LIPIDS

The broadness of the definition of lipids requires a further classification of the substances included. A slight modification of the classifications set forth by Masoro (1968) is as useful as any and simpler than most. The three major classes are simple lipids, phospholipids, and sphingolipids.

A. SIMPLE LIPIDS

Compounds that are not degraded by alkaline or acid hydrolysis or that, on hydrolysis, yield only derived lipids, i.e., substances soluble in fat solvents, or derived lipids plus glycerol, are all considered simple lipids. Thus, naturally occurring hydrocarbons (squalene), fatty acids, neutral glycerides, and lipid alcohols (cholesterol) and their esters would be included in this category.

B. PHOSPHOLIPIDS

Compounds which yield, on hydrolysis, derived lipids plus inorganic phosphate, glycerol, and, usually, a third water-soluble product are classed as phospholipids. The prototype of this category is phosphatidic acid. Other biologically important derivatives of phosphatidic acid are cardiolipin, in which two glycerides are linked via the phosphate ester, and a series of compounds in which the phosphate ester serves as a link to ethanolamine, inositol, serine, or choline (Fig. 1).

The naturally occurring phospholipids commonly contain one unsaturated fatty acid, usually esterified to the β-position of glycerol, and one saturated fatty acid usually esterified to the α-position (Hanahan, 1954). Variations, of course, do occur. One variant, a lecithin containing two saturated fatty acids deserves special mention.

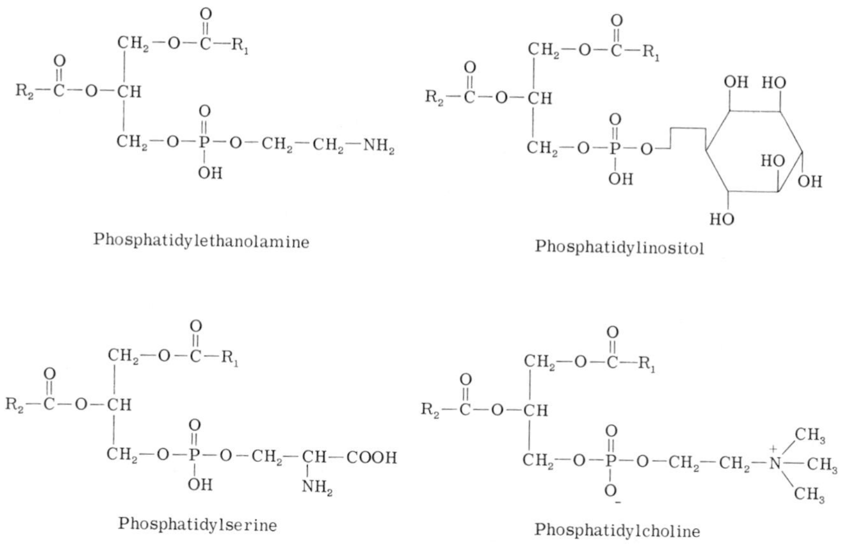

Phosphatidylethanolamine

$$\begin{array}{l}
CH_2-O-\overset{\overset{\textstyle O}{\|}}{C}-R_1 \\
R_2-\overset{\overset{\textstyle O}{\|}}{C}-O-CH \\
CH_2-O-\overset{\overset{\textstyle O}{\|}}{\underset{\underset{\textstyle OH}{|}}{P}}-O-CH_2-CH_2-NH_2
\end{array}$$

Phosphatidylinositol

$$\begin{array}{l}
CH_2-O-\overset{\overset{\textstyle O}{\|}}{C}-R_1 \\
R_2-\overset{\overset{\textstyle O}{\|}}{C}-O-CH \\
CH_2-O-\overset{\overset{\textstyle O}{\|}}{\underset{\underset{\textstyle OH}{|}}{P}}-O-\text{(inositol ring, OH HO HO OH HO)}
\end{array}$$

Phosphatidylserine

$$\begin{array}{l}
CH_2-O-\overset{\overset{\textstyle O}{\|}}{C}-R_1 \\
R_2-\overset{\overset{\textstyle O}{\|}}{C}-O-CH \\
CH_2-O-\overset{\overset{\textstyle O}{\|}}{\underset{\underset{\textstyle OH}{|}}{P}}-O-CH_2-\underset{\underset{\textstyle NH_2}{|}}{CH}-COOH
\end{array}$$

Phosphatidylcholine

$$\begin{array}{l}
CH_2-O-\overset{\overset{\textstyle O}{\|}}{C}-R_1 \\
R_2-\overset{\overset{\textstyle O}{\|}}{C}-O-CH \\
CH_2-O-\overset{\overset{\textstyle O}{\|}}{\underset{\underset{\textstyle O^-}{|}}{P}}-O-CH_2-CH_2-\overset{+}{N}(CH_3)_3
\end{array}$$

Fig. 1.   Structural formulas of some common phospholipids.

Clements (1969) has shown rather conclusively that the surfactant secreted by certain cells in the lung is dipalmityl lecithin. He has isolated this unique lecithin from the lungs of many mammals, fowl, reptiles, and amphibians. Its presence is essential for normal respiratory function.

Not all phospholipids contain two acyl fatty acids. Lysolecithin is characterized by a single fatty acid acyl group, usually on the α-carbon of glycerol. Some phospholipids contain linkages other than ester linkages to the alcohol group of glycerol. Plasmologens contain a monovinyl ether as well as mono-fatty acyl group. Although rare, phospholipids containing an ether group have been isolated in certain tissues, such as bovine red blood cells.

C. Sphingolipids

These compounds are characterized by the presence of sphingosine in the molecule (Eq. 1). Derived lipid and a water-soluble compound are the other products of

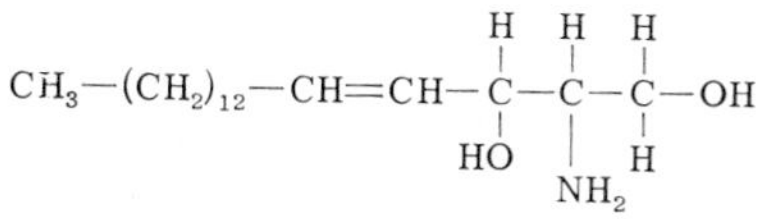

$$CH_3-(CH_2)_{12}-CH=CH-\underset{\underset{\textstyle HO}{|}}{\overset{\overset{\textstyle H}{|}}{C}}-\underset{\underset{\textstyle NH_2}{|}}{\overset{\overset{\textstyle H}{|}}{C}}-\underset{\underset{\textstyle H}{|}}{\overset{\overset{\textstyle H}{|}}{C}}-OH \qquad (1)$$

hydrolysis. Sphingomyelin, common to most mammalian tissues, is a member of this group. In this case, a fatty acid acyl group is linked to sphingosine as an amide and the primary alcoholic group forms a phosphate ester linkage with choline. Cerebrosides and cerebroside sulfates fulfill the requirements of the definition of sphingolipids. These compounds are found in high concentrations in brain tissues, but are not limited to that tissue. Cerebrosides differ from sphingomyelin only in that a mono- or oligosaccharide is linked to the primary alcohol of sphingosine as a glycoside instead of choline via a phosphate ester. Gangliosides contain sphingosine, with an acyl fatty acid on the amido group, linked with monosaccharides, hexosamines, and neuraminic acid. For example, a crystalline ganglioside containing equimolar amounts of sphingosine, stearic acid, glucose, galactose, N-acetylgalactosamine, and N-acetylneuraminic acid has been isolated from bovine brain (Kuhn and Egge, 1960). These compounds are found most commonly in the central nervous system, but gangliosides have been isolated from other tissues as well.

Decreased degradation, rather than increased synthesis, of sphingolipids has been incriminated in many lipidoses of humans, e.g., Gaucher's disease and Niemann-Pick's disease. Two recent reviews discuss the metabolic and biochemical aspects of these syndromes (Stanbury et al., 1966; Shapiro, 1967).

III. CHEMISTRY OF SOME LIPIDS

Although all types of lipid mentioned have physiological importance, the chemistry of fatty acids, glycerides, and steroids requires a more detailed description because of their wide distribution in mammalian tissues, their broad physiological importance, and their pertinence to our discussion.

A. CLASSIFICATION OF FATTY ACIDS

Naturally occurring fatty acids are straight-chained saturated or unsaturated, monocarboxylic acids containing an even number of carbon atoms. Although the most common chain lengths in nature are 16 to 18 carbon atoms, fatty acids of shorter chain lengths occur, notably in the milk of many species and in coconut oil. Fatty acids with an odd number of carbon atoms are found in small quantities throughout nature. The oil extracted from pelargoniums is rich in a saturated fatty acid containing nine carbon atoms. Propionic acid could be considered a fatty acid with an odd number of carbon atoms even though its solubility in water places it outside our definition of lipids. The importance of this organic acid in ruminant nutrition forces its inclusion in a discussion of lipid metabolism of domestic animals (Section IX,A). Branched chained and hydroxyl-containing fatty acids are also rarely found.

The free form of a fatty acid rarely occurs in animal tissues. It is common practice when referring to the fatty acid content of a tissue or diet to take for granted that the fatty acids are in an esterified form. Therefore, one must designate specifically when referring to fatty acids in the free form, not amide or ester linkages. We shall use the abbreviation FFA to refer to free fatty acids.

The abbreviation VFA is used to refer to volatile fatty acids. Although these compounds usually occur as the free acids, they are distinct from FFA both chemically and metabolically. Because of their short-chain length (C-1 to C-5), they are readily soluble in water and are steam distillable. The metabolic differences between these short-chain and the long-chain FFA will become apparent later in the chapter.

The Geneva System of nomenclature has been used to designate fatty acids on the basis of their carbon chain length and their degree of saturation. The fatty acid is regarded as an aliphatic acid derivative of a hydrocarbon in which the terminal methyl group is replaced by a carboxyl one. The name of the acid is the same as the hydrocarbon, except that the terminal "-e" is replaced by the suffix "-oic." Thus, hexadecanoic acid (palmitic) is derived from hexadecane. This nomenclature also applies to the monounsaturated fatty acids. In this case the unsaturated hydrocarbon is designated by the suffix "-ene" rather than "-ane." Thus, the fatty acid is noted by the ending "-enoic." For example, hexadecenoic acid is palmitoleic acid. When more than one unsaturated carbon–carbon bond occurs, the combining form, di-, tri- etc. is inserted before the -enoic to designate the appropriate number of unsaturated bonds.

Two systems are now in use to designate the site of the unsaturated bond within the molecule. The basis of the most common system is the number of carbon atoms away from the carboxyl group, considered C-1. In this system, palmitoleic acid is 9-hexadecenoic. In the same system, the presence of the unsaturated bond may be designated by the Greek letter δ and the site of the bond by superscripts. The number of carbon atoms away from the terminal or ω-carbon of the fatty acid is used in the second system for designating the site of the unsaturated carbon–carbon bond. In this case, palmitoleic acid is ω-7-hexadecenoic acid, oleic acid is ω-9-octadecenoic acid. This latter system is preferred by this author because it indicates whether or not a biosynthetic relationship exists between the various unsaturated fatty acids occurring naturally. In most cases, the naturally occurring, unsaturated fatty acids are in the transconfiguration. In general, the trivial name will be used in this discussion because of the general familiarity with the common fatty acids.

The polyunsaturated fatty acids, particularly linoleic acid, are required for normal function and growth of mammals, but they cannot be synthesized by the tissues of these animals. Therefore, because these fatty acids must be provided in the diet, they are referred to as essential fatty acids.

B. Chemical Reactions of Fatty Acids

Only certain chemical reactions of physiological and clinical importance will be discussed. Sunderman and Sunderman (1960) have edited a compilation of methods useful in clinical studies of lipid metabolism.

1. Solubility

The solubility of fatty acids is important from several standpoints. Since physiological environments are aqueous, it is of biochemical importance to understand the means used in nature for maintaining solutions or emulsions of fatty acids. Some of these means will be discussed in later sections of this chapter. Analytically, the solubility of fatty acids is used to isolate and purify them.

The solubility of saturated fatty acids from C-6 to C-18 in water at a variety of temperatures has been studied (Ralston and Hoerr, 1942). Solubility was inversely related to the length of carbon chain at all temperatures, caproic acid being the most soluble, about 1 gm/100 gm water, and stearic acid the least, 0.00018 to 0.0005 gm/100 gm water depending upon the temperature. Although these workers did not study the VFA, acetic, propionic, and butyric acids are known to be miscible with water in all proportions and 3.7 gm of valeric acid are soluble in 100 gm of water (Markley, 1947). We should note here that because of their solubility, fatty acids with a carbon chain length of less than eight carbons are not strictly lipids. Nonetheless, their metabolic fate is so closely tied with lipid metabolism that they will be discussed in this chapter.

Hoerr and co-workers (Hoerr and Ralston, 1944; Hoerr et al., 1946) have also studied the solubility of fatty acids in various organic solvents at various temperatures. Their results are well summarized in Deuel (1951). It will suffice here to say that the solubility of fatty acids increases with decreasing chain length and increasing degree of unsaturation. The solubility of fatty acids increases almost linearly with increasing temperature in nonpolar solvents. The relationship between solubility and temperature is less predictable as the polarity of the solvent increases.

The sodium and potassium salts of fatty acids are soluble in water and insoluble in organic solvents. Thus, extraction of lipid samples with lipid solvents after saponification, but before acidification, separates the nonsaponifiable lipids, mainly steroids and hydrocarbons, from the saponifiable ones. The same extraction of the same sample after acidification separates the fatty acids from such a mixture. The types of fatty acids that are extractable from an acidified aqueous solution will depend on the organic solvent used. For example, Abraham and associates (1961) have shown that hexane at 20°C will extract mainly fatty acids with a carbon chain of C-8 or greater. Such a separation is valuable when examining the fatty acids of tissues synthesizing short-chain fatty acids from acetate, for example, mammary glands.

2. Formation of Salts

The FFA can react with bases to produce appropriate salts. Most of the naturally occurring fatty acids exist in the salt form as fatty acid anions at physiological pH. Soaps are merely the salts of long-chain fatty acids. Sodium and potassium form water-soluble soaps, but the alkaline earth metals, such as calcium and magnesium, form insoluble soaps. Formation of the sodium salts of FFA is the basis of the determination of FFA content of body fluid, particularly plasma.

3. Formation of Fatty Acid Esters

In the presence of hydrogen ion fatty acids react with alcohol to yield esters and water:

$$R-COO^- + R_1OH \xrightarrow[H^+]{} R-\overset{\displaystyle O}{\overset{\displaystyle \|}{C}}-O-R_1 + H_2O$$

The most common ester linkages in domestic animals are between fatty acids and glycerol to form glycerides and between fatty acids and cholesterol, to yield cholesterol esters. Methyl esters of fatty acids are more volatile than the FFA and, thus, are prepared for separation of fatty acids by gas–liquid chromatography.

4. Hydrogenation and Halogenation

Unsaturated fatty acids can be converted to saturated fatty acids by the addition of 1 mole of hydrogen at the site of each double bond (Deuel, 1951). In the presence of a metal catalyst, such as platinum, hydrogenation can be accomplished using hydrogen gas under either increased pressure or increased temperature or a combination of both; this process is used extensively in the preparation of margarine from vegetable oils.

Halogenation is a comparable reaction to hydrogenation except that 1 mole of a halogen is added at each unsaturated bond (Deuel, 1951). Iodine is the most common halogen used. Chlorine and bromine are also effective. Since the degree of saturation of fatty acids is directly proportional to the amount of halogen consumed, this reaction has been used to determine the degree of unsaturation of fatty acids, namely, the iodine number of the lipid. The unsaturated fatty acids within glycerides and phospholipids can, of course, undergo the chemical reactions involving the double bond.

Halogenation is of pertinence to clinical medicine. Fatty acids in glycerides used in absorption studies are often labeled with radioactive iodine, usually ^{131}I, by means of halogenation. Lipids labeled by this means are cheaper and more easily handled and assayed than comparable ^{14}C-labeled compounds. The specific tests using these compounds will be discussed later (Tennant and Ewing, Vol. 2, Chapter 3). Whether or not fatty acids labeled with ^{131}I are handled by the organism precisely as are natural fatty acids is open to question.

C. CHEMISTRY OF GLYCERIDES

Neutral Glycerides

Of the neutral glycerides, triglycerides are by far the most common in nature. Triglycerides are compounds in which all three alcoholic groups of glycerol are esterified with the fatty acid. Hence, diglycerides and monoglycerides have an acyl fatty acid on 2 and 1, respectively, alcoholic groups of glycerol. In the case of the partial glycerides, any combination of the various alcoholic groups may be involved, but certain sites are favored over others as will be discussed later.

The term simple glycerides refers to triglycerides containing only one type of fatty acid, e.g., tripalmitin. Mixed glycerides, then, contain more than one type of fatty acid. Naturally occurring glycerides are usually of the mixed variety. The site of the fatty acid within the glyceride molecule is designated by relating the name of the fatty acid to the site where it is esterified. The center carbon of glycerol is usually referred to as the β-carbon, and the two terminal carbons as the α ones. Thus, the

$$\begin{array}{l} H_2C-O-\overset{\overset{\displaystyle O}{\|}}{C}-(CH_2-CH_2)_8-CH_3 \\ HC-O-\overset{\overset{\displaystyle O}{\|}}{C}-(CH_2)_7-CH=CH-CH_2-CH=CH-(CH_2)_4-CH_3 \\ H_2C-O-\overset{\overset{\displaystyle O}{\|}}{C}-(CH_2-CH_2)_6-CH_3 \end{array} \qquad (2)$$

following triglyceride could be referred to as β-linoleo-α-stearopalmitin (structure 2).

The fatty acids comprising the triglyceride molecule are not distributed between the three alcoholic groups of glycerol in a random manner. The position is governed by the chain length and the degree of unsaturation. The shorter and more unsaturated fatty acids tend to be found in the β position of the naturally occurring triglycerides (Desnuelle and Savary, 1963). An exception to this finding are the triglycerides of the domestic pig in that in this species palmitic acid is consistently found in the β position (Mattson *et al.*, 1964).

Neutral glycerides can be hydrolyzed either by acid or base to their constituent fatty acids and glycerol. Acid hydrolysis requires high temperature and pressure to complete the reaction. Alkaline hydrolysis is more commonly used. In this case, heating (e.g., 90°C for 90 minutes) in strong alkali results in formation of the salts of fatty acids along with glycerol.

D. Chemistry of Steroids

We will cover the complicated chemical structure of these compounds only very briefly, partly to illustrate how the same basic structure can be varied to allow a wide variety of physiological roles. For a complete presentation the reader is referred to books by Shoppee (1958) and Kritchevsky (1963). Readers specifically interested in the chemistry of steroids should be aware of the revised tentative rules for the nomenclature of steroids just published by the IUPAC Commission on the Nomenclature of Organic Chemistry and the IUPAC-IUB Commission on Biochemical Nomenclature.*

Steroids are compounds with a skeleton composed of a phenanthrene and a cyclopentane ring. The constituent carbon and the rings are designated as shown in Fig. 2. The structure of steriods is complicated in that the rings may be fused in the *trans* or *cis* configurations. The orientation of the side chains depends on whether the rings are *trans* or *cis* fused. Two series of steroids are found in nature: the normal series in which the relationship between ring A and ring B is *cis* and between rings B and C and C and D it is *trans*, and the allo- series in which all the rings are *trans* fused. Hence, in the normal series the methyl group at C-10 and the hydrogen at C-5 are in the same configuration, designated β. In the allo- series, the methyl group at C-10 is β, and the hydrogen at C-5 is α.

At first approach, it may be surprising that a group of compounds all with the same 17 carbon rings can vary so widely in their physiological roles. However, the basic structure can be varied by: (1) the configuration of the ring structures, allo-versus normal; (2) the ring structure may be broken at one bond, as in vitamin D; (3) there may or may not be an aliphatic side chain and, if present, it may vary in its structure and functional groups; (4) the ring may contain double bonds in various positions; (5) the ring may contain various side groups of various sites; and (6) these side groups can be oriented either in the α or β positions.

Certain sites on the basic pentanophenanthrene ring seem to be favored in

*Reprints are available from NAS-NRC Office of Biochemical Nomenclature, Dr. Waldo E. Cohn, Biology Division, Oak Ridge National Laboratory, Oak Ridge, Tennessee 37830.

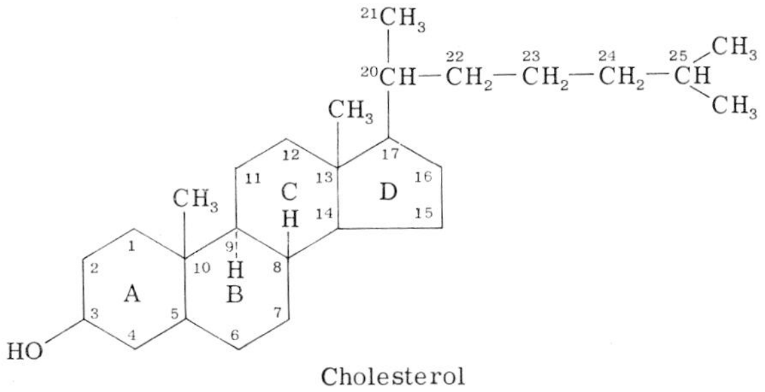

Cholesterol

Fig. 2.   Structural formula of cholesterol showing numbering of carbon atoms and designation of rings.

nature over others for the addition of methyl, alcoholic, ketonic, and aldehydic side chains. The potency of many physiologically active compounds commonly depends on the type of group, and its orientation, at C-3, C-11, and C-17.

Cholesterol can be used as a typical steroid for discussion of the physical and chemical properties of compounds comprising this group. The use of cholesterol is particularly appropriate because cholesterol is by far the most common naturally occurring steroid, owing to its implication in vascular disease and its diagnostic import, e.g., in hypothyroidism (Section VI,B).

Cholesterol is the basic steroid skeleton with a branched side chain at C-17 and secondary, β-oriented alcohol at C-3 and a double bond between C-5 and C-6 (Fig. 2).

The hydroxyl group at C-3 is often in an ester linkage with the fatty acid. The esterification reaction is catalyzed by enzymes found in liver (Goodman et al., 1964) and plasma (Glomset, 1968). The significance of the esters and reactions catalyzing their formation will be discussed later (Section VII,B).

Digitonin, a steroid saponin, also reacts with a secondary alcohol group of cholesterol to form cholesterol digitonide. This complex is virtually insoluble in organic solvents. Thus, this reaction has been used extensively for the detection, isolation, and purification of cholesterol. The reaction is specific for a β-oriented hydroxyl at C-3 so that the reaction is not limited to cholesterol. It does provide a means for separating free cholesterol from cholesterol esters.

Colorimetric reactions are also used for the detection of cholesterol. The Liebermann-Burchard reaction involves the conversion of a steroid to polymeric unsaturated hydrocarbon. In this reaction, the sample is dissolved in acetic anhydride and then treated with sulfuric acid. The intensity of the green color is proportional to the amount of cholesterol present. This reaction is not specific for cholesterol as most unsaturated steroids will undergo similar reactions.

Another colorimetric assay for cholesterol is related to the presence of the hydroxyl group as well as to the unsaturation. The basis of this assay is the color complex that results between cholesterol and $FeCl_3$ in the presence of sulfuric acid (Zak et al., 1954; Rice and Lukasiewicz, 1957). Again, this reaction is not specific for cholesterol.

A note of caution: neither of these popular colorimetric methods is specific for cholesterol. If there is doubt about the quantity of compounds other than cholesterol in a given sample that could contribute to the colorimetric assay, cholesterol can be isolated either as the dibromide or by chromatography prior to the assay.

IV. DIGESTION AND ABSORPTION OF LIPID

The general discussion in this section will apply to omnivores and carnivores only. A special section will describe recent investigations into lipid digestion and absorption in ruminants, because of the unique digestive system in this species (Section IX,A). Certainly, the generalizations developed in studies with rodents and man should be applied with caution to herbivores.

The major portion of the lipid ingested is in the form of glycerides, but some cholesterol, cholesterol ester, and phospholipid are also present in most diets. The digestion of lipid takes place in the lumen of the small intestine. There is no means of digestion of lipid in the mouth and the small amount of gastric lipase that is secreted is inactive at the normal hydrogen ion concentration in the stomach (Deuel, 1955).

The manner in which lipids are absorbed was clouded in controversy for many years (Deuel, 1955). In 1938, Frazer presented the basic concept that triglycerides may be only partially hydrolyzed to monoglycerides (MG) and FFA. Elaborating on his theory in several reviews, Frazer (1946, 1952) suggested that because of the surface properties of these compounds, they would tend to form a stable emulsion in the presence of bile acids. Further, the size of the lipid droplets formed will be small enough to allow absorption.

Recently, this concept has been verified, modified, and extended (Bergström and Borgström, 1955; Johnston, 1963; Senior, 1964). Digestion and absorption of lipids can be described in the following stages: (1) digestion of the lipid; (2) formation of the micelle suitable for absorption; (3) entry into the mucosal cell and resynthesis of triglyceride and cholesterol ester and their incorporation into chylomicrons; and (4) release of the chylomicrons into lymphatic circulation. The proximal jejunum is the major site where these events take place.

A. DIGESTION OF LIPIDS

1. Hydrolysis of Triglyceride to MG and FFA

Pancreatic lipase acts specifically on the α-ester bond of the triglyceride, thereby releasing MG and FFA (Desnuelle, 1961; Desnuelle and Savary, 1963).

Any further hydrolysis will take place only after isomerization of the remaining fatty acid moiety of the MG to the α-position, a slow reaction. Pancreatic lipase is also specific in that it acts most efficiently only at an oil–water interface. For example, triacetin, which is soluble in water, is not hydrolyzed at all by pancreatic lipase until the concentration of the lipid is increased to supersaturation so that an emulsion forms, i.e., oil droplets within the water phase (Desnuelle, 1961). This hydrolytic enzyme of the pancreas is so specific for the oil–water interphase that its kinetic properties must be expressed on the basis of interfacial area rather than on substrate concentration (Benzonana and Desnuelle, 1965).

Pancreatic lipase hydrolyzes all triglycerides with long-chain fatty acid moieties at about the same rate, if they are adequately and equally emulsified (Desnuelle and Savary, 1963). Fatty acids of short to medium chain lengths, i.e., containing 4–12 carbons, are hydrolyzed more quickly. This property of lipase is of critical importance in cases of pancreatic insufficiency. In spite of decreased secretion of pancreatic lipase in these cases, fatty acid digestion and absorption can be maintained by feeding triglyceride containing medium length fatty acids (MCT). Coconut oil is a natural source of triglycerides containing a large proportion of fatty acids with a medium chain length (Deuel, 1951).

B. Formation of a Micelle Suitable for Absorption

Although bile salts may aid in the formation of emulsions prior to hydrolysis of triglyceride, their most important role is the formation of lipid micelles suitable for absorption into the mucosal cell. The detergent properties of the bile salts promote the formation of molecular aggregates in equal solutions with the nonpolar portion directed inward and the polar group projecting outward (Roepke and Mason, 1940). Such aggregates are referred to as micelles. Lipid molecules are readily trapped and thereby concentrated in the micelle (Hofmann and Borgström, 1962). The products of hydrolysis, MG and fatty acids, are most readily accummulated in the micelle. Furthermore, MG with an unsaturated fatty acid are more soluble in the micelle than saturated MG (Mattson and Volpenheim, 1963). Such an MG is the most common one formed by the action of pancreatic lipase because the naturally occurring triglycerides commonly have an unsaturated fatty acid at the β position. These mixed micelles are probably the form in which lipid is absorbed by the mucosal cell (Johnston and Borgström, 1964). Small amounts of di- and triglyceride may also enter the micelles (Hofmann and Borgström, 1964). Quantitative studies with pig intestine reveal that the capacity for micellar absorption of lipid greatly exceeds the rate at which lipid is presented to the small intestine (Freeman et al., 1968).

Although the formation of micelles by bile salts aids in absorption of lipid, it is not indispensable for triglyceride absorption. In the absence of bile in dogs and rats 30–40% of the ingested triglyceride is absorbed (Annegers, 1954; Gallagher et al., 1965). On the other hand, absorption of cholesterol and fat-soluble vitamins is totally dependent on biliary secretion. Hence, in pancreatic insufficiency there may be a complete inability to absorb triglyceride due to lack of hydrolysis, but the presence of micelles from bile salts allows absorption of vitamins A, B, D, and K, thus preventing deficiencies of fat-soluble vitamins in the syndrome (Dawson, 1967).

C. Entry into the Mucosal Cell

A conflict has arisen between what is found biochemically and what is seen microscopically during absorption of lipids. Quantitative studies have verified that MG and FFA are the products of digestion that are absorbed and yet electron micrographs reveal droplets larger than a micelle within the mucosal cell (Palay and Karlin, 1959). It now appears that the droplets are not quantitatively related to lipid absorption and therefore may represent an event taking place after actual absorption (Strauss, 1966). After absorption, the MG and FFA are again combined to form triglycerides. This step appears to be the rate-limiting step in lipid absorption (Shapiro, 1967). Triglyceride synthesis can proceed via two pathways: (1) the glyceride-glycerol of the MG is utilized as the backbone (Clark and Hübscher, 1961), or (2) formation of a new glyceride backbone by acylation of L-α-glycerol phosphate. The fatty acids are incorporated after being "activated" to acyl CoA derivatives (Ailhaud et al., 1962). The phosphatidic acid formed in pathway (2) is dephosphorylated and the resulting diglyceride is acylated to form the final product (Coleman and Hübscher, 1962).

The lipase of the mucosal cells should be mentioned, not because of its quantitative significance, but because it may be a site for determining which pathway of triglyceride synthesis predominates and thereby provide a means of balancing available glyceride–glycerol backbone with available FFA (Dawson, 1967). In contrast to pancreatic lipase, this mucosal lipase is specific for MG (Senior and Isselbacher, 1963). Dawson (1967) has postulated that if MG is in excess over FFA available for esterification, this lipase could form more FFA from the MG. If FFA are in excess, the lipase would presumably be less likely to attack MG due to lack of available substrate. In this context, it should be noted that not all FFA absorbed is reesterified.

The enzymes of the mucosal cell responsible for activation and reesterification of the FFA prefer fatty acid with a carbon chain of 12 carbons or more (Brindley and Hübscher, 1966). Therefore, there can be a partitioning of fatty acids in the mucosal cell (Shapiro, 1967), the long-chain ones being mainly incorporated into triglyceride, the short-chain ones (less than C-10) remaining mainly as FFA. The medium-chain fatty acids can go by either pathway. The majority of the FFA enter the portal system and are carried to the liver as albumin complexes. The absorption of triglyceride with medium- and short-chain fatty acids is more rapid than triglyceride containing long-chain fatty acids because of the more rapid hydrolysis and the fact that the resulting FFA escapes the rate-limiting step of reesterification to triglyceride (Greenberger et al., 1966). This observation is of clinical importance in any malabsorption syndrome such as, short-bowel syndrome, biliary obstruction, lymphatic obstruction, and, as mentioned, pancreatic insufficiency (Isselbacher, 1967).

1. Steroid Absorption

The cholesterol resulting from the hydrolysis of the cholesterol ester in the lumen of the intestine also enters the microvillus via the micelle. In the microvillus the newly entering cholesterol displaces one previously there which then migrates to the cytoplasm of the mucosal cell (David *et al.*, 1966). The cholesterol is then reesterified and transferred to the lymph as part of the chylomicron.

2. *Phospholipid Absorption*

Phospholipids in the diet are hydrolyzed to phosphoglyceride and FFA in the lumen of the small intestine, absorbed in this form and then the phosphoglyceride is reesterified in the mucosal cell to form various diacyl derivatives.

D. FORMATION OF THE CHYLOMICRON

Within the mucosal cell the resynthesized triglyceride, phospholipid, and cholesterol ester, along with some free cholesterol and small amounts of FFA and fat-soluble vitamins, are combined with a small quantity of protein to form a particle referred to as a chylomicron. The formation of this particle is dependent on protein synthesis in the mucosal cell (Isselbacher and Budz, 1963).

It is not clear how the chylomicron leaves the mucosal cell, but reverse pinocytosis has been suggested (Shapiro, 1967). Once in the intracellular space the chylomicron diffuses through the lactyl membrane into lymph ducts and thence to the thoracic duct, to be eventually distributed throughout the circulatory system. The size of the chylomicron prevents its entrance into the capillaries of the portal system. Thus, long-chain fatty acids escape the initial filtration in the liver to which medium- and short-chain fatty acids, and most other products of the absorptive process, are subjected.

V. FATE OF DIETARY LIPIDS

A. CHYLOMICRON METABOLISM

Chylomicrons are rapidly removed from the circulation and their contents utilized by adipose tissue (Shapiro, 1965), cardiac muscle (Delcher *et al.*, 1965; Gousios *et al.*, 1963; Crass and Meng, 1966; Simpson-Morgan, 1968), liver (Belfrage *et al.*, 1965), and probably lung (Simpson-Morgan, 1968). The kinetics and the mechanism of chylomicron utilization has been investigated extensively (see Meng, 1964; Simpson-Morgan, 1967; Hallberg, 1967). Triglyceride, the major component of chylomicrons, undergoes hydrolysis to glycerol and the constituent fatty acids. These components may be utilized for synthesis of new triglycerides and phospholipids or oxidized to CO_2. Whether the initial degradation takes place on the external plasma membrane (Green and Webb, 1964; Higgins and Green, 1966) or intracellularly (Shapiro, 1965; Belfrage *et al.*, 1965) is unsettled. There is evidence for both points of view: it is possible that some tissues take up the chylomicron intact, whereas, in others, lypolysis occurs prior to entrance into the cells. It is also possible that both mechanisms operate simultaneously.

Lypolysis of the chylomicron triglyceride is catalyzed by lipoprotein lipase. This enzyme is bound in an inactive form that is released in the plasma in the active form in the presence of heparin. Because the hydrolysis of triglyceride to FFA clears the plasma, this enzymic activity has been referred to as the plasma-clearing factor. The anatomical site of binding of lipoprotein lipase is not known. The capillary endothelium has been suggested (Robinson, 1963). A congenital deficiency of lipoprotein lipase resulting in hyperlipemia of exogenous origin has been recently reported in a puppy (Baum et al., 1969). Adipose tissue contains high lipoprotein lipase activity as well. This adipose lipase is responsive to diet, increasing during feeding and decreasing during fasting (Schotz and Garfinkel, 1965).

The fate of FFA absorbed from the chylomicron varies with the tissue; in heart, it is mainly oxidized to CO_2; in adipose, it is mainly reesterified and stored as triglyceride; and in liver, a portion may be oxidized but another portion is reesterified and released back into the plasma in the form of very low density lipoprotein (VLDL) or β-lipoprotein (Section VI,C).

B. MEDIUM- AND SHORT-CHAIN FATTY ACIDS

The medium- and short-chain fatty acids are absorbed and transported to the liver via the portal system (Hashim et al., 1964, 1965; Kiyasu et al., 1952). The major portion of them are oxidized in that tissue and do not enter the peripheral circulation (Kirschner and Harris, 1961). The fate of the large quantities of VFA absorbed into the portal system in ruminants varies with each compound and will be covered in Section IX,A which is devoted to these specialized domestic animals.

C. CHOLESTEROL AND CHOLESTEROL ESTER

The cholesterol and cholesterol ester in the chylomicron are utilized almost completely in the liver. The dietary cholesterol quickly mixes with that already present part of which has been synthesized de novo in the liver. The total amount of cholesterol in mammalians is under close homeostatic control. The rate of biosynthesis in the liver is indirectly proportional to the amount of cholesterol and cholesterol ester absorbed from the gut (Siperstein and Fagan, 1964; Bortz, 1967). The output of cholesterol is also variable, increasing when the intake increases, decreasing when the intake is lessened. Cholesterol is lost from the animal in the form of bile acids and as free cholesterol and its derivatives in bile.

VI. TRANSPORT OF LIPID

None of the lipids normally found in the plasma are sufficiently soluble in water to circulate in the free form. In some cases they are associated with specific proteins which act to keep them in solution. Quantitatively, the transport of fatty acids and triglyceride is of most importance. Cholesterol and cholesterol ester are also important quantitatively in specific species (e.g., the chicken) and of clinical and diagnostic importance in all mammals. Chylomicrons are transported in the plasma especially at the height of lipid absorption. The composition and fate of these particles has been discussed (Section V,A).

A. FREE FATTY ACIDS

In reality, only a small proportion of FFA are free in the plasma; most are bound to albumin (Goodman, 1958). This albumin–fatty acid complex is formed when fatty acids are released into the circulation. Indeed, the mobilization of fatty acids is inhibited by a lack of albumin (Steinberg and Vaughan, 1965).

The FFA–albumin complex accounts for the major portion of lipid transported in the plasma. The concentration of FFA is lower than that of some other lipid components of plasma, but their turnover rate exceeds that of any other lipid faction in plasma (Fredrickson and Gordon, 1958). The concentration of FFA in most species in the postabsorptive stage is 300–600 μEq/liter of plasma. The level of FFA increases three- to fourfold during prolonged fasting (Dole, 1956) or chronic nutritional stress (Annison, 1960). The significance of FFA in ruminants will be discussed in Section IX,A.

B. LIPOPROTEINS OF PLASMA

Lipoproteins are the protein complexes which carry triglyceride, cholesterol, cholesterol ester, and phospholipid in the plasma in a soluble form. Two major classes have been isolated, usually designated α and β. The few studies in domestic animals have made clear that there are variations and that the lipoprotein complement is not the same in all species (Evans, 1964; Evans et al., 1961; Hillyard et al., 1955; Puppione, 1969). Further comparative research is needed in this area as will become obvious.

The structural basis of the lipid–protein complex is not clear, but the bonding is not primarily a covalent one (Fisher and Gurin, 1964). The following type of linkages have been suggested: electrovalent, hydrogen bonding, van der Waals, and the orientation of hydrophobic groups (Salem, 1962). It is possible that any or all of these mechanisms operate. The clinical and physiological importance is that the forces are strong enough to allow isolation of the complex and yet weak enough to allow exchange of the lipid component between plasma lipoproteins themselves and between plasma and tissue lipoproteins.

1. Methods of Isolation of Plasma Lipoproteins

The two most widely used techniques are electrophoresis and ultracentrifugation. The correspondence between the factions isolated by each of these methods is now becoming clear, at least in humans (Fredrickson et al., 1968; Noble et al., 1969). The method of electrophoretic separation is the same as that with other plasma proteins except that lipid-specific stains are used. Oil red O has been used routinely, but staining with Schiff's reagent after ozonization of the lipid has been used and gives a more intense color.* Counterstaining with any one of the usual protein stains provides a means of identifying a lipid-carrying protein in relation to the other plasma proteins. The major lipoproteins are designated by the same Greek letters as the plasma globulins moving similarly in the electrophoretic field, i.e., α, β, and pre-β. Hatch and Lees (1968) have reviewed these techniques.

Separation of the plasma lipoproteins by ultracentrifugation is based on the

---

*"Procedures, Techniques and Apparatus for Electrophoresis," Gelman Instrument Co., Ann Arbor, Michigan, p. 25.

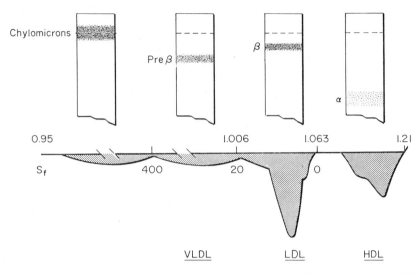

Fig. 3. Electrophoretic and ultracentrifugal patterns of the plasma lipoproteins of man. (Modified from Fredrickson, 1969.)

differences in density, mainly of the lipid component of the lipoproteins. This method has the adaptability to separate the lipoproteins into an almost limitless number of subgroups (Ewing *et al.*, 1965). Such separation is beyond the present clinical requirements, however, particularly in domestic animals. Therefore, the lipoproteins are commonly divided into four subgroups: high density lipoprotein (HDL), low density lipoprotein (LDL), very low density lipoprotein (VLDL), and chylomicron. As seen in Fig. 3, these divisions are somewhat arbitrary. The relative densities are expressed as Svedberg units (S_f) based on the flotation rate of the lipoprotein in a density gradient.

The relationship between the electrophoretic and ultracentrifugal separation are shown in Fig. 3. The type and quantity of lipid usually found in each group is shown in Table I.

The lipoproteins are synthesized predominantly in the liver Radding *et al.*, 1958;

TABLE I   LIPID COMPOSITION OF SERUM LIPOPROTEINS OF HUMANS

Density class (gm/cm³)	Electrophoretic migration	Percent lipid composition[a]			
		TG[b]	PL[b]	CE[b]	Chol[b]
< 1.006	Pre-β	63–75	16–25	13–16	4–6
1.006–1.063	β	15	26	46	13
1.063–1.21	α	8	48	40	4

[a]Estimated by Puppione (1969) from the data of Hatch and Lees (1968).

[b]TG = triglyceride; PL = phospholipid; CE = cholesterol ester; and Chol = cholesterol.

Marsh and Whereat, 1959; Windmueller and Levy, 1967). Recent evidence indicates that the intestine may contribute to the synthesis of the β-lipoprotein (Windmueller and Levy, 1968). Two apoproteins have been isolated from plasma lipoproteins from various sources (for review, see Fredrickson et al., 1967). They are designated A and B. There is also evidence that a third protein (C) exists.

Protein A is usually the only protein found with the α-lipoproteins and B with the β-lipoproteins. Protein C is found with VLDL or pre-β-lipoproteins along with small amounts of A and B (probably as contaminants). Proteins A and B have also been isolated from chylomicrons, thus suggesting that they are the protein component from these lipid-carrying particles. Both A and B apoproteins have been isolated and their amino acid sequence and properties are being investigated by several groups (e.g., Scanu, 1966; Shore and Shore, 1962; Margolis and Langdon, 1966).

The α- and β-lipoproteins normally account for about 90% of the cholesterol and phospholipids of plasma. The change in concentration of these lipids with changing conditions in the animal is insignificant when compared to that of triglyceride. Fredrickson et al. (1967) have adopted a simplifying concept, which may not be accurate in every detail but is of great help in clarifying the relationships between the lipoproteins for the clinician. In this scheme, the α- and β-lipoproteins with their constituent phospholipid and cholesterol are looked upon as stable cargo vehicles for carrying glyceride from the liver to other tissues. The glyceride-loaded lipoprotein migrates as the pre-β-lipoprotein and has the density of VLDL. The pre-β-lipoprotein is particulate and, thus, in high concentrations can result in turbidity of the plasma. The term endogenous lipid particle is used to distinguish between these particles in which glyceride content is derived mainly from the liver and the chylomicron whose glyceride component normally arises from digestion and absorption.

C. DYNAMICS OF LIPID TRANSPORT

The source, transport, and utilization of chylomicrons, exogenous lipid, has been discussed (Section V,A). Therefore, we will limit the present discussion to the mobilization, transport, and disposition of lipid arising endogenously. Adipose tissue is the main source of endogenous lipid. The lipid in adipose tissue results both from storage of lipid and synthesis in the tissue (e.g., O'Hea and Leveille, 1968). As with dietary lipid, most of this lipid is triglyceride (Vaughan and Steinberg, 1963).

Adipose tissue lipid is mobilized in the form of FFA. Glycerol is released concommitantly. Thus, hydrolysis of the ester bond is the first step in fat mobilization. This lypolytic reaction is catalyzed by the lipase of adipose tissue which differs from the lipoprotein lipase described earlier (Section V,A). This enzyme, which is sensitive to myriad hormones, catalyzes the release of one FFA leaving a diglyceride. Once formed, the diglyceride is rapidly degraded to FFA and glycerol. This series of reactions is catalyzed by a second lipase that is not responsive to hormones (Biale et al., 1965; Pope et al., 1966; Kupiecki, 1966). Increased lipolysis does not guarantee release of FFA from the tissue. If a source of lα-glycerol phosphate is available, the fatty acid moiety can be reesterified and, thereby, not be released. The latter situation is common during the absorptive state when the glucose being delivered to the adipose tissue is readily converted to phosphorylated derivatives including lα-glycerol phosphate. It should be noted that the glycerol released during lipolysis cannot be reutilized for esterification because adipose tissue lacks the enzyme, glycerokinase, that catalyzes the formation of 1 α-glycerol phosphate from glycerol. In summary, two factors will enhance the mobilization of FFA: increased lipolysis and/or decreased esterification (the reverse reaction) (Steinberg and Vaughan, 1965).

The FFA released from adipose tissue can diffuse into the plasma only if albumin is available to solubilize them (Steinberg and Vaughan, 1965). Thus, a third factor is involved in mobilization of FFA: the availability of albumin. This availability may vary with the albumin concentration in plasma and the rate of perfusion of adipose tissue.

The rate of mobilization of FFA is usually reflected in the plasma concentration. For example, an increase in the plasma concentration of FFA usually indicates increased FFA released from adipose tissue. A note of caution, however, needs to be expressed in the interpretation of plasma levels of FFA. The rate of utilization of FFA will also influence the plasma concentration. If an increased rate of release is matched by increased rate of utilization, the plasma concentration will be unaffected. The major site of FFA utilization is the liver, although most tissues can utilize these compounds for biosynthetic and oxidative purposes.

The FFA can be disposed of in the liver in a variety of ways, e.g.:

1. It may be oxidized completely to CO_2 and H_2O. If there is a block in the utilization of acetyl CoA derived from β oxidation, complete oxidation cannot occur and

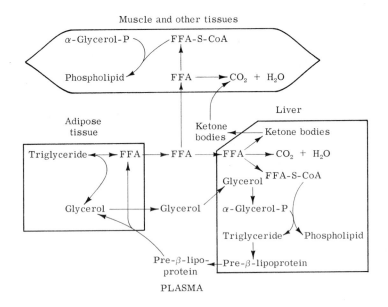

Fig. 4.   Schematic presentation of the transport and fate of endogenous lipid.

the ketone bodies, β-OH-butyrate and acetoacetate, may be formed. These ketone bodies are readily released from the liver and can be catabolized by other tissues.

2. Rather than being catabolized, the FFA may be esterified to reform triglycerides. The fate of these triglycerides is the same as those from the chylomicrons; they are incorporated into pre-β-lipoprotein and released into the blood vascular system (Fredrickson et al., 1967). The triglyceride portion of the pre-β-lipoprotein may be utilized by other tissues or returned to the adipose tissue for storage.

The transport and fate of endogenous lipid can best be summarized diagrammatically (Fig. 4).

D. Factors Affecting Fat Mobilization

In this section we will list many of the factors known to act and how they might exert their influence in fat mobilization.

1. Endocrine Factors

The catecholamines, whether secreted by the adrenal medulla or the endings of the postganglionic symphathetic nerves, markedly stimulate lipolysis in adipose tissue. The mechanism of their action appears to involve an increase in the cellular level of cyclic AMP which in turn activates the triglyceride lipase in some manner (Rizach, 1965). The hormones probably do not act during FFA release taking place normally during the postabsorbtive stage. Their role in mobilizing lipids is a part of the response to a stressor. Glucocorticoids and thyroxine have to be present for epinephrine and norepinephrine to exert their maximal effect on lipolysis (Steinberg and Vaughan, 1965).

Several peptides including ACTH, TSH, MSH, and vasopressin have lipolytic actions (Steinberg and Vaughan, 1965). The action of a given peptide is limited to certain species (Rudman et al., 1965; Raben, 1965). In each case, the site of action is triglyceride lipase and seems to involve cyclic AMP (Rizach, 1965). Another peptide, glucagon, acts similarly on adipose tissue (Kovacev and Scow, 1966). Growth hormone also stimulates lipolysis but by a different mechanism. This hormone stimulates synthesis of the enzyme adenylcyclase that catalyzes production of cyclic AMP (Fain, 1968). The physiological significance of these peptides and mobilization of lipid has yet to be established.

Thus far, only one hormone has been shown to inhibit the release of FFA from adipose tissue (Fain et al., 1966). Insulin inhibits mobilization of FFA both directly and indirectly. Insulin has been shown to lower the level of cyclic AMP which would tend to decrease triglyceride lipase activity (Butcher et al., 1966). Furthermore, the increased glucose uptake by adipose tissue in the presence of insulin will tend to enhance reesterification of FFA, thus decreasing their ultimate release (Section VI,C). Adipose tissue has been described as being exquisitely sensitive to insulin (Cahill, 1964). Thus, the action of insulin has to be given high importance in the control of lipid mobilization by adipose tissue during the feeding cycle, during high carbohydrate feeding, and during fasting.

Prostaglandins, compounds isolated recently and shown to have biological activity, appear to influence lipid mobilization by adipose tissue (Bergström and Samuelson,

1965). These compounds are synthesized in the tissues of mammalians from the essential fatty acids. Adipose tissue in the presence of prostaglandin releases more FFA than in the absence. In contrast, prostaglandin counteracts the stimulatory effects of the catecholanine on lipolysis when both groups of compounds are present. Again, the physiological importance of these observations is not established.

2.   Neural Factors

Electrical stimulation of the autonomic fibers coursing through adipose tissue results in the release of FFA into the circulation (Correll, 1963). This reaction is presumably due to the release of norepinephrine from the sympathetic fibers in the neural network. Havel (1965) stresses the day-to-day importance of the sympathetic innervation of adipose tissue as a fundamental mechanism controlling the supply of nutrients to body tissues. Nonetheless, the response of adipose tissue to sympathetic stimulation is also important in providing energy in stressful situations, such as fasting, cold exposure, and vigorous exercise (Havel, 1965). In this respect, lipolysis by adipose tissue and glycogenolysis by the liver are comparable responses to emergency situations and are elicited by similar mechanisms (cf. Sutherland, 1961; Raben, 1965).

E. ABNORMALITIES OF PLASMA LIPOPROTEINS

There have been too few studies in domestic animals to clearly establish that abnormalities and deficiencies described in man occur with significant incidence in other species. The extensive studies in man, however, provide an experimental model for conditions which might be observed in domestic animals. Studies of lipoprotein disorders have been of great value in determining the function of lipoproteins much in the same way that ablation experiments indicated endocrine function.

1.   Inherited Lipoprotein Deficiencies

Two disorders that are definitely genetically determined have been described. These are the complete lack of β-lipoprotein, abeta-lipoproteinemia, and a deficiency of α-lipoprotein sometimes referred to as Tangier disease. There appears to be some α-lipoprotein found in patients with Tangier disease, but even this small amount is probably abnormal (Fredrickson, 1966).

a. ABETA-LIPOPROTEINEMIA.   This lack of β-lipoprotein is manifest in infancy by retarded growth, steatorrhea, and abdominal distension. The acanthocytosis accompanying this syndrome was the first sign noticed (Bassen and Kornzweig, 1950). Later, the very low plasma cholesterol levels led to the demonstration of the absence of β-lipoproteins (Salt, 1960). Severe neurological defects are manifest late in childhood with signs of degeneration of the posterior lateral columns and the cerebellar tracts as well as retinal degeneration. The inability to absorb essential fatty acids and fat-soluble vitamins probably contributes to the clinical manifestations of this disease.

The electrophoretic pattern of the plasma lipoproteins from these patients indicates a complete lack of β-lipoprotein. The concentrations of cholesterol, phospholipid, and glycerides in plasma are the lowest recorded in any human disease. The lack of β-lipoprotein results in an inability to transport glyceride, either as pre-β-lipoprotein or chylomicrons. The inability to form chylomicrons means that lipids can be taken up by the mucosal cell but not released into the lymph. Blocking protein synthesis in rat intestinal mucosa produces a syndrome similar to this disease (Hatch *et al.*, 1963; Isselbacher and Budz, 1963).

When patients are fed diets high in glycerides, chylomicrons do not appear in the plasma. When fed high carbohydrate diets which normally result in the release of endogenous lipid into the plasma, no increase in the plasma concentration of glyceride nor the presence of pre-β-lipoprotein is observed (Levy *et al.*, 1966). These patients could digest and absorb MCT, but this diet could not overcome the lack of essential fatty acids. As will be discussed in a later section, glyceride formed in the liver, either as a result of a high carbohydrate diet or a diet containing MCT, might well result in a fatty liver (Section VI,F). Glyceride would accumulate due to the lack of the protein complex used to transport it to other tissues.

b. α-Lipoprotein Deficiency.   Lack of α-lipoprotein has been called Tangier disease after the first cases found, namely, two children 5 and 6 years of age in the same family living on Tangier Island in Chesapeake Bay (Fredrickson, 1966). As in abeta-lipoproteinemia the levels of plasma cholesterol and phospholipid are below normal. Glyceride concentrations in the plasma are high normal in the postabsorptive state. The deposition of cholesterol ester in all reticuloendothelial tissues provides a pathognomonic sign for this disease; the tonsils are grossly enlarged and have a unique orange color. This disease is not as serious as abeta-lipoproteinemia. There appears to be no malabsorption and the ability to release endogenous lipid is unimpaired. All the clinical signs can be related to the abnormal deposition of lipid in the body tissues.

The electrophoretic pattern of the plasma lipoproteins reveals the complete lack of an α-band and no distinct pre-β-band. The change in the protein migrating as pre-β implies that α-lipoprotein may contribute to the formation of this specific band.

2. *Hyperlipoproteinemias*

Unfortunately, in contrast to hypolipoproteinemias, these syndromes are more descriptive and provide less information on the mechanism of lipid transport as the lipoprotein complex. Increased levels of major lipoprotein fractions are observed (1) secondary to systemic disease and (2) in primary lipoproteinemia, which often has a familial occurrence. Before the advent of lipoprotein analysis, many of these conditions in both categories were referred to as hypocholesterolemia and hyperglyceridemia. These appellations are accurate, specific terms that are of valid clinical use in the absence of lipoprotein analysis.

On the basis of the lipoprotein patterns and plasma lipid analyses, Fredrickson and his co-workers (1967) have divided hyperlipoproteinemias into five categories. It is recommended, for the sake of simplicity, that an attempt be made to fit the findings of comparative studies in domestic animals into their format, at least for a start. The methods for sampling and analysis of the plasma are given in detail in their review article, and each syndrome is described with admirable conciseness.

Table II, adapted from Fredrickson *et al.* (1967), summarizes the characteristics of the plasma lipid in each category. The diseases of humans in which such a pattern may occur secondarily are also listed. This latter information may be of value in recognizing and differentiating between such diseases in domestic animals. Indeed, some of this information is already in everyday use, e.g., hypercholesterolemia secondary to hypothyroidism.

For a detailed description of each type of hyperlipoproteinemia listed in the table, the reader should refer to the original reference. Type I is characterized by the presence of chylomicrons in the plasma in high concentration at least 14 hours after a meal. The other lipoprotein fractions are low, in contrast to type V, so that type I is hyperchylomicronemia in an almost pure form. Hyperchylomicronemia is characterized by the formation of a cream layer on the plasma sample during storage in the cold. A familial disease in humans included in type I is a deficiency of lipoprotein lipase, hence, injection of heparin leads to no discernible change in the turbidity of the plasma. A similar disease has been reported in a puppy (Baum *et al.*, 1969).

Type II is characterized by an increase in the lipoproteins with β mobility on electrophoresis. In this type of hyperlipoproteinemia, the plasma cholesterol is markedly increased in the absence of a similar increase in the glycerol level. Type II lipoprotein pattern is commonly associated with hypothyroidism and obstructive liver disease, although type IV is also seen. Type II occurs familially in humans, the most common syndrome being the formation of xanthomas and atheromas. Type III varies from type II only in that the plasma glycerides are also markedly elevated.

Type IV is distinguished from types II and III by the fact that the hyperlipoproteinemia is due to endogenous lipid. Type IV can result from any of a variety of situations in which the rate of release of glycerides into the plasma exceeds their rate of removal. In general, lack of the usual close control of carbohydrate metabolism or a caloric imbalance can result in type IV hyperlipoproteinemia. Many diseases in which this is the case are listed in Table II.

The electrophoretic pattern of the lipoproteins in type IV is characterized by a marked increased in the pre-β-band and an absence of chylomicrons. The glyceride level is markedly increased and the cholesterol level increased somewhat. When the glyceride level in plasma becomes extremely high, there is a marked tailing of the pre-β-band giving the indication of the presence of chylomicrons. Dilution of the plasma with saline prior to electrophoresis will help to distinguish the pre-β and chylomicron areas in samples where this occurs.

In humans, type IV seems to have a prevalance in certain families, especially in young adulthood. It often accompanies severe obesity, disappearing when the patient returns to normal weight and avoids excessive carbohydrate consumption. Type V hyperlipoproteinemia is characterized by an increase in circulating chylomicrons and pre-β-lipoproteins as well. It is not well distinguished from type IV and may well be a combination of abnormalities such as types I and IV.

TABLE II DISEASES ASSOCIATED WITH THE HYPERLIPOPROTEINEMIAS OF HUMANS[a]

Type:	I	II	III	IV	V
Characteristic:	Chylomicronemia	Cholesterolemia	β-Lipoproteinemia	Pre-β-lipoproteinemia	Pre-β-lipoproteinemia + chylomicronemia
Diseases associated with:	Diabetes Pancreatitis Acute alcoholism	Hypothyroidism Obstructive hepatic disease Hypoproteinemia Familial xanthomatosis etc.	Familial hyper-glyceridemia + cholesterolemia	Diabetes Pancreatitis Alcoholism Glycogen storage disease Hypothyroidism Nephrotic syndrome Dysglobulinemia Gestational hormones Familial disease	Not clear; may be combination of I + IV

[a]From Fredrickson et al., 1967.

F. PLASMA LIPOPROTEINS AND FATTY LIVER

The sections on lipid transport (Section VI,C,D) outline the movement of endogenous lipid between liver and other tissues especially adipose tissue. The preceding section on lipoprotein disorders described the consequences of blocks in such movement especially after carbohydrate feeding. The relationship between liver triglycerides and plasma glycerides has been quantitated in the rat. In rats fed diets high in glucose, nearly all the triglyceride synthesized in the liver is disposed of as plasma lipoproteins, presumably as pre-β-lipoprotein (VLDL) (Baker and Schotz, 1964). Therefore, it is not surprising that any block in the synthesis of the apoproteins of the lipoproteins results in an accumulation of lipid, namely, glycerides in the liver (Lombardi, 1966; Shapiro, 1965). Ethionine, CCl_4, puromycin, and orotic acid feeding all appear to cause fatty livers by blocking synthesis of protein, particularly apolipoproteins (Smuckler and Benditt, 1965; Robinson, 1964; Farber et al., 1964; Lombardi and Ugazio, 1965; Venkataraman and Sreenivasan, 1965). Similarly, choline deficiency results in fatty liver due to the lack of synthesis of phospholipid (Zilvermit and Diluzio, 1958), a necessary component of the lipoprotein complex (Section VI,B). In all of these experimental disorders there is a fall in plasma triglycerides and a corresponding decrease in lipoprotein, particularly the VLDL.

Other disorders resulting in fatty livers are accompanied by hypertriglyceridemia. In these situations, formation and release of triglycerides by the liver are both increased. Many of these disorders have been mentioned in the section on hyperlipoproteinemia. The examples are ethanol ingestion (Isselbacher and Greenberger, 1964) and the administration of cortisone (Freidman et al., 1965; R. B. Hill and Droke, 1963). The cause of the fatty liver and subsequent hypertriglyceridemia in these studies is presumably due to mobilization of FFA derived from adipose tissue (Jones et al., 1965). The response to ethanol is complicated by the fact that ethanol is also a ready precursor of acetyl building blocks as well as a source of reducing power for fatty acid synthesis (Section VII,A). Students of the effects of alcohol on lipid metabolism in the liver are referred to the additional papers on its effects listed in the review by Shapiro (1967).

VII. BIOSYNTHESIS OF LIPID

The formation of triglycerides in various tissues has been covered throughout this chapter. The pathways for the synthesis of phospholipids (Kennedy, 1961) and sphingolipids (Brady and Koval, 1958) are known, but factors altering their synthesis are not clear. These biosynthetic pathways, then, are of little concern to the clinician. Hence, in this section, we will concentrate on fatty acid synthesis and cholesterol synthesis, and the factors that influence these pathways.

A. FATTY ACID SYNTHESIS

1. Tissues Involved in Fatty Acid Synthesis

The major tissue sites of fatty acid synthesis in the animal are adipose tissue and liver. In the lactating animal, the mammary gland also synthesizes fatty acids. In mice, and presumably all mammals, adipose tissue contributes the major portion of fatty acid synthesized within the animal (Favarger, 1965). It should be clear by now that adipose tissue is not simply a site for the passive storage of triglyceride. It actively takes up, synthesizes, and releases fatty acids. In contrast to mammals, the liver of the chicken is by far the major site of fatty acid synthesis (O'Hea and Leveille, 1968).

2. Pathway of Fatty Acid Synthesis

In all systems studied, *E. coli*, yeast, pigeon liver, rat liver, and rat mammary gland, the basic steps of fatty acid synthesis from acetyl CoA are the same (for review, see Vagelos, 1964). The first step is the formation of malonyl CoA by the addition of an active CO_2 to acetyl CoA (reaction 3). This carboxylation is catalyzed by acetyl CoA carboxylase, a biotin enzyme, and requires ATP in addition to the other reactants.

$$CH_3-\overset{O}{\underset{\|}{C}}-S-CoA + CO_2 + ATP \longrightarrow HOOC-CH_2-\overset{O}{\underset{\|}{C}}-S-CoA + ADP + P_i \qquad (3)$$

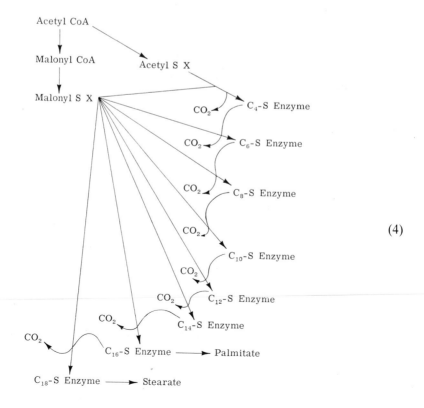

$$(4)$$

In step 2, catalyzed by a multienzyme complex, one acetyl CoA is coupled stepwise with several malonyl CoA, depending on the fatty acid formed, with the release of an equivalent number of moles of CO_2. After the addition of each two-carbon unit from malonyl CoA, there is a reduction step and a dehydration step followed by a final reduction. This multienzyme complex is called fatty acid synthetase. Studies in bacteria (Vagelos et al., 1966) and subsequently in plants (Simoni et al., 1967) have revealed that the substrates participate not as CoA derivatives but as an acyl derivative of 4-phosphopantetheine that is bound to serine of the peptides (Vagelos et al., 1966; Pugh and Wakil, 1965; Majerus, 1967). This peptide is referred to as acyl carrier protein (ACP).

Fatty acid synthetase has been isolated in pure form from pigeon liver (Hsu et al., 1964), rat liver (Burton et al., 1968), and mammary gland of lactating rats (Smith and Abraham, 1969). In all cases, it has been impossible to isolate the peptide comparable to ACP of the lower forms. On the other hand, in all cases, the multienzyme complex contains 4-phosphopantetheine. The complete set of reactions taking place on the multienzyme complex are shown in reaction 4 (Smith, 1965).

3.   Cellular Compartmentalization and Fatty Acid Synthesis

Recently, it was pointed out that in all tissues examined, the enzymes of fatty acid synthesis are in the extramitochondria, soluble portion of the cell, the cytosol. In most species, however, the major source of acetyl CoA or fatty acid synthesis is from the decarboxylation of pyruvate which takes place within the mitochondria. The question arises: how does the acetyl CoA reach the site of formation of fatty acid synthesis? Several possibilities have been suggested (Srere, 1965; Kornacker and Lowenstein, 1965). Early investigations indicated that in liver the acetyl unit was transported as acetylcarnitine (Bressler and Katz, 1965), whereas in mammary gland citrate acted as the acetyl carrier (Bartley et al., 1965). In the latter scheme, citrate cleavage enzyme played the key role in catalyzing the release in the cytosol of the same acetyl unit condensed with oxalacetic acid in the mitochondria, the reaction catalyzed by citrate-condensing enzyme. Recently, Bressler and Brendel (1966) have verified that in liver, as in mammary gland, citrate is the major carrier for acetyl units out of the mitochondria.

4.   Factors Influencing Fatty Acid Synthesis

It is well known that dietary changes are reflected in the rate of fatty acid synthesis in liver and adipose tissue (Masoro, 1962). All of these changes are the ones that would tend to maintain homeostasis. Fasting reduces lipogenesis in both liver (Lyon et al., 1952) and adipose tissue (Hausberger and Milstein, 1955), whereas ingestion of large quantities of carbohydrate markedly increases lipogenesis in both tissues (Lyon et al., 1952; Hausberger and Milstein, 1955). The carbohydrate effect may at least be partly related to the circulating level of insulin. The marked stimulating effect of insulin on lipogenesis in adipose tissue is well documented (for review, see Winegrad et al., 1964).

The lipogenic response to the ingestion of large quantities of fat is not so clearcut. There appear to be differences in the response of liver and adipose tissue.

Differences are also evident in the response elicited by rats when compared to mice. Fat feeding for 3 days depresses hepatic lipogenesis severalfold in rats (R. Hill et al., 1958). A similar response is observed in mice only if the dietary fat contains linoleate. Indeed, the degree of depression of hepatic lipogenesis in the mouse appears to be related to the linoleate content of the diet, not to the total lipid content (Allmann et al., 1965a,b). The lipogenic response of adipose tissue to fat feeding has not been tested adequately in both species to detect any differences. Long-term feeding of diets high in lipid content appears to depress lipogenesis in adipose tissue. In summary, it appears that carbohydrate feeding elicits a greater lipogenic response in adipose tissue than in liver, whereas in fat feeding liver responds to a much greater extent. Because of the difference in the quantities of these two tissues, it is difficult to say in either case which tissue is more influential in determining the lipogenic capacity of the whole animal.

The studies on lipid feeding of mice and rats make it clear that before any general conclusions can be reached, studies comparing the lipogenic responses to high fat feeding and linoleate feeding will have to be performed with several species.

It is not clear how the dietary and hormonal changes influence the enzymic activity of liver and adipose tissue. Several intracellular mediators of the dietary response have been evoked. Most of these are compounds known to alter the activity of acetyl CoA carboxylase, the rate-limiting enzyme in fatty acid synthesis (see Vagelos, 1964). Citrate (see Vagelos, 1964), ATP, magnesium (Greenspan and Lowenstein, 1967), and palmitylcarnitine (Fritz and Hsu, 1967) have been shown to activate this enzyme. Palmityl CoA has been shown to inhibit both the carboxylase (Bortz and Lynen, 1963) and the fatty acid synthetase (Porter and Long, 1958). All of these actions have been used to explain the extent of lipogenesis seen in various nutritional states. Furthermore, the ratio of palmitylcarnitine to palmityl CoA in the cell has been used to explain lipogenic responses (Fritz and Hsu, 1967). None of these suggested effectors withstands the test of actual tissue measurements at the time of a given dietary condition. The actual measurements of the effectors either do not correlate with the lipogenic responses, or are always at inhibitory levels, or the levels are too low to be effective activators. Cellular compartmentalization may explain some of these discrepancies, but, until further work is done, the cellular effectors of lipogenic responses will remain in doubt.

An aspect of fatty acid synthesis that is still not understood is the mechanism for limiting the length of the carbon chain of the fatty acids produced by the multienzyme complex (see Vagelos, 1964; Lynen et al., 1968). Understanding this mechanism is particularly important in the mammary gland of species that produce short-chain fatty acids. Two groups of workers have been examining this mechanism (Bartley et al., 1967; Smith and Dils, 1966). The possibilities of the ratio of the activity of enzymes of fatty acid synthesis or of other enzyme systems (Bartley et al., 1967) are now being investigated with the fatty acid synthetase purified from rat mammary gland (Smith and Abraham, 1969).

B. Cholesterol Synthesis

Cholesterol can be absorbed from the intestine or be synthesized by most tissues from acetate. Cholesterol is an important precursor of cholesterol ester, bile acids, and steroid hormones. The clinical chemistry of bile acids and steroid hormones is covered in Chapters 5 and 7, respectively. We will concern ourselves in this chapter with the synthesis of cholesterol and its control. The absorption and movement of cholesterol and cholesterol esters in the animal has been covered in Sections IV and VI.

1. Pathways of Cholesterol Synthesis

Cholesterol can be synthesized by many tissues of the body, but the liver appears to be the primary endogenous source. Cholesterol is synthesized from acetate in discrete stages. The first stage involves the stepwise conversion of acetyl CoA to β-OH-β-methylglutaryl CoA (HMG-CoA). These steps can take place either in the mitochondria catalyzed by the same enzymes that form acetacetate (Rudney, 1957) or extramitochondrially in which the reactants are bound to an enzyme complex (Brodie *et al.*, 1963). The second reaction, the conversion of HMG-CoA to mevalonic acid, is the rate-limiting step of cholesterol synthesis, the site of dietary control

Step 1

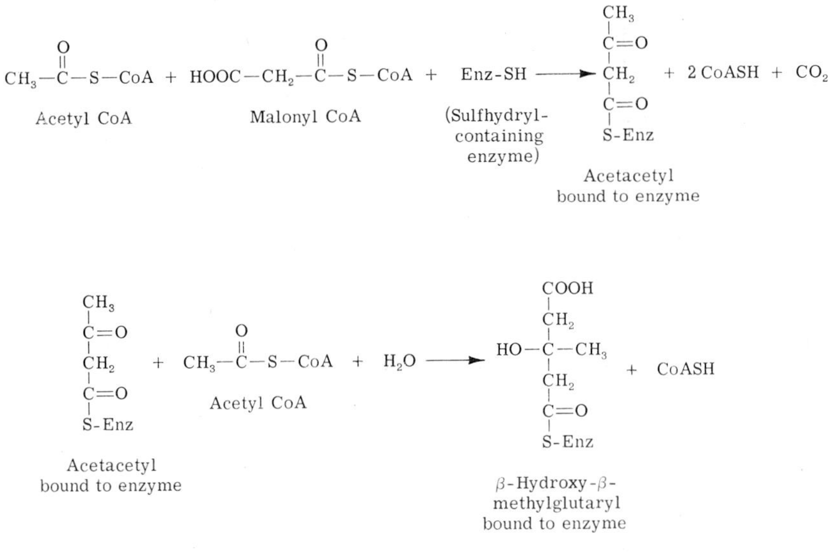

$$CH_3-\overset{O}{\overset{\|}{C}}-S-CoA \ + \ HOOC-CH_2-\overset{O}{\overset{\|}{C}}-S-CoA \ + \ Enz-SH \longrightarrow \ \begin{array}{c} CH_3 \\ | \\ C=O \\ | \\ CH_2 \\ | \\ C=O \\ | \\ S-Enz \end{array} \ + \ 2\,CoASH \ + \ CO_2$$

Acetyl CoA   Malonyl CoA   (Sulfhydryl-containing enzyme)   Acetacetyl bound to enzyme

$$\begin{array}{c} CH_3 \\ | \\ C=O \\ | \\ CH_2 \\ | \\ C=O \\ | \\ S-Enz \end{array} \ + \ CH_3-\overset{O}{\overset{\|}{C}}-S-CoA \ + \ H_2O \longrightarrow \ \begin{array}{c} COOH \\ | \\ CH_2 \\ | \\ HO-C-CH_3 \\ | \\ CH_2 \\ | \\ C=O \\ | \\ S-Enz \end{array} \ + \ CoASH$$

Acetacetyl bound to enzyme   Acetyl CoA   β-Hydroxy-β-methylglutaryl bound to enzyme

Step 2

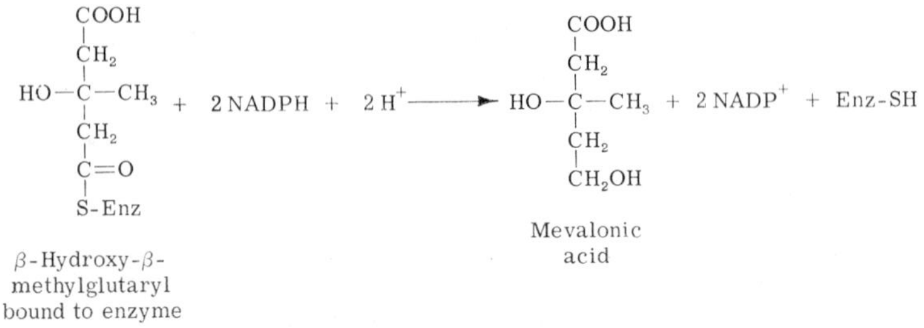

$$\begin{array}{c} COOH \\ | \\ CH_2 \\ | \\ HO-C-CH_3 \\ | \\ CH_2 \\ | \\ C=O \\ | \\ S-Enz \end{array} \ + \ 2\,NADPH \ + \ 2\,H^+ \longrightarrow \ \begin{array}{c} COOH \\ | \\ CH_2 \\ | \\ HO-C-CH_3 \\ | \\ CH_2 \\ | \\ CH_2OH \end{array} \ + \ 2\,NADP^+ \ + \ Enz-SH$$

β-Hydroxy-β-methylglutaryl bound to enzyme   Mevalonic acid

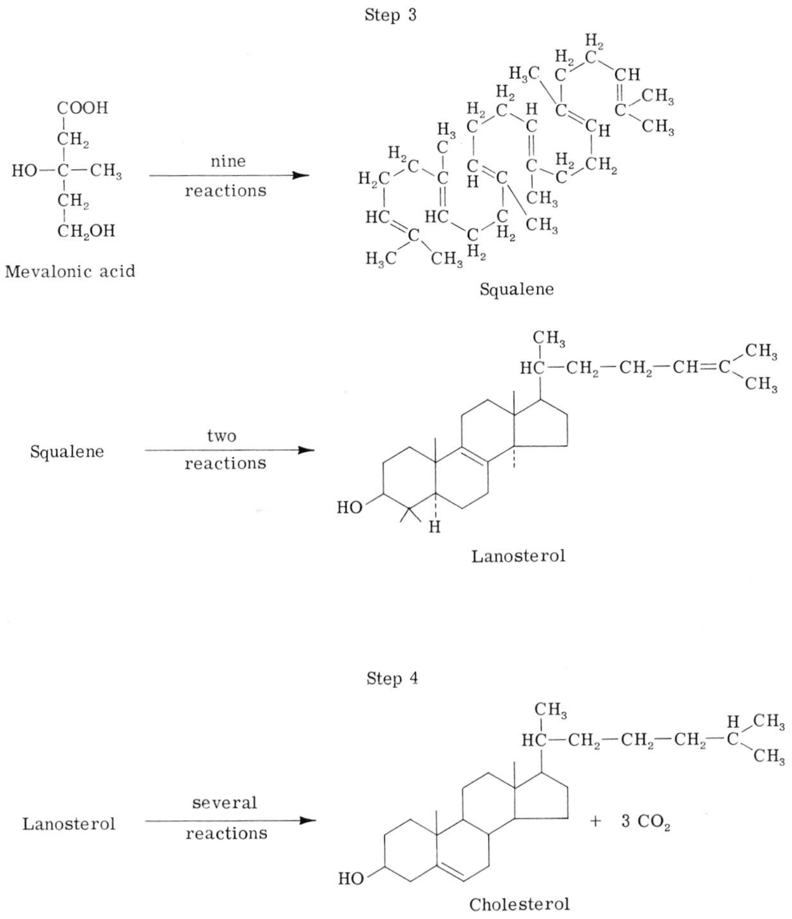

Step 3

Mevalonic acid

nine reactions

Squalene

Squalene

two reactions

Lanosterol

Step 4

Lanosterol

several reactions

$+ 3 CO_2$

Cholesterol

Fig. 5.   Reactions involved in the synthesis of cholesterol.

(Siperstein and Guest, 1959). In the penultimate stage, mevalonic acid is converted to squalene, which subsequently is cyclized to lanosterol. In the ultimate stage the lanosterol is converted to cholesterol. These reactions were reviewed by Bloch (1965) on receiving the Nobel Prize and are shown schematically in Fig. 5.

2.   Regulation of Cholesterol Synthesis

The extent of endogenous cholesterol synthesis by liver is indirectly proportional to the cholesterol content of the diet (Siperstein and Guest, 1959). The synthesis of cholesterol in other tissues, however, is not inhibited by high dietary cholesterol in the diet. In animals, such as humans, where synthesis in the liver is not a major source of plasma cholesterol (Wilson and Lindsey, 1965), this feedback control has little impact on the total body cholesterol. In contrast, it may be significant in rats in which the liver is the major site of cholesterol biosynthesis. At present, there are no definitive studies on the importance of feedback control in domestic animals.

The reduction of HMG-CoA to mevalonate is the enzymic reaction that responds to dietary manipulation (Siperstein and Guest, 1959; Bucher *et al.*, 1959). This reaction is the first one that is unique to cholesterol synthesis and is virtually irreversible.

3.   Synthesis of Cholesterol Esters

Cholesterol can be esterified with fatty acids by enzymes present in liver, adrenal cortex, intestinal mucosa, and even plasma. Indeed, most of the cholesterol in plasma, lymph, liver, and adrenal cortex is in the esterified form. Muscle, on the other hand, contains free cholesterol and almost no cholesterol esters. Hydrolysis of the cholesterol esters to free cholesterol and FFA takes place, not only in the intestinal lumen (Section IV,A), but in the liver and the adrenal gland as well.

The significance of whether cholesterol is in the free or esterified form in a tissue is not clear. It may be related to the structural characteristics of the membranes of a particular tissue.

An enzyme system has been described in plasma of humans that transesterifies the fatty acid of lecithin to cholesterol resulting in the formation of lysolecithin and cholesterol ester (Glomset, 1968). The popular abbreviation of the enzyme lecithin-cholesterol acyl transferase is LCAT. The reaction is slow, but presumably significant amounts of cholesterol ester are formed in this manner (Glomset, 1968). A lethal familial disease has been described in which LCAT is absent (Norum and Gjone, 1967). These same patients appear to have other plasma protein deficiencies, so the seriousness of the syndrome is not solely attributable to LCAT.

VIII.   OXIDATION OF FATTY ACIDS

The spiral path of long-chain fatty acids to acetyl CoA during oxidation within the mitochondria is well known. A familiar rendering is reproduced in Fig. 6. Perhaps less familiar is the form in which the fatty acid enters the mitochondria, a reaction shown to be the rate-limiting step in fatty acid oxidation (see Fritz, 1968). The acyl CoA derivative in the cytosol can arise from activation of FFA entering the cell (Section VI,C), from triglycerides and phospholipids being degraded within the cell, or from *de novo* synthesis in the case of liver and adipose tissue. In order for the fatty acid to enter the site of the oxidative spiral, it must first be converted to the acylcarnitine derivative (Fritz and Yue, 1963). The enzyme catalyzing this reaction appears to be a part of the inner mitochondrial membrane (Norum and Bremer, 1967). The activity of the palmityl CoA-carnitine transferase correlates with the rate of fatty acid oxidation, both in a variety of tissues and in a variety of nutritional states (Fritz, 1968). The intracellular effectors of this key enzyme are unknown.

The activity of the palmityl CoA-carnitine transferase has been evoked as a control point not only for fatty acid oxidation but for gluconeogenesis and ketogenesis (see Fritz, 1968). Two acetyl CoA pools within the mitochondria have been suggested, one derived from pyruvate, the other from long-chain fatty acids. Further, the acetyl CoA from fatty acids would have greater access to exert its stimulatory action

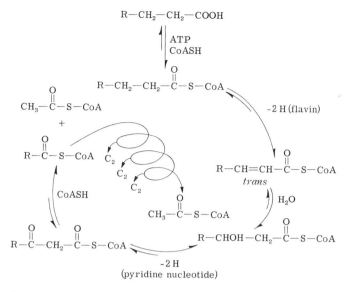

Fig. 6. Schematic presentation of β-oxidation of long-chain fatty acids to acetyl CoA. (Modified from Conn and Stumpf, 1966.)

on pyruvate carboxylase, an effect described by Utter and Keech (1963). Thus, when FFA are readily available to the liver, as in fasting, the subsequent increase in acetyl CoA derived from palmitylcarnitine could stimulate carboxylation of pyruvate to oxalacetic acid (Fritz, 1968), a rate-limiting step in gluconeogenesis (Krebs, 1964). Ketogenesis would result from the excessive production of acetyl CoA in a situation in which the availability of oxalacetic acid is limited (Krebs, 1966a,b) or from saturation of the citrate–oxalacetate condensing reaction with acetyl CoA derived from FFA (Fritz, 1968). The acetyl CoA-carnitine transferase, suggested previously as a means of transferring acetyl units out of the mitochondria (Section VII,A; Bressler and Katz, 1969), would act in this hypothesis as an intramitochondrial go-between for the two acetyl CoA pools (Fritz, 1968). Such a relationship correlates well with the observed responses. More work, however, is necessary before one can attribute all of the responses to the changes in the activity of the palmityl CoA-carnitine transferase.

IX. SPECIAL ASPECTS OF LIPID METABOLISM IN DOMESTIC ANIMALS

The paucity of material in this section reveals the lack of knowledge regarding problems relating specifically to the various domestic animals.

A. Lipid Metabolism in Ruminants

Four aspects of ruminant lipid metabolism require special mention: (1) digestion and absorption, (2) transfer of lipid into milk, (3) unique features of lipogenesis, and (4) the use of the level of FFA in plasma as a metabolic indicator.

1.   Digestion and Absorption

The small intestine of the ruminant receives mainly saturated FFA rather than triglyceride because of the extensive lypolysis and hydrogenation of dietary lipid by the microorganisms in the ruminant (Garton, 1960; Ward *et al.*, 1964). The ruminant normally receives a diet low in lipid, but it is becoming common in parts of the United States to feed them corn oil that has been used in restaurants for deep fat frying. This oil can be incorporated in the diet of fattening animals up to 5% by weight. Therefore, the recent studies by Leat and his co-workers (Leat and Hall, 1968; Leat and Cunningham, 1968; Leat and Harrison, 1967) take on more than comparative interest. If the ruminant intestine is flooded with triglyceride, is it capable of handling it?

Leat and Cunningham (1968) asked the question: If the small intestine of the ruminant receives mostly FFA, does the MG pathway still operate? In studies with isolated segments of intestine from lambs and sheep, it was shown that, as in monogastric animals, the major pathway of triglyceride absorption is via MG (Leat and Harrison, 1967).

Studies of the lipid composition of plasma and lymph of cows indicate that the fate of the lipid absorbed from the intestinal and the composition of the chylomicron in the ruminant is similar to that in monogastric animals (Leat and Hall, 1968). Hansen (1965a) has shown that isolated intestinal mucosa of lambs readily incorporates fatty acids into triglycerides and, to a small extent, cholesterol ester. In contrast, his studies with rats reveal incorporation of fatty acids into both triglyceride and cholesterol ester. Differences between the two species were also noted in the fatty acids most readily esterified (Hansen, 1965a) and which position of glycerol was preferentially esterified with a given fatty acid (Hansen, 1965b,c).

The major lipid-related material absorbed by the ruminant is, of course, VFA which enters the portal system. Of the major VFA, propionate and butyrate are utilized almost completely in the liver, but a large proportion of the acetate may be passed on to the peripheral circulation for utilization by all tissues (Annison *et al.*, 1957). A major portion of the propionate is probably utilized for gluconeogenesis (Annison *et al.*, 1963). It now seems clear that butyrate does not contribute carbon directly to glucose production, but may increase glycogenolysis in the liver of lambs (Phillips and Black, 1965), presumably by activation of phosphorylase (Phillips *et al.*, 1965). In other ruminants, the sole effect of butyrate on hepatic glucose output is via increased gluconeogenesis (Anand, 1967). Such an effect could be mediated by an increase in the level of acetyl CoA derived from butyrate. It has been shown that acetyl CoA activates pyruvate carboxylase (Utter and Keech, 1963), a key enzyme in gluconeogenesis (Krebs, 1964).

2.   Transfer of Plasma Lipid into Milk

The transfer of fatty acids and triglycerides from plasma into milk deserves mention because of the importance of milk production by ruminants. A portion of the fatty acids in milk are synthesized in the mammary gland, but another portion, especially the long-chain components, is derived from the blood (Folley and Mc Naught, 1961). Based on the arteriovenous differences across the mammary gland of lactating goats, the fatty acids of the triglycerides in chylomicrons and LDL contribute essentially all of the fatty acids in milk derived from plasma (Barry et al., 1963). The plasma concentration of FFA, however, was unchanged across the mammary gland. Earlier work in both the lactating cow (Graham et al., 1936) and the goat (Lintzel, 1934) had indicated that the mammary gland utilizes neutral lipids from the plasma. Studies with labeled fatty acids administered in the diet (Glascock et al., 1956) or as isolated chylomicrons (Lascelles et al., 1964) verified plasma lipid as a precursor of milk lipid. Plasma lipids contribute 35–75% of fatty acid in milk depending on the nutritional state of the animal (Riis, 1964; Barry, 1966; Glascock et al., 1966).

Annison and his co-workers in both the intact lactating goat (1967) and the perfused caprine mammary gland (Linzell et al., 1967) have studied the utilization of labeled acetate, stearate, oleate, and β-OH-butyrate. They also measured the arteriovenous differences across the gland of FFA, neutral glycerides, and phospholipids. FFA are indeed taken up by the gland, but a similar quantity are released so that the net difference across the gland is unchanged. The FFA are incorporated into milk fat and are not extensively oxidized. These studies verified earlier investigations showing (1) the plasma phospholipids contribute little to milk fat and (2) the fatty acids of milk with chain length of C-4 to C-14 arise almost solely from acetate. Palmitate arises from both acetate and plasma triglyceride which is almost the sole precursor of oleate and stearate. The studies with β-OH-butyrate indicate that a portion of this compound was incorporated into milk lipid as a C-4 unit. Similar evidence has recently been reported from measurements of the incorporation of labeled butyrate into the milk fat of lactating cows (Bines and Brown, 1968). There is evidence from several sources that the ruminant mammary gland forms large quantities of oleate from plasma stearate (Lauryssens et al., 1961; West et al., 1967; Annison et al., 1967).

McClymont and Vallance (1962) suggested that the depression of milk fat concentration observed after administration of glucose to cows (Vallance and McClymont, 1959) is due to the decrease in the plasma level of triglyceride and a decrease in the uptake by the gland under these conditions. Continuous infusion of triglyceride for 48 hours increased the concentration of lipid in milk (Storry and Rook, 1964). The ability of triglyceride in plasma to increase milk fat is directly correlated to the chain length of the fatty acid it contains (Storry et al., 1969).

Whether the depression in milk fat production brought about by feeding high grain diets can be attributed to the changes in circulating triglycerides (Storry and Rook, 1965) appears open to question. Varman and Schultz (1968) attribute the depression to changes in the availability of propionate and acetate from the rumen and to enzymic changes in adipose tissue and mammary gland as observed by Opstvedt et al. (1967).

3. Lipogenesis

Early tracer studies by Kleiber's group (Kleiber et al., 1952) revealed that glucose carbon is not incorporated into milk fat to any appreciable extent. The ready availability of acetate and butyrate as precursors of fatty acids seemed explanation enough for this finding. As the role of citrate cleavage enzyme in fatty acid synthesis was being established (Section VII,A), it was suggested that the reason glucose carbon failed as a precursor of fatty acids is due to a low level of citrate cleavage enzyme in ruminant tissues (Hardwick, 1966). Direct enzymic assays plus the extremely low incorporation of C-3 of aspartate into fatty acids by ruminant liver verified the minimal operation of the citrate cleavage pathway (Hanson and Ballard, 1967) in these animals.

The liver of the fetal ruminant contains citrate cleavage activity comparable to that of fetal rats and isotope studies verified the operation of the citrate cleavage pathway in these animals (Hanson and Ballard, 1968). The activity of citrate cleavage enzyme is known to be very sensitive to the dietary and hormonal changes (see Leveille and Hanson, 1966; Srere, 1965). Considering the ruminant as an animal on a high fat, low carbohydrate diet, it is not surprising that citrate cleavage activity is low when the rumen is functional. Indeed, malic enzyme, another adaptive enzyme related to lipogenesis, is also low in ruminants (Hanson and Ballard, 1968) as it is in monogastrics fed high fat, low carbohydrate diets (Leveille and Hanson, 1966).

In an attempt to show that the low activity of these two enzymes might simply be an adaptive response, we have intravenously infused nonlactating cows continuously for 4 hours with a solution of 50% glucose. The results of enzyme assays on liver biopsies taken before and after the infusion revealed that the activity of both citrate cleavage enzyme and malic enzyme increased 1.5-fold during the infusion (Bartley, 1969). Long-term carbohydrate loading studies will be required before we can conclude that the low activities of citrate cleavage and malic enzymes are solely due to an adaptive response to the nutrients absorbed from their alimentary tract.

What is the clinical significance of the low activity of these two enzymes related to lipogenesis? Under normal conditions the enzymic profile of ruminant liver, adipose tissue, and mammary gland would favor utilization of acetate for fatty acid synthesis (Ballard et al., 1969) and thereby spare glucose for its indispensible roles, i.e., the central nervous system (McClymont and Setchell, 1956), lactose production (Kronfeld et al., 1963), and support of the fetus (Kronfeld, 1958). Gluconeogenesis, mainly from propionate (Leng et al., 1967), is essential for survival of the ruminant. The magnitude of the hepatic glucose formation is difficult to measure, but Bartley and Black (1966) and Ballard and his co-workers (1969) make the point that in the ruminant the glucose entry must approximate the rate of gluconeogenesis due to the paucity of glucose from the gut. Hence, the situation can be envisioned in the ruminant in which most of the available oxalacetic acid is channeled toward glucogenesis and very little toward lipogenesis. The enzymic profile of ruminant liver and the incorporation of specific carbons into fatty acids by ruminant liver verifies such a concept (Ballard et al., 1969).

The ruminant, then, is more dependent on gluconeogenesis than the monogastric animal and any factor altering the availability of oxalacetic acid has grave consequences. The availability of this organic acid could be decreased by increased demand, in the ruminant by gluconeogenesis, or decreased supply. Krebs (1966a,b) has suggested that ketosis is due to increased gluconeogenesis. In this situation the utilization of oxalacetic acid for glucose production by the liver is so extensive that there is not enough for oxidation of acetyl CoA in the tricarboxylic acid cycle. Recently, these same workers (Baird et al., 1968) tested this hypothesis in ruminants. They found no enzymic evidence that would indicate an increase in gluconeogenesis in the ketotic ruminant. Nonetheless, they did find a decrease in the tissue level of oxalacetic acid and its immediate metabolic derivatives in the liver of these same animals. We interpret these findings to mean that the rate of gluconeogenesis is at maximal, or almost, capacity, in the ruminant, particularly those in pregnancy or lactation. Any factor which reduces the availability of oxalacetic acid will precipitate hypoglyceia and ketonemia. Treatment of this syndrome, then, should be designed to replenish the tissue level of oxalacetic acid without altering the rate of gluconeogenesis. The glucogenic amino acids, glycerol and propionate, are examples of compounds fulfilling these requirements.

The ketone bodies derived from the inability of the liver to oxidize acetyl CoA at a rate commensurate with its formation can be utilized as a source of energy by other body tissues where the supply of oxalacetic acid is not siphoned off by glucogenesis (Williamson and Krebs, 1961). Indeed, in ruminant ketosis the utilization of ketone bodies equals or exceeds that in the normal animal up to certain limits (Bergman and Kon, 1964; Leng, 1965). As in nutritionally stressed monogastric animals, the major precursor of ketone bodies in the ruminant is FFA (Fig. 4), but the cleavage of butyrate, particularly in the ruminal epithelium, contributes a portion as it does in the normal ruminant.

4. Significance of Plasma FFA in the Ruminant

Kronfeld (1965) has concluded that the responses of plasma FFA in the cow resemble those in other species. Therefore, the plasma FFA level is a sensitive clinical index of fat mobilization (Section VI,C). Kronfeld (1965) minimized the value of the plasma FFA level as such an index in bovine ketosis because cases of uncomplicated ketosis did not invariably have elevated plasma FFA. His studies in spontaneous bovine ketosis verified those of Adler et al. (1963). In contrast, measurements in pregnant sheep have indicated that the level of FFA correlated well with the severity of ketonemia (Reid and Hinks, 1962; Bergman et al., 1968). While the discrepancy may appear to be due to species differences, the recent report by Radloff and Schultz (1967) indicates that in the early stages of bovine ketosis the FFA are markedly increased.

The absolute levels of FFA observed by various workers in normal and ketotic cows, regardless of cause, do not agree, but the degree of increase does (cf. Kronfeld, 1965; Adler et al., 1963). The differences in the absolute levels may be due to differences in the methods used to extract and determine the FFA content of plasma. Using the same method as Kronfeld (the Dole method as modified by Trout et al., 1960), we have found levels similar to those reported by him and concur that levels above 650 μEq/liter are an indication of unusually high mobilization of fatty acids, derived from the triglycerides of adipose tissue.

Russel and his associates have suggested the use of the plasma concentration of FFA instead of body weight changes as an index to estimate maintenance requirements (Russel et al., 1967; Doney and Russel, 1969; Russel and Doney, 1969). The rationale of such an index is that the food intake would be controlled so that the FFA of plasma are stabilized at a level indicating neither high mobilization nor storage of lipid. Their most recent paper (Russel and Doney, 1969) critically examined the use of FFA as a maintenance index. They conclude that the relationship exists, but as one might expect, it is not a simple one and breed differences exist between FFA levels reflecting an adequately maintained animal. The true potential of this approach will require more investigation. Eventual application of such an index might aid in the prevention of ovine pregnancy toxemia and bovine ketosis.

B. EQUINE LIPEMIA

Lipemia in the equine has been observed accompanying maxillary myositis (Hadlow, 1962) and equine infectious anemia (Gainer *et al.*, 1966). When several ponies admitted to the Veterinary Medicine Teaching Hospital at the University of California exhibited lipemia, the question arose: Is the lipemia directly related to a specific equine disease or a general response to a stressor, such as inanition? To test this possibility, we (Bartley *et al.*, 1969) fasted three ponies and three burros for up to 18 days. Later on, we extended the studies to include fasted horses as well. Mature, nonlactating goats were included in the study for comparative purposes. Three blood samples were taken prior to the fast to establish baseline values. Samples were taken daily thereafter. Ethylenediaminetetracetic acid was used as anticoagulant. The following measurements were made on the plasma of each sample: FFA (Trout *et al.*, 1960), total fatty acid, total cholesterol (see Section III,D), glucose (Worthington Biochemical Corp., glucose oxidase kit), lactate (Barker and Summerson, 1941), and total ketone bodies (J. B. Lyon and Bloom, 1958). Liver function was evaluated periodically in the equine species by the rate of dye (bromsulfophthalein) clearance from the plasma and the level of transaminases in the plasma (Cornelius, 1963). To measure total fatty acids, 1 volume of plasma was heated to 90° C for 90 minutes with an equal volume 1 N NaOH, after acidification, the fatty

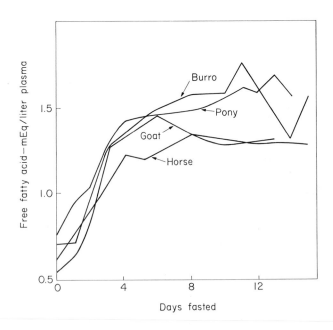

Fig. 7.   Concentration of FFA in the plasma during a prolonged fast.

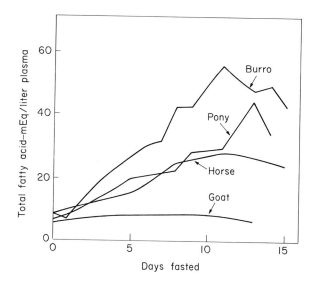

Fig. 8.   Concentration of total fatty acids in the plasma during a prolonged fast.

acids were extracted and titrated as in the FFA procedure. The total fatty acids, therefore, include FFA plus those fatty acids esterified, i.e., glycerides, phospholipids, and cholesterol esters. The other methods used are indicated by the references behind each measurement.

No consistent changes were observed in the concentration of plasma lactate or ketone bodies. The change in the plasma concentration of FFA is shown in Fig. 7. Similar increases during the fast were observed in all the species examined. The concentration increased 2- to 2.5-fold in 4 to 5 days and remained essentially at that level until placed on feed. As expected, the changes in the concentration of plasma glucose was reciprocal to that of FFA.

The most dramatic change observed was in the total concentration of fatty acids in the plasma (Fig. 8). In all the equine species, the concentration had doubled by the second day of the fast and continued to increase for at least 10 more days. The final level was three to five times that in the fed equine. In sharp contrast to the response in the equine, no discernible change was observed during the fast in the total circulating fatty acids in the goat. The total cholesterol levels followed the changes in total fatty acid concentration, but the degree of change in the equine was far less marked.

A difference was noted in the plasma from the burros and the ponies as compared to that from the horses: from the fourth day of the fast forward the plasma of the former species were visibly lipemic, whereas the plasma of the horse exhibited only slight turbidity late in the fast.

To further characterize this increase in total fatty acids and cholesterol, lipid in plasma samples was separated on thin layers of silica gel in the following solvent mixture: 85 volumes petroleum ether; 15 volumes diethyl ether and 1.5 volumes acetic acid. Lipid areas were revealed by placing the chromatogram in an atmosphere of I_2. An example of a typical chromatogram is shown in Fig. 9. Note that as the fast progressed, smaller volumes of plasma extract were applied to the plate.

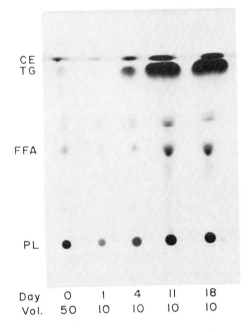

Fig. 9.   Separation by means of TLC of plasma lipid of a horse during a prolonged fast. The day refers to the day of the fast when the plasma sample was collected. The quantity of plasma lipid extract applied to the TLC plate is given as the volume in μl of plasma originally containing that lipid. CE = cholesterol ester, TG = triglyceride, FFA = free fatty acid, PL = phospholipid, which remains at the point of application. Unesterified cholesterol migrates between PL and FFA.

As the fast progressed, the glyceride areas showed the most marked increase in the equine plasma. The triglycerides of the goat showed no change on the basis of this qualitative examination. Note that, of the cholesterol present, it is clear that the majority is in the esterified form.

We have attempted to more accurately quantitate the increase in glycerides during the fast. Because most of the cholesterol was in the esterified form, we converted the total cholesterol value to microequivalents per liter of fatty acid using the assumption that the average molecular weight of the major esterified fatty acid was 300. For comparative purposes, the error in this assumption is not dangerous. This calculated value for fatty acids esterified to cholesterol and the value determined for FFA were then subtracted from the value for the total fatty acids. The net value would represent fatty acids that had been esterified as phospholipids and, mainly, glycerides. Each of these three values are plotted as histograms (Fig. 10). It is clear from the histograms and the TLC that the major lipid component is glyceride and that the major change takes place in this fraction.

A plasma particle consisting mainly of triglyceride is consistent with the pre-β particle or VLDL of other species (Section VI,B). However, electrophoretic separation of the plasma proteins on cellulose acetate followed by staining of the lipoproteins with Schiff's reagent after ozonization revealed bands moving more like the α-band of other species. Hort (1968) reported the main lipoprotein of normal

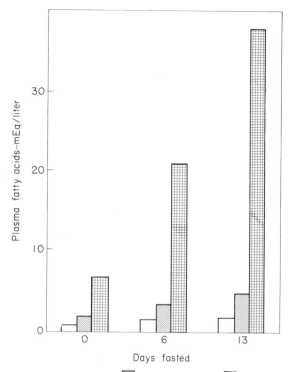

Fig. 10.   Change in concentration of FFA ☐, total cholesterol ▣, and fatty acids ▦ esterified to compounds other than cholesterol during a prolonged fast in an equine.

equines to move with the α-band on electrophoresis. Preliminary ultracentrifugal studies indicated that the lipoprotein fraction involved in the fasting lipemia is probably VLDL. More sophisticated studies by Lindgren's procedure (1967) are being planned. Until the exact identity of the lipoprotein fraction involved in this lipemia is known, we can only speculate as to the difference, if any, between the response of the ponies and the horses. A slight difference in apoproteins may exist between the equine species affecting the solubility of the lipid or there may be some chylomicron formation by the intestine of the burros and ponies as is suggested in some endogenous lipemias of humans.

How do we interpret this dramatic response to fasting in the equine? The equine probably mobilizes stored lipid in the form of FFA which are cleared in the liver as in other species (Section VI,C; Fig. 4). We suggest that the equine differs from other species thus far investigated in its ability to form VLDL. If this is the case, the equine has the ability to release large portions of mobilized lipid back into the plasma for utilization by other tissues rather than accumulating triglycerides in the liver when the capacity for handling the incoming FFA has been exceeded. Of course, some FFA would be handled as in other species: degraded to ketone bodies or oxidized completely. One would also expect some glyceride to accumulate in the liver. In times of stress, however, we predict that the equine has a greater propensity for a "fatty" plasma than for a fatty liver.

Regardless of the interpretation, the immediate, clinical significance of our observations is that the total plasma lipid concentration in the equine can be used as an index of fat mobilization as FFA are used in other species (Sections VI,A and IX,A). Hence, the plasma concentration of total lipids could be a valuable tool in gauging the metabolic response to disease and its treatment in the equine.

REFERENCES

Abraham, S., Matthes, K. J., and Chaikoff, I. L. (1961). *Biochim. Biophys. Acta* **49**, 268.

Adler, J. H., Wertheimer, E., Batana, U., and Flesh, J. (1963). *Vet. Record* **75**, 304.

Ailhaud, G., Sarda, L., and Desnuelle, P. (1962). *Biochim. Biophys. Acta* **59**, 261.

Allmann, D. W., and Gibson, D. M. (1965a). *J. Lipid Res.* **6**, 51.

Allmann, D. W., Hubbard, D. D., and Gibson, D. M. (1965b). *J. Lipid Res.* **6**, 63.

Anand, R. (1967). Ph.D. Thesis, University of California, Davis, California.

Annegers, J. H. (1954). *A. M. A. Arch. Internal Med.* **93**, 9.

Annison, E. F. (1960). *Australian J. Agr. Res.* **11**, 58.

Annison, E. F., Hill, K. J., and Lewis, D. (1957). *Biochem. J.* **66**, 592.

Annison, E. F., Leng, R. A., Lindsay, D. B., and White, R. R. (1963). *Biochem. J.* **88**, 248.

Annison, E. F., Linzell, J. L., Fazakerley, S., and Nichols, B. W. (1967). *Biochem. J.* **102**, 637.

Baird, C. D., Hibbitt, K. G., Hunter, G. D., Lund, P., Stubbs, M., and Krebs, H. A. (1968). *Biochem. J.* **106**, 683.

Baker, N., and Schotz, M. C. (1964). *J. Lipid Res.* **5**, 188.

Ballard, F. J., Hanson, R. W., and Kronfeld, D. S. (1969). *Federation Proc.* **28**, 218.

Barker, S. B., and Summerson, W. H. (1941). *J. Biol. Chem.* **138**, 535.

Barry, J. M. (1966). *Outlook Agr.* **5**, 129.

Barry, J. M., Bartley, W., Linzell, J. L,, and Robinson, D. S. (1963). *Biochem. J.* **89**, 6.

Bartley, J. C. (1969). Unpublished observations.

Bartley, J. C., and Black, A. L. (1966). *J. Nutr.* **89**, 317.

Bartley, J. C., Abraham, S., and Chaikoff, I. L. (1965). *Biochim. Biophys. Res. Commun.* **19**, 770.

Bartley, J. C., Abraham, S., and Chaikoff, I. L. (1967). *Biochim. Biophys. Acta* **144**, 51.

Bartley, J. C., Yelland, R. and Hill, H. (1969). Unpublished observations.

Bassen, F. A., and Kornzweig, A. L. (1950). *Blood* **5**, 831.

Baum, D., Schweid, A. I., Parde, D., and Bierman, E. L. (1969). *Proc. Soc. Exptl. Biol. Med.* **131**, 183.

Belfrage, P., Elovson, J., and Olivecrona, T. (1965). *Biochim. Biophys. Acta* **106**, 45.

Benzonana, G., and Desnuelle, P. (1965). *Biochim. Biophys. Acta* **106**, 121.

Bergman, E. N., and Kon, K. (1964). *Am. J. Physiol.* **206**, 449.

Bergman, E. N., Starr, D. J., and Reulein, S. S. (1968). *Am. J. Physiol.* **215**, 874.

Bergström, S., and Bergström, B. (1955). *Progr. Chem. Fats Lipids* **3**, 351.

Bergström, S., and Samuelson, B. (1965). *Ann. Rev. Biochem.* **34**, 101.

Biale, Y., Gorin, E., and Shafrir, E. (1965). *Israel J. Chem.* **3**, 112.

Bines, J. A., and Brown, R. E. (1968). *J. Dairy Sci.* **51**, 698.

Bloch, K. (1965). *Science* **150**, 19.

Bortz, W. M. (1967). *Biochim. Biophys. Acta* **135**, 533.

Bortz, W. M., and Lynen, F. (1963). *Biochem. Z.* **337**, 505.

Brady, R. V., and Koval, G. J. (1958). *J. Biol. Chem.* **233**, 26.

Bressler, R., and Brendel, K. (1966). *J. Biol. Chem.* **241**, 4092.

Bressler, R., and Katz, I. B. (1965). *J. Biol. Chem.* **240**, 622.

Brindley, D. N., and Hübscher, G. (1966). *Biochim. Biophys. Acta* **125**, 92.

Brodie, J. D., Wasson, G., and Porter, J. W. (1963). *J. Biol. Chem.* **238**, 1294.

Bucher, N. L. R., McGarrahan, K., Gould, K., and Loud, A. V. (1959). *J. Biol. Chem.* **234**, 262.

Burton, D., Haavik, A. G., and Porter, J. W. (1968). *Arch. Biochem. Biophys.* **126**, 141.

Butcher, R. W., Sneyd, J. G. T., Park, C. R., and Sutherland, E. (1966). *J. Biol. Chem.* **241**, 1651.

Cahill, G. F. (1964). *In* "Fat as a Tissue" (K. Rodahl and B. Issekutz, eds.), pp. 169–183. McGraw-Hill, New York.

Chevreul, M. E. (1823). "Recherches chimique sur le corps gras d'origine animale." Levrant, Paris (cited by Lawrie, 1928, p. 17).

Clark, B., and Hübscher, G. (1961). *Biochim. Biophys. Acta* **46**, 479.

Clements, J. A. (1969). Personal communication.

Coleman, R., and Hübscher, G. (1962). *Biochim. Biophys. Acta* **56**, 479.

Conn, E. F., and Stumpf, P. K. (1966). "Outlines of Biochemistry," 2nd ed., p. 280. Wiley, New York.

Cornelius, C. E. (1963). *In* "Clinical Biochemistry of Domestic Animals" (C. E. Cornelius and J. J. Kaneko, eds.), pp. 225–301. Academic Press, New York.

Correll, J. W. (1963). *Science* **140**, 387.

Crass, M. F., and Meng, H. C. (1966). *Biochim. Biophys. Acta* **125**, 106.

David, J. S. K., Malathi, P., and Ganguly, J. (1966). *Biochem. J.* **98**, 662.

Dawson, A. M. (1967). *Brit. Med. Bull.* **23**, 247.

Delcher, H. K., Friend, M., and Shipp, T. C. (1965). *Biochim. Biophys. Acta* **106**, 10.

Desnuelle, P. (1961). *Advan. Enzymol.* **23**, 129.

Desnuelle, P., and Savary, P. (1963). *J. Lipid Res.* **4**, 369.

Deuel, H. J. (1951). "The Lipids," Vol. 1, pp. 2–3, 59–66, 148–155, and 205. Wiley (Interscience), New York.

Deuel, H. J. (1955). "The Lipids," Vol. 2, pp. 5–6, and 144–157. Wiley (Interscience), New York.

Dole, V. P. (1956). *J. Clin. Invest.* **35**, 150.

Doney, J. M., and Russel, A. J. F. (1969). *J. Agr. Sci.* **71**, 343.

Evans, L. (1964). *J. Dairy Sci.* **47**, 46.

Evans, L., Patton, S., and McCarthy, R. D. (1961). *J. Dairy Sci.* **44**, 475.

Ewing, A. M., Freeman, N. K., and Lindgren, F. T. (1965). *Advan. Lipid Res.* **3**, 25.

Fain, J. N. (1968). *Endocrinology* **82**, 825.

Fain, J. N., Kovacev, V. P., and Scow, R. O. (1966). *Endocrinology* **78**, 773.

Farber, E., Shull, K. H., Villa-Trevino, S., Lombardi, B., and Thomas, M. (1964). *Nature* **203**, 34.

Favarger, P. (1965). *In* "Handbook of Physiology" Am. Physiological Soc. (J. Field, ed.), Sect. 5, pp. 19–23. Williams & Wilkins, Baltimore, Maryland.

Fisher, W., and Gurin, S. (1964). *Science* **143**, 362.

Folley, S. J., and McNaught, M. L. (1961). *In* "Milk: The Mammary Gland and Its Secretion" (S. K. Kon and A. T. Cowie, eds.), Vol. 1, p. 441. Academic Press, New York.

Frazer, A. C. (1938). *Analyst* **63**, 308.

Frazer, A. C. (1946). *Physiol. Rev.* **26**, 103.

Frazer, A. C. (1952). *Biochem. Soc. Symp.* (*Cambridge, Engl.*) **9**, 5–13.

Fredrickson, D. S. (1966). *In* "The Metabolic Basis of Inherited Disease" (J. B. Stanbury, J. B. Wyngaarden, and D. S. Fredrickson, eds.), 2nd ed., p. 486. McGraw-Hill, New York.

Fredrickson, D. S. (1969). *Trans. Assoc. Am. Phys.* **82**, in press.

Fredrickson, D. S., and Gordon, R. S. (1958). *J. Clin. Invest.* **37**, 1504.

Fredrickson, D. S., Levy, R. I., and Lees, R. S. (1967). *New Engl. J. Med.* **276**, 32, 94, 148, 215, and 273.

Fredrickson, D. S., Levy, R. I., and Lindgren, F. T. (1968). *J. Clin. Invest.* **47**, 2446.

Freeman, C. P., Noakes, D. E., Annison, E. F., and Hill, K. J. (1968). *Brit. J. Nutr.* **22**, 739.

Freidman, M., Van Den Bosch, J., Byers, S. O., and St. George, S. (1965). *Am. J. Physiol.* **208**, 94.

Fritz, I. B. (1968). *In* "Cellular Compartmentalization and Control of Fatty Acid Metabolism" (F. C. Gran, ed.), pp. 39–63. Academic Press, New York.

Fritz, I. B., and Hsu, M. P. (1967). *J. Biol. Chem.* **242**, 865.

Fritz, I. B., and Yue, K. T. N. (1963). *J. Lipid Res.* **4**, 279.

Gainer, J. H., Amster, R. L., Needham, J. W., and Schilling, K. F. (1966). *Am. J. Vet. Res.* **27**, 1611.

Gallagher, N., Webb, J., and Dawson, A. M. (1965). *Clin. Sci.* **29**, 73.

Garton, G. A. (1960). *Nutr. Abstr. Rev.* **30**, 1.

Glascock, R. F., Duncombe, W. G., and Reinius, L. R. (1956). *Biochem. J.* **62**, 535.

Glascock, R. F., Welch, V. A., Bishop, C., Davies, T., Wright, E. W., and Noble, R. C. (1966). *Biochem. J.* **98**, 149.

Glomset, J. (1968). *J. Lipid Res.* **9**, 155.

Goodman, D. S. (1958). *J. Am. Chem. Soc.* **80**, 3892.

Goodman, D. S., Deykin, D., and Shiratori, T. (1964). *J. Biol. Chem.* **239**, 1335.

Gousios, A., Felts, J. M., and Havel, R. J. (1963). *Metab., Clin. Exptl.* **12**, 75.

Graham, W. R., Jones, T. S. J., and Kay, H. D. (1936). *Proc. Roy. Soc.* **B120**, 330.

Green, C., and Webb, J. A. (1964). *Biochim. Biophys. Acta* **84**, 404.

Greeberger, N. J., Rodgers, J. B., and Isselbacher, K. J. (1966). *J. Clin. Invest.* **45**, 217.

Greenspan, M., and Lowenstein, J. M. (1967). *Arch. Biochem. Biophys.* **118**, 260.

Hadlow, W. J. (1962). *In* "Comparative Neuropathology" (J. R. M. Innes and L. Z. Saunders, eds.), p. 184. Academic Press, New York.

Hallberg, D. (1967). *U.S., Public Health Serv., Publ.* **1742**, 194–200.

Hanahan, D. J. (1954). *J. Biol. Chem.* **211**, 313.

Hansen, I. A. (1965a). *Comp. Biochem. Physiol.* **15**, 27.

Hansen, I. A. (1965b). *Arch. Biochem. Biophys.* **109**, 98.

Hansen, I. A. (1965c). *Arch. Biochem. Biophys.* **111**, 238.

Hanson, R. W., and Ballard, F. J. (1967). *Biochem. J.* **105**, 529.

Hanson, R. W., and Ballard, F. J. (1968). *Biochem. J.* **108**, 705.

Hardwick, D. C. (1966). *Biochem. J.* **99**, 228.

Hashim, S. A., Bergen, S. S., Krell, K., and Van Itallie, T. B. (1964). *J. Clin. Invest.* **43**, 1238.

Hashim, S. A., Krell, K., Mao, P., and Van Itallie, T. B. (1965). *Nature* **207**, 527.

Hatch, F. T., and Lees, R. S. (1968). *Advan. Lipid Res.* **6**, 1–68.

Hatch, F. T., Hagopian, L. M., Rubinstein, J. J., and Canellos, G. P. (1963). *Circulation* **28**, 659.

Hausberger, F. X. and Milstein, S. W. (1955). *J. Biol. Chem.* **215**, 483.

Havel, R. (1965). *In* "Handbook of Physiology" Am. Physiol. Soc. (J. Field, ed.), Sect. 5. pp. 575–582. Williams & Wilkens, Baltimore, Maryland.

Higgins, J. A., and Green, C. (1966). *Biochem. J.* **99**, 631.

Hill, R., Linzasoro, J. M., Chevallier, F., and Chaikoff, I. L. (1958). *J. Biol. Chem.* **233**. 305.

Hill, R. B., and Droke, W. A. (1963). *Proc. Soc. Exptl. Biol. Med.* **114**, 766.

Hillyard, L. A., Entenman, C., Feinberg, H., and Chaikoff, I. L. (1955). *J. Biol. Chem.* **214**, 79.

Hoerr, C. W., and Ralston, A. W. (1944). *J. Org. Chem.* **9**, 329.

Hoerr, C. W., Sedgwick, R. S., and Ralston, A. W. (1946). *J. Org. Chem.* **11**, 603.

Hofmann, A. F., and Borgström, B. (1962). *Federation Proc.* **21**, 43.

Hofmann, A. F., and Borgström, B. (1964). *J. Clin. Invest.* **43**, 247.

Hort, I. (1968). *Am. J. Vet. Res.* **29**, 813.

Hsu, R. Y., Wasson, G., and Porter, J. W. (1964). *J. Biol. Chem.* **240**, 3736.

Isselbacher, K. J. (1967). *U.S., Public Health Serv., Publ.*, **1742**, 30–38.

Isselbacher, K. J., and Budz, D. H. (1963). *Nature* **200**, 364.

Isselbacher, K. J., and Greenberger, N. J. (1964). *New Engl. J. Med.* **270**, 351.

Johnston, J. M. (1963). *Advan. Lipid Res.* **1**, 105.

Johnston, J. M., and Borgström, B. (1964). *Biochim. Biophys. Acta* **84**, 812.

Jones, D. P., Perman, E. S., and Lieber, C. S. (1965). *J. Lab. Clin. Med.* **66**, 804.

Kennedy, E. P. (1961). *Federation Proc.* **20**, 934.

Kirschner, S., and Harris, R. (1961). *J. Nutr.* **73**, 397.

Kiyasu, J. Y., Bloom, B., and Chaikoff, I. L. (1952). *J. Biol. Chem.* **199**, 415.

Kleiber, M., Smith, A. H., Black, A. L. Brown, M. A., and Tolbert, B. M. (1952). *J. Biol. Chem.* **197**, 371.

Kornacker, M. S., and Lowenstein, J. M. (1965). *Biochem. J.* **94**, 209.

Kovacev, V. P., and Scow, R. O. (1966). *Am. J. Physiol.* **210**, 1199.

Krebs, H. A. (1964). *Proc. Roy. Soc.* **B159**, 545.

Krebs, H. A. (1966a). *Vet. Record* **78**, 187.

Krebs, H. A. (1966b). *Advan. Enzyme Regulation* **4**, 339.

Kritchevsky, D. (1963). *In* "Comprehensive Biochemistry" (M. Florkin and E. H. Stotz, eds.), Vol. 10, Part 2, pp. 1–22. Elsevier, Amsterdam.

Kronfeld, D. S. (1958). *Cornell Vet.* **48**, 394.

Kronfeld, D. S. (1965). *Vet. Record* **77**, 30.

Kronfeld, D. S., Mayer, G. P., Robertson, J. M., and Raggi, F. (1963). *J. Dairy Sci.* **46**, 559.

Kuhn, R., and Egge, H. (1960). *Angew. Chem.* **72**, 805.

Kupiecki, F. P. (1966). *J. Lipid Res.* **7**, 230.

Lascelles, A. K., Hardwick, D. C., Linzell, J. L., and Mephan, T. B. (1964). *Biochem. J.* **92**, 36.

Lauryssens, M., Verbeke, R., and Peeters, G. (1961). *J. Lipid Res.* **2**, 383.

Lawrie, J. W. (1928), "Glycerol and the Glycols." Reinhold, New York.

Leat, W. M. F., and Cunningham, H. M. (1968). *Biochem. J.* **109**, 38.

Leat, W. M. F., and Hall, J. G. (1968). *J. Agr. Sci.* **71**, 189.

Leat, W. M. F., and Harrison, F. A. (1967). *Biochem. J.* **105**, 13.

Leng, R. A. (1965). *Res. Vet. Sci.* **6**, 433.

Leng, R. A., Steele, J. W., and Luick, J. R. (1967). *Biochem. J.* **103**, 785.

Leveille, G. A., and Hanson, R. W. (1966). *J. Lipid Res.* **7**, 46.

Levy, R. I., Lees, R. S., and Fredrickson, D. S. (1966). *J. Clin. Invest.* **45**, 531.

Lindgren, F. T., Freeman, N. K., and Ewing, E. M. (1967). *Progr. Biochem. Pharmacol.* **2**, 475.

Lintzel, W. (1934). *Lait* **14**, 1125.

Linzell, J. L., Annison, E. F., Fazakerley, S., and Leng, R. A. (1967). *Biochem. J.* **104**, 34.

Lombardi, B. (1966). "Biochemical Pathology," pp. 1–20. Williams & Wilkens, Baltimore, Maryland.

Lombardi, B., and Ugazio, G. (1965). *J. Lipid Res.* **6**, 498.

Lynen, F., Oesterhelt, D., Schweizer, E., and Willecke, K. (1968). *In* "Cellular Compartmentalization and Control of Fatty Acid Metabolism" (F. C. Gran, ed.), pp. 1–24. Academic Press, New York.

Lyon, I., Masri, M. S., and Chaikoff, I. L. (1952). *J. Biol. Chem.* **196**, 25.

Lyon, J. B., and Bloom, W. L. (1958). *Can. J. Biochem. Physiol.* **36**, 1047.

McClymont, G. L., and Setchell, B. P. (1956). *Australian J. Biol. Sci.* **9**, 184.

McClymont, G. L. and Vallance, S. (1962). *Proc. Nutr. Soc. (Engl. Scot.)* **21**, 41.

Majerus, P. W. (1967). *J. Biol. Chem.* **242**, 2325.

Margolis, S., and Langdon, R. G. (1966). *J. Biol. Chem.* **241**, 469.

Markley, K. S. (1947). "Fatty Acids: Their Chemistry and Physical Properties," p. 177. Wiley (Interscience), New York.

Marsh, J. B., and Whereat, A. F. (1959). *J. Biol. Chem.* **234**, 3196.

Masoro, E. J. (1962). *J. Lipid Res.* **3**, 149.

Masoro, E. J. (1968). "Physiological Chemistry of Lipids in Mammals." Saunders, Philadelphia, Pennsylvania.

Mattson, F. H., Volpenheim, R. A., and Lutton, E. S. (1964). *J. Lipid Res.* **5**, 363.

Mattson, F. H., and Volpenheim, R. A. (1963). *J. Lipid Res.* **4**, 392.

Meng, H. C., ed. (1964) "Lipid Transport." Thomas, Springfield, Illinois.

Noble, R. P., Hatch, F. T., Mazrimas, J. A., Lindgren, F. T., Jensen, L. C., and Adamson, G. L. (1969). *Lipids* **4**, 55.

Norum, K. R., and Bremer, J. (1967). *J. Biol. Chem.* **242**, 407.

Norum, K. R., and Gjone, E. (1967). *Scand. J. Clin. & Lab. Invest.* **20**, 231.

O'Hea, K. E., and Leveille, G. A. (1968). *Comp. Biochem. Physiol.* **26**, 111.

Opstvedt, J., Baldwin, R. L., and Ronning, M. (1967). *J. Dairy Sci.* **50**, 18.

Palay, S. L., and Karlin, L. J. (1959). *J. Biophys. Biochem. Cytol.* **5** 373.

Phillips, R. W., and Black, A. L. (1965). *Comp. Biochem. Physiol.* **18**, 527.

Phillips, R. W., Black, A. L., and Moeller, F. (1965). *Life Sci.* **4**, 521.

Pope, J. L., McPherson, J. C., and Tidwell, N. C. (1966). *J. Biol. Chem.* **241**, 2306.

Porter, J. W., and Long, R. W. (1958). *J. Biol. Chem.* **233**, 20.

Pugh, E. L., and Wakil, S. J. (1965). *J. Biol. Chem.* **240**, 4727.

Puppione, D. L. (1969). Ph.D. Thesis, University of California, Berkeley, California.

Raben, M. S. (1965). *In* "Handbook of Physiology" Am. Physiological Soc. (J. Field, ed.), Sect. 5, pp. 331–334. Williams & Wilkens, Baltimore, Maryland.

Radloff, H. D., and Schultz, L. H. (1967). *J. Dairy Sci.* **50**, 68.

Ralston, A. W., and Hoerr, C. W. (1942). *J. Org. Chem.* **7**, 546.

Radding, C. M., Bragdon, J. M., and Steinberg, D. (1958). *Biochim. Biophys. Acta* **30**, 443.

Reid, R. L., and Hinks, N. T. (1962). *Australian J. Agr. Res.* **13**, 1112.

Rice, E. W., and Lukasiewicz, D. B. (1957). *Clin. Chem.* **3**, 160.

Riis, P. H. (1964). Ph.D. Thesis, Royal Veterinary and Agricultural College, Copenhagen, Denmark.

Rizach, M. A. (1965). *In* "Handbook of Physiology" (Am. Physiol. Soc., J. Field, ed.), Sect. 5, pp. 309–311. Williams & Wilkens, Baltimore, Maryland.

Robinson, D. S. (1963). *Advan. Lipid Res.* **1**, 133.

Robinson, D. S. (1964). *In* "Lipid Transport" (H. C. Meng, ed.), pp. 194–201. Thomas, Springfield, Illinois.

Roepke, R. R., and Mason, H. L. (1940). *J. Biol. Chem.* **133**, 103.

Rudman, D., DiGirolamo, M., Malkin, M. F., and Garcia, L. A. (1965). *In* "Handbook of Physiology"

Am. Physiol. Soc. (J. Field, ed.), Sect. 5. pp. 535–540. Williams & Wilkens, Baltimore, Maryland.

Rudney, H. (1957). *J. Biol. Chem.* **227**, 363.

Russel, A. J. F., and Doney, J. M. (1969). *J. Agr. Sci.* **72**, 59.

Russel, A. J. F., Doney, J. M., and Reid, R. L. (1967). *J. Agr. Sci.* **68**, 351.

Salem, L. (1962). *Can. J. Biochem.* **40**, 1287.

Salt, H. B. (1960). *Lancet,* **II**, 325.

Scanu, A. (1966). *J. Lipid Res.* **7**, 295.

Schotz, M. C., and Garfinkel, A. S. (1965). *Biochim. Biophys. Acta* **106**, 202.

Senior, J. R. (1964). *J. Lipid Res.* **5**, 495.

Senior, J. R., and Isselbacher, K. J. (1963). *J. Clin. Invest.* **42**, 187.

Shapiro, B. (1965). *In* "Handbook of Physiology" Am. Physiol. Soc. (J. Field, ed.), Sect. 5, pp. 217–223. Williams & Wilkens, Baltimore, Maryland.

Shapiro, B. (1967). *Ann. Rev. Biochem.* **36**, 247–270.

Shoppee, C. W. (1958). "Chemistry of the Steroids." Academic Press, New York and Butterworths, London and Washington, D. C.

Shore, V., and Shore, B. (1962). *Biochem. Biophys. Res. Commun.* **9**, 445.

Simoni, R. D., Criddle, R. S., and Stumpf, P. C. (1967). *J. Biol. Chem.* **242**, 573.

Simpson-Morgan, M. W. (1967). *U.S., Public Health Serv. Publ.* **1742**, 200–205.

Simpson-Morgan, M. W. (1968). *J. Physiol. (London)* **199**, 37.

Siperstein, M. D., and Fagan, V. M. (1964). *Advan. Enzyme Regulation* **2**, 249.

Siperstein, M. D., and Guest, M. J. (1959). *J. Clin. Invest.* **38**, 1043.

Smith, S. (1965). Ph.D. Thesis, University of Birmingham, England.

Smith, S., and Abraham, S. (1969). *Federation Proc.* **28**, 537.

Smith, S., and Dils, R. (1966). *Biochim. Biophys. Acta* **116**, 23.

Smuckler, F. A., and Benditt, E. P. (1965). *Biochemistry* **4**, 671.

Srere, P. A. (1965). *Nature* **205**, 766.

Stanbury, J. B., Wyngaarden, J. B., and Fredrickson, D. S., eds. (1966). "The Metabolic Basis of Inherited Disease," 2nd ed., pp. 429–632. McGraw-Hill, New York.

Steinberg, D., and Vaughan, M. (1965). *In* "Handbook of Physiology" Am. Physiol. Soc. (J. Field, ed.), Sect. 5, pp. 335–347. Williams & Wilkens, Baltimore, Maryland.

Storry, J. E., and Rook, J. A. F. (1964). *Biochem. J.* **91**, 270.

Storry, J. E., and Rook, J. A. F. (1965). *Brit. J. Nutr.* **19**, 101.

Storry, J. E., Tuckley, B., and Hall, H. J. (1969). *Brit. J. Nutr.* **23**, 157.

Strauss, E. W. (1966). *J. Lipid Res.* **7**, 307.

Sunderman, F. W., and Sunderman, F. W., Jr. (1960). "Lipids and the Steroid Hormones in Clinical Medicine." Lippincott, Philadelphia, Pennsylvania.

Sutherland, E. W. (1961). *Harvey Lectures* **57**, 17.

Trout, D. L., Estes, E. H., and Freidberg, S. J. (1960). *J. Lipid Res.* **1**, 199.

Utter, M. F., and Keech, D. B. (1963). *J. Biol. Chem.* **238**, 2603.

Vagelos, P. R., Majerus, P. W., Alberts, A. W., Larrabee, A. R., and Ailhaud, G. P. (1966). *Federation Proc.* **25**, 1485.

Vagelos, P. R. (1964). *Ann. Rev. Biochem.* **33**, 139.

Vallance, S., and McClymont, G. L. (1959). *Nature* **183**, 466.

Varman, P. N., and Schulz, L. H. (1968). *J. Dairy Sci.* **51**, 1597.

Vaughan, M., and Steinberg, D. (1963). *J. Lipid Res.* **4**, 193.

Venkataraman, S., and Sreenivasan, A. (1965). *Indian J. Biochem.* **2**, 163.

Ward, P. F. V., Scott, T. W., and Dawson, R. M. C. (1964). *Biochem. J.* **92**, 60.

West, C. E., Annison, E. F., and Linzell, J. L. (1967). *Biochem. J.* **102**, 23.

Williamson, J. R., and Krebs, H. A. (1961). *Biochem. J.* **80**, 540.

Wilson, J. D., and Lindsey, C. A. (1965). *J. Clin. Invest.* **44**, 1805.

Windmueller, H. G., and Levy, R. I. (1967). *J. Biol. Chem.* **242**, 2246.

Windmueller, H. G., and Levy, R. I. (1968). *J. Biol. Chem.* **243**, 4878.

Winegrad, A. T., Goto, Y., and Lukens, F. D. W. (1964). *In* "Fat as a Tissue" (K. Rodahl and B. Issekuts, eds.), pp. 344–361. McGraw-Hill, New York.

Zak, B., Dickenman, R. C., White, E. G., Burnett, H., and Cherny, P. J. (1954). *Am. J. Clin. Pathol* **24**, 1307.

Zilversmit, D. B., and Diluzio, N. R. (1958). *Am. J. Clin. Nutr.* **6**, 235.

3 Plasma Proteins

George T. Dimopoullos

I. INTRODUCTION

Many of the historical developments in the metabolism, properties, and functions, of plasma proteins were covered in the first edition of this volume. Considerable data were also presented on the factors affecting their composition under a variety of conditions.

As before, the proportion of studies dealing with the plasma proteins of domestic animals to that of other species has not appeared to increase. However, there have been additional reports in this area. In any case it will again be necessary to draw on data involving the plasma proteins of other species. Appropriately, the classical designations of these substances will be used (albumin, α-, β-, and γ-globulins).

II. DIAGNOSTIC USES

Many clinical laboratories have attempted to use the changes observed in the qualitative and quantitative composition of the plasma proteins for specific diagnosis of disease. The alterations that have been observed have only served to demonstrate the state of the subject under study at that particular time. The fallacy in employing these changes as diagnostic aids is that many diseases and physiological aberrations produce similar changes in the plasma protein profile and, therefore, cannot be considered specific for any one abnormal condition. However, abrupt and major differences in any of the components can be useful insofar as to show that a pathological process is taking place. More gainful information can also be gathered when serial samples are analyzed.

The abnormalities which are observed are often compared to values which are accepted as being normal. There are many so-called normal values for the plasma proteins of different species. Differences in sex and age make the comparisons even more difficult along with the degree of abnormality, physiological state, dietary intake, and analytical procedure employed.

It is necessary that a clinical laboratory establish values which are accepted as normal for each species of animal being investigated since it is a rare occasion to find a completely normal subject. Many differences appear in the plasma proteins of healthy subjects who, for all practical purposes, are normal. The determination of normal values should be made from an accumulation of data from a significant number of apparently healthy animals which are maintained under similar conditions. It is also important that the same technique be employed throughout, and preferably the same individual should be responsible for the analyses.

Subjects who are apparently healthy and do not have their external or internal environment drastically changed can be expected to show a plasma protein profile and a total protein concentration which is relatively constant; once this balance is upset a change occurs. The total protein concentration represents the balance between biosynthesis and catabolism or mechanical loss.

The abnormalities that are observed in the plasma proteins can be grouped into a number of patterns which characterize an entire group of pathological states. These conditions are acute inflammation, chronic inflammatory and proliferative processes, liver and biliary disorders, nephrotic syndromes and carcinomas (Petermann, 1960). Within each of these disorders various degrees of severity can occur. This would only reflect the state of the subject under study and would not be indicative of a specific disease but of a condition which alters the plasma proteins because tissues responsible for their synthesis and catabolism have been affected.

Generally, the most striking change in disease is observable as a decrease in the albumin fraction. The decrease may be the result of an inhibition in the synthesis or more rapid catabolism or it may be due to an increase in the concentration of globulins. α-Globulins usually increase in concentration in such conditions as trauma, fever, infection, and a number of physiological disturbances. Changes in β-globulins indicate an abnormality in lipoprotein metabolism, but usually the factors responsible for these changes are difficult to evaluate unless the history of the subject is adequately known. Increases in the concentrations of the β-globulins are usually observed in hepatic diseases.

A change in the γ-globulins reflects the response of the reticuloendothelial system to antigens and there appears to be a correlation between concentrations of γ-globulins and antibody titers in most infections with perhaps the exception of those of viral etiology (Dimopoullos, 1961a; Petermann, 1961).

III. PLASMA PROTEINS IN INFECTIOUS DISEASES AND IMMUNOLOGICAL PHENOMENA

A. BACTERIAL INFECTIONS

The magnitude of change that occurs in the plasma proteins during infectious disease appears to depend greatly on its severity and the inherent response of the host. This was shown by Jacox and Feldmahn (1956) in experimental infections of pneumococcus in rabbits. When the infections were treated with penicillin the plasma protein profile was not as severely changed as that of untreated animals. In rabbits immunized with a killed pneumococcal vaccine a sevenfold increase occurred in the globulin concentration, whereas a decrease in the concentration of albumin was thought to be secondary and was dependent on a regulatory mechanism which functioned to keep colloid osmotic pressure within limits (Bjorneboe, 1944).

The effects of tuberculosis in mammals have been reported quite extensively. Generally, there is a decrease in the albumin/globulin ratio (A/G) which is a result of a decrease in the concentration of albumin and an increase in the globulin fractions. Seibert and Nelson (1942) and Seibert et al. (1947) observed that the increase in the concentration of α_2-globulin early in the course of the disease may have been due to destruction of tissue. However, this also occurred in advanced cases of the disease. A component with a higher electrophoretic mobility than albumin also appeared early and it was thought to show evidence of sensitization of the host to tubercular protein. It was further speculated that the increase in the concentration of γ-globulin was due to antibody formation. During the terminal stages, the concentration of the β-globulin fraction increased (Seibert and Nelson, 1942).

The above data have been further substantiated by other workers who studied tubercular guinea pigs, dogs, rabbits, rats, and humans. The findings showed that an increase occurred in the concentrations of the globulins and total serum proteins, whereas there was a decrease in the concentration of albumin and in the A/G (Ebel, 1953; Smith et al., 1954; Volk et al., 1953; Weimer and Moshin, 1953; Baldwin and Iland, 1953). Hudgins et al. (1956) and Hudgins and Patnode (1957) found the changes to be species specific.

Attempts were made to use the serum protein differences, particularly the A/G, in the diagnosis of tuberculosis of buffaloes (Reda et al., 1957). The data demonstrated that healthy buffaloes had A/G of 0.88, whereas those with pulmonary tuberculosis and generalized tuberculosis had ratios of 0.65 and 0.14, respectively. It was finally concluded, because of the nonspecific nature of the changes, that such analyses could be employed only when the animals did not react to the tuberculin test.

Twenty-four advanced cases of clinical Johne's disease were studied along with six control cows. Diagnosis was confirmed by the complement-fixation test for antibodies to *Mycobacterium johnei* and fecal smears and cultures. The concentrations of albumin and γ-globulins were consistently low, whereas β-globulins were only significantly below the control values. No significant changes were observed in the concentrations of α-globulins although they must be considered to have increased in proportion to the other serum proteins as a result of hemodilution (Patterson *et al.*, 1968).

Data obtained by Cochrane *et al.* (1965) of experimentally infected cows differed from the results obtained by Patterson *et al.* (1968). However, one must consider that the latter studies were conducted on cows which had been naturally infected and were generally in an advanced stage of the disease. The investigations of Cochrane *et al.* (1965) showed that the concentrations of albumin, α_1-, α_2-, β-, and γ-globulins did not differ significantly in sera from either infected or noninfected but presumably healthy cattle. There was only one exception of a cow which had a persistently high complement-fixing antibody titer which was also accompanied by an exceptionally high level of γ-globulin. The percentage of γ-globulin tended to be higher in sera of sheep which had been placed in contact with the infected cattle when compared to sheep not in contact with these cattle.

Patterson and Sweasey (1966) made a point of using the serum glycoproteins as a guide to prognosis in Johne's disease since the levels of protein-bound hexose above 120 mg/ml were seen only in terminal cases; however, again these changes were not specific.

The alterations in the serum proteins of chickens and turkeys with pullorum disease were studied by San Clemente (1942) and Lynch and Stafseth (1954). There was a decrease in the A/G and a relatively good relationship was found between concentrations of γ-globulin and agglutinin titers. A fraction with an electrophoretic mobility faster than albumin was observed in the sera of chickens which may have been the fast component found in the sera of laying birds (Moore, 1948; Brandt *et al.*, 1951).

The plasma protein profile of mice with acute bacterial infections was studied by Williams and Wemyss (1961) using the immunoelectrophoretic technique. Along with the expected changes, other patterns were observed in which a component could dissociate into multiple fractions.

The changes in the serum proteins in swine during the development of arthritis induced by *Erysipelothrix* demonstrated marked increases in the concentrations of total serum protein and γ-globulins (Freeman, 1964). Furthermore, affected pigs had significantly higher concentrations of β_2-globulins and decreases in albumin, α_2-, and β_1-globulins, whereas differences were not found in α_1-globulin (Papp and Sikes, 1964). An explanation for these changes has been theorized by Papp and Sikes (1964). Specifically, the organisms may cause damage to small blood vessels and allow serum proteins to escape into tissues. In addition, pathological changes may be produced in various tissues and cause normal production of serum proteins. Lastly, new enzymes may be formed or those existing may be destroyed or altered making it probable that an alteration would occur in the production and in the level of the serum proteins.

Attempts were made on the basis of plasma protein studies to differentiate non-specific from specific agglutinins to *Brucella* (Rose and Amerault, 1964). Vaccinated and nonvaccinated heifers were exposed to virulent *B. abortus* during the middle of pregnancy. In heifers which became infected there was a decrease in the A/G which persisted longer in infected nonvaccinated animals. The changes in γ-globulins roughly paralleled the serum agglutinin titers. Only minor alterations occurred in both groups of heifers which did not become infected. Use of the changes in plasma proteins proved to be of no value since they were not detectable until anti-body titers were 1:100–1:1000; most titers attributable to nonspecific agglutinins are below this range.

B. Mycotic Infections

There is very little work on the effect of mycotic infections on the plasma protein profile of domestic animals. Gorczyca and McCarty (1959) described the changes occurring in goats infected with *Candida albicans*. Although the alterations in the concentrations of total serum protein and α-globulins were variable, the concentrations of albumin and β-globulin decreased and there was an increase in γ-globulin.

C. Viral Infections

Generally, in most viral infections there is little or no change in the plasma protein picture. This lack of significant change may be due to the fact that the weight of antibodies produced is not sufficient to be evident as an increase in any of the protein fractions, although the samples may possess extremely high antibody titers (Dimopoullos, 1961a). Most of the studies that have been conducted in veterinary medicine have involved the plasma proteins in foot-and-mouth disease, vesicular stomatitis, hog cholera, Newcastle disease, infectious bronchitis, and canine distemper and hepatitis.

Wehmeyer (1954b) and Bradish *et al.* (1954b) conducted studies on the plasma proteins in experimental foot-and-mouth disease in cattle and observed little or no change. In contrast to this, Perk and Lobl (1961b) found an increase in the concentration of γ-globulin and a decrease in the albumin fraction in a naturally infected herd. Furthermore, the β- and γ-lipoproteins increased significantly and it was stated that these changes were due to alterations in hepatic function. No perceptible changes were demonstrated in the serum of guinea pigs infected experimentally with foot-and-mouth disease virus (Dimopoullos and Fellowes, 1958).

Bradish and Brooksby (1954) did not find significant changes in the plasma proteins of steers infected with vesicular stomatitis virus. The alterations which occur in equine infectious anemia have been confirmed by Gilman (1952) and Kao *et al.* (1954) as a decrease in the A/G. Hirtz (1952) emphasized that the changes could not be employed for diagnosis.

An increase in the γ-globulin fractions was observed in hog cholera during a hyperimmunization regimen (Mathews and Buthala, 1955). There was a decrease in albumin and an increase in α-globulin in pigs inoculated with virulent virus but changes did not occur in the β- and γ-globulins (Weide and King, 1962).

A number of reports have appeared on the plasma protein profile in poultry viral diseases. Gincherau and Chute (1956) and Clark and Foster (1968) studied the effects of Newcastle disease. Electrophoresis of serum samples from 3-month-old chickens of both sexes did not disclose significant changes; however, analyses by chemical precipitation methods demonstrated an increase in the concentration of globulins (Gincherau and Chute, 1956). Particular emphasis was placed on the fact that a study of isolated serum samples would be of relatively little value due to the inherent variations in individual birds. Clark and Foster (1968) vaccinated chicks at 1 day and 14 days of age and bled them when they were 28 days old. By immuno-electrophoretic analyses qualitative differences in the serum proteins of infected and normal chicks were not found; however, there was an increased amount of precipitate in the γ-globulin band in the vaccinated group. Their data on serum protein separation by paper electrophoresis indicated higher percentages of γ-globulin and lower percentages of albumin in infected chicks and there was no appreciable difference in total serum protein in both groups. The divergence in these results and those of Gincherau and Chute (1956) may be due to the use of birds of very different ages.

Serum protein profiles and neutralizing-antibody titers in chickens infected with infectious bronchitis virus were followed by Dimopoullos and Cunningham (1956). When titers were at a maximum, the concentrations of total globulins and γ-globulin were minimum. Even upon challenge a significant change in the globulins was not observed, although antibody titers increased further.

In canine distemper and infectious hepatitis it has been found that the concentration of albumin decreases, whereas there is a rapid increase in the α_2-globulin and a delay in the increase of γ-globulin (Snow et al., 1966; Beckett et al., 1964). The rapid change in the concentration of α_2-globulin corresponded to the variations observed in its glycoprotein counterpart. There appears to be a blockage in protein synthesis which is indicated by the decrease in the concentration of albumin and its passage into the interstitial spaces because of the increased permeability of the vascular system. This could account for the edema often associated with these diseases. There is also a report (Polson and Malherbe, 1952) that significant changes do not occur in canine distemper.

D. Protozoal Infections

The initial studies of the serum protein response in bovine anaplasmosis by Dimopoullos et al. (1960) and Rogers and Dimopoullos (1962) demonstrated characteristic changes. Just prior to the appearance of marginal bodies a decrease occurred in all fractions. A peak in body count was paralleled by increases in the concentration of total serum protein and α- and β-globulins. The concentration of γ-globulin was low at this time. As the number of marginal bodies decreased during the anemic phase, the concentrations of γ-globulins increased and that of α- and β-globulins returned to preinfection levels. The suggestion was made that complement-fixing antibodies were associated with the α- and β-globulins early in the disease but appeared later in the γ-globulins.

Klaus and Jones (1968) determined the differences in immunoglobulin response in both intact and asplenic calves infected with *Anaplasma marginale*. They found a delay in the synthesis of IgM in splenectomized calves and postulated that the enhanced severity of anaplasmosis resulted from a decreased sensitivity to low levels of parasite antigens which lead to a delay in synthesis of antibody. In addition, due to the absence of a spleen an impaired phagocytosis of the organism occurred.

In rabbits infected with *Eimeria stiedae*, Allen and Watson (1958) studied the serum proteins after treatment with sulfaquinoxiline. Necropsy examination showed hepatic damage which appeared to support the fact for the decrease in the albumin fraction. There was also an increase in the concentration of γ-globulins. Dunlap *et al.* (1959) found that the absolute concentrations of β- and γ-globulins increased, whereas the concentrations of albumin, α-globulins, and total serum protein did not change. There was also evidence of hepatic damage. The differences are difficult to evaluate; however, Allen and Watson (1958) did not observe the serum proteins throughout the disease and only calculated relative values.

The serum proteins of chickens infected with *Plasmodium gallinaceum* showed decreases in albumin and total serum protein concentration, whereas the α- and γ-globulins increased and no significant change occurred in the β-globulins (Rao and Cohly, 1953). These alterations were thought to be due to liver and kidney damage and normal immunological response. Schinazi (1957) found a new serum component with a mobility higher than albumin in malarial pigeons. It appeared early in infection, increased in concentration and then dissappeared. The component was associated with lipid and it was speculated that the changes were due to a result of reaction of the host to infection. Trypanosomiasis in guinea pigs (Ganzin *et al.*, 1952) and *Babesia canis* infection in dogs (Polson and Malherbe, 1952) induce increases in the globulins, particularly γ-globulins. Infection with *Entamoeba histolytica* in the dog produces decreases in the total protein concentration and albumin but there is no significant change in the level of γ-globulin (Comer *et al.*, 1956).

E. HELMINTHIC INFECTIONS

The changes occurring in the plasma proteins of animals infested with a variety of gastrointestinal parasites do not appear to differ appreciably from other infections. Leland (1961) has presented an excellent review in this area. Most of the alterations exhibit themselves as an increase or a stabilization of the total serum protein concentration. There is no direct evidence that an increase in the concentration of globulins is due to antibody formation, although, in many instances, the changes in globulins can be correlated with symptomatology (Turner and Wilson, 1962; Wilson and Turner, 1965). However, Wilson and Turner (1965) state that the increase in γ-globulins may be related to the degree of resistance and infection. It also seems likely that factors other than circulating antibodies are active in the development of resistance and are not directly related to the increases in γ-globulins.

A number of studies were conducted in sheep with a variety of parasites. In *Haemonchus* and *Trichostrongylus* infections and in fasciolosis there were decreases in total serum protein concentrations and albumin and increases in the concentrations of globulins (Kuttler and Marble, 1960; Leland *et al.*, 1959, 1960, 1961; Kóňa,

1957). When sheep were infected with *Oesophagostomum columbianum*, decreases occurred in the concentrations of albumin, α-, and β_1-globulins and the concentrations of β_2- and γ-globulins increased (Dobson, 1965).

Two confirming studies on the effects of *Ostertagia ostertagi* infection in calves have been presented. Both groups of workers (Marht *et al.*, 1964; Ross and Todd, 1965) found that there was a decline in albumin levels and a rise in γ-globulin concentration about 3 weeks after infection. When the calves were treated with antihelminthics and heavy concentrate feeding there was a rapid rise in the concentration of total protein and a slight rise in γ_2-globulin. *Trichostrongylus axei* infections of calves induced a rise in γ-globulin but no association between protective function and the elevated content of γ-globulin could be determined (Herlich and Merkal, 1963).

The turnover of bovine serum albumin in parasitized cattle has been reported (Cornelius *et al.*, 1962; Halliday *et al.*, 1968). In trichostrongylid infection the turnover rates of ^{131}I-tagged albumin were similar to controls, although increased catabolism occurred in a number of parasitized calves prior to death. Exchangeable serum albumin was less and its synthesis was also depressed. A hypercatabolic type of turnover was found in cattle who were also hypoalbuminemic. This may have been the result of abnormal leakage into the gastrointestinal tract. The divergence in results in the data above may be due to the amounts of specific activity employed. Halliday *et al.* (1968), who used 20 times less activity of ^{131}I, states that these differences could be due in part to denaturation of tracer albumin resulting from self-irradiation prior to injection.

Holmes *et al.* (1968) investigated the turnover rates of albumin and globulin in sheep with chronic fascioliosis. There was a decrease in the half-life of albumin as a result of loss into the gastrointestinal tract via the bile duct due to the feeding activities of the parasites. Similarly, plasma protein reaching the gut was largely degraded there. In the case of ^{131}I-tagged albumin the label was extensively reabsorbed and excreted in the urine and the entire process appeared to be hypercatabolic in nature. Turnover of 7 S globulin labeled with ^{125}I was also found to be higher and of the hypercatabolic type.

F. Residence of Antibodies

Antibodies for a variety of antigens have been demonstrated in all of the serum globulin fractions. Studies of their distribution has been greatly facilitated by the development of new fractionation techniques and more sensitive and critical immunological methods. In guinea pigs infected experimentally with foot-and-mouth disease virus it was demonstrated that the viral-neutralizing activity was associated with the β- and γ-globulin fractions, whereas the complement-fixing activity was present in the fast γ-globulin (Dimopoullos and Fellowes, 1958).

A shift in the location of antibody activity has also been demonstrated during the course of disease. F. Brown and Graves (1959) and F. Brown (1960) found that the precipitating antibody which was present in 7-day convalescent serum corresponded to a β-type globulin in foot-and-mouth disease. After 14 days or later in convalescence this antibody was shown to be in the γ-globulin area and both neutralizing and precipitating antibodies were demonstrated in the same fraction.

A continuation of the work on anaplasmosis initiated by Dimopoullos *et al.* (1960) by Rogers and Dimopoullos (1962) showed that acute sera possessed complement-fixing activity in the α- and β-globulin of lower mobility and in the γ-globulin of highest mobility. Antibody activity was not found in the α-globulins in convalescent sera and the activity in the β-globulins was of low titer. However, the γ-globulins possessed considerable activity in the fractions of high and intermediate mobilities. These data led to the hypothesis that the differences observed were due to structural alterations in the antibodies which developed during the course of anaplasmosis and these changes may have been responsible for the differences in net charge.

In a series of investigations by Murphy *et al.* (1965, 1966a,b), employing more sophisticated techniques of analysis, the complement-fixing and agglutinating-antibody activities were found to be associated with the γM (IgM) immunoglobulin in the early phases of the disease. A hyper-γM globulinemia was also found at the time of initial antibody synthesis. Subsequently, they demonstrated that in 4–5 days this synthesis was augmented by the production of γG (IgG) immunoglobulin which contained antibody activity only in the fraction of highest mobility.

IV. PHYSIOLOGICAL, INDUCED, AND OTHER FACTORS INFLUENCING THE PLASMA PROTEINS

A. PREGNANCY, PARTURITION, AND LACTATION

Protein metabolism is put to an extremely severe test during the development of the fetus. As a result, a variety of changes in the plasma proteins has been observed. Ewes show a decrease in the concentration of albumin during the first half of pregnancy which returns to near-normal levels at term (Dunlap and Dickson, 1955). Since albumin serves as the major amino acid pool, it may be that it decreases as a requisite to supplying protein precursors. During the latter half of pregnancy the concentration of globulins decrease markedly, in fact, more so than during the first half. This is thought to be due to the production of globulin-rich colostrum. The total serum protein concentration decreases throughout gestation.

Larson and Kendall (1957), Larson (1958), and Larson and Hays (1958) studied the alterations that occurred in the serum protein levels of the bovine species prior to parturition and found a decrease in the concentration of total serum protein of 10–30%. This was mainly due to the loss of β_2- and γ_1-globulins and to a lesser extent to a decrease in the concentration of α-globulin. The data indicated that immune β_2- and γ_1-globulins build up in the maternal blood several weeks before parturition and then leave the blood when colostrum is being formed in the mammary gland. On a quantitative basis all alterations are accounted for by the immune globulin components.

B. DEVELOPMENTAL STAGES AND EFFECTS OF AGE ON PLASMA PROTEINS

Kekwick (1959) has presented an excellent review on the serum proteins of fetal and young mammals. In the fetal stages of development it is generally accepted that the concentrations of total serum protein and albumin increase, whereas there is little change in the concentration of β-globulin. The concentrations of α-globulins are variable and there is an absence of γ-globulin (Barboriak *et al.*, 1958a,b).

The lack of γ-globulin in fetal sera has been open to question. It has been reported to be absent in sheep and goats (Barboriak *et al.*, 1958a,b) and in swine (Rutqvist, 1958; Rook *et al.*, 1951). Kniazeff *et al.* (1967) found 25% of the bovine fetal sera to contain γ-globulin. They attributed this to transplacental transfer or even possibly to fetal synthesis.

Shortly after birth and after nursing large amounts of γ-globulin appear in the serum of swine and after 24 hours up to 40% of the serum protein may consist of this fraction (Rutqvist, 1958; Rook *et al.*, 1951). In about 3 to 4 weeks the γ-globulin decreases to approximately 5% of the total serum protein and the concentrations of albumin and β-globulin increase (Rook *et al.*, 1951).

The investigations of Pierce (1955) in which studies were made on the development of the serum proteins of calves from birth to weaning demonstrated that precolostral calf serum contained no γ-globulin. Generally, in colostral-fed calves up to 80 days after birth the concentration of albumin increased but β-globulin did not change significantly. A decrease in the concentration of α-globulin was associated with the disappearance of the mucoprotein fetuin shortly after birth. In pigs the α_1-globulin disappears 7 days after birth and is possibly a fetal protein of the fetuin type (Dickerson and Southgate, 1967).

After the calf ingests colostrum γ-globulin appears in the serum within a few hours (San Clemente and Huddleson, 1943). Its absorption through the gut occurs for approximately 48 hours after birth (Polson, 1952; Ebel, 1953), after which gut permeability is altered. In colostrum-deprived calves the γ-globulin concentration increases as a result of exogenous antigenic stimuli. However, there is a decrease in the total globulin concentration up to 8 weeks of age (Hansen and Phillips, 1947).

Numerous investigations have been made on the significance of age and the concentrations of the serum proteins. Generally, there is a decrease in the concentration of albumin and an increase in the globulin fractions and total serum protein concentration with an increase in age (Larson and Touchberry, 1959; Dimopoullos, 1961b; Perk and Loebl, 1959; Garner *et al.*, 1957; Koenig *et al.*, 1949; Perk and Lobl, 1960; Forstner, 1968). In fact, direct relationships have been found between the total serum protein concentration and age (Shetlar *et al.*, 1948; Sohar *et al.*, 1956; Dimopoullos, 1961b). It is, therefore, obvious why particular emphasis has been placed on the necessity in taking the age of the animal into account when interpreting data with the exception of old subjects (Forstner, 1968).

Marshall and Deutsch (1950) studied the development of serum proteins in the chick embryo. All major electrophoretic components found in the serum of 10-day-old chick embryos were also present in adult chickens except that there was a gradual change in the relative concentration of the proteins as the embryo reached maturity. Embryonic serum also possessed components which had electrophoretic mobilities higher than albumin; these disappeared just prior to hatching. In fact, Schechtman and Hoffman (1952) found that proteins antigenically resembling α- and β-globulins could be detected in 3- and 6-day-old chick embryos.

The production of eggs requires a large amount of protein which consequently places the domestic fowl under extreme stress. Brandt *et al.* (1951) found the serum of the laying hen to contain more protein and α-globulin than the nonlayer, whereas

Tanaka and Aoki (1963) also found increases in total serum protein and in the combined β- and γ-globulin fractions. These changes were even more dramatic with advancing age. A component with a mobility higher than albumin was observed in the serum of laying hens which was thought to be related to the process of egg formation in both of the above investigations. The total serum protein and globulin concentrations were also found to be high in laying ducks and there was an increase in total serum protein with age (Perk and Lobl, 1961a).

C. Hormonal and Sexual Influences

When dogs were administered ACTH, no changes were observed in any of the serum protein fractions. Cortisone, however, tended to produce a small rise in albumin and α_2-globulin, and a small decrease in the α_1-, β_2-, and γ-globulins (Bjorneboe et al., 1952). Bossak et al. (1955) also confirmed the fact that dogs given cortisone showed a rise in the α_2-globulin and a decrease in the concentration of β-globulin. In adrenal insufficiency the concentration of globulins decreased (Lewis and Page, 1947; Page and Lewis, 1951).

Cortisone has been employed in the treatment of arthritis in swine experimentally infected with *Erysipelothrix rhusopathiae*. Clinical improvement was accompanied by a striking increase in albumin and decreases in γ-globulin (Shetlar et al., 1958).

Sexual differences in the plasma proteins of the chicken appear at the onset of sexual maturity. In fact, the serum electrophoretic patterns can be reversed by contra-sex hormones (Moore, 1948). When hens begin laying, a component having a mobility more rapid than albumin appears. Immature cockerels, pullets, and non-laying turkeys do not possess this fast component (Common et al., 1953). The electrophoretic patterns of 8-week-old cockerels can be made to appear similar to that of laying hens when the birds are administered diethylstilbestrol (Clegg et al., 1951).

Perk et al. (1960) demonstrated that under the influence of diethylstilbestrol, 10-week-old White Leghorn chickens of both sexes possessed an increased concentration of total serum protein and globulins, whereas the albumin fraction decreased. There were also major changes in the α_2- and β_3-globulins. Testosterone had no significant effects on the plasma proteins.

Administration of dienestrol diacetate to White Leghorn chickens increased the concentrations of albumin and globulins equally (Sturkie, 1951). If both DL-thyroxine and the estrogen were administered together this hyperproteinemic response was prevented. Thyroxine alone depressed the plasma protein concentration suggesting that it either inhibited the biosynthesis of protein by the liver or that it increased the oxidative destruction of these proteins.

The effect of estrogen administration in immature geese produced an increase in the β_1- and γ-globulins and a decrease in the concentration of albumin. These alterations were more pronounced in the hormone-treated group than in the laying geese (Perk et al., 1959).

Perk and Loebl (1960) studied the effects of diethylstilbestrol on the serum proteins of male calves. They found that the concentrations of total serum protein and globulins, especially the γ-globulin fraction, increased, whereas there was a decrease in the albumin.

D. Hepatic Disorders

The liver plays a major role in the biosynthesis of the majority of plasma proteins. One would anticipate that a pathological liver would be reflected in the nature of the plasma protein profile. Hepatic diseases in dogs have been studied to some extent. In hepatitis and cirrhosis there is generally a decrease in the concentration of albumin and an increase in the β-globulins (Groulade and Groulade, 1953; de Wael and Teunissen, 1954). De Wael (1956) states that these diseases can be differentiated on the basis of the changes observed in the serum proteins.

E. Gnotobiotic Environment

The qualitative and quantitative responses of the plasma proteins in animals depend greatly upon the antigenic stimuli that they are subjected to throughout their life. In the germ-free state it has been routinely confirmed that there are lower concentrations of serum globulins. When these animals are contaminated the globulins increase in concentration (Wostmann, 1959; Wostmann and Gordon, 1960). The increase in globulins after infection appears to be correlated with an increase in antibody titers and in the number of reticuloendothelial cells in the wall of the ileum (Wagner and Wostmann, 1961). In the germ-free animal the serum is usually free of antibacterial agglutinins (Wagner, 1959). Even the feeding of penicillin in the diet to conventional chicks lowers the γ-globulin concentration as compared to the untreated control group (Wostmann and Gordon, 1958).

F. Nutritional Factors and Protein Depletion

The plasma proteins are extremely sensitive to nutritional influences. Vitamins, growth factors, and related substances which affect protein, lipid, and carbohydrate metabolism would consequently be expected to make their influence felt in the plasma protein profile. For example, factors which affect protein metabolism may manifest themselves by influencing the total protein concentration of serum or plasma or the concentration of an individual protein fraction. Those substances which are intimately associated with lipid metabolism may affect the plasma lipoproteins, specifically the α- and β-globulins. In cases where carbohydrate metabolism is involved one may observe specific changes in the various plasma-bound carbohydrate components.

A direct relationship between vitamin A and albumin concentration of bovine serum has been reported by Erwin et al. (1959). When vitamin A is deficient intravenous administration of carotene returns the concentration of albumin to normal levels in 10 days.

Dietary protein depletion in rats manifests itself as decreases in the concentrations of albumin and α_1-globulin (Weimer et al., 1959a,b; Weimer, 1961). In the chick and rat the concentration of total serum protein was largely influenced by the amount of dietary protein and the changes were mainly observed in the albumin fraction (Leveille and Sauberlich, 1961; Leveille et al., 1961; Pareira et al., 1958, 1959).

Allison (1957, 1958) reported on several studies of plasma protein depletion in dogs. When protein reserves were depleted by a low nitrogen or protein-free diet a hypoproteinemic condition developed in which a decrease occurred in the concentration of albumin. Usually the plasma volume was reduced and edema occurred because of the change in osmotic pressure due to the loss of albumin. Concentrations of globulins were not decreased greatly and occasionally there was even an increase in the concentrations of these fractions. Chow *et al.* (1948) produced a hyperproteinemic condition in dogs by plasmapheresis and feeding a protein-free diet. Depletion decreased the concentrations of albumin and γ-globulin, whereas the other globulins were not affected. The dogs could be repleted by oral administration of casein or lactalbumin hydrolyzates.

Jeffay and Winzler (1958) studied the relationship of protein content of diet and turnover of serum proteins in the rat. The data indicated that serum albumin in rats maintained on a low or protein-free diet had a longer half-life and a slower replacement rate than rats maintained on adequate protein.

There is divergence of experimental data on the effects of protein malnutrition and antibody production. Bieler *et al.* (1947) and Balch (1950) found no differences in the production of antibodies in subjects suffering from such a deficiency. Benditt *et al.* (1949) observed that severe restriction of dietary protein caused impairment of antibody production. A decreased antibody response was found in protein-depleted rats (Wissler, 1947) and rabbits (Cannon *et al.*, 1943). In protein-depleted rats an increased capacity for antibody production was evident during repletion which indicated that the antibody-producing mechanisms were not permanently damaged (Wissler *et al.*, 1946).

Adult sheep on a magnesium-deficient diet showed decreases in albumin and increases in the concentrations of α_1- and γ-globulins. The concentration of total serum protein remained relatively constant (Kiesel and Alexander, 1966).

The effects of aflatoxin on the serum proteins of ducks, chickens, and swine have been reported (Annau *et al.*, 1964; J. M. M. Brown and Abrams, 1965; Németh and Juhász, 1968). The general consensus is that the animals became hypoproteinemic and changes involve most of the serum protein fractions.

G. Injury, Stress, and Blood Loss

Destruction of tissue by direct injury or through surgery upsets the dynamic equilibrium between tissue and plasma protein metabolism. Repair of tissues calls upon protein reserves and consequently the plasma proteins. Hoch-Ligeti *et al.* (1953) studied the plasma proteins of humans after a variety of surgical procedures and found a decrease in albumin and increases in the concentration of α_1- and α_2-globulins; after 4 days the components tended to return to preoperative levels.

Splenectomy of calves altered the composition of the serum proteins (Dimopoullos *et al.*, 1959a). Following surgery there was a decrease in total serum protein concentration and an increase in the globulins which persisted for about 1 month. The A/G returned to normal levels approximately 2 months after splenectomy at which time it increased. The influence of splenic tissue on globulin synthesis must be considered when evaluating these data.

Regardless of the type or cause of the injury there is always an increase in the concentration of α-globulin (Shedlovsky and Scudder, 1942). Chanutin and Gjessing (1946) stated that the destruction and disintegration of tissue was directly responsible for the increase in the concentration of α-globulin. A decrease in albumin accompanies injuries such as heat and cold, bone fractures, or turpentine abscesses. The albumin is probably lost through the capillaries.

The withdrawal of large amounts of blood would be expected to produce a call on the protein reserves and consequently alterations would be observed in the plasma proteins. When blood was withdrawn from sheep in vast quantities the albumin and total protein concentrations decreased, whereas higher globulin concentrations were observed (Kuttler and Marble, 1960). Kóňa et al. (1966) removed 1850 ml of blood daily from sheep for 10 days and observed that the concentrations of albumin and γ-globulin decreased until they were minimum at the eleventh day after which they began to return to normal levels. Similar data were obtained with chickens which were bled in large quantities (Dimopoullos and Cunningham, 1956; Sturkie and Newman, 1951). Sturkie and Newman (1951) hypothesized that this phenomenon was due to hemodilution and an increase in plasma volume.

Bradish et al. (1954a) found that no effect on the plasma proteins was exerted when 2 and $4\frac{1}{5}$ liters were withdrawn from cattle at one time.

Intake of water can affect the plasma protein composition. Cattle in a state of thirst possess higher concentrations of albumin and total protein. Two hours after watering the plasma proteins approached normal levels (Wehmeyer, 1954a).

H. Genetic Control

Several investigators have mentioned that the plasma protein profile of a particular normal subject is relatively constant over a considerable length of time (Bernfeld et al., 1953; Dole, 1944; Stockl and Zacherl, 1953). This constancy is apparently controlled genetically. In fact, Moore (1945) found that the serum protein patterns were so characteristic that it was possible to differentiate species and in some cases the strain and sex of an animal.

Various results on the influence of heredity on the plasma proteins of cattle have been reported. Perk and Lobl (1959a) studied the serum protein differences of the Damascene breed of cattle, which are heat- and thirst-resistant, and the Holstein-Friesian breed. The concentrations of α- and β-globulins were similar, although the Holstein-Friesian cattle had higher total serum protein and γ-globulin but lower A/G than the Damascene breed. The authors hypothesized that the thirst-resistance of Damascene cattle was partially due to their higher serum albumin level and as a result could retain water longer in the blood because of osmotic pressure effects. Furthermore, the Holstein-Friesian is more resistant to infections by virtue of higher γ-globulin concentrations.

Further studies on inherited serum protein variations of cattle have been reported by Smithies and Hickman (1958). They found that the differences observed in the serum proteins of two Ayrshire and Holstein-Friesian herds could be used to group the cattle into five serum types based upon the five proteins in the β-globulin region. Ashton (1957) found that the β_2-globulin could be separated into four to six components depending upon the serum type. Lewis and Page (1956) observed that fat pigs possessed higher concentrations of total serum protein and albumin than lean pigs even when the animals were on identical diets and showed similar relative gains in weight.

Genetic relationships in the serum of gallinaceous hybrids and domestic fowls were studied by Brandt et al. (1952). The serum protein components found in the hybrids were related to the components found in the serum electrophoretic patterns of the parent birds. Many of the other components which were present in the serum of hybrids were electrophoretically identical with the components found in the parent birds.

There are conditions in which one finds an almost complete absence of γ-globulin or a very marked decrease in the total globulin concentration. Agammaglobulinemia in a 3-month-old calf has been authenticated as a congenital defect (Perk and Lobl, 1962). It was inferred that the abnormality was due to an inherited malfunctioning of the cells synthesizing γ-globulin. Hypogammaglobulinemia and hypoglobulinemia are usually diagnosed in reticuloendothelial conditions, the highest incidence being in cases of lymphatic involvement (Wall et al., 1956). This decrease in the concentration of globulin is usually detected long before the diagnosis of disease is made.

I. Cancer

The demands on protein synthesis in cancer are usually greater than with normal tissues and this places great stress on the animal. In most instances the A/G decreases (Gleason and Friedberg, 1953; Ebel, 1953; Bernfeld and Homburger, 1954; Schultz et al., 1954; Roberts, 1954; de Lamirande and Cantero, 1952; Davidson and Lawrence, 1954). Allison and Wannemacher (1960) found that in rats with tumors, the greater the weight of the tumor the less serum albumin was present. In mammary carcinoma of mice, the only difference that has been observed is a decrease in the concentration of γ-globulin which may precede the development of the carcinoma (Johnson et al., 1954). Schlumberger and Wall (1957) studied the plasma proteins of parakeets with pituitary tumors and found an increase in the concentration of a protein which was tentatively identified as a globulin. Saline extracts of the tumor even showed the presence of this component.

Leukosis in chickens stimulated a number of studies on the plasma proteins. In 1944 Sanders et al. reported the presence of a component in the serum of chickens which was associated with the γ-globulin. It was termed the "L" component and represented about 10% of the total protein. Deutsch et al. (1949) immunized chickens against human γ_2-globulin which subsequently showed an increase in the γ_1-globulin concentration. It also occupied the same relative position in the γ-globulin region as did the L component of Sanders et al. (1944). It was hypothesized that the L component and the increase in the concentration of γ_1-globulin represented similar antibody responses on the part of the chicken to foreign protein. Slizewicz and Atanasiu (1953) studied sera from leukotic chickens and did not find any significant differences in the serum proteins. This may have been due to the rapid development of the disease whereby there was not sufficient time for the changes to be detected.

Dimopoullos and Cunningham (1956) found no evidence of the L component in chickens with gross manifestations of lymphomatosis at necropsy. It was hypothesized that this component may be an artifact similar to that observed in the serum electrophoretic patterns from the ascending limb of the electrophoresis cell. The component appeared to be comparable with the γ anomaly of the electrophoretic pattern of the descending limb. The L component or a similar substance was also observed in the ascending patterns of sera from chickens that did not show manifestations of lymphomatosis. All of the above data indicate that the response and the production of this substance is probably due to foreign protein, that it is nonspecific, and that the component is probably γ_1-globulin.

Electrophoretic analyses of serum proteins from paralyzed and unparalyzed chickens exposed to Marek's disease agent were conducted by Ringen and Akhtar (1968). Their data revealed that increased levels of γ-globulin in the paralyzed group appeared during the fourth week. A peak was reached around the sixth week and then declined in sharp contrast with the gradual rise in the γ-globulin concentration in the unparalyzed group.

A hyperglobulinemia produced as a result of a possible plasma cell myeloma has been reported in mink affected with Aleutian disease (Henson et al., 1961). The increase in the γ-globulin fraction was due to the 7 S component and could not be distinguished from that in normal serum (Kenyon et al., 1963). Ferrets have also been found with a condition analogous, if not identical, to Aleutian disease (Kenyon et al., 1966). Lane (1952) found that a malignant condition of the plasma cells produces an increased amount of γ-globulin in the tumor. It has been established that γ-globulin is synthesized by plasma cells (Ortega and Mellors, 1957).

Cornelius et al. (1959) studied a case of plasma cell myelomatosis in a horse and found an abnormal β-myeloma serum glycoprotein, and a decrease in the concentrations of albumin and α-globulin. In fact the glycoprotein was also found terminally in the urine.

An altered α_2-globulin concentration was found in the serum of dogs with mastocytoma (Howard and Kenyon, 1965). The substance was a glycoprotein and there appeared to be a direct correlation in its concentration and the development of the tumor. Similar increases could be produced in dogs by administering histamine dihydrochloride. It was hypothesized that the serum protein changes resulted from elaboration of histamine by the tumor mast cells.

V.   NORMAL AND ABNORMAL VALUES OF PLASMA PROTEINS

The method employed for the analysis of plasma proteins greatly influences the number of fractions which can be separated and identified. A good example of a comparative electrophoretic study, conducted by Porter and Dixon (1966), showed that mink serum proteins could be separated into four bands on paper, five bands on cellulose acetate, and twelve bands on starch gel, and 25 components could be identified by immunoelectrophoresis. Horse serum shows as many as twenty fractions by immunoelectrophoresis (Henson, 1964) and seven bands by paper electrophoresis (Hort, 1968), whereas swine serum has 22–26 components and bovine serum shows up to 36 components when separated by starch electrophoresis (Scopes, 1963).

Irfan (1967) reported data on serum electrophoretic studies from a large number of normal animals. These results and other data on normal values are listed in Tables I–VI. Additional information may be found in Sandor (1966), Spector (1956), Dittmer (1961), and Long (1961). No attempts have been made to compile data on values in disease and other pathological and physiological states simply because the changes cannot be ascribed to any specific abnormality. It must be reemphasized that the alterations observed are indicative of the status of the subject under study and should be used only to assess its condition at that time and possibly to determine prognosis. Many conditions simulate each other in the changes that are reflected in the plasma proteins. The alterations seen in unrelated abnormal states are more similar to each other than dissimilar.

TABLE I NORMAL PLASMA PROTEIN VALUES

Species	Sex	Age	No. of animals	Albumin	Relative concentrations (%)									Reference
					α-	α₁-	α₂-	β-	β₁-	β₂-	φ-	γ-	Other globulins	
Bovine	M	18–30 m	51	46.6 ±4.1	14.0 ±2.1	—	—	8.9 ±1.4	—	—	—	30.5 ±4.0		Bradish et al. (1954a)
	—	—	13	42 ±3	15 ±2	—	—	15 ±2	—	—	—	28 ±4		Decker et al. (1959)
	F	5–9 y	9	45.5 ±3.7	11.3 ±0.8	—	—	14.3 ±0.7	—	—	—	28.6 ±3.3		Perk and Lobl (1961b)
	M,F	½–12 m	—	51.2	—	3.9	10.1	11.6	—	—	—		γ₁– 8.1 γ₂– 15.1	Weber (1964)
Bovine	—	>24 m	100	43.1	11.0	4.8 ±1.2	14.1 ±2.6	12.0	—	—	—	33.9		Irfan (1967)
Ovine	—	122 d	27	51.0 ±6.5	—	—	—	7.7 ±1.7	—	—	—	22.4 ±4.9		Kuttler and Marble (1960)
Caprine	—	2–3 m	10	56.8	—	6.5	8.8	9.1	—	—	—	18.8		Irfan (1967)
	M,F	7–9 m	15	63.3	6.7	7.7	7.7	—	13.2	6.6	—	15.5		Gorczyca et al. (1960)
Porcine	—	3–6 m	10	63.0	—	7.7	—	5.6	—	—	—	16.0		Irfan (1967)
	—	5½–6½ m	79	46.0 ±5.8	20.0 ±4.0	—	—	14.5 ±1.6	—	—	—	19.5 ±4.3		Knill et al. (1958)
	—	—	17	45.0	19.0	—	—	13.0	—	—	—	23.0		Foster et al. (1950)
Equine	—	3–4 m	10	34.2	20.2	—	—	18.6	—	—	—	27.0		Irfan (1967)
	—	> 5 y	70	33.5	—	15.0	16.0	15.5	—	—	—	20.0		Irfan (1967)
	—	—	1	38.71	—	19.81	19.36	12.00	—	—	—	10.12		Kao et al. (1954)
	—	—	1	41.15	—	16.05	11.05	14.40	—	—	—	17.35		Kao et al. (1954)
	M,F	Adult	10	39.6 ±2.07	—	2.8 ±0.94	2.8 ±0.65	—	13.8 ±3.10	8.7 ±2.50	—	20.7 ±4.30	α₃– 11.6 +3.70	Hort (1968)
Chicken	—	15–18 w	1	47.4	9.0	—	—	14.4	—	—	—	19.2		Sanders et al. (1944)
	—	15–18 w	1	47.2	15.0	—	—	10.9	—	—	14.1	13.7		Sanders et al. (1944)
	F	Adult	40	46.0	22.0	—	—	8.0	—	—	—	24.0		Deutsch et al. (1949)
	—	1 m	80	42.7	—	17.4	9.5	12.3	—	—	—	9.0	α₃– 8.0	Clark and Foster (1968)

TABLE I (continued)

Species	Sex	Age	No. of animals	Albumin	α-	α₁-	α₂-	β-	β₁-	β₂-	φ-	γ-	Other globulins	Reference
Chicken (con't.)	F	40 d	8	55.34 ±5.71	24.09			(β- + γ- 20.55 ± 5.35)						Tanaka and Aoki (1963)
	F	60 d	10	56.11 ±6.64	19.84 ±3.33			(β- + γ- 24.05 ±6.08)				See col. 9		Tanaka and Aoki (1963)
	F	80 d	9	47.91 ±5.90	22.46 ±2.66			(β- + γ- 29.62 ±6.87)				See col. 9		Tanaka and Aoki (1963)
	F	100 d	10	55.03 ±4.33	15.67 ±3.10			(β- + γ- 29.34 ±3.78)				See col. 9		Tanaka and Aoki (1963)
	F	120 d	8	51.05 ±9.56	16.13 ±4.14			(β- + γ- 32.79 ±7.99)				See col. 9		Tanaka and Aoki (1963)
	F	140 d	9	43.58 ±8.20	15.26 ±3.62			(β- + γ- 40.65 ±7.41)				See col. 9		Tanaka and Aoki (1963)
	F	170 d	9	37.38 ±3.98	22.03 ±7.93			(β- + γ- 40.13 ±7.86)				See col. 9		Tanaka and Aoki (1963)
	F	210 d	6	31.33 ±2.95	22.71 ±9.94			(β- + γ- 45.58 ±9.66)				See col. 9		Tanaka and Aoki (1963)
Turkey	—	>3 m	15	35.5		13.3	7.0	13.0				31.2		Irfan (1967)
	M	Adult	23	66.5	7.9	—	—	14.4	—	—		11.2		Lynch and Stafseth (1953)
Canine	—	—	—	51.94 ±1.60	—	4.77 ±0.94	8.49 ±1.11	—	8.38 ±1.32	13.66 ±1.37	—	12.70 ±1.44		Ebel (1953)

Species	Sex	Age	No.										Reference
Rabbit	—	Adult	7	45.9 ± 1.41	10.03 ± 1.07	7.7 ± 1.16	—	10.4 ± 0.45	13.3 ± 0.39	—	4.8 + 0.30	α_3- 6.9 ± 1.06	Hahn et al. (1956)
	—	Adult	—	45.4	23.0	—	12.1	—	—	14.4	5.1		Brueckner et al. (1959)
	—	—	15	60.5 ± 3.0	4 ± 1.7	7.5 ± 2.0	—	8.5 ± 1.5	11.5 ± 1.0	—	7.6 ± 1.5		Groulade and Groulade (1953)
	—	—	16	48.74 ± 1.43	6.62 ± 0.45	6.89 ± 0.52	—	10.57 ± 0.89	14.84 ± 0.33	—	12.71 ± 0.17		de Wael and Teunissen (1954)
	—	—	20	53.5 ± 3.3	4.3 ± 0.9	5.3 ± 1.3	—	3.2 ± 0.6	4.9 ± 1.2	—	12.3 ± 1.9	α_0- 4.2 ± 1.2 β_3- 12.3 ± 1.9	Boguth (1953)
	MF	2–7 y	15	53.8	4.4	8.9	19.9	—	—	—	13.0		Irfan (1967)
		Adult	18	64.0 ± 1.63	7.21 ± 0.96	5.8 ± 1.05	12.77 ± 1.20	—	—	—	9.91 ± 1.10		Allen and Watson (1958)
	M	Adult	8	57.22	8.73	6.21	14.58	—	—	—	13.22		Hudgins et al. (1956)
Guinea pig	M	> 4 m	24	62.0	6.2	10.4	9.6	—	—	—	11.8	α_3- 8.75	Irfan (1967)
	M		8	40.19	6.45	23.70	12.26	—	—	—	8.66		Hudgins et al. (1956)
Rat	F		—	48.6 ± 1.7	13.7 ± 3.0	10.0 ± 1.3	14.4 ± 1.2	—	—	—	13.2 ± 3.0		Schultz et al. (1954)
	M		8	28.89	16.22	12.11	22.0	—	—	—	15.71	α_3- 5.02	Hudgins et al. (1956)
Mouse	M		21	53.0	—	—	19.0	—	—	—	14.0		Bueker (1961)
			5	49 ± 1.65	9.5 ± 1.0	—	15	—	—	—	9.5 ± 0.6	α_3- 7 ± 0.9	Greenberg et al. (1952)
Monkey			2	57 ± 1.05	7.5 ± 0.6	—	15 ± 1.35	—	—	11 ± 0.3	13.5 ± 1.0	α_3- 8 ± 1.4	Greenberg et al. (1952)
Goose	M	3 m	8	56.2	8.5	8.1	5.5	—	—	—	9.6	β_3- 12.0	Perk et al. (1959)
	F	3 m	8	51.5	9.7	8.0	5.3	—	—	—	12.7	β_3- 13.1	Perk et al. (1959)

TABLE II   NORMAL PLASMA PROTEIN VALUES

Species	Sex	Age	No. of animals	Albumin	α-	α_1-	α_2-	β-	β_1-	β_2-	ϕ-	γ-	Other globulins	TP[a]	Reference
Bovine	M	18–30 m	30	3.20	0.98	—	—	0.61	—	—	—	2.18		6.97 ±0.53	Bradish et al. (1954a)
	—	—	13	3.37 ±0.29	1.19 ±0.1	—	—	1.23 ±0.15	—	—	—	2.28 ±0.49		8.08 ±0.64	Decker et al. (1959)
	F	5–9 y	—	3.44 ±0.28	0.85 ±0.06	—	—	1.08 ±0.053	—	—	—	2.16 ±0.25		7.56 ±0.5	Perk and Lobl (1961b)
	F	Adult	18	3.39	1.49	—	—	1.96	—	—	—	2.35		9.20	Patterson et al. (1968)
	F	Adult	—	3.49	—	—	—	—	—	—	0.57	—		6.6	Srivastava (1959)
		Calf	—	3.19	—	—	—	—	—	—	0.57	—		5.59	Srivastava (1959)
	M,F	½–12 m	—											7.9	Weber (1964)
	F	Adult	—								0.391				Locatelli (1956)
	—	Newborn	—								0.306				Locatelli (1956)
	—	6–7 d	—								0.529				Locatelli (1956)
	—	>2 y	100											7.16	Irfan (1967)
Ovine	—	122 d	27	2.96	—	0.28	0.82	0.45	—	—	—	1.30		5.81 ±0.54	Kuttler and Marble (1960)
	—	2–3 m	10											5.46	Irfan (1967)
Caprine	M,F	7–9 m	15	3.95 ±0.26	0.42 ±0.09	—	—	—	0.83 ±0.12	0.41 ±0.07	—	0.97 ±0.18		6.25 ±0.35	Gorczyca et al. (1960)
	—	3–6 m	10											5.7	Irfan (1967)
Porcine	—	5½–6½ m	79	3.4	1.5	—	—	1.1	—	—	—	1.4		7.4 ±0.6	Knill et al. (1958)
	—	3–4 m	10											7.77	Irfan (1967)
Equine	—	—	30	3.1 ±0.34	—	—	—	—	—	—	—	—		7.1 ±0.38	Jennings and Mulligan (1953)

Species	Sex	Age	n										Reference
	—	—	—	2.60	—	1.33	1.30	0.81	—	—	0.68	6.72	Kao et al. (1954)
	—	—	2	2.99	—	—	—	—	—	—		7.81	Gilman (1952)
	M,F	Adult	10	2.87 ±0.49	—	0.02 ±0.07	0.02 ±0.05	—	1.10 ±0.07	0.63 ±0.06	1.52 α_3- 0.86 ±0.08 ±0.09	7.29	Hort (1968)
Chicken	—	> 5 y	70	—	—	—	—	—	—	—	—	7.16	Irfan (1967)
	M	18–22 m	14	1.66	—	—	—	—	—	—	—	4.00	Sturkie and Newman (1951)
	F	16–18 m	—	2.00	—	—	—	—	—	—	—	5.34	Sturkie and Newman (1951)
	F	—	9	2.50	0.64	—	—	0.23	—	—	—	5.45	Sturkie (1951)
	F	Adult	40	1.33	—	—	—	—	—	—	0.70	2.9	Deutsch et al. (1949)
	—	1 m	80	—	—	—	—	—	—	—	—	2.18	Clark and Foster (1968)
	F	40 d	8	—	—	—	—	—	—	—	—	2.81 ±0.20	Tanaka and Aoki (1963)
	F	60 d	10	—	—	—	—	—	—	—	—	2.96 ±0.40	Tanaka and Aoki (1963)
	F	80 d	9	—	—	—	—	—	—	—	—	3.14 ±0.24	Tanaka and Aoki (1963)
	F	100 d	10	—	—	—	—	—	—	—	—	3.15 ±0.15	Tanaka and Aoki (1963)
	F	120 d	8	—	—	—	—	—	—	—	—	3.53 ±0.75	Tanaka and Aoki (1963)
	F	140 d	9	—	—	—	—	—	—	—	—	3.75 ±0.62	Tanaka and Aoki (1963)
	F	170 d	9	—	—	—	—	—	—	—	—	3.43 ±0.61	Tanaka and Aoki (1963)
	F	210 d	6	—	—	—	—	—	—	—	—	4.05 ±0.81	Tanaka and Aoki (1963)
Turkey	—	3 m	15	—	—	—	—	—	—	—	—	4.08	Irfan (1967)
	M	Adult	23	—	—	—	—	—	—	—	—	4.40	Lynch and Stafseth (1953)

TABLE II (continued)

Species	Sex	Age	No. of animals	Albumin	α-	α₁-	α₂-	β-	β₁-	β₂-	φ-	γ-	Other globulins	TP[a]	Reference
Canine	—	—	20	3.36 ±0.33	—	0.27 ±0.05	0.33 ±0.88	—	0.21 ±0.04	0.31 ±0.06	—	0.78 ±0.15	α₆- 0.26±0.07 β₃- 0.78±0.10	6.3 ±0.40	Boguth (1953)
	—	—	16	—	—	—	—	—	—	—	—	—	—	5.94 ±0.09	de Wael and Teunissen (1954)
	—	2–7 y	15	—	—	—	—	—	—	—	—	—	—	6.64	Irfan (1967)
	—	—	—	—	—	—	—	—	—	—	—	—	—	6.34 ±0.24	Hahn et al. (1956)
Mouse	—	—	5	3.38	—	0.053	0.039	0.46	—	—	—	0.058	—	3.99	Gleason and Friedberg (1953)
Cotton rat	—	Adult	—	4.62	—	—	—	—	—	—	—	—	—	6.38	Dolyak and Leone (1953)
Rabbit	M	—	8	4.11	—	0.63	0.45	1.06	—	—	—	0.95	—	7.20 ±0.11	Hudgins et al. (1956)
	—	—	—	—	—	—	—	—	—	—	—	—	—	5.9 ±0.12	Weimer et al. (1954)
	—	>4 m	24	—	—	—	—	—	—	—	—	—	—	5.9	Irfan (1967)
	—	—	—	—	—	—	—	—	—	—	—	—	—	5.3 ±0.06	Weimer et al. (1954)
Guinea pig	—	—	10	2.82 ±0.05	—	0.42 ±0.03	1.38 ±0.08	—	0.35 ±0.01	0.56 ±0.03	—	0.68 ±0.05	—	—	Banerjee and Rohatgi (1958)
	M	—	8	2.28	—	0.36	1.36	0.69	—	—	—	0.49	α₃- 0.50	5.68	Hudgins et al. (1956)

Absolute concentrations (gm/100 ml)

Species	Sex	Age	N									TP	Reference
Rat	M	—	8	1.94	—	1.09	0.81	1.48	—	—	1.06 α₃- 0.34	6.71 ±0.15	Hudgins et al. (1956)
	—	—	3	2.08	—	1.23	0.83	1.08	—	—	0.73	5.95	Allison and Wannemacher (1960)
	M	3 m	8	—	—	—	—	—	—	—	—	6.92 ±0.48	Abreu et al. (1957)
	—	—	10	3.74 ±0.07	—	—	—	—	—	—	—	5.78 ±0.044	Beaton (1961)
	F	—	—	2.95 ±0.15	—	0.8 ±0.10	0.65 ±0.04	0.90 ±0.13	—	—	0.86 ±0.15		Schultz et al. (1954)
	—	—	3	2.95	—	0.04	0.012	0.23	—	—	0.097	3.33	Gleason and Friedberg (1953)
Monkey	—	—	5	3.9 ±0.15	—	—	—	—	—	—	—	6.7 ±0.2	Greenberg et al. (1952)
	—	—	2	4.4 ±0.3	—	—	—	—	—	—	—	7.45 ±0.2	Greenberg et al. (1952)
Duck	M,F	1 d	10	2.41 ±0.35	1.08 ±0.13	—	—	0.53 ±0.08	—	—	0.40 ±0.09	4.43 ±0.57	Németh and Juhász (1968)

[a]TP = total protein concentration.

TABLE III   NORMAL BOVINE PLASMA GLYCOPROTEIN VALUES

Sex	Age	No. of animals	Protein-bound nonglucosamine polysaccharide: relative concentrations (%)				Reference
			Albumin	α-	β-	γ-	
M	>2 y	35	3.7±0.6	43.0±1.0	30.2±1.0	23.1±1.0	Dimopoullos et al. (1959b)
F	>2 y	125	3.2±0.4	51.9±0.7	23.6±0.4	21.2±0.6	Dimopoullos et al. (1959b)
MF	>2 y	160	3.3±0.3	50.0±0.7	25.0±0.5	21.7±0.5	Dimopoullos et al. (1959b)
F	18–24 m	28	3.5±0.6	53.0±1.3	26.0±1.5	17.6±1.1	Dimopoullos et al. (1959b)
F	12–18 m	26	2.6±0.8	55.4±1.6	24.1±1.1	17.9±1.0	Dimopoullos et al. (1959b)
F	9–12 m	8	3.7±1.5	62.5±3.1	17.7±3.6	16.1±2.7	Dimopoullos et al. (1959b)
F	6–9 m	14	6.4±1.4	53.0±2.6	20.9±1.2	19.8±2.4	Dimopoullos et al. (1959b)
F	3–6 m	20	5.0±1.3	58.0±2.6	21.4±1.2	15.6±1.5	Dimopoullos et al. (1959b)
F	<3 m	11	3.9±1.2	63.4±1.7	19.4±1.0	13.4±1.5	Dimopoullos et al. (1959b)
—	—	13	7±4	51±6	23±4	20±5	Decker et al. (1959)

TABLE IV NORMAL PLASMA GLYCOPROTEIN VALUES

Species	Sex	Age	No. of animals	Protein-bound nonglucosamine polysaccharide: absolute concentrations (mg/100 ml)					Reference
				Albumin	α-	β-	γ-	Total	
Bovine	M	>2 y	35	4.6±0.8	53.6±1.5	37.7±1.4	29.9±1.5	124.8±2.3	Dimopoullos et al. (1959b)
	F	>2 y	125	3.8±0.4	62.7±1.2	28.3±0.6	25.6±0.8	120.4±1.5	Dimopoullos et al. (1959b)
	M,F	>2 y	160	3.9±0.4	60.7±1.1	30.4±0.6	26.3±0.7	121.3±1.3	Dimopoullos et al. (1959b)
	F	18–24 m	28	3.7±0.7	58.0±2.0	28.3±1.2	18.9±1.1	108.9±1.7	Dimopoullos et al. (1959b)
	F	12–18 m	26	2.7±0.8	62.5±2.8	26.8±1.3	20.0±1.3	112.0±2.8	Dimopoullos et al. (1959b)
	F	9–12 m	8	3.7±1.5	63.6±3.0	18.4±3.7	16.4±2.7	102.0±2.9	Dimopoullos et al. (1959b)
	F	6–9 m	14	6.9±1.4	58.6±3.7	23.2±1.8	21.9±2.1	110.6±5.1	Dimopoullos et al. (1959b)
	F	3–6 m	20	4.9±1.3	59.5±3.2	21.8±1.2	15.9±1.5	102.0±2.1	Dimopoullos et al. (1959b)
	F	<3 m	11	3.7±1.1	58.9±1.4	18.1±1.1	12.5±1.5	93.1±1.5	Dimopoullos et al. (1959b)
	—	—	13	—	—	—	—	124±12	Decker et al. (1959)
	—	—		—	—	—	—	120	Weimer and Quinn (1958)
	F	Adult	23	—	—	—	—	101.9±1.50	Patterson et al. (1968)

TABLE IV (continued)

Species	Sex	Age	No. of animals	Albumin	α-	β-	γ-	Total	Reference
				Protein-bound nonglucosamine polysaccharide: absolute concentrations (mg/100 ml)					
Porcine	M,F	200 lb (body weight)	10	—	—	—	—	163±6	Shetlar et al. (1958)
Equine	—	—	—	—	—	—	—	115	Weimer and Quinn (1958)
Rat	M	65–200 d	—	17	52	—	—	155	Shetlar et al. (1950)
	M,F	—	46	16±0.4	—	—	—	164±4	Shetlar et al. (1955)
	—	—	—	—	—	—	—	156	Weimer and Quinn (1958)
	M	3 m	8	—	—	—	—	117.4±17.9	Abreu et al. (1957)
	—	—	—	—	—	—	—	142±2.7	Weimer et al. (1954)
	—	—	—	—	—	—	—	94	Weimer and Quinn (1958)
Canine	—	—	—	—	—	—	—	80	Weimer and Quinn (1958)
Rabbit	—	—	—	—	—	—	—	77±1.8	Weimer et al. (1954)
Guinea pig	—	—	—	—	—	—	—	116	Weimer and Quinn (1958)
	—	—	—	—	—	—	—	110±1.8	Weimer et al. (1954)
	—	—	18	—	—	—	29±0.7	117±2.2	Weimer et al. (1957)

TABLE V NORMAL PLASMA GLYCOPROTEIN VALUES (MISCELLANEOUS GLYCOPROTEINS)

Species	Sex	Age	No. of animals	Absolute concentrations (mg/100 ml)				Reference
				Muco-protein polysac-charide	Portein-bound sialic acid	Sero-mucoid	Protein:polysac-charide ratio	
Rabbit	—	—	—	10±0.5	—	—	1.3±0.03	Weimer et al. (1954)
Guinea pig	—	—	—	28±0.8	—	—	2.1±0.03	Weimer et al. (1954)
Canine	—	—	—	—	—	34±0.5	—	Weimer et al. (1957)
	—	—	—	—	—	—	1.8	Weimer and Quinn (1958)
Rat	—	—	—	21±0.7	—	—	2.3±0.04	Weimer et al. (1954)
	—	—	—	—	—	8±0.4	—	Shetlar et al. (1955)
Equine	—	—	—	9.6±1.9	—	—	—	Abreu et al. (1957)
	—	—	—	—	—	—	1.6	Weimer and Quinn (1958)
Bovine	M,F	1 y	51	—	1.69±0.32	—	—	Cornelius et al. (1960)
	F	3–84 m	215	—	—	—	1.53	Dimopoullos (1961b)
	—	—	—	—	—	—	1.5	Weimer and Quinn (1958)
Ovine	M	1 y	7	—	2.87±0.45	—	—	Cornelius et al. (1960)
	F	1 y	16	—	1.86±0.53	—	—	Cornelius et al. (1960)
	M,F	6 m	35	—	2.12±0.76	—	—	Cornelius et al. (1960)
Porcine	M,F	3 m	5	—	5.51±1.07	—	—	Cornelius et al. (1960)
	M,F	200 lb (body weight)	10	—	—	12±0.7	—	Shetlar et al. (1958)
Caprine	M,F	6 m	5	—	2.26±0.70	—	—	Cornelius et al. (1960)

TABLE VI NORMAL PLASMA LIPOPROTEIN VALUES

Species	Sex	Age	No. of animals	Albumin	α-	Protein-bound lipoprotein: relative concentrations (%)						Reference
						α_1-	α_2-	β-	β_1-	β_2-	γ-	
Bovine	M	10–12 m	30	—	48.6 ±6.8	—	—	22.7 ±3.6	—	—	28.7 ±3.0	Perk and Lobl (1959b)
	F	10–12 m	8	—	67.8 ±6.2	—	—	14.2 ±3.1	13.7 ±3.28	11.4 ±1.47	18.0 ±2.1	Perk and Lobl (1959b)
	F	5 y	10	5.1 ±0.97	63.5 ±2.35	—	—	—	—	—	5.9 ±1.45	Perk and Lobl (1959b)
Ovine	M	3 m	6	50.2 ±2.67	18.3 ±3.14	—	—	9.3 ±2.13	—	—	21.0 ±3.47	Perk and Lobl (1960)
	M	10–12 m	6	44.8 ±1.97	19.3 ±2.12	—	—	19.7 ±2.01	—	—	16.1 ±2.02	Perk and Lobl (1960)
Rabbit	—	—		—	26.3	—	—	—	—	—	(β + "0"- 73.7)	Dunlap et al. (1959)
Duck	M	3 m	8	—	—	60.4 ±10.4	—	39.6 ±10.4	—	—	—	Perk and Lobl (1961a)
	F	3 m	8	—	—	61.8 ±10.8	—	38.2 ±10.6	—	—	—	Perk and Lobl (1961a)
	M	8 m	8	—	—	42.5 ±6.2	12.0 ±2.0	45.5 ±4.8	—	—	—	Perk and Lobl (1961a)
	F	8 m	8	—	—	5.0 ±2.1	19.0 ±4.3	76.0 ±6.0	—	—	—	Perk and Lobl (1961a)

There are other considerations given to the omission of tabulated data in disease. Techniques and criteria for interpretation vary and "standard" abnormal values cannot be obtained. Furthermore, the plasma proteins usually vary both qualitatively and quantitatively in successive stages of most abnormal conditions and disease states.

REFERENCES

Abreu, L. A., Abreu, R. R., and Villela, G. G. (1957). *Proc. Soc. Exptl. Biol. Med.* **94**, 375.

Allen, R. C., and Watson, D. F. (1958). *Am. J. Vet. Res.* **19**, 1001.

Allison, J. B. (1957). *J. Am. Med. Assoc.* **164**, 283.

Allison, J. B. (1958). *Voeding* **19**, 119.

Allison, J. B., and Wannemacher, R. W., Jr. (1960). *Protides Biol. Fluids, Proc. Colloq.* **7**, 281.

Annau, E., Corner, A. H., Magwood, S. E., and Jerichs, K. (1964). *Can. J. Comp. Med. Vet. Sci.* **28**, 264.

Ashton, G. C. (1957). *Nature* **180**, 917.

Balch, H. H. (1950). *J. Immunol.* **64**, 397.

Baldwin, R. W., and Iland, C. N. (1953). *Am. Rev. Tuberc.* **68**, 372.

Banerjee, S., and Rohatgi, L. (1958). *Proc. Soc. Exptl. Biol. Med.* **97**, 234.

Barboriak, J. J., de Bella, G., Setnikar, I., and Krehl, W. A. (1958a). *Am. J. Physiol.* **193**, 89.

Barboriak, J. J., Meschia, G., Barron, D. H., and Cowgill, G. R. (1958b). *Proc. Soc. Exptl. Biol. Med.* **98**, 635.

Beaton, J. R. (1961). *Proc. Soc. Exptl. Biol. Med.* **107**, 426.

Beckett, S. D., Burns, M. J., and Clark, C. H. (1964). *Am. J. Vet. Res.* **25**, 1186.

Benditt, E. P., Wissler, R. W., Woolridge, R. L., Rowley, D. A., and Steffee, C. H., Jr. (1949). *Proc. Soc. Exptl. Biol. Med.* **70**, 240.

Bernfeld, P., and Homburger, F. (1954). *Proc. Am. Assoc. Cancer Res.* **1**, 5.

Bernfeld, P., Donahue, V. M., and Homburger, F. (1953). *Proc. Soc. Exptl. Biol. Med.* **83**, 429.

Bieler, M. M., Ecker, E. E., and Spies, T. D. (1947). *J. Lab. Clin. Med.* **32**, 130.

Bjorneboe, M. (1944). *Acta Pathol. Microbiol. Scand.* **20**, 221.

Bjorneboe, M., Raaschou, F., and Sondergard, T. (1952). *Acta Endocrinol.* **9**, 318.

Boguth, W. (1953). *Naturwissenschaften* **40**, 22.

Bossak, E. T., Wang, C. I., and Adlersberg, D. (1955). *Proc. Soc. Exptl. Biol. Med.* **88**, 634.

Bradish, C. J., and Brooksby, J. B. (1954). *Biochem. J.* **56**, 342.

Bradish, C. J., Henderson, W. M., and Brooksby, J. B. (1954a). *Biochem. J.* **56**, 329.

Bradish, C. J., Henderson, W. M., and Brooksby, J. B. (1954b). *Biochem. J.* **56**, 335.

Brandt, L. W., Clegg, R. E., and Andrews, A. C. (1951). *J. Biol. Chem.* **191**, 105.

Brandt, L. W., Smith, H. D., Andrews, A. C., and Clegg, R. E. (1952). *Arch. Biochem. Biophy.* **36**, 11.

Brown, F. (1960). *J. Immunol.* **85**, 298.

Brown, F., and Graves, J. H. (1959). *Nature* **183**, 1688.

Brown, J. M. M., and Abrams, L. (1965). *Onderstepoort J. Vet. Res.* **32**, 119.

Brueckner, A. H., Taylor, H. L., Schroeder, J. P., and Loehler, A. (1959). *Proc. Soc. Exptl. Biol. Med.* **102**, 20.

Bueker, E. D. (1961). *Proc. Soc. Exptl. Biol. Med.* **106**, 373.

Cannon, P. R., Chase, W. E., and Wissler, R. W. (1943). *J. Immunol.* **47**, 133.

Chanutin, A., and Gjessing, E. C. (1946). *J. Biol. Chem.* **165**, 421.

Chow, B. F., Seeley, R. D., Allison, J. B., and Cole, W. H. (1948). *Arch. Biochem.* **16**, 69.

Clark, J. D., and Foster, J. W. (1968). *Am. J. Vet. Res.* **29**, 1293.

Clegg, R. E., Sanford, P. E., Hein, R. E., Andrews, A. C., Hughes, J. S., and Mueller, C. D. (1951). *Science* **114**, 437.

Cochrane, D., Rice, C. E., and Carriere, J. (1965). *Can. J. Comp. Med. Vet. Sci.* **29**, 209.

Comer, E. O'B., Swartzwelder, J. C., and Jones, C. A. (1956). *J. Parasitol.* **42**, 25.

Common, R. H., McKinley, W. P., and Maw, W. A. (1953). *Science* **118**, 86.

Cornelius, C. E., Goodbary, R. F., and Kennedy, P. C. (1959). *Cornell. Vet.* **49**, 478.

Cornelius, C. E., Rhode, E. A., and Bishop, J. A. (1960). *Am. J. Vet. Res.* **21**, 1095.

Cornelius, C. E., Baker, N. F., Kaneko, J. J., and Douglas, J. R. (1962). *Am. J. Vet. Res.* **23**, 837.

Davidson, D. A., and Lawrence, E. A. (1954). *Proc. Am. Assoc. Cancer Res.* **1**, 11.

Decker, B., McKenzie, B. F., and McGuckin, W. F. (1959). *Proc. Soc. Exptl. Biol. Med.* **102**, 616.

de Lamirande, G., and Cantero, A. (1952). *Cancer Res.* **12**, 330.

Deutsch, H. F., Nichol, J. C., and Cohn, M. (1949). *J. Immunol.* **63**, 195.

de Wael, J. (1956). *Ciba Found. Symp, Paper Electrophoresis* p. 22.

de Wael, J., and Teunissen, G. H. B. (1954). *Tijdschr. Diergeneesk.* **79**, 447.

Dickerson, J. W. T., and Southgate, D. A. T. (1967). *Biochem. J.* **103**, 493.

Dimopoullos, G. T. (1961a). *Ann. N. Y. Acad. Sci.* **94**, 149.

Dimopoullos, G. T. (1961b). *Am. J. Vet. Res.* **22**, 986.

Dimopoullos, G. T., and Cunningham, C. H. (1956). *Am. J. Vet. Res.* **17**, 755.

Dimopoullos, G. T., and Fellowes, O. N. (1958). *J. Immunol.* **81**, 199.

Dimopoullos, G. T., Foote, L. E., and Schrader, G. T. (1959a). *Am. J. Vet. Res.* **20**, 270.

Dimopoullos, G. T., Schrader, G. T., and Fletcher, B. H. (1959b). *Proc. Soc. Exptl. Biol. Med.* **102**, 704.

Dimopoullos, G. T., Schrader, G. T., and Foote, L. E. (1960). *Am. J. Vet. Res.* **21**, 222.

Dittmer, D. S., ed. (1961). "Blood and Other Body Fluids." Federation Am. Soc. Exptl. Biol., Washington, D.C.

Dobson, C. (1965). *Nature* **207**, 1304.

Dole, V. P. (1944). *J. Clin. Invest.* **23**, 708.

Dolyak, F., and Leone, C. A. (1953). *Trans. Kansas Acad. Sci.* **56**, 242.

Dunlap, J. S., and Dickson, W. M. (1955). *Am. J. Vet. Res.* **58**, 91.

Dunlap, J. S., Dickson, W. M., and Johnson, V. L. (1959). *Am. J. Vet. Res.* **20**, 589.

Ebel, K. H. (1953). *Zentr. Veterinärmed.* **1**, 70.

Erwin, E. S., Varnell, T. R., and Page, H. M. (1959). *Proc. Soc. Exptl. Biol. Med.* **100**, 373.

Forstner, M. J. (1968). *Zentr. Veterinärmed.* **AI**, 76.

Foster, J. F., Friedell, R. W., Catron, D., and Diechmann, M. R. (1950). *Iowa State Coll. J. Sci.* **24**, 421.

Freeman, M. J. (1964). *Am. J. Vet. Res.* **25**, 599.

Ganzin, M., Rebeyrotte, P., Macheboeuf, M., and Montezin, G. (1952). *Bull. Soc. Pathol. Exotique* **45**, 518.

Garner, R. J., Crawley, W., and Goddard, P. J. (1957). *J. Comp. Pathol. Therap.* **67**, 354.

Gilman, A. R. (1952). *Am. J. Vet. Res.* **13**, 83.

Ginchereau, M. A., and Chute, H. L. (1956). *Am. J. Vet. Res.* **17**, 531.

Gleason, T. L., and Friedberg, F. (1953). *Physiol. Zool.* **26**, 95.

Gorczyca, L. R., and McCarty, R. T. (1959). *Vet. Med.* **54**, 373.

Gorczyca, L. R., McCarty, R. T., and Lazaroni, J. A., Jr. (1960). *Am. J. Vet. Res.* **21**, 851.

Greenberg, L. D., Hoessly, U. J. P., Brooks, R., and Rinehart, J. F. (1952). *Proc. Soc. Expt. Biol. Med.* **79**, 425.

Groulade, P., and Groulade, J. (1953). *Ann. Inst. Pasteur* **85**, 508.

Hahn, P. F., Baugh, P., and Meng, H. C. (1956). *Proc. Soc. Exptl. Biol. Med.* **93**, 448.

Halliday, G. J., Mulligan, W., and Dalton, R. G. (1968). *Res. Vet. Sci.* **9**, 224.

Hansen, R. G., and Phillips, P. H. (1947). *J. Biol. Chem.* **171**, 223.

Henson, J. B. (1964). *Am. J. Vet. Res.* **25**, 1706.

Henson, J. B., Leader, R. W., and Gorham, J. R. (1961). *Proc. Soc. Exptl. Biol. Med.* **107**, 919.

Herlich, H., and Merkal, R. S. (1963). *J. Parasitol.* **49**, 623.

Hirtz, J. (1952). *Rev. Immunol.* **16**, 297.

Hoch-Ligeti, C., Irvine, K., and Sprinkle, E. P. (1953). *Proc. Soc. Exptl. Biol. Med.* **84**, 707.

Holmes, P. H., Dargie, J. D., Maclean, J. M., and Mulligan, W. (1968). *Vet. Record* **83**, 227.

Hort, I. (1968). *Am. J. Vet. Res.* **29**, 813.

Howard, E. B., and Kenyon, A. J. (1965). *Am. J. Vet. Res.* **26**, 1132.

Hudgins, P. C., and Patnode, R. A. (1957). *Proc. Soc. Exptl. Biol. Med.* **95**, 181.

Hudgins, P. C., Cummings, M. M., and Patnode, R. A. (1956). *Proc. Soc. Exptl. Biol. Med.* **92**, 75.

Irfan, M. (1967). *Res. Vet. Sci.* **8**, 137.

Jacox, R. F., and Feldmahn, A. (1956). *J. Exptl. Med.* **103**, 633.

Jeffay, H., and Winzler, R. J. (1958). *J. Biol. Chem.* **231**, 111.

Jennings, F. W., and Mulligan, W. (1953). *J. Comp. Pathol. Therap.* **63**, 286.

Johnson, R. M., Albert, S., Pinkus, H., and Wagshal, R. R. (1954). *Proc. Am. Assoc. Cancer Res.* **1**, 23.

Kao, K. Y. T., Reagan, R. L., and Brueckner, A. L. (1954). *Am. J. Vet. Res.* **15**, 343.

Kekwick, R. A. (1959). *Advan. Protein Chem.* **14**, 231.

Kenyon, A. J., Trautwein, G., and Helmboldt, C. F. (1963). *Am. J. Vet. Res.* **24**, 168.

Kenyon, A. J., Williams, R. C., Jr., and Howard, E. B. (1966). *Proc. Soc. Exptl. Biol. Med.* **123**, 510.

Kiesel, G. K., and Alexander, H. D. (1966). *Am. J. Vet. Res.* **27**, 121.

Klaus, G. G. B., and Jones, E. W. (1968). *J. Immunol.* **100**, 991.

Kniazeff, A. J., Rimer, V., and Gaeta, L. (1967). *Nature* **214**, 805.

Knill, L. M., Podleski, T. R., and Childs, W. A. (1958). *Proc. Soc. Exptl. Biol. Med.* **97**, 224.

Koenig, V. L., Perrings, J. D., and Mundy, F. (1949). *Arch. Biochem.* **22**, 377.

Kóňa, E. (1957). *Vet. Med. (Prague)* **2**, 159.

Kóňa, E., Havassy, I., Zimmerman, J., and Kaduk, J. (1966). *Vet. Med. (Prague)* **11**, 517.

Kuttler, K. L., and Marble, D. W. (1960). *Am. J. Vet. Res.* **21**, 445.

Lane, S. L. (1952). *Oral Surg., Oral Med., Oral Pathol.* **5**, 434.

Larson, B. L. (1958). *J. Dairy Sci.* **41**, 1033.

Larson, B. L., and Hays, R. L. (1958). *J. Dairy Sci.* **41**, 995.

Larson, B. L., and Kendall, K. A. (1957). *J. Dairy Sci.* **40**, 659.

Larson, B. L., and Touchberry, R. W. (1959). *J. Animal Sci.* **18**, 983.

Leland, S. E., Jr. (1961). *Ann. N. Y. Acad. Sci.* **94**, 163.

Leland, S. E., Jr., Drudge, J. H., and Wyant, Z. N. (1959). *Exptl. Parasitol.* **8**, 383.

Leland, S. E., Jr., Drudge, J. H., and Wyant, Z. N. (1960). *Am. J. Vet. Res.* **21**, 458.

Leland, S. E., Jr., Drudge, J. H., and Dillard, R. P. (1961). *J. Parasitol.* **47**, Sect. 2, 21.

Leveille, G. A., and Sauberlich, H. E. (1961). *J. Nutr.* **74**, 500.

Leveille, G. A., Fisher, H., and Feigenbaum, A. S. (1961). *Ann. N. Y. Acad. Sci.* **94**, 265.

Lewis, L. A., and Page, I. H. (1947). *Federation Proc.* **6**, No. 1.

Lewis, L. A., and Page, I. H. (1956). *Circulation* **14**, 55.

Locatelli, A. (1956). *Atti. Soc. Ital Sci. Vet.* **10**, 286.

Long, C., ed. (1961). "Biochemists' Handbook." Van Nostrand, Princeton, New Jersey.

Lynch, J. E., and Stafseth, H. J. (1953). *Poultry Sci.* **32**, 1068.

Lynch, J. E., and Stafseth, H. J. (1954). *Poultry Sci.* **33** No. 1, 54.

Marht, J. L., Hammond, D. M., and Miner, M. L. (1964). *Cornell Vet.* **54**, 453.

Marshall, M. E., and Deutsch, H. F. (1950). *J. Biol. Chem.* **185**, 155.

Mathews, J., and Buthala, D. A. (1955). *Vet. Med.* **50**, 213.

Moore, D. H. (1945). *J. Biol. Chem.* **161**, 21.

Moore, D. H. (1948). *Endocrinology* **42**, 38.

Murphy, F. A., Osebold, J. W., and Aalund, O. (1965). *Arch. Biochem. Biophys.* **112**, 126.

Murphy, F. A., Osebold, J. W., and Aalund, O. (1966a). *Am. J. Vet. Res.* **27**, 971.

Murphy, F. A., Osebold, J. W., and Aalund, O. (1966b). *J. Infect. Diseases* **116**, 99.

Németh, I., and Juhász, S. (1968). *Acta Vet. Acad. Sci. Hung.* **18**, 95.

Ortega, L. G., and Mellors, R. C. (1957). *J. Exptl. Med.* **106**, 627.

Page, I. H., and Lewis, L. A. (1951). *Am. J. Physiol.* **164**, 61.

Papp, E., and Sikes, D. (1964). *Am. J. Vet. Res.* **25**, 1112.

Pareira, M. D., Sicher, N., and Lang, S. (1958). *A. M. A. Arch. Surg.* **77**, 191.

Pareira, M. D., Sicher, N., and Lang, S. (1959). *Ann. Surg.* **149**, 243.

Patterson, D. S. P., and Sweasey, D. (1966). *Vet. Record* **78**, 364.

Patterson, D. S. P., Allen, W. M., Berrett, S., Ivins, L. N., and Sweasey, D. (1968). *Res. Vet. Sci.* **9**, 117.

Perk, K., and Lobl, K. (1959a). *Brit. Vet. J.* **115**, 1.

Perk, K., and Lobl, K. (1959b). *Am. J. Vet. Res.* **20**, 989.

Perk, K., and Lobl, K. (1960). *Brit. Vet. J.* **116**, 1.

Perk, K. and Lobl, K. (1961a). *Schweiz. Arch. Tierheilk.* **103**, 379.

Perk, K., and Lobl, K. (1961b). *Am. J. Vet. Res.* **22**, 217.

Perk, K., and Lobl, K. (1962). *Am. J. Vet. Res.* **23**, 171.

Perk, K., and Loebl, K. (1959). *Schweiz. Arch. Tierheilk.* **101**, 548.

Perk, K., and Loebl, K. (1960). *Refuah Vet.* **17**, 46.

Perk, K., Loebl, K., and Allalouf, D. (1959). *Bull. Res. Council Israel* **E7**, 201.

Perk, K., Perek, M., Loebl, K., and Allalouf, D. (1960). *Poultry Sci.* **39**, 775.

Petermann, M. L. (1960). *In* "The Plasma Proteins" (F. W. Putnam, ed.), Vol. 2, p. 310. Academic Press, New York.

Petermann, M. L. (1961). *Ann. N. Y. Acad. Sci.* **94**, 144.

Pierce, A. E. (1955). *J. Hyg.* **53**, 247.

Polson, A. (1952). *Onderstepoort J. Vet. Res.* **25**, 7.

Polson, A., and Malherbe, W. D. (1952). *Onderstepoort J. Vet. Res.* **25**, 13.

Porter, D. D., and Dixon, F. J. (1966). *Am. J. Vet. Res.* **27**, 335.

Rao, R. R., and Cohly, M. A. (1953). *Current Sci.* (*India*) **22**, 204.

Reda, H., Moustafa, E. M., and Salam, H. (1957). *Brit. Vet. J.* **113**, 504.

Ringen, L. M., and Akhtar, A. S. (1968). *Avian Diseases* **12**, 4.

Roberts, S. (1954). *Proc. Am. Assoc. Cancer Res.* **1**, 41.

Rogers, T. E., and Dimopoullos, G. T. (1962). *Proc. Soc. Exptl. Biol. Med.* **110**, 359.

Rook, J. A. F., Moustgaard, J., and Jakobsen, P. E. (1951). *Kgl. Vet.–og LandBohojskole, Ars.* pp. 81–92; see *Biol. Abstr.* **27**, 27237 (1953).

Rose, J. E., and Amerault, T. E. (1964). *Am. J. Vet. Res.* **25**, 998.

Ross, J. G., and Todd, J. R. (1965). *Brit. Vet. J.* **121**, 55.

Rutqvist, L. (1958). *Am. J. Vet. Res.* **19**, 25.

San Clemente, C. L. (1942). *Am. J. Vet. Res.* **3**, 219.

San Clemente, C. L., and Huddleson, I. F. (1943). *Mich. State Coll. Agr., Agr. Expt. Sta., Tech. Bull.* **182**, 3.

Sanders, E., Huddleson, I. F., and Schaible, P. J. (1944). *J. Biol. Chem.* **155**, 469.

Sandor, G. (1966). "Serum Proteins in Health and Disease." Williams & Wilkins, Baltimore, Maryland.

Schechtman, A. M., and Hoffman, H. (1952). *Ann. N. Y. Acad. Sci.* **55**, 85.

Schinazi, L. A. (1957). *Science* **125**, 695.

Schlumberger, H. G., and Wall, R. L. (1957). *Proc. Soc. Exptl. Biol. Med.* **96**, 43.

Schultz, J., Jamison, W., Shay, H., and Gruenstein, M. (1954). *Arch. Biochem. Biophys.* **50**, 124.

Scopes, R. K. (1963). *Nature* **197**, 1201.

Seibert, F. B., and Nelson, J. W. (1942). *J. Biol. Chem.* **143**, 29.

Seibert, F. B., Seibert, M. V., Atno, A. J., and Campbell, N. W. (1947). *J. Clin. Invest.* **26**, 90.

Shedlovsky, T., and Scudder, J. (1942). *J. Exptl. Med.* **75**, 114.

Shetlar, M. R., Foster, J. V., Kelley, K. H., and Everett, M. R. (1948). *Proc. Soc. Exptl. Biol. Med.* **69**, 507.

Shetlar, M. R., Erwin, C. P., and Everett, M. R. (1950). *Cancer Res.* **10**, 445.

Shetlar, M. R., Shetlar, C. L., and Payne, R. W. (1955). *Endocrinology* **56**, 167.

Shetlar, M. R., Shetlar, C. L., Payne, R. W., Neher, G. M., and Swenson, C. B. (1958). *Proc. Soc. Exptl. Biol. Med.* **98**, 254.

Slizewicz, P., and Atanasiu, P. (1953). *Ann. Inst. Pasteur* **85**, 505.

Smith, L. C., DesAutels, E. J., and Downey, G. J. (1954). *Proc. Soc. Exptl. Biol. Med.* **85**, 643.

Smithies, O., and Hickman, C. G. (1958). *Genetics* **43**, 374.

Snow, L. M., Burns, M. J., and Clark, C. H. (1966). *Am. J. Vet. Res.* **27**, 70.

Sohar, E., Bossak, E. T., Wang, C. I., and Adlersberg, D. (1956). *Science* **123**, 461.

Spector, W. S., ed. (1956). "Handbook of Biological Data." Saunders, Philadelphia, Pennsylvania.

Srivastava, R. K. (1959). M.V.Sc. Thesis, University of Agra, India.

Stockl, W., and Zacherl, M. K. (1953). *Z. Physiol. Chem.* **293**, 278.

Sturkie, P. D. (1951). *Endocrinology* **49**, 565.

Sturkie, P. D., and Newman, H. J. (1951). *Poultry Sci.* **30**, 240.

Tanaka, K., and Aoki, S. (1963). *Natl. Inst. Animal Health Quart.* **3**, 49.

Turner, J. H., and Wilson, G. I. (1962). *Am. J. Vet. Res.* **23**, 718.

Volk, B. W., Saifer, A., Johnson, L. E., and Oreskes, I. (1953). *Am. Rev. Tuberc.* **67**, 299.

Wagner, M. (1959). *Ann. N. Y. Acad. Sci.* **78**, 261.

Wagner, M., and Wostmann, B. S. (1961). *Ann. N. Y. Acad. Sci.* **94**, 210.

Wall, R. L., Sun, L., and Picklow, F. E. (1956). *RES Bull.* **2**, 50.

Weber, T. B. (1964). *Am. J. Vet. Res.* **25**, 386.

Wehmeyer, P. (1954a). *Acta Pathol. Microbiol. Scand.* **34**, 518.

Wehmeyer, P. (1954b). *Acta Pathol. Microbiol. Scand.* **34**, 591.

Weide, K. D., and King, N. B. (1962). *Am. J. Vet. Res.* **23**, 744.

Weimer, H. E. (1961). *Ann. N. Y. Acad. Sci.* **94**, 225.

Weimer, H. E., and Moshin, J. R. (1953). *Am. Rev. Tuberc.* **68**, 594.

Weimer, H. E., and Quinn, F. A. (1958). *Clin. Chim. Acta* **3**, 419.

Weimer, H. E., Carpenter, C. M., Redlich-Moshin, J., Little, M. S., and Nelson, E. L. (1954). *Physiol. Zool.* **27** 341.

Weimer, H. E., Redlich-Moshin, J., Quinn, F. A., and Nelson, E. L. (1957). *J. Immunol.* **78**, 1.

Weimer, H. E., Bell, R. T., and Nishihara, H. (1959a). *Proc. Soc. Exptl. Biol. Med.* **100**, 853.

Weimer, H. E., Bell, R. T., and Nishihara, H. (1959b). *Proc. Soc. Exptl. Biol. Med.* **102**, 689.

Williams, C. A., Jr., and Wemyss, C. T., Jr. (1961). *J. Exptl. Med.* **114**, 311.

Wilson, G. I., and Turner, J. H. (1965). *Am. J. Vet. Res.* **26**, 645.

Wissler, R. W. (1947). *J. Infect. Diseases* **80**, 264.

Wissler, R. W., Woolridge, R. L., Steffee, C. H., Jr., and Cannon, P. R. (1946). *J. Immunol.* **52**, 267.

Wostmann, B. S. (1959). *Ann. N. Y. Acad. Sci.* **78**, 254.

Wostmann, B. S., and Gordon, H. A. (1958). *Proc. Soc. Exptl. Biol. Med.* **97**, 832.

Wostmann, B. S., and Gordon, H. A. (1960). *J. Immunol.* **84**, 27.

Porphyrin, Heme, and Erythrocyte Metabolism: The Porphyrias*

4

J. J. Kaneko

I. INTRODUCTION

The metal-prophyrin complexes are found widespread in nature as constituents of compounds of fundamental importance in the metabolic processes of life. The photosynthetic pigment of plants, chlorophyll, is a magnesium porphyrin. The

*The work was supported in part by USPHS Grant HE-6678 from the National Heart Institute of the National Institutes of Health.

iron-porphyrin complexes are found in combination with proteins and these include the hemoglobins, myoglobins, cytochromes, and catalase. The porphyrins also exist in nature in the uncombined or free state, and it is this group with which the present chapter will principally deal.

Present knowledge of the porphyrins has its basis in the classic studies of the German physician and chemist, Hans Fischer, whose work on the porphyrins dates back to 1915. More recently, the development of more elegant methods of detection and identification of porphyrins, together with the use of isotopic tracer techniques, have given added impetus to the study of porphyrin biosynthesis and metabolism. This has resulted in the present clearer understanding of the mechanisms of porphyrin biosynthesis and the biochemical bases for the disorders of porphyrin metabolism.

II.   STRUCTURE OF THE PORPHYRINS

The parent nucleus of the porphyrins is a cyclic tetrapyrrole, which consists of four pyrrole nuclei with their α (adjacent to the N) carbon atoms linked together by methene ($-C=$) bridges. This compound is called porphin and is shown in Fig. 1. The various synthetic and naturally occurring porphyrins are derivatives of porphin, distinguished from each other by the type and position of the radicals substituted for the hydrogen atoms at positions 1 through 8. For convenience in discussing the substitutions, the simplified representation of the porphin nucleus, as shown in Fig. 1, is used.

The classification of the prophyrins is based upon the synthetic porphyrin, etioporphyrin (ETIO), in which two different radicals are substituted. The substituted radicals are 4-methyl and 4-ethyl groups. The number of structural isomers

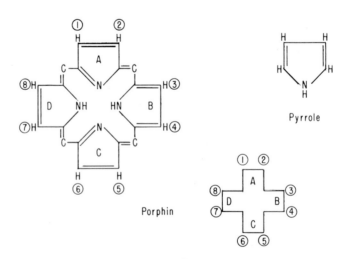

Fig. 1.   Schematic representation of the porphin nucleus.

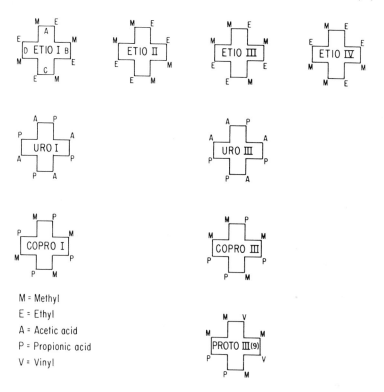

Fig. 2.   The isomeric porphyrins. See text for abbreviations.

possible with these eight radicals are the four shown at the top of Fig. 2. The porphyrins which occur in nature are only those in which the positioning of their substituted radicals correspond to isomers I and III of etioporphyrin. This observation led to reference by Fischer of a "dualism" of porphyrins in nature, which is in essential agreement with present concepts of the biosynthesis of the porphyrin isomers as proceeding along parallel and independent paths.

The uroporphyrins also contain two different radicals, acetic and propionic acid, and four each of these are arranged to correspond to either isomer I or III (Fig. 2). Therefore, these are designated uroporphyrin I (URO I) or uroporphyrin III (URO III). Similarly, the coproporphyrins contain four methyl and four propionic acid groups and are designated coproporphyrin I (COPRO I) and coproporphyrin III (COPRO III). The protoporphyrin of heme (iron–protoporphyrin, the prosthetic group of hemoglobin) corresponds to the series III isomer. In this case, however, three different radicals instead of two are substituted. These consist of four methyl, two propionic acid, and two vinyl radicals. With three different radicals, a total of fifteen isomers is possible, but the protoporphyrin of heme is the only naturally occurring isomer known. This isomer was designated protoporphyrin IX because it was ninth in the series of protoporphyrin isomers listed by Fischer. The arrangement of the methyl groups of this isomer, as shown in Fig. 2, corresponds to that of a type III etioporphyrin isomer and should therefore be more properly termed protoporphyrin III (9) [PROTO III (9)].

Other naturally occurring or artifically prepared porphyrins are derivatives of PROTO III (9). If the two vinyl groups are hydrogenated to ethyl groups, the product is mesoporphyrin III (9). If the two vinyl groups are converted to hydroxy-ethyl groups, the product is hematoporphyrin III (9). Deuteroporphyrin III (9) results if the two vinyl groups are replaced by hydrogen atoms. It should be noted that protoporphyrin and deuteroporphyrin occur in feces but these are considered to be result of intestinal bacterial action upon ingested meat.

III. BIOSYNTHESIS OF THE PORPHYRINS

Present knowledge of the pathway for heme biosynthesis has its basis in the demonstration by Shemin and Rittenberg (1946a) that the nitrogen atom of glycine

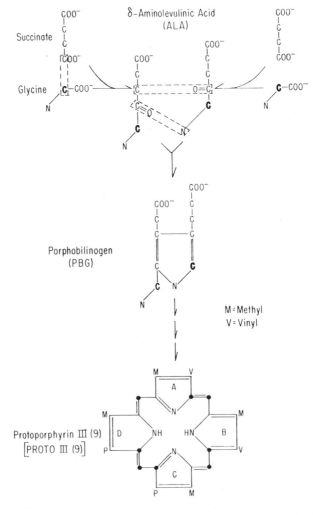

Fig. 3.   The synthesis of protoporphyrin (adapted from Shemin *et al.*, 1955).

TABLE I   SURVIVAL TIME OF ERYTHROCYTES OF VARIOUS DOMESTIC ANIMALS

Isotope	Species	Survival time (days)	Reference
^{15}N	Cat	77	Valentine et al. (1951)
	Rabbit	65–70	Neuberger and Niven (1951)
^{14}C	Horse	140–150	Cornelius et al. (1960)
	Cow	135–162	Kaneko (1963, 1969)
	Cat	66–79	Kaneko et al. (1966)
	Sheep	64–118	Kaneko et al. (1961)
	Goat	125	Kaneko and Cornelius (1962)
	Pig	62	Bush et al. (1955)
	Dog	86–106	Cline and Berlin (1963)

is incorporated into the heme of hemoglobin. The concentration of the isotopic nitrogen (^{15}N) which was observed in heme indicated that the nitrogen atoms of glycine were direct precursors of the nitrogen atoms of the porphyrin ring. These findings were rapidly followed by extensive investigations which have almost completely elucidated the mechanisms of heme biosynthesis. The subject has been extensively reviewed, the most notable being those of Eales (1961), Tschudy (1965), Levere (1968), and Schmid (1966).

It is now known that in addition to contributing the nitrogen atoms, the methyl carbon atom (C-2) of glycine is also incorporated into the porphyrin ring. These supply 8 of the 34 carbon atoms of protoporphyrin: one for each of the four methene bridges and one for each of the pyrroles (Fig. 3). The carboxyl carbon atom of glycine is not incorporated into the molecule. The direct incorporation of the nitrogen atom and the methyl carbon atom of glycine into the heme of hemoglobin has been the basis for a useful technique with which to "tag" the erythrocyte and measure its survival time. In their original studies, Shemin and Rittenberg (1946b) observed that after administering ^{15}N-glycine, the concentration of ^{15}N in the heme of hemoglobin rose rapidly, remained constant for a time and then fell. Statistical analysis of the data indicated a survival time of about 120 days for the human erythrocyte. On a similar basis, glycine labeled at the methyl carbon atom has been employed for studies of the survival time of the erythrocytes of a number of domestic animals (Table I).

The remaining carbon atoms of protoporphyrin are supplied by a tricarboxylic acid (TCA) cycle intermediate, succinyl CoA. A schematic outline of the current concept of porphyrin biosynthesis is shown in Fig. 4.

A. δ-Aminolevulinic Acid (ALA)

The initial step in the synthetic pathway involves the enzymic condensation of glycine with succinyl CoA (Fig. 3, 4) to form δ-aminolevulinic acid (ALA). This reaction requires the presence of vitamin B_6 as pyridoxal phosphate (Gibson et al., 1958), a finding of interest, for anemia is known to occur in pyridoxine deficiency. A pyridoxal-PO_4–glycine complex combines with succinyl CoA (Kikuchi et al., 1958). This condensing reaction which is catalyzed by the enzyme ALA synthetase

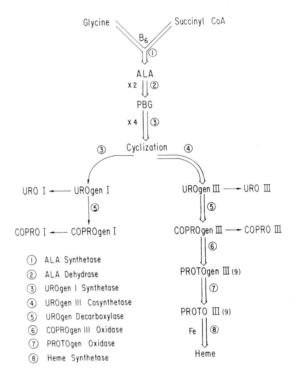

Fig. 4.   Pathways of porphyrin biosynthesis. See text for abbreviations. Note that enzymes 3 and 4 are required to form the heme of hemoglobin.

(ALA-syn) occurs in the mitochondria. The ALA is then transferred into the cytoplasm (Sano and Granick, 1961). The enzyme, ALA-syn, is the rate-controlling enzyme for heme synthesis (Granick, 1966). Its formation is also known to be induced by the chemicals used in the experimental production of porphyria (Granick and Urata, 1963). The inducible synthesis of the enzyme, ALA-syn, and its suppression by negative feedback inhibition by heme is the basis for the mechanism controlling heme synthesis as proposed by Granick and Levere (1964).

B. PORPHOBILINOGEN (PBG)

The enzymic condensation of two molecules of ALA (Figs. 3 and 4) to form the precursor pyrrole, porphobilinogen (PBG), is also known. This compound has been isolated from the urine of patients with the hepatic type of porphyria (Westall, 1952), and its structure (Fig. 3) as established by Cookson and Rimington (1953) is compatible with the mechanism shown in Fig. 4. This step and all those leading to coproporphrinogen (Fig. 4) occurs in the cytoplasm of the cell. The enzyme catalyzing this reaction, ALA-dehydrase, has been reported to contain copper (Iodice et al., 1958), and copper is a known requirement for hemoglobin synthesis (Anderson and Tove, 1958). Although the anemia of copper deficiency is well known, the mechanism for the role of copper in hemoglobin synthesis remains unclear (Cartwright and Wintrobe, 1964). Studies of the anemia of copper deficiency in swine have indicated a close similarity to iron-deficiency anemia and have led to the conclusion that copper deficiency affects iron metabolism in one or more ways (Bush *et al.*, 1956). This enzyme, ALA-dehydrase, is blocked by lead and the determination of ALA in the urine is now commonly used to detect exposure to lead and lead poisoning.

C. PORPHYRINOGENS AND PROTOPORPHYRIN

The earlier assumptions that the formation of the uroporphyrins was the next step in the biosynthesis of heme were soon found to be untenable. The next intermediate is now known to be the reduced form of uroporphyrin, uroporphyrinogen (UROgen). It is now known that the oxidized forms, the uroporphyrins, are side-reaction products of the biosynthetic reactions which lead to protoporphyrin formation (Fig. 4).

The mechanism of cyclization of the four molecules of PBG to form the UROgens continues to be obscure. Several hypotheses have been advanced (Bogorad and Granick, 1953; Shemin *et al.*, 1955; Granick and Mauzerall, 1958), but the mechanism is still unestablished. The observations of Bogorad (1958a,b) on plant extracts provide an indication of the enzymic complexity of this step. Uroporphyrinogen synthesis appears to be the result of the combined action of at least two enzymes, porphobilinogen deaminase (PBG-D) now called uroporphyrinogen I synthetase (UROgen I-syn) and uroporphyrinogen isomerase (UROgen-Is) now called uroporphyrinogen III cosynthetase (UROgen III-cosyn). UROgen I-syn (PBG-D) first catalyzes the condensation of PBG to di- or tripyrroles, which are then cyclized in the presence of the second enzyme, UROgen III-cosyn (UROgen-Is), to yield UROgen III. If UROgen I-syn (PBG-D) is the only enzyme present in the system, type I uroporphyrinogen is formed. A system of this type has now been demonstrated in animal tissues (Levin and Coleman, 1967). UROgen I-syn and UROgen III-cosyn were isolated from extracts of spleens from anemic mice and, in the presence of both enzymes, UROgen III was produced.

The 8-carboxyl group UROgens (I or III) formed are next progressively decarboxylated in a stepwise manner (de Viale and Grinstein, 1968), the principal product being the 4-carboxyl group (COPROgen (I or III). The decarboxylating enzyme involved in this step is nonspecific so that it catalyzes the decarboxylation of either the type I or III isomer to the corresponding COPROgen. In the next step, however, the COPROgen-decarboxylating enzyme (COPROgen-oxidase) is specific for COPROgen III and does not decarboxylate COPROgen I. This enzyme catalyzes the transformation of two of the propionic acid groups to two vinyl groups, and the resulting product is protoporphyrinogen III (PROTOgen III), a 2-carboxyl porphyrinogen. The specificity of this decarboxylating enzyme for COPROgen III would explain the occurrence of only type III isomers in nature. Further oxidation of PROTOgen III then results in the formation of protoporphyrin III (9). Protoporphyrin III (9) then combines with 4 moles of iron to form the heme moiety of hemoglobin.

The scheme as outlined (Fig. 4) portrays the current concept of heme biosynthesis which places the uro- and coproporphyrins outside the mainstream of the synthetic pathway. The scheme in Fig. 4 indicates that the mechanism of cyclization remains to be clarified. It should also be noted that the mechanism of heme biosynthesis is an aerobic process associated with the mitochondria. The TCA cycle is an aerobic cycle and therefore a lack of oxygen would preclude the synthesis of succinyl CoA and hence of heme. The conversion of COPROgen III to PROTO III (9) and the incorporation of iron into PROTO III (9) to form heme are also oxygen-requiring systems.

Iron can be incorporated with relative ease by a nonenzymic method into PROTO III (9). Conditions which help to maintain iron in its ferrous (2^+) form such as the presence of reducing agents (ascorbic acid, cysteine, glutathione), or anaerobiosis enhance both enzymic and nonenzymic iron incorporation (Labbe and Hubbard, 1961). The enzymic iron incorporation, however, is more than ten times that of the nonenzymic incorporation. The enzyme heme synthetase (HS) (Fig. 4), also called ferrochelatase, is localized in the mitochondria.

Mitochondria are a requirement for the initial synthesis of ALA and also for the final conversations of COPROgen to heme. The presence of mitochondria in the developmental stages and their absence in the mature nonnucleated erythrocyte would account for the cessation of hemoglobin synthesis upon maturation. A control mechanism for heme biosynthesis has been proposed by Granick and Levere (1964) which is based upon the operon concepts of Jacob and Monod (1963). Heme is central to this mechanism because it is thought to control its own synthesis by repressing the synthesis of ALA-syn and also to inhibit the activity of ALA-syn by feedback inhibition. The overall mechanism and compartmentalization of hemoglobin synthesis in the developing erythrocyte is shown in Fig. 5.

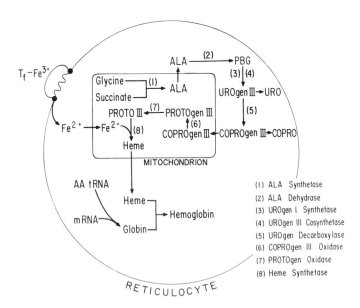

Fig. 5. Summary of hemoglobin synthetic mechanisms in the reticulocyte showing mitochondrial and cytoplasmic separation of activities.

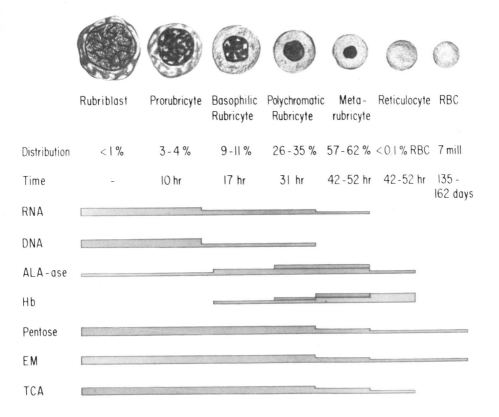

	Rubriblast	Prorubricyte	Basophilic Rubricyte	Polychromatic Rubricyte	Meta- rubricyte	Reticulocyte	RBC
Distribution	< 1 %	3 - 4 %	9 - 11 %	26 - 35 %	57 - 62 %	< 0.1 % RBC	7 mill.
Time	–	10 hr	17 hr	31 hr	42 - 52 hr	42 - 52 hr	135 - 162 days
RNA							
DNA							
ALA-ase							
Hb							
Pentose							
EM							
TCA							

Fig. 6. Summary of metabolic activities of the erythrocytic maturation series. Maturation progresses from left to right. Adapted from various sources. Figures for distribution and duration are from bone marrow of normal cows (Rudolph, 1968).

IV. METABOLISM OF THE ERYTHROCYTE

The metabolism of the erythrocyte has received considerable attention in recent years (Bartlett and Marlow, 1951; Prankerd, 1961; Harris, 1963; Bishop, 1964) largely due to interest in erythrocyte preservation and survival and to the discoveries of inherited erythrocyte enzyme deficiencies. An unexplained anemia of Basenji dogs may be the first of this type of inherited erythrocytic enzyme defect in dogs (Tasker et al., 1969; Ewing, 1969). The current concept of erythrocyte metabolism is summarized in Figs. 6 and 7.

A. DEVELOPING ERYTHROCYTE AND RETICULOCYTE

The developing erythrocyte is a cell comparable in all respects to cells of other tissues and is uniquely occupied with the synthesis of hemoglobin. It contains the nucleus, cytoplasmic particles, and all the enzymic machinery of other cells. During maturation, it respires actively, synthesizes protein and hemoglobin, replicates, and differentiates. Near the end of maturation, it ceases replication and loses its nucleus to become a reticulocyte which continues to respire and to synthesize hemoglobin. Protein synthesis in the reticulocyte occurs on preformed RNA. When it matures, it has lost its ribosomal reticulum (ribonucleoprotein). These changes during the course of maturation are summarized in Fig. 6.

B. MATURE ERYTHROCYTE

The mature erythrocyte, lacking a nucleus, ribosomes, and mitochondria, restricts its metabolism to anaerobic glycolysis (E-M) and the pentose cycle (P-C) pathways. Heme and hemoglobin synthesis ceases and there is no cytochrome or TCA cycle activity. The limited metabolism of the erythrocyte still permits it to survive for a life span characteristic for the species (Table I).

The primary function of the mature erythrocyte is to transport oxygen and this requires that hemoglobin be in its functional reduced state and that the erythrocyte maintains its structural integrity. These tasks are accomplished by erythrocyte

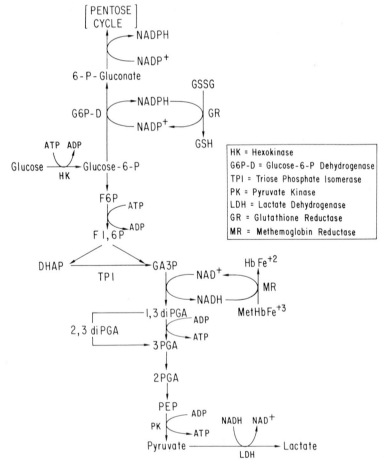

Fig. 7. Summary of carbohydrate metabolism in the mature erythrocyte and the principal mechanisms for reduction of oxidized glutathione and methemoglobin. The complete pentose cycle is shown in Fig. 6 of Chapter 1. See text for abbreviations.

metabolism which depends solely upon glucose utilization. These pathways are summarized in Fig. 7. Glucose enters the cell freely, is dependent on the glucose concentration in the surrounding medium and is independent of insulin. Glucose is first phosphorylated to glucose-6-phosphate (G-6-P) by the rate-limiting hexokinase reaction (Chapman *et al.*, 1962) to initiate glucose catabolism by the mature erythrocyte. The G-6-P formed is then oxidized either by the E-M or P-C pathways.

The enzymic oxidation of G-6-P by G-6-P dehydrogenase (G-6-P-D) in the initial step of the P-C generates NADPH (TPNH) which is the major cofactor in the enzymic reduction of glutathione by glutathione reductase (GR) (Fig. 7).

$$\text{Oxidized glutathione (GSSG)} \xrightarrow[\text{NADPH}]{\text{GR}} \text{reduced glutathione (GSH)}$$

GSH metabolism is important in erythrocyte function but its exact role is unknown. The P-C is the oxygen-utilizing pathway of glucose metabolism in the erythrocyte and under normal conditions, accounts for about 10% of its glucose metabolism (Murphy, 1960). Therefore, the capacity of the mature erythrocyte to use oxygen is limited.

The major pathway for glucose oxidation is the anaerobic E-M pathway in which G-6-P is catabolized to lactate. The E-M pathway provides for at least two other major functions of the erythrocyte. Generation of NADH (DPNH) provides for the reduction of the methemoglobin (MetHb) which is constantly being formed. The reaction catalyzed by the NADH (DPNH)-linked MetHb reductase (MR) is the major reducing mechanism under normal conditions (Fig. 7).

Secondly, the maintenance of cell integrity is associated with the maintenance of ion (Na$^+$, K$^+$) concentration gradients across the erythrocyte membranes. Sodium moves freely into the cell and must be "pumped" out against a concentration gradient (Hoffman, 1962). Potassium is "pumped" in and diffuses out of the cell. The energy for this "pump" is supplied by "high energy" phosphate in the form of ATP which is generated in the E-M pathway. Therefore, metabolic pathways are available for the generation of cofactors (NADPH, NADH) and ATP which are required for the survival of a functional erythrocyte.

The E-M pathway of the erythrocyte differs from that of other tissue cells in that there is high concentration of 2,3-diphosphoglycerate (2,3-diPGA) and glucose-1,6-diphosphate (G-1,6-P) in the erythrocyte. The high concentration of 2,3-diPGA may serve as a phosphate sink and a ready source of phosphate for the synthesis of ATP (Bishop, 1964). Carbohydrate and phosphate storage in the erythrocyte are minimal and the erythrocyte depends upon a constant and ready source of glucose for its energy requirements. When erythrocytes are incubated *in vitro*, structural and degenerative changes occur rapidly in association with depletion of glucose in the medium. Glucose in whole blood is utilized at about 10% per hour at room temperature and is almost completely utilized in 5–6 hours when incubated at 37° C. These metabolic changes are slowed when blood is stored at 4° C with a supply of glucose and with pH controlled. Under these conditions, erythrocytes can be stored for several weeks as is done using the acid–citrate–dextrose (ACD) solutions and may be enhanced by the addition of adenosine or inosine (Gabrio *et al.*, 1956).

In the young erythrocyte, certain of its enzyme activities are high. As the erythrocyte ages, its metabolic activity gradually decreases in association with decreases in these enzyme activities. Among those known to decrease with age are hexokinase (HK), glucose-6-phosphate dehydrogenase (G-6-P-D), pyruvate kinase (PK), triosephosphate isomerase (TPI), and lactate dehydrogenase (LDH) (Fig. 7). When the metabolism is reduced to a point where the energy requirements of the erythrocyte are not being met, it undergoes destruction to complete its life span.

V. DETERMINATION OF THE PORPHYRINS

The principal method now employed for detection of porphyrins in biological materials in the clinical laboratory is based upon the characteristic red fluorescence observed when acidic solutions of the porphyrins are exposed to ultraviolet light. The color of the fluorescence cannot be used to distinguish between the uroporphyrins and the coproporphyrins and therefore these must be separated prior to examination for fluorescence. The separation procedures take advantage of the solubility differences of the porphyrins in various organic solvents. In general, the following solubility properties are principally employed in the separation of the uroporphyrins from the coproporphyrins:

1. The coproporphyrins are soluble in diethyl ether, but the uroporphyrins are not, and therefore these remain in the aqueous phase.
2. Both uroporphyrin and coproporphyrin are soluble in strong acid (usually 1.5 N HCl). Coproporphyrins may, therefore, be extracted from the organic phase with 1.5 N HCl. The uroporphyrins in the aqueous phase may be adsorbed with Al_2O_3 and subsequently eluted with 1.5 N HCl.

The acidic solutions of the porphyrins obtained may then be observed visually for fluorescence or determined quantitatively in a sensitive fluorometer. The most suitable condition for the excitation of fluorescence is the use of ultraviolet light in the near-visible range upon aqueous solutions of the porphyrins at pH 1–2. Further means of identification include spectrophotometric examination, melting points of their methyl esters, and paper chromatography. The methods for the quantitative determination of the porphyrins in biological materials have been presented in detail (Schwartz *et al.*, 1960) and should be consulted. The following simplified screening procedures may be employed as guides for further laboratory examinations.

A. QUALITATIVE TEST FOR URINARY PORPHYRINS

The urine for porphyrin examination should remain alkaline, for in acid urine, the porphyrins readily precipitate. This may be accomplished by the addition of about 0.5 gm Na_2CO_3 to the collecting bottle for each 100 ml of urine. This step may be omitted when dealing with normally alkaline urines. The alkaline urine can be stored at 4° C for several days prior to examination. All contact of the urine with metal should be avoided and the unfiltered urine should be used. The following simplified procedure is outlined schematically in Fig. 8.

1. Place 5 ml urine in a 250 ml separatory funnel and add 5 ml of acetate buffer (4 parts glacial acetic acid:1 part saturated sodium acetate) and adjust to pH 4.6–5.0.

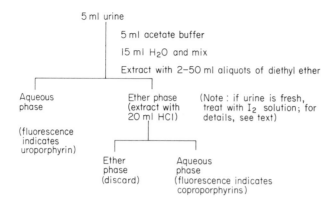

Fig. 8.   Qualitative test for porphyrins.

2. Add 15 ml cold distilled water.
3. Extract with two 50 ml aliquots of diethyl ether (or until the ether phases show no fluorescence) and pool. The coproporphyrin will go into the ether phase.
4. Much of the porphyrins present in urine are in the form of their nonfluorescent precursors. Storage of the urine for 24 hours will enhance their conversion to the fluorescing pigments. If fresh urine is being examined, the ether phase should be gently shaken with 5 ml of fresh 0.005% I_2 solution (prepared by diluting 0.5 ml of a stock 1% I_2 in alcohol solution to 100 ml with distilled water). This will also convert the precursors to the porphyrins.
5. Extract the pooled ether phases with 20 ml 5% HCl (1.5 N) and examine for fluorescence. Fluorescence indicates the presence of coproporphyrin.
6. Uroporphyrins are insoluble in ether. Therefore, fluorescence in the aqueous urinary phase indicates the presence of uroporphyrins.

B. QUALITATIVE TEST FOR FECAL PORPHYRINS

The qualitative test as described for urine may also be applied to fecal samples after prior extraction with strong acid. The following procedure is satisfactory (Sunderman and Sunderman, 1955). A 5-gm portion of a fecal sample is emulsified with 10 ml 95% alchohol. Then 25 ml of conc. HCl and 25 ml water are added to the emulsion and the mixture is allowed to stand overnight at room temperature. It is then diluted to 200 ml with water, filtered, and the filtrate is examined for porphyrins as described for urine.

C. QUALITATIVE TEST FOR PORPHOBILINOGEN

The qualitative test for porphobilinogen developed by Watson and Schwartz (1941) is considered to be a reliable procedure since false positives are not commonly encountered. The test consists of mixing 3 ml of fresh urine and 3 ml of Ehrlich's aldehyde reagent (0.7 gm p-dimethylaminobenzaldehyde, 150 ml conc. HCl and 100 ml H_2O) which is commonly used for the urine urobilinogen test. Then, 6 ml of saturated sodium acetate are added and again mixed. Next, 5 ml chloroform are added, shaken vigorously, and allowed to separate. The porphobilinogen aldehyde formed in the test is insoluble in chloroform and will remain in the aqueous supernatant phase. If the pink color is due to urobilinogen, it will be extracted into the chloroform phase. Porphobilinogen is found characteristically in the urine of patients with the hepatic form of porphyria, a form which has not been reported in domestic animals.

VI. THE PORPHYRIAS

A. CLASSIFICATION

By convention, the term porphyria is used to define those disease states having a hereditary basis and which exhibit increased urinary and/or fecal excretion of the uroporphyrins or their precursors. In addition, increased amounts of coproporphyrins are usually found in the urine and feces. The term porphyrinuria is used to define those acquired conditions in which the principal, if not the sole, porphyrins excreted are the coproporphyrins. The excretion of increased amounts of coproporphyrin has been observed in a wide variety of conditions in man, conditions which include infections, hemolytic anemias, liver disease, and lead poisoning. The detection of coproporphyrinuria has been especially useful as a screening test for exposure to lead.

The classification of the porphyrias has undergone revision periodically and doubtless will continue to do so until the precise defects in the various forms are known. There is general agreement as to the use of the term "erythropoietic porphyria" to describe the hereditary conditions manifested by involvement of the erythropoietic tissue. The confusion exists in the classification of the disorders described as subgroups of the hepatic forms. These have been variously classified on the basis of their clinical manifestations, genetics, and on the basis of the principal porphyrin compound(s) excreted (Eales, 1961). For the present purpose, the modified classification suggested by Tschudy (1965) and given in Table II will be used.

Methods are presently available for the experimental production of the two

TABLE II CLASSIFICATION OF THE PORPHYRIAS

I. Erythropoietic porphyrias
    A. Congenital erythropoietic porphyria (porphyria erythropoietica)
    B. Erythropoietic protoporphyria

II. Hepatic porphyrias
    A. Acute intermittent porphyria (Swedish porphyria)
    B. Mixed porphyria (variegate porphyria, South African porphyria, cutanea tarda)
        1. Principally cutaneous manifestations
        2. Principally acute intermittent manifestation
        3. Combination of signs
    C. Symptomatic porphyrias
        1. Idiosyncratic: associated with alcoholism, liver disease, systemic disease, drugs, etc.
        2. Acquired: hexachlorobenzene induced porphyria and hepatoma

major types. In lead or phenylhydrazine poisoning, a type of porphyrinuria is produced which exhibits some of the characteristics of the hereditary erythropoietic form of man and cattle (Schwartz *et al.*, 1952). A hepatic type may be produced by means of Sedormid (allylisopropylacetylcarbamide) (Schmid and Schwartz, 1952) or dihydrocollidine (Granick and Urata, 1963).

B. PORPHYRIA OF CATTLE

1. Introduction

One of the characteristic findings in bovine erythropoietic porphyria is a reddish-brown discoloration of the teeth and bones. Discolorations of this type have been observed in cattle after slaughter since the turn of the century, and these cattle are presumed to have had the disease. The first living cases were encountered in South Africa in a herd of grade Shorthorn cattle and the findings described by Fourie (1936) and Rimington (1936). Since that time, erythropoietic porphyria has been reported in Denmark (Jorgensen and With, 1955), England (Amoroso *et al.*, 1957), United States (Ellis *et al.*, 1958; Rhode and Cornelius, 1958), and Jamaica (Nestel, 1958). The disease is now known to occur in Holsteins and Jamaican cattle in addition to the Shorthorn breed.

The simple Mendelian recessive hereditary nature of the disease was established by study of the genealogy of the affected cattle and by breeding experiments (Fourie, 1939). The affected homozygous animals are characterized by discoloration of the teeth and urine, photosensitivity of the lighter areas of the skin, and generalized lack of condition and weakness. The condition is present at birth and severely affected calves must be kept out of sunlight if a reasonable state of health is to be maintained.

The predominating symptoms of teeth and urine discoloration and the photosensitization of the severely affected animal are readily apparent, and a tentative diagnosis can be confirmed by the red fluorescence of the teeth and urine when examined in the dark with Woods light. The symptomatology of affected animals, however, may vary from minimal to severe and with age and time of year (Fourie and Roets, 1939). The discoloration of the teeth may vary in the same animal, usually being more pronounced in the young and less apparent in older animals. Since porphyrin deposits occur in the dentine, examination of the occlusal surface should also be included. The degree of photosensitization will vary with the extent of porphyrin deposition and exposure to sunlight and may be so slight as to escape recognition. At times, loss of condition may be the only outward symptom for which the veterinarian may be called upon to examine the animal. Marked variations in the urinary excretion of the porphyrins also occur. These may range from minimal to thousands of micrograms in the same animal. The variations observed in this condition provide an indication of the dynamic state of flux of porphyrin metabolism in the living animal and the porphyrin deposits constitute a part of this dynamic state.

2. Distribution of Porphyrins

In Table III are listed some normal values for the porphyrins found in animals. It should be noted that these values are only approximations at best and were

TABLE III   NORMAL VALUES FOR PORPHYRINS

	Urine (μg%/100 ml)		Feces (μg/gm)		RBC (μg/100 ml cells)		Plasma (gm/100 ml)		Bone marrow (μg/100 ml cells)		
	URO	COPRO	COPRO	PROTO	COPRO	PROTO	COPRO	PROTO	URO	COPRO	PROTO
Cattle[a]	1.09 ± 0.92 (0.80–1.60)	4.06 ± 1.96 (2.05–6.15)	3.12 ± 0.96 (1.11–4.28)	0.75 ± 0.30 (0.15–1.25)	Trace	Trace	Trace	Trace	1	5	100
Swine[b]		104[e]				118	—	—			
Rabbit[c]	25[e]	41[e]	25[e]		2.6	83.3	—	—	Trace	4.5	87.5
Dog[d]	50[e]			50[e]		35	—	—			

[a]Jorgensen (1961b); Watson et al. (1959); Amoroso et al. (1957); Kaneko (1969). (Data in parentheses are minimal and maximal values.)

[b]Cartwright and Wintrobe (1948).

[c]Schmid et al. (1952); Schwartz et al. (1952).

[d]Schwartz et al. (1960).

[e]μg/day.

obtained from relatively few animals. The figures given, however, do provide an indication of the very low concentrations of the free porphyrins found normally in the body. As such, the finding of porphyrins in greater than trace amounts should not be ignored. Table IV gives porphyrin concentrations in porphyric cows and calves (Kaneko and Mills, 1969, 1970).

a. URINE. It has been emphasized that porphyrin excretion may vary over wide limits. Jorgensen (1961a,b), in an extensive study of 52 cases, found values for urinary uroporphyrins between 6.3 and 3900 $\mu g\%$ and coproporphyrins between 2.1 and 8300 $\mu g\%$. At concentrations of 100 $\mu g\%$ or more a reddish discoloration is discernible in the urine. At 1000 $\mu g\%$ or more intense red fluorescence of the urine is readily observed when examined in the dark with Woods light. The principal porphyrins excreted are URO I and COPRO I and only a small fraction is of the type III isomers. The percentage of each appearing in the urine is not constant. In contrast to earlier reports, Jorgensen (1961b) observed a greater excretion of COPRO I than URO I.

Porphobilinogen is not characteristically present in bovine porphyria urine and earlier reports of its presence (Ellis *et al.*, 1958; Jorgensen and With, 1955) have not been confirmed (Jorgensen, 1961b). Normally colored, nonfluorescent urine of a porphyria cow has consistently given a definite pink Ehrlich reaction but, unlike porphobilinogen aldehyde, the pigment is soluble in chloroform (Kaneko, 1969). The nature of this pigment is at present unknown. Upon heating on a steam bath for an hour or standing at room temperature for several days, a definite red fluorescence is apparent upon exposure to uv light. Quantitative porphyrin determinations of this urine have yielded values at 135 $\mu g\%$ and 87 $\mu g\%$ for uroporphyrin and coproporphyrin, respectively. Watson *et al.* (1959) have also described a similar experience with bovine porphyria urine.

b. BILE AND FECES. The bovine fecal porphyrins may be derived from two sources: bile and chlorophyll. The porphyrin derived from chlorophyll is, however, generally excluded by the usual analytic method. Essentially, the only porphyrin found in the bile and feces of porphyria cattle is coproporphyrin I, and its concentration is similarly found to vary over wide limits (Table IV). Fecal coproporphyrin varied between 1.9 and 11,800 $\mu g/gm$, and biliary coproporphyrin between 320 and 13,600 $\mu g\%$ (Jorgensen, 1961b). Only small amounts of COPRO III have been observed in feces. This preponderance of COPRO I in feces was also observed by Watson *et al.* (1959), who reported the presence of small amounts of URO I as well.

c. PLASMA AND ERYTHROCYTES. Normally, only traces of free porphyrins are found in the plasma and in the erythrocytes. In bovine porphyria plasma Watson *et al.* (1959) observed variable amounts which were, in general, equally URO I (1–27 $\mu g\%$) and COPRO I (4.2–25 $\mu g\%$). A striking difference as compared to the human disorder was the high level of free protoporphyrin in the erythrocytes of the porphyria cow. The significance of this high level remains unclear. The isomer type of this protoporphyrin, although undetermined, is probably PROTO III (9) which was not used for heme synthesis. Elevated protoporphyrin levels are commonly found in iron-deficiency and hemolytic anemias and in heavy metal poisoning. Presumably, a real or relative lack of iron could account for the accumulation of free protoporphyrin in the erythrocyte (Watson, 1957). Serum iron levels, however, are normal or elevated in porphyria (Watson *et al.*, 1959; Kaneko, 1963; Kaneko

TABLE IV PORPHYRINS IN BLOOD AND EXCRETA OF NORMAL, PORPHYRIC, AND PORPHYRIA CARRIER CATTLE[a]

Animals[b]	Red blood cells		Plasma		Urine		Feces	
	Copro-porphyrin	Protopor-phyrin	Copro-porphyrin	Protopor-phyrin	Copro-porphyrin	Uropor-phyrin	Copro-porphyrin	Protopor-phyrin
Normal mature cows (N = 10)	Trace	Trace	Trace	Trace	4.06 (2.05–6.15)	1.09 (0.80–1.60)	312 + 96 (111–428)	75 ± 30 (15–125)
Mature porphyric cows								
1184	3.0	61	15.3	1.8	410	378	5670	46
652 (N = 3)	3.4	64	4.5	1.6	313	336	1900	12
2026 (N = 2)	3.1	457	8.9	1.5	498	487	2090	62
718	89.7	36	—	—	1450	1280	—	—
Mature porphyria carrier cows								
1140	Trace	Trace	Trace	Trace	Trace	Trace	292	88
1141	Trace	Trace	Trace	Trace	Trace	Trace	273	92
Porphyric calves: 2–6 months old								
1857 (N = 3)	2.9	104	1.5	Trace	13	70	796	144
1801 (N = 3)	7.8	252	38.4	2.6	1430	1144	12	72
1959	18.6	288	Trace	Trace	480	265	22	99
Porphyria carrier calf: 5 months old								
1802	Trace	Trace	Trace	Trace	Trace	Trace	495	40

[a] Values are expressed in μg/100 ml or μg/100 gm; mean values ± standard deviation (data in parentheses are minimal and maximal values). From Kaneko and Mills,1970.

[b] N = Number of animals or number of determinations per animal.

and Mattheeuws, 1966), and it would appear that a cause other than iron deficiency accounts for the high protoporphyrin level. Alternately, the possibility has been considered (Schmid, 1966) that the protoporphyrin conceivably could be the type I isomer, a finding which would be a unique instance of its natural occurrence.

d. Tissue. The range of concentration of porphyrins in various tissues of porphyric cattle are given in Table V. The deposition of porphyrins throughout the bones and soft tissues is readily apparent at postmortem of severe cases by the generalized discoloration. A reddish-brown discoloration is most apparent in the teeth, bones, and bone marrow. Greatest discoloration of soft tissues occurs in the lungs and spleen in which characteristic flourescence may be observed with ultraviolet light. The high concentrations of porphyrins in splenic tissue is consistent with the hemolytic type of anemia observed in porphyria. Discoloration of skin, muscle, heart, liver, and kidney may also be observed but only a part is due to porphyrins. The discoloration is presumably due to porphyrin precursors and/or derivatives.

3. Hematological Findings

The hematological picture of the majority of reported cases is one of increased erythrogenesis in response to an anemic process of the type seen in hemolytic anemias. In general, the degree of response is related to the severity of the anemia associated with erythropoietic porphyria. The anemia is normochromic and, depending on the degree of response, may be macrocytic. There is associated reticulocytosis, polychromasia, anisocytosis, basophilic stippling, and an increased number of metarubricytes. A consistent monocytosis has been observed (Rhode and Cornelius, 1958; Kaneko, 1963) but has remained unexplained. The hematological

TABLE V   TISSUE PORPHYRINS (μg/100 gm) IN BOVINE ERYTHROPOIETIC PORPHYRIA

Tissue	URO	COPRO	PROTO	Total porphyrins
Bone marrow	Tr–162	Tr–1890	Tr–394	Tr–2396
Bones	6000	Tr	Tr	6000
Teeth	18550	Tr	Tr	18550
Spleen	0–10	Tr–342	Tr– 60	7–400
Liver	0–Tr	16–340	42– 65	66–403
Lung	0–79	0– 37	Tr– 20	20–130
Kidney	0	Tr–117	5– 16	5–133
Lymph node	0	0– 40	1– 7	1–49
Intestine	0	Tr– 65	7– 77	18–104
Stomach	0	Tr– 58	12– 82	12–111
Bile	0–690	112–12, 205	0–856	112–13,750
Adrenal	0–6	Tr–202	19–170	19–378
Ovary	0	65	1	66
Testes	0	0	9– 14	9–14
Skin	0	0	0	0
Muscle	0	10	30	40
Brain and spinal cord	0	23	57	80

TABLE VI   HEMATOLOGICAL FINDINGS IN TWO CASES OF BOVINE ERYTHROPOIETIC PORPHYRIA

Case No.	#652	#718
RBC	7,550,000	2,350,000
Hemoglobin	11.0	6.3
PCV	31	18
MCV	41	79.5
MCHC	35.3	35.0
Icterus index	5	15
Reticulocytes	0.6%	37.4%
Nucleated erythrocytes	3/100 WBC	23.5/100 WBC
Anisocytosis	Moderate	Marked
Polychromasia	Slight	Marked
Basophilic stippling	—	Marked
Poikilocytosis	Moderate	Moderate
WBC (corrected)	14,650	16,300
Band	—	1
Neutrophils	37.5	30.5
Lymphocytes	41	38.5
Monocytes	10.5	24
Eosinophils	9.5	4.5
Basophils	1.5	0.5
Unclassified		1
Bone Marrow M:E ratio	0.64	0.098

data in Table VI are representative of the findings in two cases over an 18-month period. Bone marrow hyperplasia is shown by the markedly depressed M:E ratio. As previously mentioned, bone marrow is also a principal site of porphyrin deposition. Watson et al. (1959) reported high concentrations of uroporphyrins in bone marrow of a porphyria cow (Table V).

The presence of porphyrins in the nucleated cells of the erythrocytic series is clearly evident by examination of unstained bone marrow smears with the fluorescent microscope. These have been designated as fluorocytes. This was originally observed by Schmid et al. (1955) in the bone marrow of a human patient and was an important contribution to the localization of the metabolic lesion in the metarubricyte (normoblast as used by Schmid et al., 1955). They also reported that fluorescence was observable in only one type of metarubricyte and that these were morphologically abnormal. The nuclei of the abnormal metarubricytes contained inclusions. Similar nuclear abnormalities have been observed in bovine porphyria marrow (Watson et al., 1959). Schmid et al. (1955) concluded that there were two separate populations of erythrocytes, one normal and one which contains free porphyrins.

The presence of two populations of cells was reported in humans but was attributed to the intermittent hemolytic crises which occurred (Gray et al., 1950). Tschudy (1965) has also pointed out that a single population of erythrocytes is more likely to be present rather than two separate lines of cells. Runge and Watson (1969), in their studies of fluorescing bovine porphyric bone marrow cells after bleeding, have also concluded that their data are compatible with a single line of cells.

The hemogram of the newborn porphyric calves also have important differences from that seen in older porphyric calves and cows. There is a striking erythrogenic response in the neonatal porphyric calf which persists for the first 3 weeks of life. Nucleated erythrocyte counts during the first 24 hours of life have ranged from 5000 to 63,500 per mm^3. Reticulocyte counts were lower than might be expected (6.4%) and increased to a peak of only 12.5% at 4 days (Kaneko and Mills, 1970). This may be a result of a postulated maturation defect as well as hemolysis (Smith and Kaneko, 1966; Rudolph, 1968).

4.   Mechanism of the Anemia

An anemia with evidence of an erythropoietic response is a well-established occurrence in erythropoietic porphyria. Morphologically, the anemia is compatible with that of a hemolytic process. Erythrocyte porphyrins are high in porphyria and if these erythrocytes with high porphyrin concentration were more susceptible to destruction, a shortening of life span would be expected. Erythrocyte life span is indeed shortened in bovine (Kaneko, 1963) and in human (Gray et al., 1950) porphyria. There is also general agreement that this shortening is associated with hemolysis but the mechanism of the hemolysis remains obscure.

In vivo ^{59}Fe metabolism studies are completely compatible with a hemolytic type of anemia and a degree of bone marrow hemolysis, i.e., ineffective erythropoiesis, also occurs (Kaneko, 1963; Kaneko and Mattheeuws, 1966). Plasma iron turnover and transfer rates, erythrocyte iron uptake, and organ uptakes were increased in keeping with a hemolytic process. More recently, it has been found that erythrocyte survival in bovine porphyria is inversely correlated with the erythrocyte coproporphyrin concentration (Kaneko, 1969). The shortest abnormal erythrocyte survival time of 27 days was associated with the highest erythrocyte coproporphyrin concentration. It would be reasonable to expect to find an association between one or more of the plasma or erythrocyte porphyrins and erythrocyte survival. The porphyrins are presumed in some way to alter the erythrocyte and make it more susceptible to destruction or removal from the circulation.

The mechanism of the cell alteration has also been studied in erythrocytes, reticulocytes, and in the developing erythrocyte. A number of erythrocytic enzymes associated with erythrocyte survival were determined and only the GSH stability was found to be abnormal in porphyric cows (Kaneko and Mills, 1969a, 1969b). Porphyria-carrier cows also exhibited the same instability and this phenomenon may prove to be a convenient biochemical test for the detection of the carrier state.

The porphyric reticulocyte has also been shown to have a biochemical defect. This defect is expressed as an increase in porphyrin synthesis, a marked decrease in heme synthesis and a delay in the maturation of the reticulocyte (Smith and Kaneko, 1966). The $T_{\frac{1}{2}}$ for the maturation of the reticulocyte was 50 hours in comparison to the normal of 3–10 hours. This delay in reticulocyte maturation is thought to be the result of the defect in heme synthesis since the rate of heme synthesis appears to control the rate of maturation of the reticulocyte (Schulman, 1968).

A similar delay in maturation of the metarubricyte (Fig. 6) to reticulocyte was observed in the bone marrow cells of porphyric cows (Rudolph, 1968) but there was no effect on the younger cells of the erythrocytic series. Thus, it appears that the more mature cells of the erythrocytic series (metarubricyte, reticulocyte, erythrocyte) are the ones noticeably affected by the high porphyrin content. This is not surprising since heme and hemoglobin synthesis are most active in the later stages (Fig. 6). Ultimately, the sum total of these changes may alter the cells making them more susceptible to hemolysis and this hemolysis, either intra- or extravascular, would occur with cells of the bone marrow or of the peripheral blood. On exposure to sunlight, an enhancement of a photohemolysis of the type observed in erythropoietic protoporphyria (Harber et al., 1964) might further aggravate the hemolysis.

This mechanism might also explain the striking erythrogenic response of the neonatal porphyric calf. If porphyrins do not cross the placental barrier—and this is not known—they would be stored in the fetus and exert a profound hemolytic effect in the fetus.

The newborn calf would therefore exhibit a marked rate of erythrogenesis. At birth, porphyrins are high and fall to a steady-state level in about 3 weeks in porphyric calves (Kaneko, 1969). This is comparable to the rate of clearance of porphyrin-^{14}C in urine which fell to 0.1% of the initial level in 3 weeks (Kaneko, 1969). Furthermore, 3 weeks is also the time at which the erythrogenic response has stabilized at a steady-state level for the particular neonatal calf (Kaneko and Mills, 1970).

In summary, these findings suggest that a high porphyrin content induces a defect in heme synthesis. This biochemical defect is thought to be morphologically expressed as a maturation defect and the defective and altered cell may be more susceptible to intra- or extravascular hemolysis. This would be compatible with the observed hemolytic type of anemia with shortened life span, the degree of which depends upon the severity of the porphyria.

5.   Detection of the Carrier State

The hereditary nature of bovine erythropoietic porphyria is of the simple autosomal recessive type. As such, carrier animals have thus far been detected only by progeny study and testing. Recently, two potentially useful biochemical methods for detection of the carrier state have been reported. The finding of GSH instability in mature porphyria-carrier cows has already been mentioned (Kaneko and Mills, 1969a, 1969b). Levin (1969) has recently observed an intermediate level of UROgen III-cosyn activity in the blood of the heterozygous carriers of porphyria. The establishment of either or both of these biochemical methods of detection of the carrier state would be extremely valuable contributions.

6.   Metabolic Basis of Bovine Erythropoietic Porphyria

The present status of knowledge concerning the mechanisms for heme biosynthesis and the biochemical nature of the porphyrins found in high concentrations in the tissues and excreta provide for a reasonable explanation of the metabolic defect in erythropoietic porphyria. Certain features of the biosynthetic mechanism are particularly important in attempting to explain this porphyria in terms of enzymic derangement. These may be briefly summarized:

1. There appears to be an anatomical separation (or compartmentation) of the enzymes involved in heme biosynthesis. Some of the enzymes are found in association with the mitochondrial and others are found in the soluble fraction.
2. The mitochondrial systems are involved in:
   a. the initial synthesis of ALA;
   b. the synthesis of protoporphyrin III (9) from COPROgen III;
   c. heme formation, i.e., incorporation of iron into protoporphyrin III (9).
3. The soluble enzymes catalyze the intervening steps which lead to the formation of PBG, UROgens, and COPROgens.
4. Mitochondria are present only in the immature erythroid cells. This would include the nucleated cells and the reticulocytes. The most active hemoglobin formation occurs in the metarubricyte and ceases upon reaching maturity.

The metabolic defect is localized in the erythropoietic tissue of the porphyric animal and the probable site is within the developing erythroid cells. These are considered to be the mitochondria-containing cells, principally the metarubricytes, and would exclude the mature, nonnucleated erythrocyte.

The precise nature of the enzymic defect awaits complete clarification of the steps involved in heme biosynthesis, mainly the mechanism for the cyclization of four molecules of PBG to form uroporphyrinogen. The action of the UROgen I-syn and UROgen III-cosyn systems in heme biosynthesis of animals would offer an explanation for erythropoietic porphyria. Accordingly, the formation of the type III isomer requires the combined action of both enzymes, and if UROgen I-syn is acting alone, the type I isomer is formed. Thus, the level of activity of each of these enzymes would exercise a degree of control over which of the two independent pathways for isomer synthesis is traversed. In the homozygous state for porphyria, the formation of type I isomers could occur by excess UROgen I-syn, deficiency of UROgen III-cosyn, or, more likely, a combination of both resulting in a real or relative increase in UROgen I-syn activity. A decrease in UROgen III-cosyn in porphyric cows and humans has been reported (Levin, 1968; Romeo and Levin, 1970).

Total deficiency of UROgen III-cosyn is obviously incompatible with life. Also, there is wide variation in severity of the disease between animals but the degree of severity is quite constant in each animal kept under standard conditions. This provides an indication of the variability in the homozygous state between animals and further attests to the interaction of several enzyme systems. A summary of a proposed metabolic basis for bovine erythropoietic porphyria is given in Fig. 9. Central to this proposal is the genetically controlled UROgen III-cosyn deficiency and the resultant failure of heme feedback repression which is currently speculative.

C. PORPHYRIA OF SWINE

The occurrence of porphyria in swine was first recognized by Clare and Stephens (1944) in New Zealand. This was later followed by its recognition in Denmark and a number of accounts of the studies conducted with these swine have been published (Jorgensen and With, 1955; Jorgensen, 1959).

In contrast to the bovine form, the disease in swine is inherited as a dominant characteristic. Except in the very severe cases, there appears to be little or no

Metabolic Basis of Bovine Erythropoietic (Congenital) Porphyria

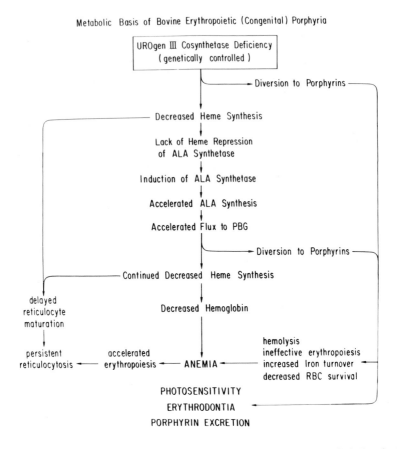

Fig. 9.   A speculative summary of the metabolic basis of Bovine Erythropoietic Porphyria.

effect upon the general health of the pig. Photosensitivity is not seen even in the white pigs. The predominant feature in the affected pig is a characteristic reddish discoloration of the teeth which usually fluoresce when examined with uv light. Porphyrin deposition in the teeth of the newborn pig appears to be so consistent as to be pathognomic. On occasion, darkly discolored teeth may not fluoresce, but porphyrins may be extracted from these with 0.5 N HCl (With, 1955). Similar, though less apparent, deposition occurs in the bones. The porphyrins, which have been found in concentrations of up to 200 μg/gm, are comprised principally of URO I. The liver, spleen, lungs, kidneys, bones, and teeth also are discolored by another dark pigment, the nature of which is unknown (Jorgensen, 1959).

The urine of the affected pig is discolored only in the more severely affected pig. The 24-hour excretion of uroporphyrins ranged between 100 and 10,000 μg and for coproporphyrin, only 50 μg. These were both the type I isomers. PBG is absent in the urine. Close similarities in this pattern of porphyrin excretion to that found in bovine porphyria are apparent but the localization of the defect in erythropoietic tissue remains unestablished.

D. Porphyria of Cats

The occurrence of porphyria in cats was reported in a young male kitten (Tobias, 1964). One of its three littermates was affected and kittens from a previous litter were also reported to have had the same unusually colored teeth. The kitten's teeth were brown and under ultraviolet light, fluoresced red. Its urine was amber colored and was qualitatively positive for uroporphyrin, coproporphyrin, and porphobilinogen. There was no evidence of anemia or photosensitization. These cats had been kept indoors all their lives.

One of these cats was the propositus for a porphyric cat colony (Glenn et al., 1968). Study of the inheritance of the porphyria in these cats indicates it to be of a simple Mendelian autosomal dominant trait analogous to that seen in swine. Further biochemical studies are currently being conducted by this group.

E. Erythropoietic Protoporphyria

This disorder of porphyrin metabolism is found only in humans. It was first reported in 1961 (Magnus et al., 1961) and now well recognized (Redeker, 1963; Harber et al., 1964). It appears to be inherited as a dominant autosomal trait. Major signs of erythropoietic porphyria such as anemia, porphyrin excretion, and erythrodontia are absent. Photosensitivity of the skin appears to be the only clinical manifestation of the disease and this is associated with the plasma protophorphyrin concentration. In the laboratory, the most striking findings are the high concentrations of PROTO III (9) in the erythrocytes and feces.

The nature of the biochemical defect is at present unknown. PROTO III (9) might accumulate if iron incorporation (Fig. 4) were defective but iron metabolism is normal in this disease. It has also been suggested that if the iron incorporating enzyme heme synthetase (HS) Fig. 4 (also called ferrochelatase) were to become rate-limiting and ALA-syn increased, PROTO III (9) might then accumulate. There is the additional possibility that erythropoietic protoporphyria may be a combination of both an erythropoietic and a hepatic porphyria.

F. Hepatic Porphyrias

This group of disorders has thus far been observed only in man and constitutes the most common type of porphyria seen. They are probably inherited as dominant traits. The salient features of this group of porphyrias are summarized in Table VII together with those of erythropoietic porphyria and erythropoietic protoporphyria. As the name implies, the metabolic defect in hepatic porphyria is involved with hepatic porphyrin metabolism. Further subdivisions are based upon the principal clinical manifestations of this disturbance.

In the intermittent acute type, paroxysmal attacks, which may be precipitated by barbiturates or alcohol, occur intermittently in an otherwise chronic condition. Attacks are manifested by extreme abdominal pain and/or nervous involvement, which are often the presenting symptoms. Photosensitivity is not a feature of this form. The principal urinary finding is the excretion of large amounts of ALA and PBG. An explanation for the biochemical defect in hepatic porphyria must explain

TABLE VII   SUMMARY OF THE PORPHYRIAS

	Erythropoietic porphyrias		Hepatic porphyrias	
	Congenital erythropoietic porphyria	Erythropoietic protoporphyria	Acute intermittent porphyria	Mixed porphyria
Heredity				
Cattle	Recessive			
Cat, pig	Dominant			
Man	Recessive	Dominant	Dominant	Dominant
Site of defect	Hematopoietic tissue	Hematopoietic tissue	Liver	Liver
Clinical anemia	Yes	No	No	No
Photosensitivity	Yes	Yes	Yes	Yes
Abdominal pain	No	No	Yes	Yes
Erythrodontia	Yes	No	No	No
Urine color	Reddish brown	Normal	Normal	Normal
Porphyrin	URO I, COPRO I	Normal	ALA, PBG	ALA, PBG, URO, COPRO
Liver	—	—	ALA, PBG	ALA, PBG, URO, COPRO
Bone marrow	URO I, COPRO I, PROTO	PROTO	Normal	Normal
RBC	COPRO I, PROTO	PROTO	Normal	Normal
Plasma	URO I, COPRO I	PROTO	Normal	Normal

this excess in ALA and PBG. From experimental animal studies, it is known that the enzyme ALA synthetase is an inducible enzyme in liver (Granick and Urata, 1963) and also the rate-limiting enzyme in porphyrin synthesis. This would mean that when the ALA-syn level is high, excess ALA and PBG would be formed and excreted. This has been demonstrated in human hepatic porphyria (Tschudy, 1965). The biochemical basis for this genetically related induction of ALA-syn, however, is not yet known.

The cutaneous form has been subgrouped because photosensitivity is the predominant symptom. ALA and PBG may be present in the urine but, more commonly, a mixture of porphyrins, both I and III, is found. The mixed or combined form, which is rarely seen, exhibits the symptoms of both the cutaneous and the intermittent acute forms.

REFERENCES

Amoroso, E. C., Loosmore, R. M., Rimington, C., and Tooth, B. E. (1957). *Nature* **180**, 230.
Anderson, R. L., and Tove, S. B. (1958). *Nature* **182**, 315.
Bartlett, G. R., and Marlow, A. A. (1951). *Bull. Scripps Metab. Clin.* **2**, 1.
Bishop, C. (1964). *In* "The Red Blood Cell" (C. Bishop and D. M. Surgenor, eds.), p. 148. Academic Press, New York.
Bogorad, L. (1958a). *J. Biol. Chem.* **233**, 501.
Bogorad, L. (1958b). *J. Biol. Chem.* **233**, 510.
Bogorad, L., and Granick, S. (1953). *Proc. Nat. Acad. Sci. U.S.* **39**, 1176.
Bush, J. A., Berlin, N. I., Jensen, W. N., Brill, A. B., Cartwright, G. E., and Wintrobe, M. M. (1955). *J. Exptl. Med.* **101**, 451.
Bush, J. A., Jensen, M. M., Athens, J. W., Ashenbrucher, H., Cartwright, G. E., and Wintrobe, M. M. (1956). *J. Exptl. Med.* **103**, 701.
Cartwright, G. E., and Wintrobe, M. M. (1948). *J. Biol. Chem.* **172**, 557.
Cartwright, G. E., and Wintrobe, M. M. (1964). *Am. J. Clin. Nutr.* **14**, 224.
Chapman, R. G., Hennessey, M. A., Waltersdorph, A. M., Huennekens, F. M., and Gabrio, B. W. (1962). *J. Clin. Invest.* **41**, 1249.
Clare, H. T., and Stephens, E. H. (1944). *Nature* **153**, 252.
Cline, J. J., and Berlin, N. I. (1963). *Am. J. Physiol.* **204**, 415.
Cookson, G. H., and Rimington, C. (1953). *Nature* **171**, 875.
Cornelius, C. E., Kaneko, J. J., Benson, D. C., and Wheat, J. D. (1960). *Am. J. Vet. Res.* **20**, 1123.
de Viale, L. C. S. M., and Grinstein, M. (1968). *Biochim. Biophys. Acta* **158** 79.
Eales, L. (1961). *Ann. Rev. Med.* **12**, 251.
Ellis, D. J., Barner, R. D., Madden, D., Melcer, I., and Orten, J. M. (1958). *Mich. State Univ. Vet.* **18**, 89.
Ewing, G. O. (1969). *J. Am. Vet. Med. Assoc.* **154**, 503.
Fourie, P. J. J. (1936). *Onderstepoort J. Vet. Sci. Animal Ind.* **7**, 535.
Fourie, P. J. J. (1939). *Onderstepoort J. Vet. Sci. Animal Ind.* **13**, 383.
Fourie, P. J. J., and Roets, G. C. S. (1939). *Onderstepoort J. Vet. Sci. Animal Ind.* **13**, 369.
Gabrio, B. W., Donohue, D. M., Huennekens, F. M., and Finch, C. A. (1956). *J. Clin. Invest.* **35**, 657.
Gibson, K. D., Laver, W. G., and Neuberger, A. (1958). *Biochem. J.* **70**, 71.
Glenn, B. L., Glenn, H. G., and Omtvedt, I. T. (1968). *Am. J. Vet. Res.* **29**, 1653.
Granick, S. (1966). *J. Biol. Chem.* **241**, 1359.
Granick, S., and Levere, R. D. (1964). *Progr. Hematol.* **4**, 1.
Granick, S., and Mauzerall, D. (1958). *J. Biol. Chem.* **232**, 1119.
Granick, S., and Urata, G. (1963). *J. Biol. Chem.* **238**, 821.
Gray, C. H., Muir, I. M. H., and Neuberger, A. (1950). *Biochem. J.* **47**, 542.
Harber, L. C., Fleischer, A. S., and Baer, R. L. (1964). *J. Am. Med. Assoc.* **189**, 191.

Harris, J. W. (1963). "The Red Cell: Production, Metabolism and Destruction: Normal and Abnormal." Harvard Univ. Press, Cambridge Massachusetts.

Hoffman, J. F. (1962). *Circulation* **26**, 1201.

Iodice, A. A., Richert, D. A., and Schulman, M. P. (1958). *Federation Proc.* **17**, 248.

Jacob, F., and Monod, J. (1963). *In* "Cytodifferentiation and Macromolecular Synthesis" (M. Locke, ed.), p. 30, Academic Press, New York.

Jorgensen, S. K. (1959). *Brit. Vet. J.* **115**, 160.

Jorgensen, S. K. (1961a). *Brit. Vet. J.* **117**, 1.

Jorgensen, S. K. (1961b). *Brit. Vet. J.* **117**, 61.

Jorgensen, S. K., and With, T. K. (1955). *Nature* **176**, 156.

Kaneko, J. J. (1963). *Ann. N.Y. Acad. Sci.* **104**, 689.

Kaneko, J. J. (1969). Unpublished data.

Kaneko, J. J., and Cornelius, C. E. (1962). *Am. J. Vet. Res.* **23**, 913.

Kaneko, J. J., and Mattheeuws, D. R. G. (1966). *Am. J. Vet. Res.* **27**, 923.

Kaneko, J. J., and Mills, R. (1969a). *Federation Proc.* **23**, 453.

Kaneko, J. J., and Mills, R. (1969b). *Am. J. Vet. Res.* **30**, 1805.

Kaneko, J. J., and Mills, R. (1970). *Cornell Vet.* **60**, 52.

Kaneko, J. J., Cornelius, C. E., and Heuschele, W. P. (1961). *Am. J. Vet. Res.* **22**, 683.

Kaneko, J. J., Green, R. A., and Mia, A. S. (1966). *Proc. Soc. Exptl. Biol. Med.* **123**, 783.

Kikuchi, G., Kumar, A., Talmage, P., and Shemin, D. (1958). *J. Biol. Chem.* **233**, 1214

Labbe, R. F., and Hubbard, H. (1961). *Biochim. Biophys. Acta* **52**, 130.

Levere, R. D. (1968). *Advan. Clin. Chem.* **11**, 133.

Levin, E. Y. (1968). *Science* **161**, 907.

Levin, E. Y. (1969). Personal communication.

Levin, E. Y., and Coleman, D. L. (1967). *J. Biol. Chem.* **242**, 4248.

Magnus, I. A., Jarrett, A., Prankerd, T. A. J., and Rimington, C. (1961). *Lancet* **II**, 448.

Murphy, J. R. (1960). *J. Lab. Clin. Med.* **55**, 286.

Nestel, B. L. (1958). *Cornell Vet.* **48**, 430.

Neuberger, A., and Niven, J. S. F. (1951). *J. Physiol. (London)* **112**, 292.

Prankerd, T. A. J. (1961). "The Red Cell." Blackwell, Oxford.

Redeker, A. G. (1963). *J. Lab. Clin. Med.* **9**, 235.

Rhode, E. A., and Cornelius, C. E. (1958). *J. Am. Vet. Med. Assoc.* **132**, 112.

Rimington, C. (1936). *Onderstepoort. J. Vet. Sci. Animal Ind.* **7**, 567.

Romeo, G., and Levin, E. Y. (1970). *Proc. Notl. Acad. Sci. U.S.* (in press).

Rudolph, W. G. (1968). M.S. Thesis, University of California, Davis, California.

Runge, W., and Watson, C. J. (1969). *Blood* **32**, 119.

Sano, S., and Granick, S. (1961). *J. Biol. Chem.* **236**, 1173.

Schmid, R. (1966). *In* "The Metabolic Basis of Inherited Disease" (J. B. Stanbury, J. B. Wyngaarden, and D. S. Fredrickson, eds.), p. 939. McGraw-Hill, New York.

Schmid, R., and Schwartz, S. (1952). *Proc. Soc. Exptl. Biol. Med.* **81**, 685.

Schmid, R., Hanson, B., and Schwartz, S. (1952). *Proc. Soc. Exptl. Biol. Med.* **79**, 459.

Schmid, R., Schwartz, S., and Sundberg, R. D. (1955). *Blood* **10**, 416.

Schulman, H. M. (1968). *Biochim. Biophys, Acta* **155**, 253.

Schwartz, S., Keprios, M., and Schmid, R. (1952). *Proc. Soc. Exptl. Biol. Med.* **79**, 463.

Schwartz, S., Berg, M. H., Bossenmaier, I., and Dinsmore, H. (1960). *Methods Biochem. Anal.* **8**, 221.

Shemin, D., and Rittenberg, D. (1946a). *J. Biol. Chem.* **166**, 621.

Shemin, D., and Rittenberg, D.(1946b). *J. Biol. Chem.* **166**, 627.

Shemin, D., Russell, C. S., and Abramsky, T. (1955). *J. Biol. Chem.* **215**, 613.

Smith, J. E., and Kaneko, J. J. (1966). *Am. J. Vet. Res.* **27**, 931.

Sunderman, F. W., Jr., and Sunderman, F. W. (1955). *Am. J. Clin. Pathol.* **25**, 1231.

Tasker, J. B., Severin, G. A., Young, S., and Gillette, E. L. (1969). *J. Am. Vet. Med. Assoc.* **154**, 158.

Tobias, G. (1964). *J. Am. Vet. Med. Assoc.* **145**, 462.

Tschudy, D. P. (1965). *J. Am. Med. Assoc.* **191**, 718.

Valentine, W. N., Pearce, M. L., Riley, R. F., Richter, E., and Lawrence, J. S. (1951). *Proc. Soc. Exptl. Biol. Med.* **77**, 244.

Watson, C. J. (1957). *A.M.A. Arch. Internal Med.* **99**, 323.

Watson, C. J., and Schwartz, S. (1941). *Proc. Soc. Exptl. Biol. Med.* **7**, 393.

Watson, C. J., Perman, V., Spurell, F. A.. Hoyt, H. H., and Schwartz, S. (1959). *A.M.A. Arch. Internal Med.* **103**, 436.

Westall, R. G. (1952). *Nature* **170**, 614

With, T. K. (1955). *Biochem. J.* **60**, 703.

5   Liver Function

Charles E. Cornelius

I. INTRODUCTION

The diagnosis of liver disorders in clinical veterinary medicine today has been greatly facilitated by the recent development of numerous new laboratory procedures. The multiplicity of hepatic functions and their measurement magnifies the complexity of the organ. No single test provides a clear impression of the functional status of the liver.

The *dissociation* of liver function has continually challenged the clinical investigator. The ability of the liver to lose certain functions to a greater degree than others attests to this complexity (Hargreaves, 1968).

No single test for liver function is universally accepted since the organ in various disease conditions may lose specific biochemical functions in a different sequence. Lesions placed strategically may spare parenchymal metabolic processes but blockade biliary channels. Generalized or mixed types of lesions are more common and usually affect structural elements unevenly. The dissociation of functions may be partial or complete in that one function, i.e., intrahepatic biliary obstruction, may only partially disturb parenchymal cell metabolism, or in others, i.e., certain non-inflammatory degenerative liver diseases, may produce little intrahepatic obstruction and allow a free outflow of bile.

To the clinician, the recognition of the *association* of liver functions is of prime importance. That many mechanisms of liver function are interlocked but not evenly impaired is well known. This unequal involvement of different functions is no longer attributed to a lack of sensitivity of different tests, but to the fact that some tests as performed are unduly sensitive and many times are affected by pathological processes which are not primarily hepatic. Lichtman (1953) has suggested that more emphasis be placed on the quantitative association of tests rather than their qualitative dissociation of partial function.

The known functions of the liver are so numerous that well over 100 standard liver function tests have been devised for man (Knisely, 1951) with nearly 100 tests now available for domestic animals. Of the many tests introduced during the last 40 years, few have survived. Only those procedures which have been of great value in diagnosis or prognosis and quite practical in the average clinical laboratory are presently used. Certain excellent tests are ignored owing to the necessity for the use of more complex reagents or apparatus.

Unfortunately, no one test can be relied on to totally differentiate the various forms of icterus. A thorough knowledge of normal hepatic function and pathology should preclude any such thoughts. The use of a limited battery of tests, appropriate to the clinical situation and which can be interpreted on the basis of past experience, is the most desirable. This battery of tests can be summarized in terms of the percent of the average expected function for this species and referred to as the "liver profile," in which each specific function is expressed in bar-graph form (%) for rapid clinical appraisal of hepatic function.

Attempts to relate gross structural changes with functional failure have been at times disappointing because there is usually more than one anatomical unit of the liver involved. The four anatomic units of the liver are (Lichtman, 1953): (1) the parenchymal mass; (2) the bile duct, canalicular or cholangiolar unit; (3) the vascular, hemodynamic unit; and (4) the reticuloendothelial unit. Since clinical signs are ultimately derived from the alterations in the pathological anatomophysiological units, the choice of test procedures and their interpretation must be related to these basic structural components.

II. INDICATIONS AND LIMITATIONS OF LIVER FUNCTION TESTS

A. INDICATIONS

1. *Primary liver disorders with or without icterus* such as infectious hepatitis, leptospirosis, suppurative hepatitis, diffuse hepatic fibrosis, acute toxic necrosis, hepatic hemangioma, hepatoma, intrahepatic bile duct adenoma, and carcinoma, etc.

2. *Secondary liver disorders*, such as the infiltrative and degenerative lipidoses accompanying hypothyroidism, diabetes mellitus, pancreatic atrophy or fibrosis, and starvation; also chronic passive congestion in cardiac decompensation; metastatic hepatic malignancies; secondary amyloidosis; equine encephalomyelitis, etc.

3. *Differential diagnosis of icterus* from hemolytic crisis, intrahepatic cholestasis, and extrahepatic obstruction of the bile duct system.

4. *Anemias* of undetermined origin. Normocytic, normochromic anemias from chronic progressive hepatic fibrosis (dogs) as well as the anemias associated with hemorrhages in prothrombin deficiency.

5. *Prognosis* of hepatic disease, evaluation of therapy, and estimation of residual damage after recovery. Following the trend of a disease, evaluating the degree of hepatic insufficiency, and the measurement of hepatic integrity to evaluate preoperative surgical risk, are all indicated in rational veterinary medicine.

6. *Specific research investigations* such as testing the toxicity of drugs, estimating residual damage from experimental hepatotoxins, assessing parasitic hepatic migrations, etc. (Cornelius, 1957).

B. LIMITATIONS

Liver function tests must be closely correlated with the clinical signs as well as with the histopathological findings from biopsy. The concept that the clinical diagnosis of hepatic disease can be made from the laboratory bench is quite erroneous. Many tests have been discredited as much from overenthusiasm on the part of their proponents as from the negativism of their critics.

Standard objections against each and every liver function test are as follows (Lichtman, 1953; Maclagan, 1956).

1. Extensive damage is required to impair function owing to the great reserve power of the liver.

2. There are so many functions, that testing one does not indicate the state of the whole organ.

3. The test lacks sensitivity.

4. Specific hepatic functions are affected greatly by many different pathological conditions of an extrahepatic nature.

Refutations of these specific objections, respectively, are needed:

1. A great reserve power exists when viewed from its ability to function after removal of a large proportion of the organ surgically; however, pathological conditions affecting all the hepatic cells may produce profound effects rapidly. *Because of the rapid regenerative ability of the liver, interpretations of all function tests must be viewed in terms of short time intervals.*

2. Since many hepatic functions are available for measurement, the clinician may use specific functions which are disturbed early. Owing to the severity of their change from normal, he may obtain a quantitative index of liver cell pathology.

3. Criticism concerning the sensitivity of tests usually arises when results appear normal even though liver damage is great. Since each test is quite different, a distinct understanding of the procedure, its dependencies, and the possible laboratory inaccuracies must be known. Many times the criticisms concerning the hypersensitivity of tests is only the result of an attempt to either correlate abnormal hepatic function tests of a previous date to the autopsy findings of a regenerated liver or substantiate a tentative clinical diagnosis.

4. One must agree that the liver can be affected secondarily to many other primary conditions. The observation of this is of considerable interest in itself, even if at times it confuses the diagnostician. However, unless an animal shows unequivocal clinical signs of liver disease such as icterus or the amine-like odor of massive liver degeneration (Watson, 1944), the diagnosis of latent hepatopathy may still be largely dependent upon a liver function test or biopsy.

It has been known for some time that there is no strict correlation between structure and function of hepatic cells. Conspicuous alterations are not always correlated with aberrant liver function tests when viewed by light microscopy. In many instances of frank hepatic disease, however, a good correlation is found. Electron micrographs may demonstrate changes in cellular microbodies unobservable with microscopy at $900 \times$, which positively correlate with certain biochemical tests (Schaffner, 1966). Regeneration of hepatic tissue, found concurrently with processes of tissue destruction as observed in the postnecrotic scarring syndrome, may outstrip the degenerative processes. Liver dysfunction may precede the development of, or remain following the disappearance of, alteration in structure. Tests of liver function have been found to detect early changes before any histopathological lesions can be observed from biopsy examinations. Virus particles many times affect the metabolism of liver cells before producing their destructive processes.

III. CLASSIFICATION OF LIVER FUNCTION TESTS

Only established liver function tests in domestic animals will be discussed in detail in this chapter, whereas some other procedures without proper clinical evaluation or of questionable significance will be only briefly mentioned.

The established liver function tests may be arbitrarily grouped as: tests measuring the hepatic uptake, conjugation, and excretion of organic anions; serum enzyme tests; specific biochemical tests; liver biopsy; and miscellaneous tests.

IV. TESTS MEASURING THE HEPATIC UPTAKE, CONJUGATION, AND EXCRETION OF ORGANIC ANIONS

A. BILE PIGMENTS

1. Unconjugated and Conjugated Bilirubin in Serum

a. GENERAL.   Open-chain tetrapyrrolic compounds played a central metabolic role in the early course of evolution (Lester and Troxler, 1969). Bile pigments in mammals are waste products and have a less central metabolic role than observed previously in unicellular and plant organisms. Bilirubin was first crystallized from ox gallstones in 1864 and Kuster later discovered its relationship to hemoglobin in 1899 (With, 1954). The great pathologist Virchow early recognized the relationship of "hematoidin" in the tissues to degraded hemoglobin. As early as 1883, Ehrlich discovered that after the addition of sulfanilic acid, hydrochloric acid, and sodium nitrite to serum containing bile pigments, a violet pigment of azobilirubin was formed (With, 1954). Van den Bergh and Müller (1916) concluded that two forms of bilirubin existed in the serum of some clinical cases of icterus in man since the addition of alcohol was not needed to produce the diazo reaction color in the "direct reaction." The "indirect reaction" required the presence of alcohol for color development and was found primarily in cases of hemolytic crisis. The present use of the van den Bergh test calls for the addition of alcohol to the mixture of acidic diazobenzene–sulfonic acid and serum in order to measure the total bilirubin in the serum. Next, the "direct reacting" pigment is measured at a 1-minute reaction interval. The calculated difference between the total and "direct reacting" pigment gives an "indirect reacting" bilirubin value. Normal values for the serum bilirubin concentrations in the various domestic animals are presented in Table I.

Prior to 1953, innumerable conflicting reports appeared concerning the interpretation of the van den Bergh reactions. Lemberg and Legge (1949) were forced to conclude that "there are few fields of biochemistry in which so much has been done with so little success." Cole and co-workers (Cole and Lathe, 1953; Cole et al., 1954), by means of reverse phase partition chromatography, were able to separate the serum pigments giving the "direct and indirect reactions." Schmid (1956), with ascending paper chromatography, found that in obstructive icterus the "direct reacting" pigment was a glucuronide conjugate of bilirubin. In hemolytic icterus the "indirect reacting" serum bilirubin was in a free and unconjugated state (see Fig. 1). This free bilirubin was observed to be relatively insoluble and nonpolar at the pH of blood and therefore required alcohol in the reaction to render it soluble for diazotization. The use of the terms conjugated and free bilirubin in place of "direct and indirect reacting bilirubin," respectively, is presently recommended. So-called "biphasic" serum reactions were due to a mixture of conjugated and free bilirubin.

In past years, differences in the direct and indirect reacting bilirubin was explained as due to a greater water afinity of conjugated bilirubin. Solubility in water cannot explain this difference since neither low concentrations of unconjugated bilirubin or "solubilized" unconjugated bilirubin in a taurocholate micellar solution will react directly. Strong evidence could suggest that hydrogen bonding within the bilirubin molecule between the carbonyl oxygen and pyrrole ring nitrogens is more likely the explanation. It has been proposed that any access of diazotized sulfanilate to the central methene group would be greatly diminished by steric interference (Fog and Jellum, 1963).

Grodsky and Carbone (1957), using liver homogenates, and Schmid et al. (1957), using hepatic microsomal preparations, observed that glucuronic acid was transferred to bilirubin in its activated form of uridine diphosphoglucuronic acid (UDPGA). The enzyme UDPGA transferase, which is present in the hepatic microsomes, is a nonspecific enzyme active in the transfer of the two glucuronic acid

TABLE I NORMAL LEVELS OF SERUM BILIRUBIN IN DOMESTIC ANIMALS[a]

Species	Author	Total bilirubin (mg/100 m)			Conjugated bilirubin (direct-reacting) (mg/100 ml)		
		Mean	σ^b	Range	Mean	σ^b	Range
Dog	Lopez Garcia et al. (1943)	—	—	(0–0.2)	—	—	—
	Karsai (1954)	—	—	(0.28–0.35)	—	—	(0.06–0.12)
	Berger (1956)	0.10	±0.10	—	0.0	—	—
	Klaus (1958)	0.10	—	(0–0.3)	0.07	—	(0–0.14)
	L. F. Müller (1960)	0.25	±0.10	(0.07–0.61)	0.14	—	—
	Van Vleet and Alberts (1968)	0.22	—	(0.05–0.55)	—	—	—
	Hoe and Harvey (1961b)	—	—	(0.0–0.6)	—	—	—
Cat	Lopez Garcia et al. (1943)	—	—	(0.15–0.20)	—	—	—
Horse	W. Grassnickel (1926)	—	—	(1.9–3.1)	—	—	—
	Zink (1932)	—	—	(2.0–4.0)	—	—	—
	Meyer (1938)	—	—	(1.0–4.5)	—	—	—
	Natscheff (1939)	—	—	(0.5–2.1)	—	—	—
	Doring (1940)	—	—	(0.8–1.6)	—	—	—
	Royer et al. (1941)	—	—	(0.5–3.0)	—	—	—
—	Rudra (1946)	—	—	(1.0–7.4)	—	—	—
	Muzzo (1949)	1.25	±0.07	(0.81–2.07)	0.37	±0.02	(0.18–0.72)
	Beijers et al. (1950)	—	—	(1.1–1.2)	—	—	—
	Benndorf (1955)	—	—	(0.47–1.02)	—	—	—

	Reference						
Cow	Berger (1956)	1.10	±0.40	—	0.50	±0.20	—
	Klaus (1958)		0.99	(0.50–1.50)	0.15		(0.02–0.4)
	Eikmeier (1959)	1.94		—	0.87		—
	Cornelius et al. (1960a)	2.7		(0.2–6.2)	0.10		(0–0.4)
	Zink (1932)			(0.2–0.5)			
	Berger (1956)	0.20	±0.10	—	0.10	±0.10	—
	Natscheff (1939)	0.14	±0.017	(0.0–0.5)			
	Muzzo (1949)	0.31	±0.168	(0.0–0.54)			
	Garner (1953)	0.21		(0–1.4)			
	Klaus (1958)			(0.01–0.47)	0.18		
	Hansen (1964)	0.19	±0.07	(0.0–0.41)			(0.04–0.44)
Calf	Zink (1932)			(0.3–1.0)			
	Nabholz (1938)			(0.1–0.9)			
	Natscheff (1939)			(0.5–1.9)			
Sheep	Berger (1956)	0.7	±0.50	—	0.4	±0.30	—
	Zink (1932)			(0–0.2)			
	Natscheff (1939)			(0.1–0.5)			
	Muzzo (1949)	0.10	±0.007	(0.0–0.18)			
	Berger (1956)	0.20	±0.2	—	0.10	±0.10	—
	Klaus (1958)	0.19		(0–0.39)	0.12		
	Cornelius et al. (1968)			(0.2)			(0–0.27)
	Hansen (1964)	0.23	±0.09	(0.1–0.42)			
	Roberts (1968)			(0–0.3)			

TABLE I (continued)

Species	Author	Total bilirubin (mg/100 ml)			Conjugated bilirubin (direct-reacting) (mg/100 ml)		
		Mean	σ[b]	Range	Mean	σ[b]	Range
Goat	Berger (1956)	—	—	(0–0.1)	—	—	—
Chimpanzee	Deinhardt et al. (1962)	—	—	(0.0–0.4)	—	—	(0.0–0.1)
	Wisecup et al. (1969)	0.17	±0.05	—	—	—	—
	Havens and Ward (1945)	—	—	(0.07–0.89)	—	—	—
Rhesus monkey	Anderson (1966)	0.38	±0.28	—	0.80	±0.28	—
Squirrel monkey	Minette and Shaffer (1968)	0.50	—	—	0.20	—	—
	Rosenblum and Cooper (1968)	0.20	±0.3	(0.0–1.9)	—	—	—
Marmoset monkey	A. W. Holmes et al. (1967)	0.21	—	(0–2.6)	0.10	—	(0.0–2.1)
	Deinhardt and Deinhardt (1966)	0.20	—	(0–0.4)	0.10	—	(0–0.3)
Howler monkey	Katz et al. (1968)	0.75	±0.06	—	0.17	±0.03	—
Baboon	Pena and Goldzieher (1967)	0.30	±0.17	—	—	—	—
Pig	Zink (1932)	—	—	(0–0.3)	—	—	—
	Lopez Garcia et al. (1943)	—	—	(0.3–0.8)	—	—	—
	Muzzo (1949)	0.09	±0.008	(0.0–0.18)	—	—	—
	Mühe (1951)	—	—	(0.2–0.5)	—	—	—
	Berger (1956)	0.20	±0.2	—	0.10	±0.10	—
	Sisk et al. (1968)	—	—	(0.01–0.23)	—	—	—

[a] Conjugated bilirubin values may vary slightly according to the length of time (1.5 or 15 minutes) allowed by each author for the diazo reaction to proceed. Some free bilirubin may react directly after 5 minutes of interaction and falsely increase the conjugated pigment values.

[b] σ = Standard deviation.

moieties to the carboxyl groups of the two propionic acid side chains of bilirubin (see Fig. 1). Early observations that hepatectomized dogs contained bilirubin conjugates "direct reacting") in their serum caused considerable doubt concerning the interpretation of the van den Bergh test. The exact nature of the bilirubin conjugates in the serum of most domestic animals with hepatic disease is not known.

Gunn (1938), a Canadian geneticist, observed that a strain of rats developed jaundice and severe kernicterus shortly before birth. A similar syndrome of *congenital nonhemolytic jaundice* (Crigler and Najjar, 1952) was reported in human infants with serum free bilirubin levels of 25–45 mg/100 ml. Both syndromes are transmitted as simple autosomal recessives and are due to a deficiency of glucuronyl transferase in the liver. Another bile pigment disease called *Gilbert's syndrome* or *constitutional hepatic dysfunction* has been reported in human adults between 15 and 25 years with free bilirubin levels of between 1 and 6 mg/100 ml. Arias and London (1957) reported that hepatic glucuronyl transferase is also greatly reduced in these patients and that inheritance is most likely dominant with incomplete penetrance. Recent studies (Barrett *et al.*, 1968) indicate a lower fractional transfer of bilirubin from plasma to liver exists in Gilbert's syndrome. A Southdown mutant sheep with a similar hepatic uptake defect for bilirubin has been recently studied (Cornelius and Gronwall, 1965), and resembles Gilbert's syndrome in man. *Chronic idiopathic jaundice* (Dubin and Johnson, 1954) in man is characterized by a tender liver, chronic intermittent bilirubinemia (both free and conjugated bilirubin), impaired sulfobromophthalein (BSP) excretion, normal serum transaminase activity, and an unidentified melanin hepatic pigment. An identical syndrome in Corriedale sheep has recently been observed (Cornelius *et al.*, (1965a, 1968). A reduced transport maxima for bilirubin and BSP are characteristic signs of this lethal disease. Another inherited condition in man, *chronic familial nonhemolytic jaundice*, was first recognized by

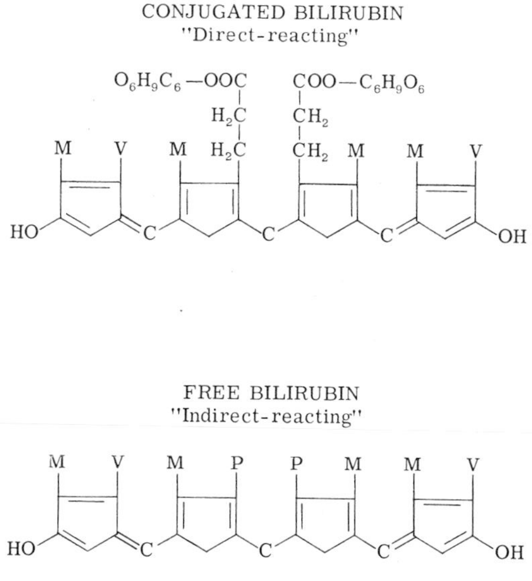

Fig. 1.   Chemical structure of free bilirubin and bilirubin diglucuronide.

Rotor *et al.* (1948) in the Philippine Islands and later studied chromatographically by Schiff *et al.* (1959). Clinical findings included: a greatly delayed BSP excretion; all other function tests normal; chronic, mild, intermittent icterus (both free and conjugated bilirubin); no abnormal liver pigments; and normal life span.

Isselbacher and McCarthy (1958) have presented evidence that a small percentage of excreted bilirubin can also be conjugated as an alkali-stable ethereal sulfate derivative. This conjugation is similar to that observed in the conjugation of corticosteroids, estrogens, morphine, and serotonin, which are all excreted as either glucuronides or ethereal sulfate derivatives. That bilirubin is excreted into the bile mainly as a glucuronide derivative is recognized in man (Schmid, 1956), dog (Talafont, 1956), guinea pig (Schmid *et al.*, 1957), rat (Grodsky and Carbone, 1957), and horse, pig, and cat (Cornelius *et al.*, 1960a). Azo derivatives isolated from freshly secreted bile of the bull and sheep were indistinguishable chromatographically (Fig. 2) from the azo derivatives of bilirubin glucuronide of rat and canine bile (Cornelius *et al.*, 1960a). Little bilirubin or biliverdin was detected in freshly collected hepatic duct bile from sheep or pigs. This finding was interpreted as presumptive evidence that free bilirubin or biliverdin commonly observed in the gallbladder bile of sheep, cattle, and pigs results from the hydrolysis of bilirubin

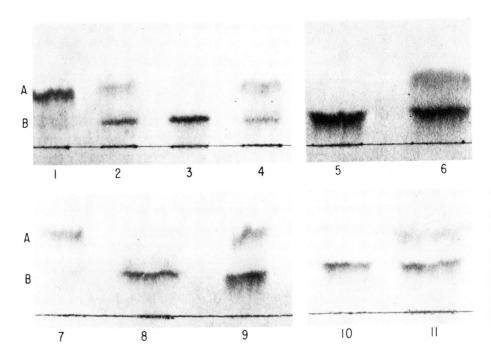

Fig. 2.   Ascending paper chromatograms—methyl ethyl ketone, propionic acid, and water (75:25/30)—of hydroxypyrromethene azo derivatives of commercial free bilirubin (CFB) and polar, water-soluble bilirubin glucuronide (BG) in several species: 1, CFB; 2, mixture of CFB and canine BG; 3, canine BG; 4, mixture of CFB and rat BG; 5, feline BG from hepatic duct bile; 6, ovine free bilirubin and BG from gall bladder bile; 7, CFB; 8, canine BG; 9, porcine free bilirubin and BG from gall bladder bile; 10, equine BG; and 11, mixture of CFB and equine BG. (Cornelius *et al.*, 1960a.)

conjugates previously present in the gallbladder. Subsequent reoxidation of a percentage of the resulting free bilirubin to biliverdin occurs in these species and imparts the green color to their bile. A recent study on bile pigments in chickens revealed that hepatoenteric duct bile contained 70% as much biliverdin as bilirubin (Lind *et al.*, 1967). Chromatographic analysis of bile pigment extracted from a gallstone in a calf revealed the presence of only free bilirubin (Cornelius *et al.*, 1960a). Free bilirubin, which is nonpolar and relatively insoluble in alkaline bile, is known to precipitate with biliary glycoproteins in man to form biliary calculi. Various cases of biliary lithiasis have been reported in many domestic animals: dogs (Schlotthauer, 1945), cow (Ford, 1955), and horse (Sastry, 1945).

   b. Classification of Icterus.   The various types of icterus may be classified as follows.

i. Prehepatic or Hemolytic Icterus.   This condition is characterized by the presence of an indirect van den Bergh reaction due to the presence of increased amounts of free bilirubin from excessive erythrocyte hemolysis or overproduction by the liver. Recent studies on the turnover of hepatic nonhemoglobin hemoproteins such as catalase, peroxidase, tryptophan pyrrolase, and the mitochondrial cytochromes suggest that their overproduction could account for unexplained hyperbilirubinemias in certain disorders (Lester and Troxler, 1969).

ii. Hepatic Icterus.   This condition can be identified primarily by a direct van den Bergh reacting pigment (bilirubin conjugates) which regurgitates into the serum from intrahepatic functional or mechanical obstruction of biliary canaliculi. In addition, some indirect reacting pigment (free bilirubin) will be present from decreased hepatic uptake of free bilirubin from the blood or increases in hepatic β-glucuronidase (Acocella *et al.*, 1968) due to hepatic cell insufficiency (the horse is an exception; see Section IV,A,1,e).

iii. Obstructive Icterus (extrahepatic).   This condition is characterized by a direct reaction due to serum bilirubin diglucuronide. Bilirubin conjugates gain entrance to the blood by extensive regurgitation via hepatic lymphatics from bile duct obstruction. Some unconjugated bilirubin will also be present in the serum.

   c. van den Bergh test.   Following the biochemical clarification of the van den Bergh test in recent years, the clinician can now more rationally differentiate between the types of icterus present. (See Figs. 3–6 for simplified graphic illustrations of the types of icterus and of the enterohepatic circulation of bile pigments.)

   The qualitative test is no longer used extensively as a practical diagnostic procedure. The quantitative test which measures the unconjugated (indirect reacting) and conjugated bilirubin (direct reacting) may be determined by routine methods (Malloy and Evelyn, 1937; Ducci and Watson, 1945).

   A host of modifications of the 1-minute method of reading the direct reaction have been suggested in human medicine. Sherlock (1958) has recommended reading the conjugated bilirubin (direct reacting) photoelectrically after 30 minutes and the total bilirubin in 50% methyl alcohol also at 30 minutes. A preponderance of unconjugated bilirubin indicates hemolytic icterus, but if more than half is conjugated, the icterus may be either hepatocellular or obstructive. Powell (1944) has modified the procedure of Malloy and Evelyn (1937) since turbidity from protein precipitation occurs when over 0.4 ml serum is used in the case of low bilirubin concentrations.

d. DOG.   The interpretation of the van den Bergh test in the dog more closely approximates that of man than that of the other domestic animals. However, the low renal threshold (F. Rosenthal and Meier, 1921; Mills and Dragstedt, 1938) observed in the dog for bilirubin conjugates is responsible for lower serum levels of bilirubin in intrahepatic cholestasis or extrahepatic obstruction of the biliary system. High levels of preponderantly free bilirubin are indicative of hemolytic diseases in the dog. If greater than 50% of the total bilirubin is of the conjugated variety, hepatocellular disease is most likely present. Extrahepatic obstruction of the bile duct system is accompanied by even a greater percentage of conjugated bilirubin in the serum, but minor amounts of unconjugated bilirubin are usually present. The presence of unexplained amounts of serum unconjugated bilirubin in intrahepatic cholestasis may result from either increased hepatic deconjugation of bilirubin glucuronide (Acocella *et al.*, 1968), or different net fractional clearance rates for bilirubin and its conjugate from serum during the process of active transport. This unconjugated bile pigment, however, may result from the lack of hepatic uptake of bilirubin, the exact cause of which is unknown at present.

Because of the low renal threshold for the regurgitated bilirubin glucuronide in the serum, slight elevations in concentration are quite indicative of hepatocellular disease. Needless to say, an elevated presence in the urine is quite a sensitive and practical clinical test. Hoe and Harvey (1961b) also observed that dogs showing bilirubinuria many times were without hyperbilirubinemia.

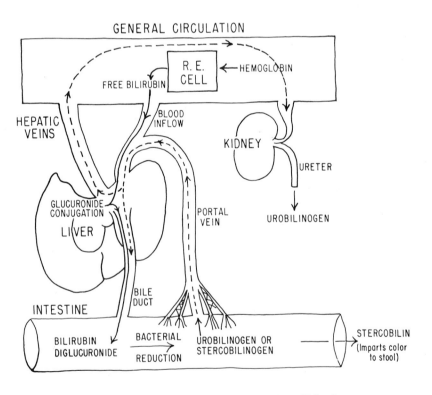

Fig. 3.   The normal enterohepatic circulation of bile pigments.

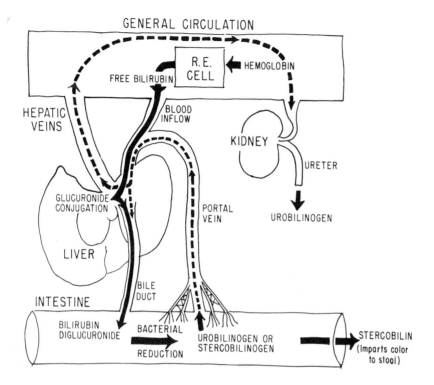

Fig. 4.   Hemolytic crisis. Observe the increase in the quantity of free bilirubin in the serum (unable to pass the renal filter), stercobilin in the stool (imparts a darker color to the stool), and urinary urobilinogen. Increased urinary urobilinogen may be due partly to secondary liver damage (less reexcreted into the bile and hence lost to the serum and urine) in addition to the increased quantity of bile pigments metabolized owing to erythrocyte hemolysis. If secondary liver damage is extensive from hemosiderosis or bile pigment overload, some bilirubin glucuronide may be regurgitated and lost to the urine (not in diagram).

Brouwers (1941), Hoerlein and Greene (1950), Gornall and Bardawill (1952), and Karsai (1954), studied serum bilirubin levels in canine diseases. Total bilirubin levels as high as 4.0 mg/100 ml were observed in dogs with leptospirosis. A detailed study by Hoe and Harvey (1961b) on bilirubin in 300 canine sera revealed that exceedingly low values are found in nearly all healthy canine sera with 63% less than 0.2 mg/100 ml and 35% exhibiting no measurable bilirubin. A considerable range was reported for dogs with jaundice. A Labrador with cirrhosis revealed a serum level of 1 mg/100 ml while a poodle with the same condition had levels of 20 mg bilirubin/100 ml serum. The level of serum bilirubin does not always correlate with the degree of hepatic damage when renal parenchymal disease is present. In experiments with various hepatotoxic halogenated hydrocarbons, the serum bilirubin levels increased proportionately with hepatic necrosis. Although serum bilirubin values can occasionally be quite elevated in prolonged extrahepatic obstruction or intrahepatic cholestasis (19.6 mg/100 ml; Malherbe, 1959; Van Vleet and Alberts, 1968), most hepatocellular diseases are accompanied by serum bilirubin levels of less

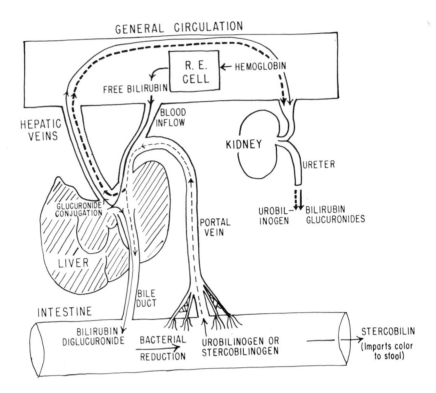

Fig. 5. Hepatocellular pathology. Observe the presence of bilirubin glucuronide and increased amounts of urobilinogen in the urine. Increased urinary urobilinogen is due to the inability of the altered hepatic cells to quantitatively reexcrete this pigment into the bile. Free bilirubin may also be elevated in the serum owing to a decreased hepatic uptake of the pigment.

than 4 mg/100 ml. Similar hepatic diseases in man would be accompanied by substantially higher serum bilirubin concentrations. Snell *et al.* (1925) observed that only traces of bilirubin could be detected in canine serum 24 hours after common duct ligation with the gallbladder *in situ*; in 48–72 hours the serum contained 2–4 mg/100 ml of bilirubin and it appeared in the urine. Bilirubinemia increased for the first 2 weeks and then reached a plateau. In dogs with cholecystectomy and common duct ligation, increases in serum bilirubin appeared within 30 minutes (0.3 mg/100 ml). Four hours after ligation, it had reached 2.2 mg/100 ml and 13.4 mg/100 ml at the end of 17 days of stasis. Similar findings have been observed in cats. Others (Van Vleet and Alberts, 1968) have reported serum bilirubin levels to peak at near 4 mg/100 ml by 5–6 days and subside thereafter.

Numerous investigations on the fate of intravenously injected free bilirubin in dogs have been made. Early studies by Tarchanoff (1874) revealed that free bilirubin, injected intravenously into dogs with biliary fistulas, was excreted into the bile and not the urine. Appelmans and Bouckaert (1926) observed that hyperbilirubinemia in dogs following the injection of 15 mg of free bilirubin disappeared more slowly in those with ligated bile ducts or with phosphorus poisoning. Intravenously injected free bilirubin is rapidly removed from the serum of the dog during the first 3 hours and cannot be totally accounted for in the bile. Berman *et al.* (1941) infused 5–12 mg free bilirubin/kg body weight to dogs with functional nephrectomy. Serum bilirubin levels were elevated to 9–13 mg/100 ml and at 1 hour after autopsy, only 34–40 mg/100 ml total injected bilirubin could be accounted for in blood and bile. Bilirubin loading experiments in dogs generally suggest that the removal of injected bilirubin is determined by the amount of functional liver tissue. Following the intravenous injection of free bilirubin, measurable biliary pigments began rising in concentration at 30 minutes after injection, reaching a peak at 2.5 hours and subsiding by 5–6 hours (Stroebe, 1932). With more exacting techniques, Cantarow *et al.* (1948) claimed to recover 60–100% of the intravenously injected bilirubin by 4 hours. Li *et al.* (1944) were able to produce chronic hyperbilirubinemia and icterus of 4 weeks duration by repeated injections of 50 mg bilirubin dissolved in canine plasma. No demonstrable injury occurred in the bilirubin loading experiments of Snapp *et al.* (1947), who repeatedly injected 300 mg every 3 days into dogs. Cytotoxic effects from albumin-bound free bilirubin can be produced by injecting 10 mg bilirubin/100 mg body weight. Such serum concentrations (60–70 mg/100 ml) never occur in adult mammals owing to the high clearing capacity of the liver. More recent studies reveal that 10–20% of all bilirubin originates from non-erythroid sources and accounts for the rapid penetrance of isotope into bilirubin following the administration of aminolevulinic acid-^{14}C (S. H. Robinson *et al.*, 1966).

The injection of BSP and other organic anions are well known to interfere with the excretion of bilirubin. The biochemical nature of this competition and its sites have not been elucidated. The icteric index of the dog is normally less than 6 units and is generally correlated directly with the total serum bilirubin

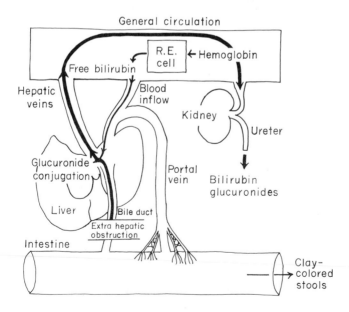

Fig. 6. Extrahepatic obstruction. Observe regurgitation to the serum and subsequently the urine of all bilirubin diglucuronide conjugated in the liver. Urinary urobilinogen and fecal stercobilin are absent.

levels. Distinct elevations indicate an increase in the total serum bilirubin level.

e. HORSE. The interpretation of the van den Bergh test or quantitative values of unconjugated and conjugated serum bilirubin in the horse is quite different from other species. It is well known that the greater part of bilirubin found in the serum of horses with either hemolytic or hepatic icterus is free bilirubin (Eikmeier, 1959; Cornelius *et al.*, 1960a; Benedek, 1961). It is not uncommon to find serum levels up to 25 mg/100 ml of free bilirubin in equine hepatopathy with less than 2 mg/100 ml of direct-reacting pigment. The serum bilirubin from a series of horses with hepatic lesions was recently examined chromatographically which confirmed the "indirect reacting" pigment to be free bilirubin. Bierthen (1906) and Benedek (1956) have reported that the bile of the horse fails to react with routine bile pigment tests, whereas Cornelius *et al.* (1960a) observed that bile collected via biliary cannulation contained bilirubin as a glucuronide derivative as in man. V. H. Grassnickel (1959) and Eikmeier (1959) concluded that icterus of the equine scleral conjunctiva cannot be used as a symptom of damaged liver parenchyma or aberrant bilirubin metabolism. Since icterus and hyperbilirubinemia do not always coincide in time, it was concluded that the yellow coloration of the conjunctiva of a healthy horse could be due to bilirubin storage. The measurement of conjugated and total bilirubin levels in horses with and without yellow coloration revealed no difference in their serum concentrations. The serum icteric index in the horse and the cow varies directly with the amounts of carotenoids and xanthophylls present in the diet. The icteric index of the normal horse is usually between 7.5 and 20 and that of the cow between 5 and 25. For this reason, the use of the icteric indices in such herbivores in estimating the bilirubin level is quite unsatisfactory. Its use in sheep is feasible due to the lack of serum carotenoids; however, xanthophyll elevations in liver disease can be confusing (Roberts, 1968).

Elevations in the serum free bilirubin may be observed secondarily to many environmental and pathological conditions in horses. Lopuchovsky and Jantosovic (1958) observed bilirubin levels to be elevated as follows: cardiac insufficiency, 2.76–6.27 mg/100 ml; constipation, 2.8–7.8 mg/100 ml; gangrenous pneumonia, 5.12 mg/100 ml; hemolytic diseases, 6.8–8.3 mg/100 ml; and primary hepatic disorders, 5.19–26.14 mg/100 ml, with the majority of levels over 20 mg/100 ml. Another investigator found serum bilirubin levels in horses with pneumonia and other infectious diseases to be between 10 and 50 mg/100 ml (Zenglein, 1930). In colic-constipation syndromes of horses, the serum free bilirubin is usually markedly elevated. The suggestion by many investigators that this is presumably due to occlusion of the biliary passages is questionable. Starvation of only a few days' duration is also accompanied by hyperbilirubinemia.

A recent study by Gronwall and Mia (1969) revealed that plasma bilirubin levels increased in the horse within 12 hours of last feeding and increased between 2 and 4 days to levels eight times prestarvation values. Infusion of bilirubin resulted in a more rapid rise in plasma-unconjugated bilirubin levels in starved horses; in addition, a decreased removal capacity was present. Conjugated bilirubin increased only slightly following starvation or bilirubin infusion. The fractional transfer of unconjugated bilirubin-^{14}C from the "rapidly mixing pool" to the "storage pool" (primarily liver) was decreased in starved horses. This redistribution of bilirubin into the "rapidly mixing pool" which includes the plasma and an apparent reduction in the volume of distribution of this pool, accounted in part for the un-conjugated hyperbilirubinemia observed.

Elevation in the serum free bilirubin has been observed in a case of equine hemolytic anemia to be as high as 80 mg/100 ml (Bendixen and Carlström, 1928). In equine infectious anemia, serum bilirubin levels between 25 and 75 mg/100 ml are not uncommon (Zenglein, 1930). Icterus and hyperbilirubinemia are common findings in equine encephalomyelitis; however, degenerative changes are observed in the liver (Chernyak and Rozhov, 1953). The observation of high serum bilirubin levels in a horse should be accompanied by other function tests which are more organ-specific to determine if a serious hepatopathy truly exists.

f. CATTLE. Serum bilirubin levels are only slightly increased in diffuse and severe hepatic disease in the cow. The test may be occasionally helpful but is not always a sensitive indicator of hepatic dysfunction. An extensive outbreak of severe hepatosis occurred in cattle from the ingestion of toxic herring meal in Norway (Hansen, 1964). All cattle with acute "toxic hepatosis" had livers with extensive centrolobular necrosis and damage to the hepatic veins. Chronic cases were typified by a nonportal fibrosis with obliterating changes in the central and sublobular veins. All cattle with the acute form had plasma values for total bilirubin higher than the "upper normal limit"; values for fifteen cattle were recorded at 1.49 ± 0.86 mg/100 ml as compared to levels of 0.19 ± 0.07 in normal animals. A recent study by Ford and Ritchie (1968) on ragwort intoxication in calves concluded that any interference with the liver's ability to remove bilirubin was a terminal change. The elevation of bilirubin levels in the serum of cattle, sheep, pigs, and dogs following starvation or near-starvation conditions has been reported by Berger (1956) and Zink (1932). Nineteen cattle with severe hepatic degeneration and fourteen cattle following experimental carbon tetrachloride had total bilirubin levels between 0.2 and 2.5 mg/100 ml with no immediate "direct-reacting" bilirubin conjugates at a measurable concentration (Benedek, 1961). Similar hepatopathy in man would routinely be associated with levels greater than 10 mg/100 ml. Garner (1953) observed a positive correlation between the icteric indices and plasma carotenoid concentration. No correlation between the icteric indices and the serum bilirubin level was noted. The levels of serum bilirubin shown in the following tabulation were observed in bovine icterus (Garner, 1953).

Clinical	No.	Total bilirubin (mg/100 ml)		
		Mean	Standard deviation	Range
Normal cattle	102	0.31	±0.17	0–1.4
Mild diffuse hepatic lesions	17	0.53	±0.03	0–2.4
Severe diffuse hepatic lesions	10	0.54	±0.03	0–1.2
Localized liver lesions	5	1.0	—	0–2.7
Biliary obstruction	2	0.3, 0.3	—	—
Hemolytic icterus	2	2.3, 7.7	—	—

Beijers (1923) observed a hyperbilirubinemia in newborn calves, similar to that reported in human infants, but never observed visible icterus. In another study of 322 newborn calves, 24 had observable icterus (Metzger, 1927). The causes of neonatal jaundice are under extensive study today on many animal species. Species differences are great. The near-term fetal liver of the dog is relatively mature and contains considerable glucuronyl transferase for conjugation of bilirubin at birth. Unlike the canine placenta, the monkey placenta is a prime excretory organ for bilirubin excretion into the maternal circulation and hepatic glucuronyl transferase activities are low. Certainly the dependence on placental transfer and excretory immaturity in certain species are major contributory factors to the development of neonatal jaundice in certain species (Lester and Troxler, 1969). A thorough investigation of the development of the hepatic uptake, conjugation, and excretory mechanisms will be necessary to elucidate the causative factors in neonatal jaundice in each species in question.

g. PRIMATES. Following the innoculation of squirrel monkeys with *Leptospira icterohaemorrhagiae* organisms, total serum bilirubin levels were elevated to 10.4 mg/100 ml by the tenth day with 50% direct-reacting (Minette and Shaffer, 1968). Studies by Deinhardt *et al.* (1967) on the transmission of human viral hepatitis to marmoset monkeys showed that hyperbilirubinemia occurred in about 20% of the effected animals and found it not to be a sensitive indicator of this experimental hepatic injury. A mild nutritional Laennec's cirrhosis in the rhesus monkey, characterized by lipidic infiltration and cirrhosis, was not accompanied by clinical jaundice and serum bilirubin values remained at normal levels (Gaisford and Zuidema, 1965). No differences in bilirubin levels have been observed in morphine-addicted rhesus monkeys as questionably reported to be present in man (Brooks *et al.*, 1963). Venoocclusive disease in monkeys receiving monocrotaline intraperitoneally was characterized by marked elevations in 8 of 18 experimental animals having serum bilirubin levels over 1.0 mg/100 ml (average of 2.8 mg/100 ml) on the fourteenth day of the experiment. All monkeys which survived exhibited serum bilirubin levels below 1.0 mg/100 ml (Allen *et al.*, 1969).

Limited studies and observations on bilirubin metabolism in nonhuman primates to date suggest a close similarity to humans in the interpretation of serum bilirubin levels in all types of icterus.

h. OTHER SPECIES. The interpretation of the van den Bergh quantitative test is much the same in sheep, goats, and swine as cattle. Major elevations in total bilirubin are usually found only in hemolytic crisis. Increased concentrations in the serum bilirubin conjugates are indicative of severe hepatic involvement or extrahepatic obstruction. Lopez Garcia *et al.* (1943) observed that sheep, swine, and dogs did not tolerate complete biliary occlusion well and died as early as 3 weeks in some instances. Sheep receiving as many as 5000 metacercariae (fascioliasis) were ill by 4–9 weeks and died by the twelfth week. During the course of the disease, bilirubin was elevated only terminally to 1.0 mg/100 ml but sera became discolored with a yellow-orange pigment postulated to be xanthophyll (Roberts, 1968). The interpretation of icteric indices in sheep with hepatopathy has been confusing at best at most veterinary medical centers. Hansen (1964) suggests that the use of serum bilirubin levels in sheep must not be overlooked since, if elevations in concentration remains or increases, prognosis is grave. Complete biliary occlusion is well tolerated in man and monkey; reports have been published of case histories of over 300 days of complete bile duct obstruction without profound symptoms. Centrilobular necrosis occurs in swing livers secondary to complete obstruction in contrast to peripherolobular degeneration in the dog. Beijers (1923) has observed hyperbilirubinemia in newborn lambs, pigs, and goats as previously reported in human infants. A dose level of over 300 μg/kg of aflatoxins to young swine is highly toxic and results in progressive increases in the total serum bilirubin concentrations (Sisk et al., 1968). Elevations in bilirubin occur also following starvation, pregnancy, parasitic obstruction of the bile ducts (Ascaris lumbricoides in pigs; Thysanosoma actinioides in lambs), ingestion of hepatotoxins, and infectious hepatopathy.

Two different lines of mutant sheep were recently observed. Southdown mutants (Cornelius and Gronwall, 1968) with congenital photosensitivity and hyperbilirubinemia are characterized by elevations in serum bilirubin ranging from 0.5 to 1.9 mg/100 ml of which over 60% is unconjugated. In addition, the plasma removal rate of bilirubin is greatly delayed. This Southdown mutant exhibits a hepatic *uptake* defect for bilirubin and other organic anions and resembles Gilbert's syndrome in man (Mia et al., 1969).

A Corriedale ovine mutant (Cornelius et al., 1965a) possesses an organic anion *excretory* defect for bilirubin and certain other organic anions. This mutant is characterized by hyperbilirubinemias of 1.6 ± 0.1 mg/100 ml of which over 60% is bilirubin glucuronide. Livers contain a melanin pigment in the pericanalicular dense bodies and are brownish-black in color. These sheep are nearly identical in all respects to human patients with Dubin-Johnson syndrome. Experimental complete extrahepatic bile duct obstruction in chickens results in only a hyperbilirubinemia, although the bile contains 70% as much biliverdin as bilirubin. All chickens exhibited marked hepatic fibrosis and ductal hyperplasia within 30 days (Lind et al., 1967).

2. Bile Pigments in the Urine

a. BILIRUBIN CONJUGATES. *i. General.* Since free bilirubin apparently does not normally pass the renal filter in most species, only conjugated bilirubin complexes are generally detected in the urine due to their glomerular filtration. The renal threshold for these bilirubin conjugates is directly related to their usefulness in clinical medicine. The low renal threshold for conjugated bilirubin in the dog allows for its use as an extremely sensitive test for early hepatocellular changes (i.e., acute leptospirosis) as well as bile duct obstruction. Naunyn (1868) observed that simple inanition regularly caused bilirubinuria in the dog. The disappearance of bilirubinuria in dogs (with ligated bile ducts) in 24 hours following the administration of nephrotoxins (HgCl$_2$ and uranyl acetate) was reported by Nonnenbruch (1919). Bilirubinuria in hepatic diseases with accompanying renal malfunction may be difficult to interpret because of shifts in the renal threshold for bile pigments. Extrahepatic obstructions due to calculi, parasites, or tumors occluding the common bile duct, account for bilirubinurias of the greatest magnitude. Care should be exercised in interpreting its presence in canine urine since it may be present in a low concentration in any febrile state. The presence of a 1+ reaction on commercial pill tests* is a common finding in many febrile diseases. A 2–3+ reaction is generally considered of diagnostic significance in the dog when specific gravity is between 1.020 and 1.035. The concentration of this bile pigment in the urine is directly proportional to the degree of biliary obstruction, whether intra- or extrahepatic in nature. Hoerlein and Greene (1950) observed increased bilirubin concentrations in the urine of sixteen dogs to be proportional in most instances to severity of BSP retention and elevation of the serum bilirubin level. Urinalysis on eleven canine cases of various types of liver diseases without concomitant kidney damage, revealed bilirubinurias of varying degrees somewhat predicted on the basis of the liver pathology (Hoe and O'Shea, 1965). Sixty percent of normal dogs excrete detectable bilirubin in their urine (Anonymous, 1959). Hoe and Harvey (1961b) have observed, as expected, that many dogs with significant bilirubinuria many times show no bilirubinemia. Gardiner and Parr (1967) observed that the urinary bilirubin levels in two sheep with experimental lupinosis were significantly increased just following the first significant rise in plasma bilirubin levels.

In a group of 78 cattle with traumatic reticulitis, 20 tested positive for bilirubinuria with the methylene blue test; two of three cattle with acetonemia and accompanying hepatic lipidosis were also positive for bilirubin in the urine (Heidrich, 1954). In the same study, only 60% of all cattle with established hepatopathy exhibited bilirubinuria. Since as high as 25% of normal cattle have been reported to have traces of bilirubin in the urine in one study (Kühle, 1926), the interpretation of bilirubinurias in the bovine species requires a careful evaluation. Bilirubinuria must be closely correlated with a careful clinical examination and other more sensitive liver function tests for the cow (i.e., BSP clearance, serum arginase, SGOT). Bilirubin concentration in the urine may be quite instructive concerning the quantitative regurgitation of bile pigments in obstructive processes.

Bilirubin conjugates are not normally found in the urine of the horse, sheep, pig, and cat. Bierthen (1906) observed that bilirubin was nearly always absent from normal equine urine. Cases of equine hemolytic anemia with free serum bilirubin levels as high as 180 mg/100 ml have been observed without bilirubinuria (Beijers *et al.*, 1950). Two horses with extensive hepatopathy and total bilirubin levels of 19.6 mg/100 ml (8.8 mg/100 ml conjugated bilirubin) and 17.8 mg/100 ml (0.8 mg/100 ml of conjugated bilirubin), respectively, continuously excreted 4+ bilirubinurias when measured with the rapid diazo tablet test. Twelve horses with other primary diseases routinely excreted 1+ bilirubinurias (Cornelius and Mia, 1962). Since it is known that such horses have elevations in the free bilirubin and not conjugated bilirubin of the serum, an extremely low renal threshold for bilirubin conjugates could possibly exist in the horse. This has not been established experimentally. An intriguing observation has been the existence of considerable indirect-reacting bilirubin in the urine of the dog and horse. Further studies are needed to clarify if unconjugated bilirubin truly exists in the urine of these two species or whether other diazo-positive pigments are present. Chronic hemolytic diseases with secondary hemosiderosis and/or hepatic necrosis from anemia are nearly always

*Ictotest, Ames Co., Elkhart, Indiana.

accompanied by bilirubinuria from hepatic regurgitation of bilirubin conjugates in all species.

ii. Methods for the Estimation of Urinary Bilirubin Conjugates. The demonstration of conjugated bilirubin in urine is quite helpful in veterinary practice. Most methods used extensively in clinical laboratories are developed for both qualitative and semiquantitative determinations. If freshly voided urine is placed in a bottle and vigorously shaken, the presence of a greenish-yellow foam is suggestive of bilirubinuria. This *foam test* is quite sensitive and easily performed; however, marked increases in the urinary urobilinogen may give a false positive test.

*iii. Diazo Tablet Test.** This rapid and sensitive test is based on the use of a stable diazonium compound which couples with bilirubin under specific conditions. The diagnostic tablet is composed of *p*-nitrobenzene diazonium *p*-toluene sulfonate, sulfosalicylic acid, and sodium carbonate.

iv. Gmelin-Rosenbach Test. In this test, nitric acid is added dropwise (2 drops) to filter paper impregnated with urine. If bilirubin is present, the nitrous acid present oxidizes the bile pigment to colored derivatives: biliverdin (green), bilicyanine (blue), and choletelin (yellow). A modification of this test calls for the addition of 10 ml of 10% barium chloride to 20 ml of urine. After standing for a few minutes, the precipitated bilirubin is filtered and tested with the nitric acid as above. The positive reaction usually shows green on the periphery, then in order toward the center, blue, violet, red, and yellow. The absence of green excludes the presence of bile pigment (Hepler, 1949). This test is many times unsatisfactory in the cow due to the presence of false positive reactions.

v. Harrison's Spot Test. After the precipitation of the urinary bilirubin conjugates with 10% barium chloride as performed above, add 1 or 2 drops of Fouchet's reagent (25 gm trichloracetic acid, 100 ml distilled water, and 10 ml of 10% ferric chloride). A positive reaction is indicated by a blue or green color (Hepler, 1949).

vi. Quantitative Methylene Blue Test. According to Fellinger and Menkes (1933), this test presents an easily performed and accurate quantitative determination of urinary bilirubin. By measuring the number of drops of 0.2% methylene blue to change the initial green color to a definite blue color, a quantitative estimate can be made. Two hundred drops of a 0.2% solution are needed for every milligram of bilirubin. The changing of methylene blue to a green color in the presence of bilirubin may be from an admixture of pigments and not a specific chemical reaction with bilirubin. The test agrees well with other chemical tests for urinary bilirubin and does not react with urobilinogen. The presence of 2 drops of blood hemolyzed in 10 ml of water will, however, give a slightly positive test (Gradwohl, 1956). The test has worked well in hospital laboratories for domestic animals (Krispien, 1952; El-Gindy, 1957).

b. URINARY UROBILINOGEN. *i. General.* This urinary pigment may represent a group of substances rather than a single chemical entity. This heterogeneity, however, may be partially due to an artifact induced for mass spectral analysis. The use of the term urobilinogen in the text of this chapter will in most cases

---

*Ictotest, Ames Co., Elkhart, Indiana.

refer to all "urobilinoids" reacting positively with Ehrlich's reagent. Unless a specific chemical structure is noted (i.e., *l*-stercobilin), the reader should consider the general use of urobilinogen by various authors to refer to a mixture of pigments resulting from the enteric reduction of bilirubin by the bacterial flora. The presence of the "urobilinogen group" in urine signifies the presence of an open bile duct with the simultaneous occurrence of an enterohepatic circulation of bile pigments. Members of this group are produced by bacterial reduction and deconjugation of bilirubin in the intestine. Ten to twenty percent is partially absorbed into the portal circulation and recycled in part (see Fig. 3). The remainder of this reduced pigment is lost to the feces as "stercobilin," which imparts part of the normal color to the stool. Urobilinogen is excreted into the bile intact and unaltered in contrast to bilirubin which must be conjugated to a polar derivative for excretion. The dipyrranes (bilifuscins and pentodyopent compounds) are also important degradation products of hemoglobin and account for much of the color of normal stool. These dipyrranes and possibly tissue cytochromes may possibly be related chemically to the poorly identified "urochromes" which account for most of the color of urine. In addition, the colorless urobilinogen is oxidized by light to the highly colored urobilin by central bridge unsaturation which imparts color to the urine. The presence of clay-colored stools is presumptive evidence for total biliary obstruction; however, in chronic, diffuse, and progressive fibrosis of the liver, clay-colored stools may also occasionally be present due to advanced intrahepatic obstruction in the presence of an open bile duct. A small portion of the "urobilinogen group," which is reabsorbed from the intestine, passes unchanged through the liver and enters the general circulation where it is excreted into the urine. The absence of urinary urobilinogen at one sampling need not indicate bile duct closure since diurnal variations are common. Diuresis encountered in chronic renal diseases may excessively dilute the urobilinogen below the sensitivity of the test in urinalysis (Cornelius, 1957). Urine urobilinogen excretion partly depends on renal function, the state of hydration, and urine pH. It may be advisable in certain cases under study to carefully regulate hydration and the urinary pH.

In hepatocellular damage, there is a defect in the re-excretion into the bile of the urobilinogen from the portal blood; this results in the escape of a greater percentage of these pigments into the circulation and the urine. Royer (1943) found the blood concentration of urobilinogen, injected into the portal vein of dogs, to be five times as high as in hepatic vein blood. Since in experimental hepatic necrosis, equal concentrations of urobilinogen in both the portal and hepatic veins were observed, the escape of large amounts of urobilinogen to the urine would be expected. In hemolytic anemias, greater amounts occur in the urine from both secondary hepatic insufficiency and a quantitative increase in the enterohepatic circulation of bile pigments. Stools are correspondingly darker owing to the increased concentration of stercobilin in hemolytic diseases from increased amounts of circulating pigments. Royer and Biasotti (1932) observed great increases in the concentration of urobilinogen in canine urine following acute hemolysis.

Watson (1959) recently studied the urobilin(ogen) group of pigments in urine, bile, and feces in normal humans and in a variety of pathological circumstances, especially in hemolytic and hepatic states. The three important members of this group were *i*-urobilin, *d*-urobilin, and *l*-stercobilin. Optical activity measurement was of great value in confirming the presence of *d*-urobilin when accompanied by considerable amounts of *i*-urobilin. *i*-Urobilin was found to be preponderant in the urine of certain normal individuals while *l*-stercobilin was observed in others. A considerable amount of new biochemical information is now available in this rapidly growing field of knowledge. Similar findings were observed in hemolytic and hepatic diseases. Fecal urobilin composition also varied greatly. Following broad spectrum antibiotics, which greatly reduce the urine and fecal urobilinogen by suppression of enteric coliforms and clostridia (Sborov *et al.*, 1951), a great preponderance of *d*-urobilin is observed in the urine, feces, and bile (Watson, 1959). These findings are only compatible with an enteric source of all three members of the urobilin(ogen) group.

Incomplete studies are available concerning the metabolism of urobilinoids in man and animals. These have been extensively reviewed by With (1954). Berger (1956) reported to have isolated only stercobilin from the urine of herbivora (horse, cow) and found no urobilin present. In hepatic diseases, both bilirubin conjugates and urobilin were found in addition to the stercobilin. Another study on elevations in the urinary urobilinoids in 100 slaughtered cattle, revealed a 93% correlation with histopathological studies on hepatic tissues. In only 7 of 100 animals with elevated urobilinogen levels were no histopathological changes observed. The author concluded from extensive clinical studies in cattle, horses, and dogs that elevations in the urinary urobilinogen were good diagnostic signs of hepatopathy (Montemagno, 1954). Wester (1912) found only a slight increase in the urinary urobilinoid level following the injection of 3 liters of blood intraperitoneally into cows. This and other studies in dogs have shown that urobilinuria never reaches a high degree after hemorrhagic exudations and hematomas.

Clinical reports concerning the use of the urinary urobilinogen test in hepatic disease in small animals have been conflicting. Early studies on normal and CCl_4-poisoned dogs revealed that various grades of hepatopathy resulted in the excretion of proportional increases in the urobilinogen of the urine. The elevation of urinary urobilinogen did not correlate directly with dye retention tests (phenoltetrachlorphthalein) and suggested a dissociation of specific liver functions (Wallace and Diamond, 1925). No marked abnormalities in the urinary urobilinogen were observed following mild hepatic damage in cats and rabbits, experimentally poisoned with selenium (Smith *et al.*, 1940). Gornall and Bardawill (1952) reported normal levels of urinary urobilinogen in dogs of 0–2 mg/100 ml using Watson's technique. Following CCl_4 poisoning, urobilinogen levels both increased and decreased and led the authors to conclude that the test was of little use in the dog. Others observed that the time required after experimental liver damage (with xylidine) for the urine urobilinogen to increase varied considerably (Svirbely *et al.*, 1946). Most well-controlled studies in which fresh 24-hour urine volumes were available indicate that an absolute increase occurs in the urinary urobilinogen in domestic animals with hepatopathy. The near impossibility in veterinary medicine for the procurement of 24-hour urine aliquots in clinic cases for quantitative estimations subjects urinalysis to questionable semiquantitative methods of measuring urobilinogen. Urobilinogen is rapidly oxidized to urobilin if urine samples are neglectfully left standing at room temperature and exposed to light. Since urobilin does not react in the Ehrlich test, clinical interpretations on such samples may be misleading.

Changes in the specific gravity of urine in the maintenance of water balance will vary the urobilinogen concentration considerably.

ii. Estimation of Urinary Urobilinogen.   Urobilinogen and its colored oxidation product, urobilin, are of equal clinical significance and the choice of tests for the qualitative determinations is a matter of convenience. Fresh urine samples primarily contain the colorless urobilinogen which converts slowly to the brown urobilin upon standing. This change can be accelerated by oxidation of urobilinogen with iodine followed by the spectroscopic examination for urobilin or by Schlesinger's test using zinc acetate (Todd *et al.*, 1953). Watson's quantitative method which depends on the reduction of all urobilin to urobilinogen in a 24-hour sample with ferrous hydroxide is quite accurate and used by most investigators (Watson *et al.*, 1944). In addition, the fresh specimen may be tested for urobilinogen with Ehrlich's aldehyde reagent, preferably followed by saturated sodium acetate to subdue interfering pigments.

Ehrlich's semiquantitative test

1. To 2 ml of fresh urine in a test tube, add 2 ml of modified Ehrlich's reagent (0.7 gm *p*-dimethylaminobenzaldehyde, 150 ml concentrated HCl, and 100 ml distilled water).

2. Immediately mix, and add 4 ml of saturated sodium acetate after 15 and before 30 seconds.

The resulting cherry pink color, which becomes more prominent upon heating, can be reported semiquantitatively from 1 to 4+. Any pink color which results following the addition of Ehrlich's reagent suggests the presence of urobilinogen even though the final dilution with sodium acetate may excessively dilute the color. The color may be observed most sensitively by viewing down from the top of the test tube. A green color which develops immediately in icteric animals may result from the oxidation of bilirubin to biliverdin. Ehrlich's reaction is best performed in urine after precipitation and removal of excessive bilirubin by adding either a small amount of crystalline lead acetate or 1.0 ml of a 10% solution of calcium or barium chloride to 4 ml of urine. A rapid but not always successful method for detecting urobilinogen in the presence of excess bile pigments is the simple deletion of Ehrlich's reagent from the control tube using 2 ml of urine with saturated sodium acetate to volume. Excessive amounts of protein may also interfere by clouding the tube; these may be removed by filtering following protein precipitation with equal volumes of 0.3% sulfosalicylic acid.

Since porphobilinogen is found in the urine in cases of acute intermittent porphyria and also reacts with Ehrlich's reagent to produce a cherry red color, it must be differentiated from urobilinogen. A few milliliters of chloroform may be added and mixed thoroughly. The red aldehyde chromogen of porphobilinogen or indole is completely extracted into the chloroform.

3.   Fecal Bile Pigments

a. FECAL BILIRUBIN.   Bilirubin appears in the feces in conditions preventing its reduction to urobilinogen such as the diarrheas, in the newborn receiving milk, or from the suppression of bacterial action, i.e., the clinical use of broad spectrum antibiotics. Little bilirubin is reabsorbed from the intestinal mass. Gmelin's or

Harrison's test may be used to test qualitatively for the presence of bilirubin. In Gmelin's test, simply add a few drops of nitric acid (containing nitrous acid) to a smear of feces on a piece of white porcelain; the play of colors, green, blue, violet, red, and yellow, indicates a positive reaction. In stools with excessive chlorophyll or bacterial pigments, an aqueous extract can be tested. Fouchet's reagent (Harrison test) can be added to a 1:20 dilution of stool and the presence of a blue color indicates the presence of bilirubin.

b. Fecal Stercobilin. Compounds of the urobilinoid group similar to those observed in the urine are found in the stool, with stercobilin(ogen) usually predominating. A daily visual inspection for stool color of the icteric patient is quite important since stercobilin and various dipyrranes gives the stool its characteristic color. In contrast to the situation in urine, most of the bile pigments are in their highly colored and oxidized form. They are elevated considerably following hemolytic processes and decreased in bile duct obstruction. Quantitative fecal stercobilin determinations cannot be recommended for routine practice since reproducible methods are quite lengthy. They should be used only in the investigation of cases of obscure icterus when one questions the presence of hemolytic manifestations.

Schmidt Test. Rub a pea-sized amount of fresh feces into a petri dish and mix with a 5% aqueous solution of mercuric chloride. Cover the dish and observe after several hours, perferably 24 hours. Urobilinoids give a pink color, while bilirubin is oxidized to a green biliverdin color. The absence of any color after 24 hours indicates the absence of bile pigments. Excessive lipids may be extracted with ether.

B. Foreign Dyes

Halogenated phthalein dyes were first used in the study of liver function by Rowntree *et al.* (1913), who measured the fecal excretion of phenoltetrachlorphthalein following its parenteral administration. Subsequently, it was shown by S. M. Rosenthal and White (1925) that intravenously administered BSP is removed almost exclusively by the liver. The uptake, conjugation, and excretion by the liver of foreign dyes is a measure of both hepatic biochemical integrity and blood flow. Owing to the large number of rate-limiting steps in their excretion, they are among the most sensitive indicators of hepatic dysfunction. Delay in their removal from the blood may be due to hepatic necrosis and/or fibrosis with a reduced parenchymal mass and subsequent depressed hepatic blood flow. Since competition for hepatic uptake between many foreign dyes and bilirubin occurs with subsequent delay of their clearance from the plasma, these tests offer certain problems in interpretation in the presence of icterus with high levels of serum bilirubin. Foreign dyes which have been used in veterinary medicine are BSP (Bromsulphalein)*, rose bengal, indocyanine green, and phenoltetrachlorphthalein.

1. *Sulfobromophthalein (BSP)*

The BSP clearance rate from plasma is widely used at present as an index of hepatic function in domestic animals. Both Brauer *et al.* (1955) and Wirts and

*Hynson, Wescott and Dunning, Inc., Baltimore, Maryland.

Cantarow (1942) early showed that the pigment is taken up quite rapidly and concentrated by the liver with subsequent excretion into the bile. Wheeler and coworkers (1960a) have demonstrated that the rate of hepatic uptake continues to increase in proportion to the dose and plasma concentration with the rate of excretion by the liver reaching a maximum when BSP is infused at high concentrations. Experimental data suggest that uptake, conjugation, and excretion of BSP are controlled by independent mechanisms. The major portion of BSP is conjugated in the liver with glutathione via the mercaptide linkage of the cysteine moiety (Grodsky et al., 1959) and excreted into the bile. The maximum secretion rate for free BSP in rats was 3–7 μg/min/gm liver, while the maximum secretory capacity of the BSP conjugate was not reached even when 60 mg BSP/kg body weight was administered. It would appear that the uptake of BSP from the blood is a dynamic process which proceeds somewhat independent of its conjugation with glutathione. Philp et al. (1961) concluded that conjugation is one limiting step which affects the hepatic secretory rate of this dye. Gronwall and Cornelius (1966) recently presented evidence that a concentration maximum exists for BSP in the bile of sheep at approximately 15 mg/ml. The BSP excretory rate is therefore related proportionately to the bile flow rate when the concentration maximum for BSP in bile has been reached.

Probably the most exciting new diagnostic procedure to be recently developed is a method by Wheeler et al. (1960a,b) in which BSP is infused at three different rates and both the hepatic storage (S) and transport maximum (T_m) for BSP can be indirectly calculated from analyzing multiple peripheral blood samples. This method allows for the independent calculation of S and T_m without any concern about hepatic blood flow or hepatic vein BSP concentrations. Since many clinical disorders are characterized by differences in their BSP storage and T_m, this technique should be of great use in veterinary medicine. The technique has already proven useful in studying ovine mutants with hyperbilirubinemia (Cornelius et al., 1965a, 1968). All students of liver function should become familiar with this new clinical technique. Numerous compounds known to interfere and compete with BSP uptake have been reported: cholic acid derivatives, bilirubin, and 17-substituted testosterones (Heaney and Whedon, 1958). The BSP clearance test is difficult to interpret in cases of severe bilirubinemia.

a. Dog. Extensive experimental studies have been made concerning BSP clearance in dogs (Moses et al., 1948; Brauer et al., 1955; Larson and Morrill, 1960). The superiority of the BSP test in the dog over many other liver functions has been suggested by Drill and Ivy (1944), Svirbely et al. (1946), and Hoerlein and Greene (1950).

The rate of BSP disappearance and hence percentage retention in dogs is independent of dosage between 5 and 20 mg BSP/kg (Moses et al., 1948). The use of 5 mg/kg is generally accepted (Fig. 7). It is demonstrated in Fig. 7 why the BSP test in the dog is considerably less sensitive than the new infusion technique of Wheeler et al. (1960b). After the single injection of 5 mg BSP/kg, certain dogs will have less than 5% dye retention by 10–15 minutes and allow for the clinician to miss minor hepatic damage. Using the Wheeler "indirect" technique for measuring BSP S and T_m, average values of 25 mg BSP stored per mg/100 ml plasma/10 kg and 1.9 mg/min/10 kg, respectively, were reported for the dog (Wheeler et al.,

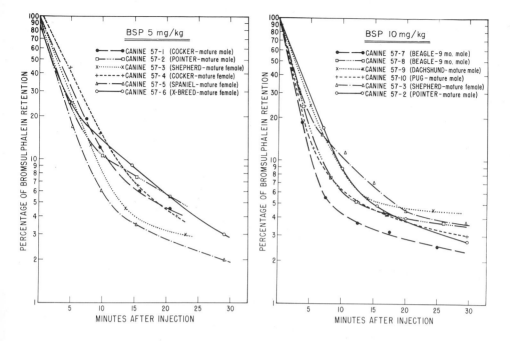

Fig. 7. Percentage retention of sulfobromophthalein (Bromsulphalein; BSP) in dogs following the injection of 5 and 10 mg/kg body weight. Note similarity of retention at both levels. (Cornelius, 1957).

1960b). The use of BSP in cats has been mainly limited to experimental studies, i.e., studies in the alteration of BSP retention in relation to morphological changes in the liver and bile passages following total biliary stasis (Cantarow and Stewart, 1935).

i. Method:

1. Weigh the dog and divide his weight *in pounds* by the factor 22. This figure provides the number of milliliters of the BSP solution (50 mg/ml) to inject in order to give 5 mg/kg body weight.
2. Inject the dye solution into the cephalic vein slowly, taking care to prevent any perivascular infiltration which may cause sloughing.
3. At 30 minutes after injection, remove 5 ml of heparinized blood from the opposite cephalic vein.
4. Centrifuge blood and pipet 0.5 ml of the unhemolyzed plasma into two cuvettes. Add 2.5 ml of distilled water to each tube.
5. Add 3 ml of 0.1 N HCl to the blank tube (colorless) and 3 ml of 0.1 N NaOH to the other tube to produce maximum BSP color.
6. Read unknown against the blank at 565 mμ on a standard curve as recommended by Hepler (1949).
7. Percent retention can be calculated by multiplying the 30-minute concentration (mg/100 ml) by the factor 10.

Rapid office kit. A comparator box with permanent standards can be obtained commercially* for rapid determinations in the veterinary hospital. In using this kit, pipet the plasma into 2 small tubes and add 1 or 2 drops of 10% sodium hydroxide to one tube to bring out the color of the remaining dye. To the other (blank tube) add a few drops of 5% HCl to ensure the absence of any BSP color. Place the latter tube as a blank in front of the standard. By comparing the alkalinized serum to the standards, a colorimetric estimation of the percent of retained dye can easily be made.

ii. Interpretation.   Less than 5% BSP retention at 30 minutes is generally accepted to be the normal range for dogs. Most studies, however, agree that up to 10% retention at 30 minutes after injection will only rarely be found in dogs with no apparent hepatic injury (Svirbely *et al.*, 1946). Similar findings were observed by Drill and Ivy (1944). Others (Hoerlein and Greene, 1950) have reported a trace to no BSP present at 30 minutes, using the commercial comparator blocks. Differences in methods have caused a wide variation of dye retention values for normal dogs. Larson and Morrill (1960) have recently proposed the use of the 45-minute retention value using a Beckman Model B spectrophotometer and the procedure of Hepler (1949). BSP retentions in normal control dogs using this procedure were less than 1.5% at 45 minutes. Richards *et al.* (1959) have recently shown experimentally that the BSP test can be modified in the dog to allow for the prediction of the rate of transfer of dye between blood, liver cell, and bile from a graph of the fall in the plasma BSP concentration.

Delayed BSP retention in dogs has been reported in a variety of diseases affecting the liver: leptospirosis (Hoerlein and Greene, 1950); Harvey, 1967; Van Vleet and Alberts, 1968), hepatic lipidoses with centrilobular necrosis, periportal fibrosis, focal hepatitis, carbon tetrachloride poisoning, infectious hepatitis (Larson and Morrill, 1960), xylidine intoxication (Svirbely *et al.*, 1946), diabetes mellitus with hepatic lipidoses and degeneration, leukemia with hepatic metastasis, diffuse hepatic fibrosis, secondary hepatic degeneration associated with ascites, ulcerative duodenitis, gastroenteritis, coccidial hemorrhagic enteritis, thallium and tetrachlorethylene intoxication (Nielsen, 1952), and diseases of the uterus (Lettow, 1961). Larson and Morrill (1960) concluded in an extensive study on 85 dogs that although BSP retention and hepatic damage were at times inconsistently related, it still remained as one of the most sensitive tests to measure acute viral and toxic hepatitis in the dog. In 63 bitches with hormonal uterine diseases, histological examination of the liver in nearly all cases showed some degree of degenerative or inflammatory changes; 52% of these bitches had severe secondary hepatic degeneration (Lettow, 1961). Delayed BSP clearance is usually observed in conditions such as cardiac decompensation, shock, and severe dehydration which cause a lowered hepatic blood flow and hence less BSP extraction. Findings concerning the effects of fever, per se, on BSP clearance in animals are not in agreement. Smith *et al.* (1940) studied BSP removal for the estimation of liver damage in cats with selenium poisoning and observed no dye retention at 30 minutes in all cases.

Although the BSP test in the dog appears to be one of the most sensitive of all tests to detect latent liver damage, correlation of dye retention, and hepatic lesions

---

*Hynson, Wescott and Dunning, Inc., Baltimore, Maryland.

are not always consistent when either one is of a mild nature. In this test, the hepatic blood flow, the complex process of cellular BSP uptake, conjugation, and excretion, and the patency of the bile duct are all assessed. The absence of elevations in the serum glutamic pyruvic transaminase (SGPT) from hepatic necrosis, associated with delayed BSP retention, indicates the presence of fibrosis or a reduced hepatic blood flow. Lesions impeding primarily the hepatic arterial flow in the dog have been reported to affect the dye clearance more than those restricting the portal flow (Andrews *et al.*, 1956). This observation has not been substantiated.

The measurement of the hepatic blood flow by the BSP method was first proposed by Bradley *et al.* (1945) in man by measuring the hepatic extraction of BSP. Myers (1947) found similar flow values using either urea or BSP in man. Both Sherlock *et al.* (1950) and Cohn *et al.* (1948) questioned the validity of the technique and suggested that the high rate of extrahepatic BSP removal invalidated its use. The average hepatic blood flow values for 49 dogs using hepatic vein catheterization were 42 ml/kg/min or 140 ml/100 gm liver/min. Such estimates were slightly high owing to extrahepatic loss of BSP (Werner and Horvath, 1952). In this method, the infusion rate of BSP was such to maintain a constant level (P, mg/100 ml) and this rate was considered equivalent to removal (R) of BSP. By applying the Fick principle, the estimated hepatic blood flow (EHBF) was calculated using the formula of Bradley and associates (1945):

H = BSP concentration in mg/100 ml of efferent hepatic blood

$$\text{EHBF} = \frac{R}{0.01(P - H)} \times \frac{1}{1 - \text{hematocrit}}$$

b. HORSE.   Due to the rapid removal of injected BSP from equine blood, the fractional clearance (K) of BSP/min has recently been proposed as the BSP method of choice for the horse (Cornelius and Wheat, 1957; Karsai, 1960). Others have proposed the use of methods which obtain the percentage of BSP retention at 15–30 minutes after injection (Aktan, 1954; Morgan, 1959a). Advantages of the BSP clearance test over the percentage retention test are: that sampling can be completed within 12 minutes after injection; plasma samples can be taken any time between 5 and 12 minutes after injection; plasma volume can be calculated; and quantitative assessment of liver function can be made in terms of the kinetics of BSP disappearance from the plasma. Some disadvantages of any test which requires the calculation of percentage retention are: the animal must be weighed; an exact quantity of dye must be injected; the plasma sample must be taken at one critical time only; and the influences of plasma volume and estimated hepatic blood flow are not assessable.

i. *BSP Clearance Method.*   The dye is available in 1-gm ampules for use in large domestic species (Cornelius, 1958).

Inject 1 gm intravenously.

Following an approximate 5-minute period, two heparinized blood samples are taken before 12 minutes, preferably about 4 minutes apart, i.e., 5 and 9 or 6 and 10 minutes postinjection. However, the two samples can be taken at any recorded time after injection. The BSP concentrations of the two samples are determined spectrophotometrically as follows: 2 ml of plasma is transferred to 12 × 105 mm cuvettes containing 3 ml of 0.1 N NaOH. The blank consists of 2 ml plasma, 3 ml 0.1 N NCl, and 1 ml water. Any spectrophotometer with a wavelength of 565 mμ

can be used for the BSP determinations. Standard curves for BSP determinations should be made using 2 ml equine plasma.

BSP concentrations of the two samples (mg/100 ml) are next plotted on semilog paper and the $T_{1/2}$ for BSP clearance calculated as shown in Fig. 8. The $T_{1/2}$ is that time required for the BSP concentration to be halved in the plasma. BSP clearance can be expressed clinically in $T_{1/2}$ units (minutes).

Fractional clearance (K) or the percent of dye cleared from the plasma per minute can easily be calculated from the following formula:

$$K = \frac{\ln 2}{T_{1/2}} \qquad \ln 2 = 0.692$$

Fractional clearance (K) can also be calculated by using the following kinetic relationships:

$$K = \frac{c}{V} = 2.3 \times \frac{\log P_1 - \log P_2}{t_2 - t_1}$$

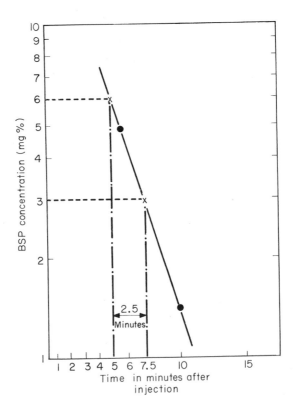

Fig. 8. Method of calculating $T_{1/2}$ values for sulfobromophthalein (Bromsulphalein; BSP) clearance test in the horse. (Cornelius, 1958.) Procedure: (1) Bled at 6 and 10 minutes after injection. (2) Plotted points (●) of 4.9 and 1.4 mg%. Line drawn through points. (3) Time ($T_{1/2}$ observed, e.g., from 6 mg% to 3 mg%. (4) $T_{1/2}$ = 2.5 minutes. Horse has normal liver. (Normals = 2.81 ±0.5 minutes.)

where c = clearance (units in ml plasma/min); V = plasma volume; P = plasma BSP concentration (mg/100 ml); and t = time of sampling (minutes).

True hepatic plasma flow can only be calculated if the plasma volume (V), fractional clearance (K), and efficiency (N) of dye extraction from the circulating plasma are known. Dobson and Jones (1952), using colloidal chromic phosphate, performed similar techniques in hepatic blood flow studies. Since no extraction efficiency (N) for the hepatic removal of BSP in horses and cattle is known, clearance (c) may be used only in comparative studies between normal and diseased animals. In the presence of hepatic injury, hepatic plasma flow may be overestimated due to an unpredictable extent from increased extrahepatic dye uptake.

ii. Plasma Volume. This can be readily determined since BSP is bound primarily to albumin in the circulating blood. The two concentrations of BSP are plotted on semilog coordinates and a line drawn through them to intersect the ordinant at 0 time. This ordinant intercept (X_0) represents the concentration of BSP at the time of injection in the plasma if mixing had been complete and instantaneous. Since the number of milliliters of BSP injected (i) and its concentration (X_i) are known, the plasma volume (V) can be accurately calculated from the BSP clearance test:

$$V = \left[X_i/X_o - 1 \right] i$$

Since normal horses have an average of 51 ml plasma/kg body weight (Dukes, 1946), the clinician can note whether hypovolemia exists. If dehydration and subsequent hypovolemia are present, the presence of a delayed BSP clearance should be expected due to subnormal hepatic plasma flow.

iii. Normal Values. Average half-times ($T_{1/2}$) for normal mature horses are 2.8 ± 0.5 minutes with a range of 2–3.7 minutes. Average fractional clearance (K) was 0.25 ± 0.05 of dye removed per minute with a range of 0.19–0.38 during the first 12 minutes. This exponential clearance was not altered in the same horse by the use of doses of BSP between 2 and 6.3 mg/kg. The same horse, tested at yearly intervals under different weight conditions, had nearly dentical $T_{1/2}$ values (Cornelius and Wheat, 1957). Olsen and Phillips (1966) reported similar fractional BSP clearances for normal horses, 0.21 (0.1–0.47). Following the first 12 minutes after intravenous injection, a slower clearance may be observed when sufficient dye remains for detection. Morgan (1959a) has reported that less than 10% retention at 15 minutes after injection is normally expected in horses of approximately 900 lb when 5 mg/kg of BSP is administered intravenously.

iv. Clinical Observations. Delayed BSP excretion in the horse has been reported in hepatic fibrosis, chloroform poisoning (Aktan, 1954); hepatic hemosiderosis, extensive lipidosis, CCl_4 intoxication (Cornelius and Wheat, 1957); and cirrhosis and impaction (Petrovic, 1958; Morgan, 1959a). Following the oral administration of both phenothiazine and carbon disulfide to a group of horses, fractional BSP clearance was lower at (0.15–0.223) but not associated with abnormal clinical symptoms (Olsen and Phillips, 1966). BSP clearance tests are quite useful in horses since a mild icterus is quite a common finding secondary to many clinical diseases. BSP clearance tests are quite specific diagnostically in horses with symptoms of hepatoencephalopathy. Hepatic involvement can easily be distinguished from equine encephalomyelitis or "wobbles," if a severe hypovolemia from dehydration is not present. To determine whether delayed BSP clearance is from hepatic necrosis rather than fibrosis, serum enzymes such as arginase, glutamic dehydrogenase, or sorbitol dehydrogenase may be measured (Section V,C).

c. Cow.   The BSP clearance technique is quite a sensitive test in cattle to detect hepatic necrosis or fibrosis. Early studies on cattle, in which the percentage retention of dye remaining at 45 minutes was calculated, were in disagreement. Vardiman (1953) reported that the BSP retention test was only dependable in the

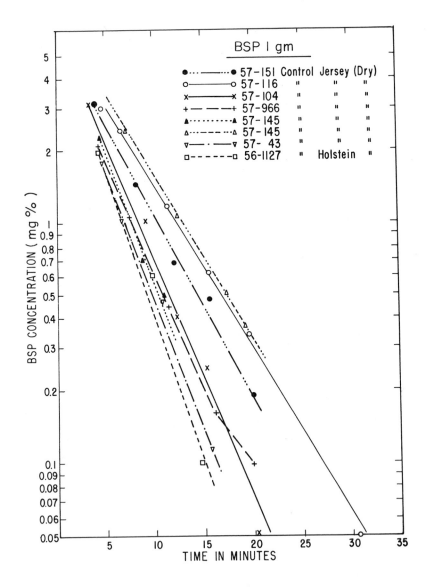

Fig. 9.   Sulfobromophthalein (Bromsulphalein; BSP) clearance in mature, nonlactating dairy cows after the administration of 1 gm BSP intravenously. (Cornelius *et al.*, 1958a.)

last stages of chronic fibrosis from chronic *Senechio* ingestion in the bovine. Jasper (1947) found greater dye retention in cows in late parturition and with ketosis. Extensive studies on BSP retention in cows by Freese (1952) in Germany indicated the retention test was useful diagnostically in animals with advanced fascioliasis, bacterial septicemias, and "toxic" hemoglobinemias.

Advantages of the BSP clearance technique as compared to the dye retention method have been discussed in the previous equine section. The BSP clearance test can be performed identically as described for the horse by injecting intravenously 1 gm BSP (Cornelius *et al.*, 1958a) or 1 mg/lb body weight (Mixner and Robertson, 1957).

The use of 1 gm of BSP in cattle ranging in weight from 500 to 1200 lb results in a measurable concentration during the first 20 minutes in the plasma and removes the problem of securing the weight of the animal. The veterinary practitioner should obtain at least two heparinized blood samples between 5 and 20 minutes after injection and plot the concentrations (ordinate) on semilog paper at each sampling time (abscissa). $T_{1/2}$ values can be calculated rapidly. Spectrophotometric procedures similar to those recommended for the horse are indicated. Methods for correcting for hemolysis are available (Frey and Frey, 1949; Anderson and Mixner, 1960); however, the use of heparin to simply wet the syringe to prevent coagulation will remove such problems in the laboratory.

i. Normal Values.   Average half-time ($T_{1/2}$) values for mature nonlacting dairy cows 3.3 ±0.5 minutes with a range of 2.5–4.1 during the first 20 minutes after injection. Fractional clearance (K) is 0.22 ±0.03 of dye removed per minute with a range of 0.17–0.28 (Fig. 9). $T_{1/2}$ and K values for yearling steers and heifers were 4.5 ±0.3 minutes and 0.15 ±0.1/min, respectively (Cornelius *et al.*, 1958a). Mixner and Robertson (1957) reported similar average fractional clearance (K) values for BSP in lactating cows (weighing on an average 558 kg) to be 0.19/min with a range of 0.16–0.24. Bull calves weighing 49 kg on average had mean BSP K values of 0.15/min with a range of 0.11–0.20. Differences in the fractional clearance of BSP between yearling and mature cattle may be attributable to developmental differences in gastrointestinal mass and the associated splanchnic blood flow. Hanson reported BSP $T_{1/2}$ values in 27 normal cattle to be 3.4 ± 0.5 minutes (2.8–4.4) using 2 mg BSP/kg body weight.

ii. Clinical Observations.   Extremely low BSB fractional clearance (increased $T_{1/2}$) was observed in two cows with suppurative hepatitis following acute coliform mastitis (0.07 and 0.13 BSP cleared per minute); extensive fascioliasis with hepatic fibrosis (0.05/min); and hepatic abscesses (*Spherophorus necrophorus*) (0.14/min) (Fig. 10). Hepatopathy was confirmed by biopsy and microscopic examination (Cornelius *et al.*, 1958a). BSP clearance is markedly depressed in ketotic cows (average $K = 0.09$/min with a range of 0.05–0.11) as compared to normal lactating cows, 1–4 weeks postpartum (Robertson *et al.*, 1957). Hansen (1964) observed a delayed clearance of BSP ($T_{1/2} = 11.7$–69.3 minutes) in cattle in Norway with acute hepatosis from toxic herring meal.

d. SHEEP.   Owing to the extremely rapid clearance of BSP from the plasma in sheep, the use of a percentage retention method may be preferable (Cornelius *et al.*, 1958b; Arendarcik, 1959). The major disadvantage of the clearance technique in sheep is that sampling must be performed quite rapidly since BSP disappears

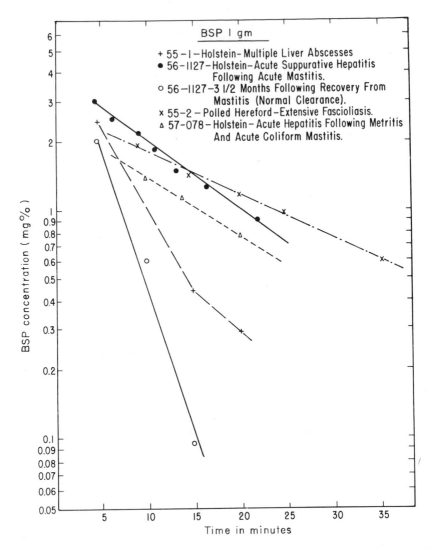

Fig. 10.   Sulfobromophthalein (Bromsulphalein; BSP) clearance in cattle with hepatic diseases. Notice the change in BSP clearance in Cow 56–1127 after recovery from suppurative hepatitis associated with acute coliform mastitis. (Cornelius *et al.*, 1958a.)

exponentially for only 7 minutes after dye injection. The percentage retention of BSP in the serum of normal mature sheep at 10 minutes after injection is approximately 6 ± 2%. Mean fractional clearance (K) using either 2 or 5 mg/kg BSP between 3 and 7 minutes after injection was 0.35 ±0.06/min, with a range of 0.25–0.44/min. The mean $T_{1/2}$ value was 2 ±0.3 minutes with a range of 1.6–2.7 minutes (Cornelius *et al.*, 1958b); 5 mg/kg body weight is recommended. Mean fractional BSP clearance in normal sheep on summer pasture was recently reported to be 0.31 ± 0.06 with a range of 0.195–0.484. Ewes on autumn pastures in England exhibited slightly lower clearance values (Forbes and Singleton, 1966).

The $T_{1/2}$ value for BSP removal from the plasma between 15 and 30 minutes after injection in twelve ewes with severe ketosis was 20 $\pm$ 17 minutes with a range between 7 and 62 minutes. These ewes had BSP retentions between 13 and 64% at 15 minutes after the injection of 2 mg BSP/kg. It was of interest that all ewes retaining over 20% BSP at 15 minutes after injection succumbed despite various therapeutic measures. All ewes dying from ketosis exhibited friable, yellow livers with severe lipidosis and necrosis. The slow clearance of BSP by sheep with clinical ketosis is probably the result of both an impediment to hepatic blood flow from extensive lipidosis and the presence of biochemical lesions associated with cellular necrosis (Cornelius et al., 1958b). Sheep with acute hepatosis from toxic herring meal revealed BSP half-time values ranging from 3.2–46.2 minutes (Hansen, 1964). The BSP fractional clearance test has also been useful in assessing the degree of hepatic damage (fascioliasis) from migrating metacercaria (Roberts, 1968).

Congenital photosensitivity and hyperbilirubinemia in Southdown sheep is characterized by an inherited defect in the hepatic uptake of phylloerythrin, bilirubin, and BSP. Mean BSP half-time values average 43.4 $\pm$ 5.8 and are quite diagnostic since no structural changes are present in the liver. Average hepatic storage (S) and transport maximum (T_m) in two Southdown mutants as calculated by the method of Wheeler et al. (1960b) were 0 mg/mg/100 ml/kg and 0.025 mg/min/kg, respectively. Hepatic S and T_m were 1.79 $\pm$0.86 mg/mg/100 ml/kg and 0.235 $\pm$0.019 mg/min/kg, respectively, in eight normal Southdown sheep (Cornelius and Gronwall, 1968).

Mutant Corriedale sheep (Dubin-Johnson syndrome) with a hepatic excretory defect for BSP exhibited normal hepatic S but hepatic T_m values were 19–25% that of normal sheep. BSP was retained in the plasma primarily as a glutathione conjugate in Corriedale mutants, whereas Southdown mutants' sera contained only unconjugated BSP (Cornelius et al., 1965a). A delay in BSP clearance increased with age in Corriedale Dubin-Johnson mutants (Cornelius et al., 1968).

e. SWINE.   Prinz and Fiesel (1957) have investigated BSP clearance in pigs in protein deficiency and following chloroform poisoning. BSP retention in normal swine weighing 30 kg was: 5 minutes, 5.3 $\pm$2.0%; 10 minutes, 1.4 $\pm$0.9%; and 15 minutes, 0.6 $\pm$0.6%. Following 3–5 months on a protein-deficient diet, the following BSP retention ranges were observed after injection: 5 minutes, 10.5–16.7%; 10 minutes, 1.7–6.0%; and 15 minutes, 0.6–2.6%. BSP retention values returned to normal following protein supplementation. Chloroform narcosis increased the BSP retention three to four times in the protein-deficient syndrome.

BSP half-times in four normal pigs were approximately 2 minutes before receiving aflatoxin and increased to over 19 minutes by 6 hours following toxin introduction through gastric fistulas (Cysewski et al., 1968).

f. FOWL.   Methods for measuring BSP clearance in chickens and turkeys have been described; 20 mg/kg body weight has been the recommended dose. A sexual difference was observed in chickens. Males caponized by stilbesterol possessed a female type of clearance. Androgens caused a clear reversion to the male or more rapid clearance curve (Campbell, 1957). Studies in turkeys revealed that the rate of transfer of BSP between blood, liver, and bile can be predicted from a graph of the fall of plasma BSP alone. The BSP test appears to be quite a sensitive indicator of hepatopathy in the fowl (Clarkson, 1961). Additional studies by Clarkson and

Richards (1967) calculated the transfer rates of BSP between plasma and liver in unanesthetized turkeys by following the fall in plasma BSP concentration after a single injection.

g. PRIMATES.   A listing of data concerning BSP clearance in various primate species is presented in Table II.

Increased BSP retention was reported by Deinhardt et al. (1962) in studies with human infectious hepatitis in chimpanzees. Retentions of up to 15% at 40 minutes was observed. BSP studies on free-ranging Howler monkeys with hepatic pigmentation did not suggest that an excretory defect for such organic anions exists as in Dubin-Johnson syndrome in man and Corriedale sheep. In two Howler monkeys with pigmented livers, hepatic T_m and S were observed to be within a range previously reported in normal man and dog (Katz et al., 1968). Rhesus monkeys have been studied extensively using BSP to measure hepatic disorders; such conditions have included nutritional cirrhosis with retentions up to 45% (Gaisford and Zuidema, 1965); and veno-occlusive disease with up to 65% retention (Allen and Carstens, 1968).

2.   Rose Bengal

This rose-colored dye was first used by Delprat (1923) to measure liver function in man. The dye is primarily removed by the liver (Glaser et al., 1959) and excreted into the bile in an unconjugated state. The danger of photosensitivity following its use is its primary disadvantage. Results with rose bengal are interpreted as being similar to those with BSP, although clearance rates are quite different. Bromsulphalein inhibits the removal of rose bengal from the blood (Cohen et al., 1953). Shaw (1933) first proposed the use of rose bengal in sheep with extensive fascioliasis with fibrosis and hepatic lipidosis from ketosis. Garner (1952a) administered 2 mg rose bengal/kg body weight to cattle and questionably concluded that the test as performed was unreliable even in severe diffuse fibrosis and lipidosis. Since clearance procedures were not used for rose bengal in cattle as recommended in the section of BSP (Section IV,B,1,C), the true value of rose bengal for cattle is not presently known. Svirbely and associates (1946) concluded that in the dog the rose bengal test was nearly as sensitive as BSP in assessing experimental hepatic necrosis from xylidine intoxication; 5 mg dye/kg body weight was injected and the percentage retention at 30 minutes was measured spectrophotometrically. The percentage retention at 30 minutes in normal dogs was usually less than 10% with values up to 73% reported in advanced cirrhosis. A simple modified method for the dog using rose bengal and Sahli hemometer tubes does not require a spectrophotometer. The method is based on the premise that a normal canine liver removes one-half of the dye present in the plasma 2 minutes after injection (M. J. Burns and Clark, 1963). Smith et al. (1940) intravenously injected 5 mg/kg rose bengal into a series of normal cats and in cats with chronic selenium poisoning. Samples were taken at 15, 30, and 60 minutes after injection and the percentage retention calculated following spectrophotometric measurements of plasma at 565 mμ. The authors adopted the 30-minute plasma sample as the ideal time for comparative purposes. Normal cats had average rose bengal retentions (%) of: 15 minutes, 33%; 30 minutes, 8%; and 60 minutes, 3%. Percent retention of rose bengal in cats with chronic selenosis ranged between 9 and 58% at 30 minutes.

TABLE II BSP CLEARANCE IN PRIMATES: NORMAL VALUES

Monkey	Author	Percent retention (5 mg/kg)	Fractional clearance (%/min)
Rhesus	Anderson (1966)	—	17.6 ±4.2
	Allen and Carstens (1968)	<5%/30 min	—
	Gaisford and Zuidema (1965)	0.9–3.1%/45 min	—
	T. O. King and Gargus (1967)	0.7 ±1.8%/30 min	—
	Vogin et al. (1966)	0–3.6%/30 min	—
Cebus	G. V. Mann et al. (1952)		81.3 ±8.2%/15 min
African Green	Pridgen (1967)	♂. 5.7 ±3.3% (1.5–19.7)/30 min	
	(10 mg/kg; injected dose)	♀. 5.5 ±6.4% (1.3–33.0)/30 min	
Howler	Katz et al. (1968)	2–8%/20 min	27 (17–46)
Chimpanzee	Deinhardt et al. (1962)	0–3%/30 min	—
	Wisecup et al. (1969)	21.1 ±9.5/10 min	—
		4.7 ±2.6/20 min	—

^{131}I-labeled rose bengal has been extensively used in man for the detection of liver insufficiency (Taplin *et al.*, 1955; C. H. Brown and Glasser, 1956; Moertel and Owen, 1958; Mena *et al.*, 1959). In this method, small doses of radioactive-labeled rose bengal are traced by external scintillation probes placed over the area of the liver. J. R. Holmes (1960) has proposed the use of ^{131}I-labeled rose bengal to assess liver function in sheep. In this test 20 μCi of ^{131}I in 3 ml of 1% rose bengal were administered intravenously. A scintillation probe with a lead shield was connected to a rate meter and recorder operating at a rate of 6 in./hr. The probe was centered at right angles to the body on the right side, 3.5 in. behind and immediately above the point of the elbow. The crystal was directed at the hepatic tissue (which is slightly more dorsal) and not the gallbladder. Counts were recorded for 1.5–2 hours post-injection. J. R. Holmes (1960) observed maximum activity by 27 minutes on an average in seven experiments with a range of 13–55 minutes. As much as 80 ml of CCl$_4$ were required per os to produce liver lesions in mature sheep observable by this technique (see Fig. 11). Preliminary observations indicate the test may be useful in measuring hepatic insufficiency in ruminants.

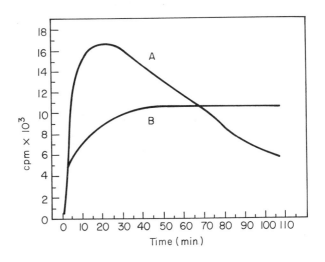

Fig. 11.   Count-rate curve following the intravenous injection of 20 μCi ^{131}I-rose bengal to sheep. (A) an average of four normal tests; (B) after 80 ml of CCl$_4$. (J. R. Holmes, 1960.)

3.   Phenoltetrachlorophthalein

This dye has been used very little in domestic animals (Garner, 1952a; Kowatsch, 1947). S. M. Rosenthal (1922) first proposed the use of this dye in measuring liver function in man. Garner (1952a) injected 5 mg/kg into normal cattle and in cattle with hepatopathy and concluded that the percent retention test as performed was without merit. If samples had been taken between 5 and 20 minutes for the calculation of fractional clearance (K) in this study, the test might have been quite similar to the BSP test. Since the BSP test in domestic animals has proved quite effective, no effort has been made to restudy the clearance of both phenoltetrachlorophthalein and rose bengal.

4. Indocyanine Green

Fox and co-workers (1957) first introduced indocyanine green (ICG) for the measurement of blood flow and detection of cardiac malformations by indicator-dilution techniques. In recent studies on hepatic function using this dye, the following advantages over other protein-binding dyes such as BSP are apparent (Hunton *et al.*, 1961): nearly complete recovery from bile (Wheeler *et al.*, 1958), single exponential plasma removal pattern (Cherrick *et al.*, 1960), distribution is limited to the intra-vascular volume (Fox *et al.*, 1959), no apparent uptake by extrahepatic tissues (Rapaport *et al.*, 1959), no excretion into the urine (Hunton *et al.*, 1960), no entero-hepatic circulation (Rapaport *et al.*, 1959), and no lymphatic reabsorption (Hunton *et al.*, 1960).

a. DOG. *General.* The use of ICG is recommended in the dog since its re-moval rate is exponential for the first 15 minutes after injection. This is not true for BSP. Average fractional clearance or the plasma removal rate per minute (K) is 7.6%/min ($T_{1/2}$ = 9.1 minutes) following the administration of 1 mg/kg body weight (Hunton and co-workers, 1960). Individual dogs ranged from 5.5 to 9.8%/min. Ketterer *et al.* (1960) reported fractional clearance (K) of 6.9±1.0%/min at the 0.4–0.6 mg/kg injection level. Doses near 9.0 mg/kg body weight will decrease the amount of dye removed per minute (K) to approximately one-third the normal clearance. Three days following the single oral dose of 2.5 ml CCl_4/kg body weight, the plasma disappearance rate in a dog was reduced to 1.5%/min (Hunton *et al.*, 1960). Van Vleet and Alberts (1968) prefer the BSP retention test over ICG clearance due to the simplicity of the BSP procedure.

b. METHOD (Ketterer *et al.*, 1960). The technique as summarized below for the dog can be performed with any spectrophotometer with wavelengths in the infrared range.

1. Inject intravenously 0.5 mg/kg body weight of ICG.

2. Three blood samples should be taken from the opposite radial vein at any time between 3 and 15 minutes postinjection.

3. Centrifuge heparinized blood samples and read the plasma dye concentrations directly at a wavelength of 805 mμ in a Beckman DU spectrophotometer. Since this tricarbocyanine dye is colorimetrically unstable in dilute aqueous solutions, small amounts of plasma must be added to all tubes in preparing the standard curve.

4. Plot the dye concentration on graph paper with semilogarithmic coordinates as recommended in the section on BSP (Section IV,B,1) and calculate the $T_{1/2}$ directly. The fractional clearance (K) or percent removed per minute can then be calculated from the equation:

$$K = \frac{\ln 2}{T_{1/2}} \qquad \ln 2 = 0.692$$

c. HEPATIC BLOOD FLOW AND PLASMA VOLUME (VOLUME OF DISTRIBUTION) IN THE DOG. Estimated hepatic blood flow values for 13 anesthetized dogs were found to be on an average 36.9 ± 11.0 ml/min-kg using ICG. Extraction ratios for the dye by canine liver varied between 10.2 and 24.7% with an average of 18.0%. Formulas for use in calculations following the single injection method are as follows (adapted from Ketterer *et al.*, 1960):

$$\text{Fractional clearance } (K) = \frac{\ln Ct_1 - \ln Ct_2}{t_2 - t_1 \text{ (minutes)}}$$

Volume of distribution (ml plasma or volume) =

$$= \frac{\text{mg injected}}{\text{extrapolated concentration at 0 time (mg/ml)}}$$

Plasma clearance (*c*) (ml/min) =
     volume of distribution (ml) × fractional clearance (% cleared/min)

$$\text{Extraction ratio} = \frac{\text{arteriohepatic venous concentration difference (mg/ml)}}{\text{arterial concentration (mg/ml)}}$$

$$\text{Estimated hepatic plasma flow (ml/min)} = \frac{\text{plasma clearance (ml/min)}}{\text{extraction ratio}}$$

The great advantages of ICG in studying hepatic problems in the dog are quite obvious. The practitioner can obtain from this test, in addition to the removal rate of the dye, the plasma volume, and an *estimated* hepatic blood flow using the average extraction ratio of 18% observed by Ketterer and associates (1960).

   d. OTHER SPECIES.   The normal plasma disappearance rates (*K*) for ICG in rats and rabbits are greater than 30%/min, but are not truly single exponential functions. The average disappearance rate (*K*) in man at the 0.25 mg/kg dose with sampling at 5 and 10 minutes is 25.9%/min.

   Fractional clearances (%/min) for ICG in unanesthetized rhesus monkeys are: 36.5 ± 2.6 in females and 52.9 ± 4.9 in males. The slopes of clearance curves were exponentially linear for 12 minutes after injection. Pentabarbital anesthesia significantly delayed the clearance of dye (Vogin *et al.*, 1966). Mutant sheep with congenital photosensitivity and hyperbilirubinemia exhibit delayed ICG clearance ($T_{1/2} = 32.4 \pm 5.0$ minutes) as compared to normal Southdown sheep ($T_{1/2} = 4.8 \pm 0.5$ minutes) (Cornelius *et al.*, 1968).

V.   SERUM ENZYME TESTS

   Variations in the concentration of certain serum enzymes as measured by their biochemical activity occur primarily as a result of three processes involving the liver: (1) their elevation due to the escape of enzymes from disrupted hepatic parenchymal cells with necrosis or altered membrane permeability [glutamic pyruvic transaminase (SGPT); glutamic oxalacetic transaminase (SGOT); arginase; TPN-linked isocitric dehydrogenase (SICD); sorbitol dehydrogenase (SD); glutamic dehydrogenase (GD); ornithine carbamyl transferase (OCT); and lactic dehydrogenase (LDH)]; (2) their elevation due to the lack of biliary excretion in obstructive icterus [alkaline phosphatase (SAP)]; and (3) their decrease in concentration in the serum due to impaired synthesis by the liver (choline esterase). Enzymes which increase in concentration in the blood following hepatic necrosis (group 1) must also be divided into two groups: (a) enzymes which are "liver-specific" in that high concentrations are present primarily in hepatic tissue (SGPT in dog, cat, and primates; SD and GD in sheep and cattle; SD in horses; arginase and OCT in all ureotelic animals); and (b) enzymes which are in high concentrations in other tissues in addition to liver (SGOT, LDH and SICD). SGOT, LDH and ICD are not "liver specific," but may be of use diagnostically to measure the level of liver necrosis if all tissues other than liver are known to be free of pathology. The liver-specific enzymes are the most sensitive and reliable tests available to detect mild to severe hepatic necrosis. They are excellent for prognostication and in the evaluation of therapy. A prediction of which enzymes can serve as diagnostic agents is possible only through thorough analytical studies on the enzyme composition of specific tissues or organs (Nagode *et al.*, 1966). The International Enzyme Commission recommends that serum levels of enzyme activity be expressed as micromoles per minute per liter. Unfortunately, much of the published work is expressed in other more popular units.

A. SERUM GLUTAMIC PYRUVIC TRANSAMINASE (SGPT)

1. Interpretation

The use of serum transaminase activities in the diagnosis of disease was pioneered by the investigations of Wroblewski and LaDue (1955, 1956a,b) in which they observed elevations in human cardiac infarction and hepatic necrosis. SGOT activity was early found to be elevated in experimental hepatic necrosis in the horse, cow, pig, dog (Cornelius *et al.*, 1959b), and cat (Cornelius and Kaneko, 1960), but also elevated in diseases involving the cardiac (myocardial infarction) and skeletal systems (muscular dystrophy, azoturia) in these species. Considerable GOT activity was found in almost all tissues analyzed in mammals, while high GPT concentrations have been observed only in canine, feline, and human hepatic parenchymal cells (Cornelius *et al.*, 1959b). Since the livers of mature horses, cattle, sheep, and pigs do not contain significant levels of GPT, only very small elevations in SGPT occur from hepatic necrosis in these species (see Fig. 12). Significant elevations in the SGPT activity are liver-specific only in small animals as well as all primates studied to date.

2. Methods

Normal values for SGPT activities in various species are presented in Table III. SGPT and SGOT activities are usually determined by the methods of Wroblewski and Cabaud (1957) and Cabaud *et al.* (1956), respectively. A rapid kit method for the measurement of SGPT and SGOT is available commercially* and expresses the enzyme activities as Sigma-Frankel units. Both methods give comparable results. In both techniques the assay for transaminase activity is based on the transfer of

*Sigma Chemical Co., St. Louis, Missouri, Technical Bulletin 55.

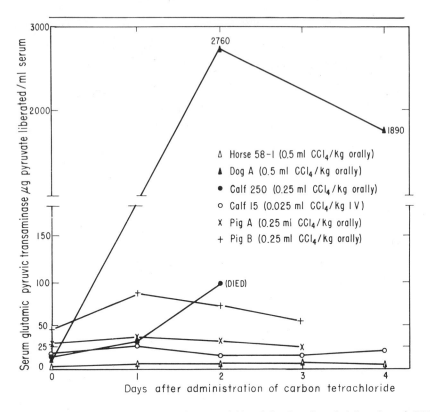

Fig. 12. Serum glutamic pyruvic transaminase activities following the administration of CCl₄ to certain domestic species. Observe the only significant elevation in activity occurring in the dog. (Cornelius *et al.*, 1958b.)

the α-amino group of either aspartic acid or alanine to α-ketoglutaric acid. The oxalacetate that results in the determination of GOT activity is converted to pyruvic acid by aniline citrate. In both procedures a pyruvate-dinitrophenylhydrazone is next prepared and measured colorimetrically at either 490 mμ without the extraction procedure (Sigma Chemical Co.). Units are usually expressed either as μg of pyruvic acid liberated in 20 minutes at 25° C/ml serum or as Sigma-Frankel units. The Sigma-Frankel unit is defined as the enzyme activity necessary to produce a decrease in the optical density at 340 mμ of 0.001/min/ml serum under the conditions of Karmen (1955) at 25°C/cm light path.

3. Pathological Findings

Dal Santo (1959), Malherbe (1960), and Hoe (1961) observed significant elevations in SGPT activity in dogs with infectious hepatitis. No such increases were observed in dogs with distemper and this test appeared to be quite helpful in the differential diagnosis of certain cases where clinical symptoms were questionable. Significant elevations in SGPT have been reported in the following primary and secondary

TABLE III   SERUM GLUTAMIC PYRUVIC (SGPT) AND OXALACETIC TRANSAMINASE (SGOT) ACTIVITIES IN DOMESTIC ANIMALS

Species	Age or wt	Units		Reference
		SGPT	SGOT	
Dog	9–12 mo	21±11	20±7	Cornelius et al. (1959b)
	—	<30	<40	Hoe and Jabara (1967)
	>5 yr	21.9±5.6	22.4±5.2	Crawley and Swenson (1965)
	—	20.5(5–50)	22.8(3–80)	Van Vleet and Alberts (1968)
	—	5–23	20–48	J. M. Hamilton et al. (1966)
	—	18.0±2.3	27.0±4.4	Hoe and Harvey (1961b)
Cat	—	15.6±9.9	19.0±4.8	Cornelius and Kaneko (1960)
Cow	—	43.2±0.7	169.6±3.2	Boyd (1962)
	2–10 yr	24.1±5.0	68.7±17.5	Hansen (1964)
	7–27 days	16±8	56±14	Cornelius et al. (1959b)
	1–97 wk	2±3	25±6	Cornelius et al. (1959b)
	—	18±12	24±17	Roussel and Stallcup (1966)
Horse	1–11 yr	8±6	158±37	Cornelius et al. (1959b)
	2.5 yr	—	228±66	Wolff et al. (1967)
	—	0.213±0.264	6.14±1.69 (μm/100 ml/min)	Freedland et al. (1965)
Sheep	1 yr (penned)	17.4±5.1	74.7±13.6	Hansen (1964)
	1 yr (pastured)	—	95.0±6.1	Young et al. (1965)
	—	—	122.3±5.1	Young et al. (1965)
	—	23.2±1.8	164±23	Boyd (1962)
Swine	1–3 yr	27±8	31±14	Cornelius et al. (1959b)
	—	—	29	Cysewski et al. (1968)
Chickens	6 mo	0	370±186	Cornelius et al. (1959b)
Chimpanzee	5–20 kg	36.9±16.4	47.5±13.8	Hartwell et al. (1968)
	2–12 yr	16.9±6.2	20.3±4.9	Wisecup et al. (1969)
	—	19.6±16.8	30.7±18.2	Sadun et al. (1966)
	6 mo–10 yr	—	10–35	Deinhardt et al. (1962)
	Juvenile	31.6±3.1	31.4±4.0	K. F. Burns et al. (1967)
	Juvenile anesthetized	30.1±9.5	47.6±15.1	Krushak and Hartwell (1968)

TABLE III (continued)

Species	Age or wt	Units		Reference
		SGPT	SGOT	
Baboon				
African	—	18 ±12	34 ±8.9	Pena and Goldzieher (1967)
Domestic	—	17 ±7	30 ±11	Pena and Goldzieher (1967)
Kenya	—	29 ±11	10 ±4	Pena and Goldzieher (1967)
Kenya	8.5–26.9 kg	33.2 ±7.3	51 ±5.5	K. F. Burns et al. (1967)
Monkey				
Rhesus	3.3–8.0 kg	37.9 ±19.1	20.4 ±9.9	Brooks et al. (1963)
	—	27.5	39.7	F. A. Robinson and Ziegler (1968)
	2.8–5.3 kg	13.1 ±5	27 ±6.5	Anderson (1966)
Squirrel	—	117 ±75	138 ±62	Rosenblum and Cooper (1968)
Marmoset	—	—	98.7 (48–204)	Deinhardt and Deinhardt (1966)
	Mature	20.2 ±8.3	143 ±33	K. F. Burns et al. (1967)
	—	—	113 (62–106)	A. W. Holmes et al. (1967)
Howler	—	12–27	140–400	Maruffo et al. (1966)
	—	35 ±8 (Karmen)	786 ±10 (Karmen)	Katz et al. (1968)
African Green	—	38 ±9.2	61 ±9.8	Pridgen (1967)
		47 ±13.3	54 ±9.9	Pridgen (1967)

hepatic diseases in the dog: intrahepatic cholestasis (Malherbe, 1959), complicated *Babesia canis* infections (Malherbe, 1960), hepatic neoplasia, fatty degeneration of the liver, leptospirosis (Hoe and Harvey, 1961a), CCl_4 poisoning (Kutas and Karsai, 1961; Frankl and Merritt, 1959; Cornelius *et al.*, 1959b), suppurative hepatic necrosis, severe anemia from a ruptured splenic hemangioma, arsenic poisoning, extensive lipidosis from hypothyroidism, hepatic necrosis secondary to pyometra, and extensive hepatic malignancies (Cornelius, 1957). No significant elevations are usually observed in distemper, uremia, chronic peritonitis, hypothyroidism, osteodystrophy, lymphatic, leukemia, or pneumonias.

An extensive study by Hoe and Jabara (1967) concluded that the SGPT and SAP tests were more effective in diagnosing liver diseases in the dog than the SGOT, SICD, SLDH, and serum α-hydroxybutyrate dehydrogenase tests. Hoe and O'Shea (1965) were able to detect hepatic damage in 80–100% of the cases of severe fatty change, malignant neoplasia, hepatoma, cirrhosis, and hepatitis in dogs. The detection of chronic passive congestion of the liver was not possible with the SGPT test. The use of the SGPT test to detect infectious canine hepatitis has been well confirmed (Beckett *et al.*, 1964; J. M. Hamilton *et al.*, 1966).

An ascitic dog was examined at the University of California Veterinary Hospital with a total bilirubin level of 4.5 mg/100 ml of which 3.4 mg/100 ml was of the conjugated "direct-reacting" type. The total serum protein was quite low (3.5 gm/100 ml) with an albumin; globulin ratio of only 0.3:1. A constant bilirubinuria was also observed. SGOT and SGPT activities were within the normal range and confirmed histopathologically by a lack of hepatic necrosis at autopsy. The liver, however, was nearly twice its normal size due to a diffuse infiltration of *Histoplasma capsulatum* within the Kupfer cells. If elevations in SGPT activity are observed in any disease studied, it may be concluded that hepatic necrosis is occurring.

SGPT data from our laboratory as correlated with conventional microscopic examination of livers at autopsy are arbitrarily interpreted as follows for the dog:

Normal values   10–50 units
Moderate necrosis   50–400 units
Severe liver necrosis 400 units

Elevations above 1000 units are not uncommon in severe hepatic necrosis. Dogs can be tested daily for prognosis and for the evaluation of therapy. The use of the BSP test in conjunction with the SGPT test in dogs is highly recommended. BSP clearance will be delayed in hepatic fibrosis or necrosis, whereas the SGPT activity will be elevated only in necrosis. The nature of the type of hepatic pathology that is present can therefore be determined by the simultaneous use of both BSP retention and SGPT activity.

The use of the SGPT test should be confined to primates, dogs, cats, and smaller animal species since large animals contain little hepatic GPT activity. Elevated SGPT activity has been reported in many different conditions in primates: human viral hepatitis research in marmosets (Deinhardt and Deinhardt, 1966) and chimpanzees (Deinhardt *et al.*, 1962), Leptospiral infections in squirrel monkeys (Minette and Shaffer, 1968), hepatic hemangioma in a rhesus monkey (Woodruff and Johnson, 1968), veno-occlusive disease in the rhesus monkey (Allen *et al.*, 1969), morphine addiction in the rhesus monkey (Brooks *et al.*, 1963), and malarial infections in baboons (Sadun *et al.*, 1966).

B. Serum Glutamic Oxalacetic Transaminase (SGOT)

Elevations in the activity of SGOT can be associated with alterations in cell necrosis of many tissues. Pathology involving the skeletal or cardiac muscle and/or the hepatic parenchyma allows for the leakage of large amounts of this enzyme into the blood.

Normal SGOT activities are presented in Table V. Considerable SGOT activity was observed in nearly all tissues analyzed in the horse, cow, pig, dog, and chicken (Cornelius et al., 1959b). Since all major tissues contain high concentrations of GOT, the finding of significant elevations in SGOT need not indicate hepatic necrosis unless diseases of other large organ systems can be ruled out. SGOT, however, can be used successfully in large animals prognostically to evaluate the degree of liver necrosis once other tests, such as the BSP clearance and serum and urine bilirubin determinations, have established hepatic involvement. Since SGPT determinations are of little help in diagnosing hepatic necrosis in large domestic animals due to its absence in high concentrations in their livers, SGOT has been at times used in its place. It must be remembered, however, that SGOT is not liver-specific and that other enzymes such as SD or GD, arginase or OCT are far more liver-specific in domestic animals.

Elevations in SGOT activity were noted by Rudolph et al. (1957) in dogs following surgical ligation of pulmonary or mesenteric vessels and in myocardial infarction. Elevated SGOT levels occur in necrosis of either heart or liver and suggests that these two organs may each contribute considerable amounts of enzyme to the serum. Significant elevations of SGOT have been observed in muscular dystrophies of nearly all animal species (Cornelius et al., 1959c; Blincoe and Dye, 1958). No discussion of SGOT activities in liver disorders in the dog, cat, or primate will be attempted since the SGPT test is the test of choice in these species.

Considerable information is available concerning elevations in the SGOT activity associated with liver diseases in species other than the dog. Elevations in SGOT activities have been observed in: postparturient state in the cow (Lupke, 1965); ragwort intoxication in calves (Ford and Ritchie, 1968); toxic hepatosis in cattle and sheep consuming contaminated herring meal (Hansen, 1964); extrahepatic bile duct obstruction in swine (Bicknell et al., 1967); aflatoxicosis in swine (Cysewski et al., 1968); halothane and chloroform anesthesia in the horse (Wolff et al., 1967; Thorpe et al., 1968); carbon tetrachloride poisoning in the horse (Freedland et al., 1965); pasture conditions for sheep (Young et al., 1965); sporidesmin intoxication in sheep (Mortimer, 1962); metacercariae (fascioliasis) migrations in sheep (Roberts, 1968); and in predicting copper poisoning in sheep (MacPherson and Hemingway, 1969).

C. Serum Arginase

Elevations in the serum arginase level have been used as a liver-specific test for hepatic necrosis in man (Ugarte et al., 1961). Arginase is only found in significant concentrations within the liver of ureotelic mammals such as man, dog, sheep, cattle, and rat (Cornelius et al., 1963). The finding of extremely high arginase activities in the livers of various mammals as compared to all other tissues examined suggests that

TABLE IV   SERUM ARGINASE ACTIVITIES IN SOME MATURE
MAMMALS[a]

| Species | Units/ml | | |
	Mean	σ	Range
Horses	0.64	±1.1	0–4.2
Nonlactating cows	0.34	±0.08	0–0.17
Lactating cows	0.50	±0.35	0.08–1.8
Wethers	0.30	±0.57	0–2.7
Ewes	0.37	±0.29	0–1.1
Dogs	0.03	±0.01	0–0.28
Rats	1.28	±0.98	0–4.2
Men	0.04	—	0–0.11

[a]Cornelius et al. (1963).

significant elevations in plasma arginase activity would indicate a necrotic process occurring within the liver per se. Normal values for serum arginase in the various species are presented in Table IV. A new and sensitive method using gel filtration for the determination of arginase activity in serum is now available (Cornelius and Freedland, 1962).

Following a single oral dose of CCl_4 to the horse, calf, sheep, and dog, the serum arginase activity rose rapidly followed by recovery to the normal range within 3–4

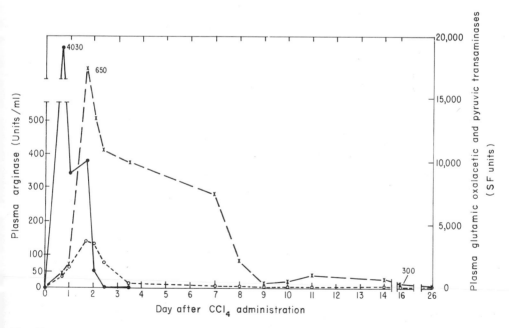

Fig. 13.   Serum arginase, glutamic oxalacetic transminase, and glutamic pyruvic transaminase activities in the dog following the administration of CCl_4 orally (1.5 ml CCl_4/kg orally). Observe rapid return of arginase to its normal activity and prolonged elevation in SGPT activity. (●) Arginase. (○) GOT. (×) GPT.

days. The SGPT (dog) and SGOT (horse, calf, sheep) activities remained significantly elevated for over 1 week in all animals, during the same CCl$_4$-poisoning experiments (see Fig. 13). There appeared to be a more rapid disappearance of the serum arginase, a mitochondrial enzyme, as compared to the transaminases which are in the hyaloplasmic fraction of cells. Preliminary clinical and experimental data suggest that if both serum arginase and transaminase activities are continuously elevated, a progressive hepatic necrosis is most likely present. If normal serum arginase and elevated transaminase activities are observed following significant elevations of both enzymes, prognosis is favorable as hepatic necrosis is subsiding.

Numerous clinical cases with suspected liver necrosis were observed and examined for plasma enzyme activities at the university veterinary hospital in California. A severly icteric dog in the recovery phase of accidental arsenic ingestion had a plasma arginase level of only 1.68 units/ml with a plasma GOT activity still elevated at 1090 S_f units. Two dogs with progressive and acute hepatic necrosis from *Leptospira canicola* infections had significant elevations in both serum arginase and GPT activities. Elevated activities of both arginase and SGPT were observed in a dog with progressive hepatic necrosis from a metastatic hepatic malignancy. Similar findings have been observed in equine, bovine, and ovine hepatopathy. Elevated serum arginase and SGOT activities in two icteric sheep with progressive necrosis were observed after their admission to the hospital. Of special interest was the extremely rapid return of serum arginase activity to a normal level in one sheep upon clinical recovery, whereas the SGOT activity still remained significantly elevated. These preliminary findings suggest that the simultaneous measurement of serum arginase and transaminase activities in mammals with hepatic necrosis may allow for the prediction of the nature of the lesion, i.e., either a progressive necrosis or regeneration. The determination of serum arginase activity is a good liver-specific enzyme test for *active* hepatic necrosis in horses, cattle, sheep, and pigs. Significant elevations in serum arginase hepatic necrosis were observed in horses following chloroform anesthesia, whereas halothane anesthesia produced only minor enzyme elevations (Wolff *et al.*, 1967).

D. Serum TPN-Linked Isocitric Dehydrogenase (SICD)

In clinical cases of human hepatic disease (Sterkel *et al.*, 1958), SICD has been used as a liver function test in differentiating intrahepatic and extrahepatic obstructive icterus in man. Elevation in the serum activity of this enzyme following CCl$_4$-poisoning parallels changes in transaminase activities in man and animal. Increased SICD and SGOT activities were observed in four horses with hepatic abscesses, hepatic centrilobular necrosis with extensive lipidosis, portal fibrosis and necrosis, and hemolytic anemia (Cornelius, 1961). All tissues examined (liver, kidney, and heart and skeletal muscle) of cow, horse, sheep, dog, cat, chicken, and guinea pig contain considerable SICD activity and suggest a similarity to the distribution of GOT activities. Since a variety of tissues contain significant SICD, its elevation in the serum may not indicate only the presence of hepatic disease.

Elevations in the SICD activity has been studied in chloroform and halothane anesthesia in the horse (Wolff *et al.*, 1967), carbon tetrachloride poisoning in the horse (Freedland *et al.*, 1965), sheep, and cow (Boyd, 1962), in various hepatopathies in the dog (Hoe and Jabara, 1967), and in human viral hepatitis studies in marmoset monkeys (Deinhardt and Deinhardt, 1966). Hoe and Jabara (1967) observed that no correlation could be found between elevated SGOT and SICD activities with liver disease in the dog and concluded that SGPT and SAP tests were more diagnostic. SICD activity determinations can be performed by the method of S. K. Wolfson and Williams-Ashman (1957), in which 1 W-Wa unit is defined as the amount which forms 1 mμmole TPNH/ml serum-hr at 25° C under the conditions of the test. Normal activities for SICD in domestic animals are presented in Table V.

E. Serum Ornithine Carbamyl Transferase (OCT)

OCT catalyzes the reaction between ornithine and carbamyl phosphate. The enzyme is highly concentrated in the liver like GPT and can be measured either by the microdiffusion technique of Reichard and Reichard (1958) or a colorimetric procedure developed by Brown and Grisolia (1959). OCT is quite liver-specific like SGPT, but does not provide any more information than the SGPT test. This liver-specific enzyme may be particularly useful in large animals, whose livers do not contain high concentrations of GPT (Cornelius *et al.*, 1959b). Holtenius and Jacobson (1965) found high concentrations of OCT only in liver tissue of cattle and suggested its measurement in serum to be an effective diagnostic procedure for bovine hepatic necrosis. High serum levels are observed in necrotic processes such as in hepatitis and active cirrhosis. Minor elevations may be observed in intrahepatic cholestasis.

Elevations in the serum OCT activities have been reported in a variety of liver disorders: *Senecio jacobea* intoxication in calves (Ford and Ritchie, 1968), acute toxic hepatosis in cattle in Norway (Hansen, 1964), severe hepatic lipidosis in cattle

TABLE V   SERUM TPN-LINKED ISOCITRIC DEHYDROGENASE ACTIVITIES IN DOMESTIC ANIMALS[a]

Species	Age (years)	W-WA units/ml[b]		
		Mean	σ	Range
Horses	1–18	600	±200	291–1075
Steers and non-lactating dairy cows	1–6	817	±130	622–1036
Lactating dairy cows	2	1004	±167	565–1314
Wethers	1–2	276	±166	78–659
Rams	1–2	225	±130	26–528
Ewes	1–8	276	±110	106–482
Dogs	1–7	178	± 99	27–437
Cats	< 1	321	±190	118–703
Chickens	6 weeks	558	±129	275–770
Turkeys	23 weeks	524	±102	391–742

[a]Cornelius (1961).

[b]One W-WA unit = the amount which forms 1 nmole TPNH/ml serum-hr at 25°C under conditions of the test.

(SGOT of no use) (Holtenius and Jacobson, 1965), chloroform anesthesia in the horse (Thorpe *et al.*, 1968), and aflatoxicosis in swine (Cysewski *et al.*, 1968).

Average normal serum levels for serum OCT are: swine, 210 units (Cysewski *et al.*, 1968), and cattle and sheep, 5.1 ± 2 and 4.0 ± 3.9, respectively (Hansen, 1964).

F. Serum Glutamic (GD) and Sorbitol (SD) Dehydrogenases

Due to the lack of GPT activity in the livers of large domestic animals, recent research has focused on finding liver-specific enzymes for diagnostic purposes. Two of the more promising enzymes are SD in the horse and GD in cattle and sheep.

SD and GD are highly concentrated in the livers of horses (Freedland *et al.*, 1965). Following CCl$_4$ poisoning, the sera of horses contained a 600-fold increase in SD activity and a 75-fold increase in GD activity. Due to ease of measurement, time specificity and subcellular localization, SD appears at present to be the enzyme of choice for the diagnosis of hepatic necrosis in the horse (Freedland *et al.*, 1965). This usefulness of the SD test in horses has been confirmed by Thorpe *et al.* (1968) in hepatic function studies following chloroform anesthesia.

SD is also primarily confined to canine liver and may be used for measuring liver necrosis in the dog (Zinkle *et al.*, 1969). The many advantages in using one enzyme test such as SD for all animal species in a clinical pathology laboratory is obvious.

Boyd (1962) and Ford and Ritchie (1968) have effectively utilized the GD and SD tests in measuring hepatic necrosis following CCl$_4$ and ragwort intoxication.

G. Serum Alkaline Phosphatase (SAP)

The measurement of AP activity has been called an "empirical" test by Maclagan (1956) since the reason for elevated values is not conclusively known. Early theories suggested a simple retention of the enzyme because of a failure of biliary excretion (Armstrong *et al.*, 1934). The additional complication of steatorrhea which accompanies duct occlusion and its effect on bone metabolism through insufficient calcium absorption may result in elevated phosphatase activities from parathyroid stimulation. Later, other investigators observed elevated serum activities in human hepatitis, hepatic fibrosis, and amyloidosis; however, higher values were usually observed in extrahepatic obstructive icterus. Since serum alkaline phosphatase activity is also elevated in rickets, osteomalacia, osteogenic sarcoma, and secondary hyperparathyroidism, the interpretation of SAP activity in relation to the liver presupposes that these other conditions do not exist. High values are occasionally observed in hepatocellular damage due to intrahepatic cholestasis in addition to extrahepatic bile duct obstruction.

AP hydrolyzes organic phosphates such as those of glucose or glycerol to yield inorganic phosphate and the organic moiety. It is most active at a pH near 9.5 but is also quite active at the pH of blood, 7.4. It is determined by estimating the phosphate liberated from glycerol phosphate (Bodansky, 1933, 1937) or the phenol liberated from phenylphosphate (E. J. King and Armstrong, 1934). Another method occasionally used clinically is the measurement of the *p*-nitrophenol liberated from its phosphate complex (Bessey *et al.*, 1946). To convert the millimolar alkaline phosphatase unit of Bessey-Lowrey to King-Armstrong units, the former is multiplied by a factor of 2.5. Conversion of units by such factors is not recommended. The Bodansky test is generally the accepted method of choice in most clinical hospitals in the United States.

1. Dog

Normal SAP values in the adult dog have been reported to be < 4 Bodansky units (Svirbely et al., 1946); < 8 King-Armstrong units (Hoe and O'Shea, 1965); and 0.22 (0.05–0.55) Sigma units/ml (Van Vleet and Alberts, 1968). A comparison of mean values of AP in the dog by four different methods has been recently made by Harvey (1967). Armstrong et al. (1934) observed that the SAP activities increased 30- to 100-fold 6 days after experimental obstruction of the bile duct in the dog. Freeman et al. (1938) found normal AP levels of approximately 5 King-Armstrong units/ml serum in dogs and observed values in experimental obstruction of 100 units/ml and in leptospirosis of 20 units/ml. Increases have also been reported in the dog by: Svirbely et al. (1946) in xylidine poisoning, Drill and Ivy (1944) in CCl_4 poisoning, and Hoe (1969) in hepatic neoplasm, hepatitis, and fatty degeneration.

The SAP test is a sensitive test to detect liver damage and roughly correlates with BSP retention. Significant elevations occur both in intrahepatic cholestasis from hepatic necrosis and in extrahepatic bile duct obstruction. The elevations in hepatocellular damage are usually 6–10 Bodansky units with levels above 10 units in total obstruction (Bloom, 1957).

2. Primates

SAP levels in primates have been reported as follows: rhesus monkey, 9.5 ±5.1 Bessey-Lowry (B-L) units (Anderson, 1966), squirrel monkey, 21.8 ± 10.7 B-L units, mmole units/liter (Rosenblum and Cooper, 1968), chimpanzee, 11.4 Bodansky units (Wisecup et al., 1969), Tamarin marmoset monkey, 29.8 (11.7–75.9), and cotton top marmoset monkey 11.9 (3.6–39.9) B-L units (A. W. Holmes et al., 1967), and African green monkey, 30 ± 14 Bodansky units (Pridgen, 1967).

3. Cattle and Sheep

The wide range of SAP activities in normal cattle and sheep prohibits its use as an indicator of liver insufficiency or obstructive icterus in these species. Garner observed an average of 11.8 King-Armstrong units/100 ml of serum with a range of 4.7–62.4 units in 294 Zebu cattle. Although the enzyme activity of the serum of each cow remains fairly constant over a long period of time, a great range of activities (0.3–114.3 King-Armstrong units/100 ml) is observed in cattle (Allcroft and Folley, 1941). In both sheep and cattle, the serum phosphatase activities progressively decreased with age until maturity was reached. Slightly elevated levels are observed in pregnancy. Serum values for sheep range greatly with reported values between 3 and 166 (Allcroft and Folley, 1941) and 14 and 427 (Ford, 1958) King-Armstrong units/100 ml. Leaver reported normal values for sheep to be 14 ± 7 (5–33) King-Armstrong units and reported no increase in SAP activity in both bile duct obstruction or in sporodesmin poisoning which is known to produce intrahepatic bile duct obstruction. Sheep, therefore, like cats (Wilkinson, 1962) present a very small rise in SAP activity in bile duct obstruction.

H. Serum Choline Esterase

Serum choline esterase (serum esterase) is a nonspecific enzyme which hydrolyzes acetylcholine and many other esters. It is a mucoprotein synthesized by the liver and migrates electrophoretically as an α_2-globulin. McArdle (1940) first reported low values of this serum enzyme in chronic hepatic insufficiency in man. Its level was found to reflect the nutritional state as similarly found in the case of serum albumin. It has been concluded that this test is of only limited value in both man and animals.

Brauer and Root (1947) observed a twofold increase in serum choline esterase activity after repeated poisoning with CCl_4 during a 30-day period. Male and female dogs had normal serum values of 101 ± 4 and 105 ± 4 mmoles/liter/hr, respectively. Using the method of Ammon (1934), it was shown that the canine liver contained five to seven times the amount of choline esterase activity which circulates in the blood plasma. Since this mucoprotein simply represents one more protein synthesized by the liver, the intravenous infusion of albumin depresses its synthesis and hence serum concentration. Ferreira Neto (1958) questioned the reliability of this test and suggested elevations in its activity in the dog appeared to be due to gastrointestinal lesions. It was concluded that wide variations in the normal values of serum choline esterase in dogs makes this test quite unreliable (Hoe and Harvey, 1961a). Kutas and Karsai (1961) also concluded that esterase values were not diagnostic in dogs, horses, and cattle with experimental hepatic necrosis. Deinhardt et al. (1962) reported values in 81 normal chimpanzees to be 0.9–1.35 units.

Few other enzymes have been studied in domestic animals with liver disease. Serum procaine esterase has been studied in horses with liver disease (Humlicek and Kruska, 1960).

I. Other Serum Enzymes

Lactic dehydrogenases (LDH) are found in high concentrations in various tissues of the body such as GOT and ICD; the measurement of LDH activity is not organ-specific unless isoenzyme analysis is performed. Elevations in the serum activity of LDH have been reported in a variety of hepatic disorders: CCl_4 intoxication in the dog (Zinkle et al., 1969) and in ruminants (Boyd, 1962); various hepatopathies and malignancies in the dog (Hoe and Jabara, 1967), and acute lupinosis in sheep (Gardiner and Parr, 1967). Many other serum enzymes have been studied such as malic dehydrogenase in sheep (Young et al., 1965) and leucine aminopeptidase in the monkey (Anderson, 1966). Only through extensive clinical investigations will the true value of any enzyme be known.

VI. SPECIFIC BIOCHEMICAL TESTS

A. Carbohydrate Metabolism Tests

Hepatic physiologists have been stressing the importance of the liver in many biochemical processes ever since Claude Bernard first demonstrated the participation of the liver in carbohydrate metabolism. The ability of normal liver to metabolize increased amounts of glucose, galactose, levulose, and lactic and pyruvic acids in a consistent fashion has resulted in a number of liver function tests. These tests are not used extensively at the present time in veterinary medicine; however, their use in the *liver profile* may at times be interesting. Although the glucose tolerance test and the determination of blood lactic and pyruvic acid levels may be abnormal in hepatic insufficiency (Lichtman, 1953), these tests have little specific diagnostic value and have not been studied adequately in the domestic animals to warrant their discussion. Experimental evidence, however, suggests that the galactose tolerance test may be successful in detecting hepatic alterations because only the liver can utilize galactose in significant amounts in certain species. The test, however, fails to reveal lesser degrees of liver damage, and is quite time-consuming in execution and analysis.

1. Galactose Tolerance Test

The use of this sugar was first suggested as a test for man by Bauer (1906). Its utilization primarily by the liver was shown by Sachs (1899), Blumenthal (1905), and Bollman *et al.* (1931). Owing to a series of problems encountered in the oral test proposed by Bauer, it is now performed in man and animals by injecting galactose intravenously at an amount that the average normal liver can completely remove in approximately 1 hour. Any galactose above the expected values at 1 hour may imply liver pathology. Bassett and Althausen (1941) recommend the injection of 0.5 gm galactose and sampling at 60 and 75 minutes for galactose analysis in man. Drill and Ivy (1944) suggest for the dog an intravenous injection of 1.0 ml of 50% galactose/kg.

The test is somewhat difficult to interpret in the dog; however, advanced hepatopathy can be detected. Markiewicz (1956) found this test to be better than the Takata-Ara reaction in detecting liver disease in 20 clinical canine cases. The BSP test was quite superior to the galactose test in its ability to detect early changes as well as its adaptability for close standardization (Drill and Ivy, 1944).

Cow. Garner (1952b) administered 0.5 gm/kg body weight to cattle which had been fasted overnight. Blood samples were taken prior to and at 0.5, 1, 1.5, and 2 hours after injection. Galactose levels were determined by the Harding-Nelson method described by E. J. King and Garner (1947) after removal of the glucose by fermentation with a suspension of washed baker's yeast for 15 minutes at 37° C. Galactose was observed to persist in the blood for considerably longer periods of time in normal cattle than in humans. The galactose disappearance curves in cattle with diffuse liver damage were quite elevated as compared to curves in control cattle. It was concluded that both the galactose tolerance and adrenaline response test with certain modifications could be applied to the detection of bovine hepatopathy (Garner, 1952b). Galactose and glucose tolerance, as well as pyruvic and lactic acid metabolism have also been studied in normal horses and in equine hepatopathy (Forenbacher, 1957).

2. Levulose Tolerance Test

Since levulose is metabolized by both liver and muscle, it cannot be used as a specific index of liver disease. The test as used in man (Lichtman, 1953) originally consisted of determining the presence or absence of levulose in the urine and blood after the oral administration of 100 gm. This test failed to give reliable results since the kidney threshold for this hexose in man is extremely low. The usual finding of little hyperglycemia (< 125 mg/100 ml) within 1 hour following the ingestion of 50 gm of levulose in normal individuals differed considerably from the marked hyperglycemia observed in cases of liver insufficiency. Stiebale (1942) studied levulose tolerance in normal dogs and following the administration of hepatotoxins (phosphorus and CCl_4). He concluded that the test showed diagnostic promise. Levulose was present only in the urine (Seliwanoff's reaction) in advanced liver disease. Blood glucose curves climbed to 30 mg/100 ml above the fasting level or remained elevated for over 4 hours following levulose administration to dogs with liver insufficiency. The test has not been used extensively owing to the availability of other simple and more specific function tests.

B. Protein Metabolism Tests*

Although none of the alterations in the serum proteins are entirely specific for liver damage, the combination of an absolute low albumin and/or a high γ-globulin level are quite typical. Hyperplasia of the immunocytic variety of liver cells is associated with a marked increase in serum γ-globulin.

The concentrations of the plasma proteins depend upon a multitude of factors (Hargreaves, 1968). These include: the extent, duration, severity and primary nature of the damage, current rates of synthesis, catabolism, hepatic release, and distribution. In addition, each of the above factors can be affected by circulatory, inflammatory, reparative, degenerative, metabolic, and regenerative processes occurring in the specific liver disease. It is, therefore, impossible to define a typical plasma protein pattern in certain types of liver disease, but changes in certain types of patterns are characteristic of specific hepatopathies.

Paper electrophoresis or the rapid fractionation procedure of serum proteins by W. G. Wolfson et al. (1948) may be used. The original Tiselius (1930) free electrophoresis techniques were somewhat elaborate and not suited well for clinical application; however, the recent development of paper and other supporting media for electrophoresis has changed this situation with the method now being a routine procedure in all laboratories. Since all domestic animals may vary in their total serum protein concentration between 5 and 8 gm/100 ml owing to individual differences and variations in water balance, a differential fractionation is needed to allow for the detection of changes in the absolute quantities of certain specific serum proteins. Total serum protein values are rarely of aid for clinical interpretations unless values fall below 5 gm/100 ml, which are usually observed only in late stages of disease processes.

1. Serum Albumin

The fall in serum albumin concentration from the failure of hepatic parenchymal synthesis is not an early change and therefore is found more commonly in chronic

---

*See Chapter 3 on Proteins for a more detailed outline on serum proteins.

conditions such as diffuse fibrosis or subacute hepatitis. Since only 12% (Fink *et al.*, 1944) and 5% (Cornelius *et al.*, 1963) of the serum albumin is synthesized per day in the dog and cow, respectively, a longer time lapse is required than for many tests to detect hepatic insufficiency. In portal fibrosis, the characteristic change is usually a diminution in the serum albumin level and an elevation in the γ-globulin. As might be expected, the changes in albumin are less conspicuous in acute hepatitis, but an elevation in the γ-globulins is a consistent finding. High β-lipoproteins have been observed primarily in biliary obstruction. Apart from liver disease, low albumin levels are found in domestic animals with nephritis, nephrosis, malnutrition, circulatory diseases, deficient protein digestion and absorption from pancreatic disorders, and a host of other chronic diseases resulting in cachexia.

2. Serum Globulins

The serum globulin level is elevated in both hepatitis and diffuse fibrosis. Although the cause for the fall in serum albumin is understood, the reason for the increase in γ-globulins is still not clear. Since elevations are usually greater in hepatitis and cholangitis and are sometimes absent in degenerative conditions such as chloroform poisoning, it may in part represent an antibody reaction to infective organisms. Hyperglobulinemias associated with chronic diffuse fibrosis have been interpreted by many as the terminal stage of an infective condition. Tissue breakdown may result in the formation of homologous tissue antibodies which increase the total serum γ-globulin level (Sherlock, 1958). Since the elevation in γ-globulin is from an increased production and not due to delayed removal (Havens *et al.*, 1954), the increased numbers of plasma cells in the bone marrow may represent part of the source of γ-globulin in addition to Kupfer cell proliferation. Many disease conditions may cause an elevation in the γ-globulin level, such as lymphocytoma, acute bacterial and protozoan infections, chronic bacterial endocarditis, osteomyelitis, and a number of diseases of the bone marrow and reticuloendothelial system. The γ-globulin peak in hepatopathy shows a wide base electrophoretically which is quite different from the sharp peak observed in multiple myeloma.

Polson and Malherbe (1952) and Groulade and Groulade (1960) have studied the serum protein fractions in dogs with hepatopathy. Hypoalbuminemia was nearly always observed but only associated occasionally with increased γ-globulin levels. Hoe and Harvey (1961b) carried out electrophoretic analyses on 140 dogs suffering from various diseases. Serum albumin decreased in most cases studied, whereas α_2-globulins deviated from the normal range in a nonspecific manner. β_1-Globulin increased in neoplasia but decreased in all cases of jaundice and the majority of diabetes mellitus cases. β_2-Globulins increased in all cases of jaundice as did the γ-globulins. In cirrhosis, a poor separation occurred between the β and γ zones. In canine hepatitis, a decrease in serum albumin, a rapid increase in α_2-globulin, and a delayed increase in γ-globulin is observed (Beckett *et al.*, 1964). Similar changes in the serum albumin and globulin have been reported in calves receiving ragwort (Ford and Ritchie, 1968); sporodesmin poisoning in sheep (Leaver, 1968; Mortimer, 1962); and venoocclusive disease in monkeys (Allen and Carstens, 1968).

An extensive electrophoretic study on average values for serum proteins in cattle with various liver diseases was made by Venturoli (1958) and presented in Table VI.

TABLE VI   SERUM PROTEINS IN BOVINE HEPATOPATHY[a]

	Albumin (%)	Globulin (%)			Total protein (gm/100 ml)	Albumin/ globulin (ratio)
		α	β	γ		
Normal cattle	43.5	14.5	13.5	27.0	6.4	0.77
Parasitic liver diseases	34.7	14.8	15.8	35.3	6.1	0.52
Hepatic *Echinococcus*	33.7	15.7	15.0	35.8	6.2	0.51
Foreign body invasion	29.9	13.6	18.7	37.8	6.5	0.42
Hepatic tuberculosis	22.9	14.2	17.7	45.1	8.3	0.29

[a]Venturoli (1958).

3. Flocculation Tests

A large number of empirical tests arising as the result of some serum protein abnormality have been extensively used due to their simplicity in diagnosing human liver disease. Since the albumin:globulin ratios may be less than 1.0 in domestic animals, false positive reactions may occur in these tests since they were developed for use on human sera with albumin:globulin ratios greater than 1.5. The chemical or paper electrophoretic fractionation of serum proteins is recommended as a more direct method to assess the status of the serum proteins in liver disorders in domestic animals. The earliest of these empirical tests was the formol gel test which was developed by Napier (1921) for humans with kala-azar, a tropical disease caused by the Leishman-Donavan parasite. Other such tests are the Weltman coagulation band, Takata-Ara, cephalin-cholesterol, colloidal gold, thymol turbidity, colloidal red, cadmium sulfate, zinc sulfate, and ammonium sulfate (Maclagan, 1956). All of these flocculation tests resemble one another, differing mainly in the precipitating reagent used and in the pH of the test. With abnormal sera, a precipitate, turbidity, or flocculation occurs, whereas no such results are present in normal sera. At the time of the development of many of these empirical tests, the mechanism of the reaction was not known. Only recently has electrophoretic techniques of human serum protein fractionation helped clarify these mechanisms. Since some flocculation tests are dependent upon increased serum γ-globulin levels (zinc sulfate, ammonium sulfate), they are usually positive in acute hepatitis and active fibrosis in man. Other tests depend on a variety of different factors such as pH denaturation (Takata-Ara), lyophobic colloids (cephalin cholesterol), α-globulins (another cephalin-cholesterol reaction), and lipoprotein disruption (thymol turbidity). No two tests are exactly the same in their mechanism of precipitation.

Since albumin:globulin ratios may be lower in domestic animals (Deutsch and Goodloe, 1945) and may cause false positive reactions, the empirical turbidometric and flocculation tests have not been used extensively in veterinary clinical laboratories. These tests as used in some investigations in domestic animals are summarized in Table VII. No two tests agree exactly in their mechanism of precipitation.

It is quite interesting that a few of these empirical tests appear to correlate positively with liver damage in animals. The Takata-Ara test can be used in cattle with advanced hepatopathy, but is quite unreliable in the dog. An investigation by

Hoe and Harvey (1961b) in dogs revealed the Kunkel test could be used semiquantitatively while the Takata-Ara and thymol turbidity tests were less specific. The thymol turbidity on the other hand has been recommended for the dog but not for the cow. Data concerning these tests at present are really insufficient for their proper evaluation in animals. Since more specific information concerning the serum proteins can readily be gained by their fractionation, the flocculation tests cannot be recommended at present in veterinary clinical medicine.

4. Serum Glycoproteins

Since the site of much of the total protein-bound hexose production is the liver, it has been observed that the plasma glycoprotein level decreases in rabbits and

TABLE VII A PARTIAL LIST OF REFERENCES ON SOME FLOCCULATION TESTS IN DOMESTIC ANIMALS

Test	Species	Reference
Takata-Ara	Dog	Karsai (1954); Ferreira Neto (1958); Garner (1952c); Shibanai et al. (1956); Janecek et al. (1957); Bodya (1960); Boda (1960a); Hoe and Harvey (1961b)
	Horse	Janecek et al. (1957)
Thymol turbidity	Dog	Gornall and Bardawill (1952); Karsai (1954); Hoe and Harvey (1961b)
	Cow	Garner (1952c)
	Sheep	Mortimer (1962)
	Chimpanzee	Deinhardt et al. (1962)
	Monkey	Anderson (1966) Evans et al. (1953) A. W. Holmes et al. (1967) Deinhardt and Deinhardt (1966)
Zinc sulfate	Dog	Gornall and Bardawill (1952)
	Sheep	Leaver (1968) Mortimer (1962)
Formol-Gel	Cattle	Garner (1952c)
Cadmium turbidity	Cattle	Garner (1952c)
Cephalin-cholesterol	Cattle	Schaffer (1949) Garner (1952c)
	Sheep	Mortimer (1962)
	Monkey	Evans et al. (1953)
	Chimpanzee	Wisecup et al. (1969) Deinhardt et al. (1962)
Colloidal gold	Cattle	Garner (1952c)
Iodine	Sheep	Mortimer (1962) Ford and Ritchie (1968)

man in parenchymatous liver disease (Stary, 1957). The existence of highly soluble carbohydrate-protein conjugates in mammalian serum was first reported by Freund (1892). A few limited investigations on the levels of the plasma glycoproteins in domestic animals have been reported. Mayer (1942) analyzed a glycoprotein fraction isolated from horse serum with 60% ethanol which was present in a concentration of 10.1 mg/100 ml. Weimer and Winzler (1955) have isolated and analyzed an acidic glycoprotein, called *orosomucoid*, from pooled ox and horse serum; this is the major constituent of the seromucoid fraction in mammals. The seromucoid fraction is routinely isolated by precipitation with 5% phosphotungstic acid in 2 N HCl following initial deproteinization by 0.6 M perchloric acid. The seromucoid can then be estimated in terms of its protein tyrosine, hexose, hexosamine, or sialic acid content. Cornelius *et al.* (1959a) reported an increase in both the seromucoid fraction and urinary glycoproteins of sheep in experimental urolithiasis. Elevations in the protein-bound polsaccharides have been reported in dogs with various skin diseases (Tradati and Abbate, 1958), bacterial or sterile abscesses, and following extensive surgery (Shetlar *et al.*, 1949). Marked elevations of the seromucoid fraction in the blood of the various mammals appear to parallel the degree of tissue inflammation or destruction (Cornelius *et al.*, 1960b).

Boda (1959) observed decreases in the serum mucoproteins in certain cattle with liver diseases and suggested that elevated levels of mucoproteins prevent the colloidal reaction of the Takata-Ara test (Boda, 1960b). Other cattle with hepatic lesions exhibited high or normal levels (Boda, 1959). No decrease in the blood seromucoid level was observed in two horses with subacute hepatitis. One horse with generalized plasma cell myelomatosis had a slightly elevated plasma level in contrast to the reduced level frequently observed in man (Cornelius *et al.*, 1960b).

5. *Amino Acid Tolerance Tests*

Deamination rates of injected amino acids such as tyrosine and arginine by the liver have been used as liver function tests in man and animals. In addition, increases in the amino acid concentration in the blood and urine may also be indicative of hepatic failure. Experimental studies have shown that approximately 85% of the effective hepatic parenchyma must be lost before these tests are of diagnostic significance (F. C. Mann, 1927). In infectious hepatitis in man, increased amounts of cystine in the plasma and urine seem to be quite a sensitive index of hepatic cell failure. Karsai (1954) noted in dogs that deamination was incomplete in hepatic diseases and this resulted in increases in amino acids in the serum and urine. The presence of tyrosine and leucine crystals in the urine was indicative of both hepatic malfunction and extensive parenchymal destruction. Millon's reagent was used to detect the urinary tyrosine in this study. A positive test was observed only in dogs with severe hepatic dysfunction and the test was best used to assess the severity of hepatic cell destruction.

Gornall and Bardawill (1952) performed both the tyrosine tolerance test (6 gm to fasted dogs, with postinjection samples hourly for 7 hours) and the arginine tolerance test (1.5 gm to fasted dogs). Fasting normal dogs had blood tyrosine and arginine levels of 1.1–1.9 and 1.6–2.2 mg/100 ml, respectively. Forty-eight hours after the administration of 5 ml of CCl_4, the fasting levels were above 2 mg/100 ml for tyrosine and within the normal range for arginine. The tolerance tests as performed gave little evidence of being useful. Others (Goettsch et al., 1942; Doggart et al., 1958) have confirmed the presence of increased blood and urine levels of various amino acids using paper chromatography in severe liver damage in dogs. Peredereev (1959) found similar results using a glycine tolerance test in cows.

The hippuric acid test is not presently used in canine veterinary medicine since any administered phenol derivatives such as benzoic acid are conjugated primarily by the kidney. Elevations in the serum "phenol body" concentration are diagnostic for renal insufficiency in the dog. A liver function test based on hippuric acid synthesis in cows following sodium benzoate administration has been studied by Cerkasov (1959).

6. Prothrombin Time

Low plasma prothrombin levels can occur from two causes in liver disease. A damaged liver may be unable to synthesize prothrombin in the presence of adequate metabolites; or in the presence of inadequate bile, fat-soluble vitamin K, which is needed for prothrombin synthesis, is unabsorbed from the intestine. Both abnormalities may exist in advanced diffuse hepatic fibrosis. In localized postnecrotic scarring of the liver following extensive necrosis, there is usually sufficient regenerated hepatic tissue remaining for the normal synthesis of prothrombin. If clotting is delayed in the presence of clinical icterus, an injection of vitamin K (50 mg) may decrease the coagulation time if extrahepatic obstruction of the bile duct is present. No response to vitamin K therapy may suggest the presence of diffuse parenchymal insufficiency.

METHOD.   Prothrombin time may be estimated by the laboratory method of Quick (1938). The coagulation time, however, can be rapidly and simply performed at the time of physical examination by use of clean capillary glass tubes, 1 mm in diameter. In this method, the buccal surface of the upper lip is punctured with a scalpel and a drop of fresh blood (free of tissue juices) is drawn into the tube by capillary attraction. The tube is broken at 15-second intervals and examined for the presence of fibrin, which normally occurs by 1–1.5 minutes. A normal control animal should also be tested to account for the effects of abnormally high or low environmental temperatures. Coagulation times upward of 2 minutes by this method should be interpreted as prolonged. The test is quite diagnostic in acute viral hepatitis of puppies.

Gornall and Bardawill (1952) reported normal prothrombin times in dog of 7.4–8.6 seconds. Five dogs had increased prothrombin times from 11 to 24 seconds after the oral administration of CCl_4, returning to normal within 10 days. Prothrombin estimations were sensitive indicators of liver injury in dogs during the acute phase. This test was not found to be as sensitive as the BSP or AP tests in detecting liver damage (Drill and Ivy, 1944; Svirbely et al., 1946). The test has been studied extensively in the dog (V. Müller, 1959; Gorisek, 1954; Florio et al., 1959). Gorisek (1958) observed that the severity of the prothrombin level was related to the severity of liver damage in horses and was quite helpful in prognostication. Mortimer (1962) observed that the prothrombin time was prolonged in sheep

21 days after dosing with sporidesmin. Horses with acute and subacute hepatitis, hepatic necrosis with regeneration, and diffuse fibrosis (as confirmed by biopsy) had 76, 56, and 77% of the normal prothrombin level, respectively.

7. Blood Uric Acid

In the dog, hepatectomy is followed by an elevation in the blood and urine uric acid. The end product of purine metabolism is allantoin in all dogs except the Dalmation, whose incomplete renal tubular reabsorption of uric acid allows for its excretion. A membrane transport defect for this anion accounts for this difference. Since the dog converts uric acid to allantoin in the liver, its elevation above 1 mg/100 ml in the blood has been recommended as an indicator of liver disease in this species. Normal blood values for the dog are between 0.1 and 1 mg/100 ml (Bloom, 1957). Since methods for accurate uric acid determinations are quite tedious (H. Brown, 1945), this test has not been used greatly and appears to be of doubtful value for the measurement of liver insufficiency in the dog. Ott (1956) indicated that blood uric acid levels were significantly elevated in hepato-cellular jaundice, but normal in hemolytic and obstructive jaundice. Malherbe (1959) and Morgan (1959b) have concluded that the BSP test is much more sensitive than uric acid determinations in canine hepatopathy. Hoe and Harvey (1961a) have shown in extensive studies with dogs that only 75% of clinical cases with the highest ranges of uric acid were dogs suspected of liver dysfunction. While 100% of jaundiced canine cases showed slight elevations in AP activity, only 86% had elevated uric acid levels.

8. Blood Ammonia

Ammonia concentrations in the peripheral blood and cerebrospinal fluid are usually elevated in hepatic coma (Silen and Eiseman, 1960). In normal individuals, the liver rapidly and efficiently removes ammonia by transamination. Ammonia is derived from bacterial action in the gastrointestinal tract and reaches the liver through the portal circulation. In hepatic cellular insufficiency, the removal of gastrointestinal ammonia is incomplete and may be aggravated by the ingestion of large quantities of nitrogenous foods (Webster and Davidson, 1957). Diagnosis may be based on an elevated ammonia level in the blood, but its determination is quite difficult and subject to error. Therapy is aimed at the removal of large amounts of protein from the diet and the inhibition of bacteria by antibiotics in the intestinal tract. Hepatic insufficiency associated with central nervous system symptoms has been recognized in the horse in all parts of the world (Stenius, 1941; Boiteux, 1958; Innes, 1953; Jalkanen, 1953; Forenbacher et al., 1959). Intermittent hepatic coma has been observed in horses at 3 weeks following the ligation of the common bile duct. Blood ammonia levels of 700 μg/100 ml were observed (Cornelius et al., 1965b).

C. LIPID METABOLISM TESTS

1. Serum Free and Esterified Cholesterol

As early as 1862 (Flint, 1862), attempts were made to differentiate the types of icterus by the levels of cholesterol in the serum. The origin of cholesterol esters in the blood has been a constant source of controversy. Thannhauser and Schaber (1926) reported that in cases of liver disease in man, the serum cholesterol ester values were below those of the free cholesterol. In acute generalized hepatopathy, cholesterol esters were greatly depressed or absent. Adler and Lemmel (1928) evaluated this conception on an extensive scale in human subjects with liver disease. Their conclusions were that the esterification of cholesterol with fatty acids is primarily a function of the liver parenchyma. Increases in the serum total cholesterol level in obstructive jaundice may be due to overproduction by the liver (Byers *et al.*, 1951) and not retention of cholesterol normally excreted into the bile (see Chapter 2 on Lipid Metabolism). Of greatest clinical importance in hepatocellular damage is the ratio of free cholesterol to cholesterol esters in the serum. In both chronic and acute hepatocellular disease, esterification is significantly depressed, giving a higher free cholesterol ester ratio than observed in the normal mammal.

Limited data suggest that esterification is also depressed in liver disease of domestic animals (Romagnoli, 1954; Piccotin, 1956; Darraspen *et al.*, 1959; Done *et al.*, 1960). Normal dogs had total cholesterol and cholesterol ester values of 166 ± 32 and 115 ± 70 mg/100 ml, respectively (70 ± 8% as cholesterol ester). Dogs with liver diseases exhibited average total and esterified cholesterol values of 187 and 75 mg/100 ml, respectively (42% as cholesterol ester). This study showed a 40% drop in cholesterol ester in canine hepatopathy (Piccotin, 1956). Hoe and Harvey (1961a) found normal average total serum cholesterol values in kennel dogs and household pets to be 186 ± 14 and 258 ± 36 mg/100 ml, respectively. In both groups the percent ester was quite similar at 65 ± 12 and 62 ± 3, respectively. The diet of household scraps containing a high concentration of cholesterol and other lipids most likely accounted for the higher levels in the household group. It was concluded in this study that although a dog with a normal ester ratio (60–80%) would most likely not have liver involvement, the converse would not be true. High blood cholesterol levels also occur in other diseases such as hypothyroidism, diabetes mellitus, and advanced nephrosis. The ratio of blood cholesterol to phospholipids in dogs with hepatopathy has also been reported by Darraspen *et al.* (1959). Romagnoli (1954) reported total average blood cholesterol levels of 50 mg/100 ml (range = 24–75 mg/100 ml) in healthy sheep. Sheep with livers affected moderately by *Echinococcus* and *Fasciola* infections had blood cholesterol levels within this normal range. Livers severely affected with these parasites had elevated cholesterol values averaging 76 mg/100 ml. Total cholesterol and cholesterol ester levels in 35 normal cattle were observed to be on an average 140 and 103 mg/100 ml, respectively (73 ± 6% as cholesterol ester). Fifty-eight cattle with various liver diseases showed a significant decrease in the percent of cholesterol ester. Total cholesterol and cholesterol ester levels in bovine hepatopathy averaged 161 and 85 mg/100 ml, respectively (54 ± 12% as cholesterol ester) (Piccotin, 1956).

PHOSPHOLIPIDS. These are formed primarily in the liver and disappear from the mammal following hepatectomy (Fishler *et al.*, 1943). Since their estimation in the blood is technically difficult, most studies have involved the isolation of the total lipids and the measurement of lipid phosphorus. High serum levels have been reported in human obstructive jaundice, of either an intrahepatic or extrahepatic nature. Increased levels have occasionally been reported in acute hepatitis. (See Chapter 2 for further details.)

VII. LIVER BIOPSY

Although liver biopsy is not usually referred to as a liver function test, its omission in this chapter would be a serious oversight. In the study of an animal with known liver disease, the diagnosis may still remain doubtful in spite of careful clinical and laboratory studies. Examination of liver biopsy samples in these cases may prove invaluable. This technique is usually not needed in the differential diagnosis of icterus since clinical history and laboratory tests will usually suffice. In routine hospital practice concerning jaundiced human patients with liver disease, only 15% of these patients require biopsy for diagnosis. Indications for needle biopsy are: (1) suspected portal fibrosis with nearly normal liver function tests; (2) hepatic malignancies; (3) metabolic diseases—lipidosis, amyloidosis, and glycogen storage disease; (4) obscure hepatomegaly; (5) extremely rare cases of icterus when laboratory tests are confusing; (6) vitamin A determinations; and (7) heavy metal intoxications, i.e., by molybdenum, selenium, arsenic. etc. Liver biopsy is not without risk, particularly in unskilled hands; complications may include biliary peritonitis from a punctured gallbladder or dilated bile duct; hemorrhage resulting from rupture of a large vessel or a low prothrombin level; hepatitis, pleuritis, or peritonitis from bacterial contamination; and puncture of other viscera. The use of a small biopsy sample may not reflect the status of the whole organ unless the lesions are uniformly of a diffuse nature. References to the methods of liver biopsy in the various domestic animals are presented in Table VIII.

TABLE VIII REFERENCE LIST TO LIVER BIOPSY METHODS IN DOMESTIC ANIMALS

Species	References
Dog	Chandrasekharan, and D'Sousa (1951); Knowles (1952); Romagnoli (1958); Chapman (1965); Van Vleet and Alberts (1968).
Horse	Wittfogel (1939); Isaksson (1951); Konrad (1958); Wolff et al. (1967).
Swine	Jones et al. (1956).
Sheep	Dick (1952); F. J. Hamilton (1957).
Fowl	Grueul (1959).
Cattle	Garner (1950); Loosmore and Allcroft (1951); Udall et al. (1952); Whitehair et al. (1952); Seghetti and Marsh (1953); Moller and Simesen (1959); Simesen and Moller (1959); Nikov (1960); Schultz et al. (1960).

VIII. MISCELLANEOUS LIVER FUNCTION TESTS

A. CHOLECYSTOGRAPHY

Roentgenological studies on the liver and biliary system have been increasing in veterinary medicine. Present studies suggest their use should be further investigated. No attempt will be made to cover these important techniques in this chapter and the reader should consult standard procedures available in radiological and X-ray texts in veterinary medicine.

B. Chloral Hydrate Clearance

The ability of the canine liver to detoxify chloral hydrate by glucuronic acid conjugation and subsequent urinary excretion has been studied by Mukerji and Ghose (1939, 1940a,b). Chloral hydrate can be measured by the procedure of Friedman and Calderone (1934). After the oral administration of 100–200 mg choral hydrate/kg to dogs, 1.0-ml blood samples are collected at approximately 45 minutes after injection and hourly to ascertain the time of maximal blood concentration. Following the oral administration of 100 mg/kg to dogs, the average blood concentrations at 45 minutes were on an average (mg/100 ml): normal dogs, 1.32; recent CCl_4 administration, 1.94; and prolonged CCl_4 administration, 3.55. Following the 200 mg/kg dose, chloral hydrate values were on an average 3.32, 4.52, and 8.25 mg/100 ml, respectively, at 45 minutes after administration. The test appeared sensitive in canine hepatic necrosis.

TABLE IX SUMMARY OF CLINICAL AND LABORATORY FINDINGS IN ICTERUS AND LIVER DISEASE[a]

Test	Hemolytic icterus (without secondary liver damage)	Hepatocellular damage	Extrahepatic obstruction of bile duct
1. Clinical icterus	+	+ or −	+ (after a few days)
2. Stool color	Dark	N	Clay
3. Urine color	Dark (white foam)	Dark (yellow-green foam)	Very dark (yellow-green foam)
4. Serum free bilirubin (Indirect van den Bergh)	+	+ or − [b]	−
5. Serum bilirubin conjugates (direct reaction)	−	+ [c]	+
6. Urine bilirubin conjugates	−	+	+
7. Urine urobilinogen	Increased	Increased	Absent
8. Prothrombin time	N	Increased	Increased (if prolonged)
9. Dye retention (BSP, rose bengal, ICG)	N to increased [d]	Increased	Increased (due to obstruction)
10. Serum albumin	N	Decreased	N
11. γ-Globulin	N	Increased	N
12. Total serum cholesterol	N	Variable	Occasionally increased
13. Serum cholesterol ester (%)	N	Decreased	N
14. Blood uric acid	N	Increased	N
15. Blood ammonia (hepatic coma)	N	Increased	N
16. Galactose tolerance	−	+	−
17. Serum enzymes (SGPT, SD, GD, OCT, arginase)	N	Greatly increased	N [e]

[a]Key to symbols: +, positive test; −, negative test; N, normal results.

[b]Always positive in the horse, and up to 40% of the total bilirubin in other species.

[c]May be negative in the horse.

[d]May be increased due to competition with serum bilirubin, if elevated.

[e]SGPT and SGOT may be slightly increased after a few days of complete obstruction.

REFERENCES

Acocella, G., Tenconi, L. T., Armas-Merino, R., Raia, S., and Billing, B. H. (1968). *Lancet* **00**, 68.

Adler, A., and Lemmel, H. (1928). *Deut. Arch. Klin. Med.* **158**, 173.

Aktan, V. F. (1954). *Monatsh. Veterinaermed.* **9**, 97.

Allcroft, W. M., and Folley, S. J. (1941). *Biochem. J.* **35**, 254.

Allen, J. R., and Carstens, L. A. (1968). *Am. J. Vet. Res.* **29**, 1681.

Allen, J. R., Carstens, L. A., and Katagiri, G. J. (1969). *Arch. Pathol.* **87**, 279.

Ammon, R. (1934). *Klin. Wochschr.* **13**, 1422.

Anderson, D. R. (1966). *Am. J. Vet. Res.* **27**, 1484.

Anderson, R. R., and Mixner, J. P. (1960). *J. Dairy Sci.* **43**, 1465.

Andrews, W. H., Magraith, B. G., and Richards, T. G. (1956). *J. Physiol.* (*London*) **131**, 669.

Anonymous, Atlas Newsletter, Small Animal Digest. (1959). *Vet. Med.* **54**, 307.

Appelmans, R., and Bouckaert, J. P. (1926). *Rev. Med.-Chir. Maladies Foie* **1**, 294.

Arendarcik, J. (1959). *Vet. Casopis* **8**, 515.

Arias, I. M., and London, I. M. (1957). *Science* **126**, 563.

Armstrong, A. R., King, E. J., and Harris, R. I. (1934). *Can. Med. Assoc. J.* **31**, 14.

Barrett, P. V. D., Berk, P. D., [N. S.] Menken, M., and Berlin, N. I. (1968). *Ann. Internal Med.* **68**, 355.

Bassett, A. M., and Althausen, T. L. (1941). *Am. J. Digest. Diseases* **8**, No. 11, 432.

Bauer, R. (1906). *Wien. Med. Wochschr.* **56**, 2537.

Beckett, S. D., Burns, M. J., and Clark, C. H. (1964). *J. Am. Vet. Med. Assoc.* **25**, 1186.

Beijers, J. A. (1923). Proefschrift, University of Utrecht.

Beijers, J. A., Van Loghem, J. J., and Van der Hart, M. (1950). *Tijdschr. Diergeneesk.* **75**, 955.

Bendixen, H. C., and Carlström, B. (1928). *Maanedsskr. Dyrlaeg.* **40**, 129.

Benedek, G. (1956). *Magy. Allatorv. Lapja* **11**, 361.

Benedek, G. (1961). *Acta Vet. Acad. Sci. Hung.* **11**, 293.

Benndorf, E. (1955). Inaugural Dissertation, University of Leipzig.

Berger, H. J. (1956). *Zentr. Veterinaermed.* **3**, 273.

Berman, A. L., Snapp, E., and Ivy, A. C. (1941). *Am. J. Physiol.* **132**, 176.

Bessey, O. A., Lowry, O. H., and Brock, M. J. (1946). *J. Biol. Chem.* **164**, 321.

Bicknell, E. J., Brooks, R. A., Osburn, J. A., and Whitehair, C. K. (1967). *Am. J. Vet. Res.* **28**, 943.

Bierthen, E. (1906). Inaugural Dissertation, University of Bern.

Blincoe, C., and Dye, W. B. (1958). *J. Animal Sci.* **17**, 224.

Bloom, F. (1957). *North Am. Vet.* **38**, 17.

Blumenthal, F. (1905). *Beitr. Chem. Physiol. Pathol.* **6**, 329.

Boda, K. (1959). *Vet. Casopis* **8**, 290.

Boda, K. (1960a). *Folia Vet.* **4**, 21.

Boda, K. (1960b). *Folia Vet.* **4**, 29.

Bodansky, A. (1933). *J. Biol. Chem.* **101**, 93.

Bodansky, A. (1937). *J. Biol. Chem.* **120**, 167.

Bodya, K. (1960). *Veterinariya* **37**, No. 7, 56.

Boiteux, R. D. (1958). *Rev. Militar Remonta Vet. Rio de Janeiro* **17**, 13.

Bollman, J. L., Power, M. H., and Mann, F. C. (1931). *Proc. Staff Meetings Mayo Clinic* **6**, 724.

Boyd, J. W. (1962). *Res. Vet. Sci.* **3**, 256.

Bradley, S. E., Ingelfinger, F. J., Bradley, G. P., and Curry, J. J. (1945). *J. Clin. Invest.* **24**, 890.

Brauer, R. W., and Root, M. A. (1947). *Am. J. Physiol.* **149**, 611.

Brauer, R. W., Pessotti, R. L., and Krebs, J. S. (1955). *J. Clin. Invest.* **34**, 35.

Brooks, F. P., Deneau, G. A., Potter, H. P., Reinhold, J. G., and Norris, R. F. (1963). *Am. J. Gastroenterol.* **44**, 287.

Brouwers, J. (1941). *Ann. Med. Vet.* **85**, 266.

Brown, C. H., and Glasser, O. (1956). *J. Lab. Clin. Med.* **48**, 454.

Brown, H. (1945). *J. Biol. Chem.* **158**, 601.

Brown, R. W., and Grisolia, S. (1959). *J. Lab. Clin. Med.* **54**, 617.

Burns, K. F., Ferguson, F. G., and Hampton, S. H. (1967). *Am. J. Clin. Pathol.* **48**, 484.

Burns, M. J., and Clark, C. H. (1963). *J. Am. Vet. Med. Assoc.* **142**, 1007.

Byers, S. O., Friedman, M., and Michaelis, F. (1951). *J. Biol. Chem.* **188**, 637.

Cabaud, P., Leeper, R., and Wroblewski, F. (1956). *Am. J. Clin. Pathol.* **26**, 1101.
Campbell, J. G. (1957). *J. Endocrinol.* **15**, 339.
Cantarow, A., and Stewart, L., (1935). *Am. J. Pathol.* **11**, 561.
Cantarow, A., Wirts, C. W., Snapp, W. S., and Miller, L. L. (1948). *Am. J. Physiol.* **154**, 507.
Cerkasov, D. P. (1959). *Sb. Cesk. Akad. Zemedel. Ved, Vet. Med.* **4**, 97.
Chandrasekharan, K. P., and D'Sousa, B. A. (1951). *Indian Vet. J.* **28**, 16.
Chapman, W. L. (1965). *J. Am. Vet. Med. Assoc.* **146**, 126.
Chernyak, N. Z., and Rozhov, D. I. (1953). *Sb. Tru. Leningr. Nauch.-Issledovatel. Vet. Inst.* **5**, 81.
Cherrick, G. R., Stein, S. W., Leevy, C. M., and Davidson, C. S. (1960). *J. Clin. Invest.* **39**, 592.
Clarkson, M. J. (1961). *Res. Vet. Sci.* **2**, 143.
Clarkson, M. J., and Richard, T. G. (1967). *Res. Vet. Sci.* **8**, 48.
Cohen, E. S., Giansiracusa, J. E., Strait, L. A., Althausen, T. L., and Karg, S. (1953). *Gastroenterology* **25**, 232.
Cohn, C., Levine, R., and Kolinsky, M. (1948). *Am. J. Physiol.* **155**, 286.
Cole, P. G., and Lathe, G. H. (1953). *J. Clin. Pathol.* **6**, 99.
Cole, P. G., Lathe, G. H., and Billings, B. H. (1954). *Biochem. J.* **57**, 514.
Cornelius, C. E. (1957). "7th Gaines Symposium," p. 20. Kankakee, Illinois.
Cornelius, C. E. (1958). *Iowa State Coll. Vet.* **20**, No. 3, 155.
Cornelius, C. E. (1961). *Cornell Vet.* **51**, 559.
Cornelius, C. E., and Freedland, R. A. (1962). *Cornell Vet.* **52**, 344.
Cornelius, C. E., and Gronwall, R. R. (1965). *Federation Proc.* **24**, No. 2.
Cornelius, C. E., and Gronwall, R. R. (1968). *Am. J. Vet. Res. Assoc.* **29**, No. 2, 291.
Cornelius, C. E., and Kaneko, J. J. (1960). *J. Am. Vet. Med. Assoc.* **137**, No. 1, 62.
Cornelius, C. E., and Mia, A. S. (1962). Unpublished data.
Cornelius, C. E., and Wheat, J. D. (1957). *Am. J. Vet. Res.* **18**, 369.
Cornelius, C. E., Theilen, G. H., and Rhode, E. A. (1958a). *Am. J. Vet. Res.* **19**, 560.
Cornelius, C. E., Holm, L. W., and Jasper, D. E. (1958b). *Cornell Vet.* **48**, No. 3, 305.
Cornelius, C. E., Moulton, J. E., and McGowan, B., Jr. (1959a). *Am. J. Vet. Res.* **20**, 863.
Cornelius, C. E., Bishop, J. A., Switzer, J., and Rhode, E. A. (1959b). *Cornell Vet.* **49**, No. 1, 116.
Cornelius, C. E., Law, G. R. J., Julian, L. M., and Asmundson, V. S. (1959c). *Proc. Soc. Exptl. Biol. Med.* **101**, 41.
Cornelius, C. E., Kilgore, W. W., and Wheat, J. D. (1960a). *Cornell Vet.* **50**, 47.
Cornelius, C. E., Rhode, E. A., and Bishop, J. A. (1960b). *Am. J. Vet. Res.* **21**, 1095.
Cornelius, C. E., Douglas, G. M., Gronwall, R. R, and Feedland, R. A. (1963). *Cornell Vet.* **53**, 181.
Cornelius, C. E., Arias, I. M., and Osburn, B. I. (1965a). *J. Am. Vet. Med. Assoc.* **146**, 709.
Cornelius, C. E., Gazmuri, G., Gronwall, R. R., and Rhode, E. A. (1965b). *Cornell Vet.* **55**, 110.
Cornelius, C. E., Osburn, B. I., Gronwall, R. R., and Cardinet, G. H. (1968). *Am. J. Digest. Diseases* [N. S.] **13**, 1072.
Crawley, G. J., and Swenson, M. J. (1965). *Am. J. Vet. Res.* **26**, 1468.
Crigler, J. E., and Najjar, V. A. (1952). *Pediatrics* **10**, 169.
Cysewski, S. J., Pier, A. C., Engstrom, C. W., Richard, J. L., Dougherty, R. W., and Thurston, J. R. (1968). *Am. J. Vet. Res.* **29**, 1577.
Dal Santo, F. (1959). *Acta Med. Vet.* **5**, 579.
Darraspen, E., Floria, R., Cottereau, P., Lescure, F., and Campredon, G. (1959). *Rev. Pathol. Gen. Comparee* **59**, 1349.
Deinhardt, F., and Deinhardt, J. (1966). *Symp. Zool. Soc. London* **17**, 127.
Deinhardt, F., Courtois, G., Dherte, P., Osterrieth, P., Nenane, G., Henle, G., and Henle, W. (1962). *Am. J. Hyg.* **75** 311.
Deinhardt, F., Holmes, A. W., Capps, R. B., and Popper, H. (1967). *J. Exptl. Med.* **125**, 673.
Delprat, G. D. (1923). *A.M.A. Arch. Internal Med.* **32**, 401.
Deutsch, H. F., and Goodloe, M. B. (1945). *J. Biol. Chem.* **161**, 1.
Dick, A. T. (1952). *Australian Vet. J.* **28**, 234.
Dobson, E. L., and Jones, H. B. (1952). *Acta Med. Scand.* **144**, Suppl. 273, 1.
Doggart, J. R., McCredie, J. A., and Welbourn, R. B. (1958). *Vet. Record* **70**, 279.
Done, J., Mortimer, P. H., and Taylor, A. (1960). *Res. Vet. Sci.* **1**, 76.
Doring, J. (1940). Innaugural Dissertation, Tierarztliche Hochschule, Hannover.

Drill, V. A., and Ivy, A. C. (1944). *J. Clin. Invest.* **23**, 209.

Dubin, I. N., and Johnson, F. B. (1954). *Medicine* **33**, 155.

Ducci, H., and Watson, C. J. (1945). *J. Lab. Clin. Med.* **30**, 293.

Dukes, H. H. (1946). "The Physiology of Domestic Animals." Cornell Univ. Press (Comstock), Ithaca, New York.

Eikmeier, H. (1959). *Berlin. Muench. Tieraerztl. Wochschr.* **72**, 48.

El-Gindy, H. (1957). *Vet. Med. J. (Giza)* **3**, No. 3, 45.

Evans, A. S., Evans, B. K., and Sturtz, V. (1953). *Proc. Soc. Exptl. Biol. Med.* **82**, 437.

Fellinger, K., and Menkes, K. (1933). *Wien. Klin. Wochschr.* **46**, 133.

Ferreira Neto, J. M. (1958). Thesis, Cornell University.

Fink, R. M., Enns, T., Kimball, C. P., Silberstein, H. E., Bale, W. F., Madden, S. C., and Whipple, G. H. (1944). *J. Exptl. Med.* **80**, 455.

Fishler, M. C., Entenman, C., Montgomery, M. L., and Chaikoff, I. L. (1943). *J. Biol. Chem.* **150**, 47.

Flint, A. (1862). *Am. J. Med. Sci.* **44**, 305.

Floria, R., Cottereau, P., Marie, C., and Marie, F. (1959). *Bull. Soc. Sci. Vet. Lyon* **61**, 139.

Fog, J., and Jellum, E. (1963). *Nature* **198**, 88.

Forbes, T. J., and Singleton, A. G. (1966). *Brit. Vet. J.* **122**, 55.

Ford, E. J. H. (1955). *Vet. Record* **67**, 634.

Ford, E. J. H. (1958). *J. Anat.* **92**, 447.

Ford, E. J. H., and Ritchie, H. E. (1968). *J. Comp. Pathol.* **78**, 207.

Forenbacher, S. (1957). *Vet. Arhiv.* **27**, 185.

Forenbacher, S., Marzan, B., and Topolnik, E. (1959). *Vet. Arhiv.* **29**, 322.

Fox, I. J., Brooker, L. G. S., Heseltine, D. W., Essex, H. E., and Wood, E. H. (1957). *Proc. Staff Meetings Mayo Clinic* **32**, 478.

Fox, I. J., Swan, H. J. C., and Wood, E. H. (1959). *In* "Intravascular Catheterization" (H. A. Zimmerman, ed.), p. 609. Thomas, Springfield, Illinois.

Frankl, H. D., and Merritt, J. H. (1959). *Am. J. Gastroenterol.* **31**, 166.

Freedland, R. A., Hjerpe, C. A., and Cornelius, C. E. (1965). *Res. Vet. Sci.* **6**, 18.

Freeman, S., Chen, Y. P., and Ivy, A. C. (1938). *J. Biol. Chem.* **124**, 79.

Freese, U. (1952). Inaugural Dissertation, Tierarztliche Hochschule, Hannover.

Freund, E. (1892). *Zentr. Physiol.* **6**, 345.

Frey, A., and Frey, M. (1949). *Am. J. Clin. Pathol.* **19**, 699.

Friedman, M. M., and Calderone, F. A. (1934). *J. Lab. Clin. Med.* **19**, 1332.

Gaisford, W. D., and Zuidema, G. D. (1965). *J. Surg. Res.* **5**, 220.

Gardiner, M. R., and Parr, W. H. (1967). *J. Comp. Pathol.* **77**, 51.

Garner, R. J. (1950). *Vet. Record* **62**, 729.

Garner, R. J. (1952a). *J. Comp. Pathol. Therap.* **62**, 306.

Garner, R. J. (1952b). *J. Comp. Pathol. Therap.* **62**, 292.

Garner, R. J. (1952c). *J. Comp. Pathol. Therap.* **62**, 300.

Garner, R. J. (1953). *J. Comp. Pathol. Therap.* **63**, 247.

Glaser, W., Gibbs, W. D., and Andrews, G. A. (1959). *J. Lab. Clin. Med.* **54**, 556.

Goettsch, E., Lyttle, J. D., Grim, W. M., and Dunbar, P. (1942). *J. Biol. Chem.* **144**, 121.

Gorisek, J. (1954). *Vet. Arhiv* **24**, 69.

Gorisek, J. (1958). *Deut. Tieraerztl. Wochschr.* **65**, 268.

Gornall, A. G., and Bardawill, C. J. (1952). *Can. J. Med. Sci.* **30**, 256.

Gradwohl, R. B. H. (1956). "Clinical Laboratory Methods and Diagnosis, A Testbook on Laboratory Procedures, with Their Interpretation," 5th ed., 2 vols. Mosby, St. Louis, Missouri.

Grassnickel, V. H. (1959). *Berlin. Muench. Tieraerztl. Wochschr.* **72**, 444.

Grassnickel, W. (1926). Inaugural Dissertation, University of Berlin.

Grodsky, G. M., and Carbone, J. V. (1957). *J. Biol. Chem.* **226**, 449.

Grodsky, G. M., Carbone, J. V., and Fanska, R. (1959). *J. Clin. Invest.* **38**, 1981.

Gronwall, R. R., and Cornelius, C. E. (1966). *Federation Proc.* **25**, 576.

Gronwall, R. R., and Mia, A. S. (1969). *Physiologist* **12**, 241.

Groulade, P., and Groulade, J. (1960). *Rev. Med. Vet.* **111**, 686.

Grueul, E. (1959). *Deut. Tieraerztl. Wochschr.* **65**, 437.

Gunn, C. H. (1938). *J. Heredity* **29**, 137.

Hamilton, F. J. (1957). *Australian Vet. J.* **33**, 273.

Hamilton, J. M., Cornwell, H. J. C., McCusker, H. B., Campbell, R. S. F., and Henderson, J. J. W. P. (1966). *Brit. Vet. J.* **122**, 255.

Hansen, M. A. (1964). *Nord. Veterinar Med.* **16**, 323.

Hargreaves, T. (1968). "The Liver and Bile Metabolism." Appleton, New York. p. 241.

Hartwell, W. V., Kimbrough, R. D, and Love, G. J. (1968). *Am. J. Vet. Res.* **29**, 1449.

Harvey, D. G. (1967). *J. Small Animal Pract.* **8**, 557.

Havens, W. P., Jr. and Ward, R. (1945). *Proc. Soc. Exptl. Biol. Med.* **60**, 102.

Havens, W. P., Jr., Dickensheets J., Bierly, J. N., and Eberhard, T. P. (1954). *J. Immunol.* **73**, 256.

Heaney, R. P., and Whedon, G. D. (1958). *J. Lab. Clin. Med.* **52**, 169.

Heidrich, K. M. (1954). Inaugural Dissertation, Tierarztliche Hochschule, Hannover.

Hepler, O. E. (1949). "Manual of Clinical Laboratory Methods," 4th ed., p. 110. Thomas, Springfield, Illinois.

Hoe, C. M. (1961). *Vet. Record* **73**, 153.

Hoe, C. M. (1969). "A Textbook of Veterinary Clinical Pathology," Chapter 3, p. 75. Academic Press, New York.

Hoe, C. M., and Harvey, D. G. (1961a). *J. Small Animal Pract.* **2**, 22.

Hoe, C. M., and Harvey, D. G. (1961b). *J. Small Animal Pract.* **2**, 109.

Hoe, C. M., and O'Shea, J. D. (1965). *Vet. Record* **77**, 1164.

Hoe, C. M., and Jabara, A. G. (1967). *J. Comp. Pathol.* **77**, 245.

Hoerlein, B. F., and Greene, J. E. (1950). *North Am. Vet.* **31**, 662.

Holmes, A. W., Passovoy, M., and Capps, R. B. (1967). *Lab. Animal Care* **17**, 41.

Holmes, J. R. (1960). *Cornell Vet.* **50**, No. 3, 308.

Holtenuis, J. M., and Jacobson, S. O. (1965). *Nord. Veterinar Med.* **17**, 415.

Humlicek, O., and Kruska, K. (1960). *Sb. Vysoke Skoly Zemedel. Brne* **B8**, 16.

Hunton, D. B., Bollman, J. L., and Hoffman, H. N. (1960). *Proc. Staff Meetings Mayo Clinic* **35**, 752.

Hunton, D. B., Bollman, J. L., and Hoffman, H. N. (1961). *J. Clin. Invest.* **40**, No. 9, 1648.

Innes, J. R. M. (1953). *North Am. Vet.* **34**, 29.

Isaksson, A. (1951). *J. Am. Vet. Med. Assoc.* **118**, 320.

Isselbacher, K. J., and McCarthy, E. A. (1958). *Biochim. Biophys. Acta* **92**, 658.

Jalkanen, J. I. (1953). *Finsk Veterinaer tidskr.* **59**, 211, 215, and 222.

Janecek, A., Neuman, V., and Kucera, K. (1957). *Sb. Vysoke Skoly Zemedel. Brne* **B5**, 285.

Jasper, D. E. (1947). Thesis, University of Minnesota.

Jones, E. W., Ullrey, D. E., and Gallup, W. D. (1956). *Cornell Vet.* **46**, 360.

Karmen, A. (1955). *J. Clin. Invest.* **34**, 131.

Karsai, F. (1954). *Magy. Allatorv. Lapja.* **9**, 271.

Karsai, F. (1960). *Acta Vet. Acad. Sci. Hung.* **10**, 263.

Katz, S., Gilardoni, A., Genovese, N., Wikinski, R. W., Cornelius, C. E., and Malinow, M. R. (1968). *Lab. Animal Care* **18**, 626.

Ketterer, S. G., Wiegand, B. D., and Rapaport, E. (1960). *Am. J. Physiol.* **199**, 481.

King, E. J., and Armstrong, A. R. (1934). *Can. Med. Assoc. J.* **31**, 376.

King, E. J., and Garner, R. J. (1947). *J. Clin. Pathol.* **1**, 30.

King, T. O., and Gargus, J. L. (1967). *Lab. Animal Care* **17**, 391.

Klaus, H. (1958). *Arch. Exptl. Veterinaermed.* **12**, 725.

Knisely, M. H. (1951). *Trans. 10th Josiah Macy Jr. Conf. Liver Injury, New York, 1900* p. 48.

Knowles, R. P. (1952). *Vet. Med.* **47**, 140.

Konrad, J. (1958). *Veterinarstvi* **8**, 714.

Kowatsch, O. (1947). Inaugural Dissertation, Tierarztliche Hochschule, Vienna.

Krispien, H. (1952). *Tieraerztl. Umschau* **7**, 118.

Krushak, D. H., and Hartwell, W. V. (1968). *J. Am. Vet. Med. Assoc.* **153**, 866.

Kühle, E. (1926). Inaugural Dissertation, University of Berlin.

Kutas, F., and Karsai, F. (1961). *Acta Vet. Acad. Sci. Hung.* **11**, 277.

Larson, E. J., and Morrill, C. C. (1960). *Am. J. Vet. Res.* **21**, 949.

Leaver, D. D. (1968). *Res. Vet. Sci.* **9**, 265.

Lemberg, R., and Legge, J. W. (1949). "Hematin Compounds and Bile Pigments; Their Constitution, Metabolism, and Function," Monograph, p. 546. Wiley (Interscience), New York.

Lester, R., and Troxler, R. F. (1969). *Gastroenterology* **56**, 143.

Lettow, E. (1961). *Zentr. Veterinaermed.* **8**, 353.

Li, T. W., Snapp, F. E., Hough, V. H., and Ivy, A. C. (1944). *Federation Proc.* **3**, 29.

Lichtman, S. S. (1953). "Diseases of the Liver, Gallbladder and Bile Ducts," Vol. I. Lea & Febiger, Philadelphia, Pennsylvania.

Lind, C. W., Gronwall, R. R., and Cornelius, C. E. (1967). *Res. Vet. Sci.* **8**, 280.

Loosmore, R. M., and Allcroft, R. (1951). *Vet. Record* **63**, 414.

Lopez Garcia, A., Zelasco, J. F., and Pedace, E. A. (1943). *Anales Inst. Invest. Fis. Apl. Pathol. Humana (Buenos Aires)* **5**, 13.

Lopuchovsky, J., and Jantosovic, J. (1958). *Vet. Casopis* **7**, 327.

Lupke, H. (1965). *Nord. Veterinaermed.* **17**, 467.

McArdle, B. (1940). *Quart. J. Med.* **9**, 107.

Maclagan, N. F. (1956). *In* "Diseases of the Liver: A Symposium" (L. Schif, ed.), p. 125. Lippincott, Philadelphia, Pennsylvania.

MacPherson, A., and Hemingway, R. G. (1969). *Brit. Vet. J.* **125**, 213.

Malherbe, W. D. (1959). *J. S. African Vet. Med. Assoc.* **30**, 113.

Malherbe, W. D. (1960). *J. S. African Vet. Med. Assoc.* **31**, 159.

Malloy, H. T., and Evelyn, K. A. (1937). *J. Biol. Chem.* **119**, 481.

Mann, F. C. (1927). *Medicine* **6**, 419.

Mann, G. V., Watson, P. L., and Adams, L. (1952). *J. Nutr.* **47**, 213.

Markiewicz, K. (1956). *Med. Veterynar.* (Poland) **12**, 724.

Maruffo, C. A., Malinow, M. R., Depaoli, J. R., and Katz, S. (1966). *Am. J. Pathol.* **49**, 455.

Mayer, K. (1942). *Z. Physiol. Chem.* **275**, 16.

Mena, I., Kivel, R., Mahoney, P., Mellinkoff, S. M., and Bennet, L. R. (1959). *J. Lab. Clin. Med.* **54**, 167.

Metzger, E. (1927). *Arch. Pathol. Anat. Physiol.* **263**, 703.

Meyer, K. (1938). Inaugural Dissertation, Tierarztliche Hochschule, Hannover.

Mia, A. S., Gronwall, R. R., and Cornelius, C. E. (1969) *Physiologist* **12**, 301.

Mills, M. A., and Dragstedt, C. A. (1938). *A. M. A. Arch. Internal Med.* **62**, 216.

Minette, H. P., and Shaffer, M. F. (1968). *Am. J. Trop. Med. Hyg.* **17**, 202.

Mixner, J. P., and Robertson, W. G. (1957). *J. Dairy Sci.* **40**, 914.

Moertel, C. G., and Owen, C. A., Jr. (1968). *J. Lab. Clin. Med.* **52**, 902.

Moller, T., and Simensen, M. G. (1959). *Nord. Veterinaermed.* **11**, 719.

Montemagno, F. (1954). *Atti. Soc. Ital. Sci. Vet.* **8**, 667.

Morgan, H. C. (1959a). *J. Am. Vet. Med. Assoc.* **135**, 412.

Morgan, H. C. (1959b). *Am. J. Vet. Res.* **20**, 372.

Mortimer, P. H. (1962). *Res. Vet. Sci.* **3**, 269.

Moses, C., Critchfield, F. H., and Thomas, T. B. (1948). *J. Lab. Clin. Med.* **33**, 448.

Mühe, G. (1951). Inaugural Dissertation, Hannover.

Mukerji, B., and Ghose, R. (1939). *Nature* **144**, 636.

Mukerji, B., and Ghose, R. (1940a). *Indian J. Med. Res.* **27**, 757.

Mukerji, B., and Ghose, R. (1940b). *Indian J. Med. Res.* **27**, 765.

Müller, L. F. (1960). *Zentr. Veterinaermed.* **7**, 183.

Müller, V. (1959). *Tieraerztl. Umschau* **14**, 367.

Muzzo, J. P. (1949). *Rev. Fac. Med. Vet. Univ. Nacl. Mayor San Marcos, Lima, Peru* **4**, 9.

Myers, J. D. (1947). *J. Clin. Invest.* **26**, 1130.

Nabholz, A. (1938). Inaugural Dissertation, University of Zurich.

Nagode, L. A., Frajola, W. J., and Loeb, W. F. (1966). *Am. J. Vet. Res.* **27**, 1385.

Napier, L. E. (1921). *Indian J. Med. Res.* **9**, 830.

Natscheff, B. (1939). *Jahrb. Vet. Med. Fak. Sofia* **14**, 323.

Naunyn, B. (1868). *Arch. Anat. Physiol. Wiss. Med.* p. 401.

Nielsen, I. M. (1952). *Nord .Veterinaermed.* **4**, 1192.

Nikov, S. I. (1960). *Monatsch. Veterinaermed.* **15**, 379.

Nonnenbruch, W. (1919). *Mitt. Grenzg. Med. Chir.* **31**, 470.

Olsen, R. E., and Phillips, T. E. (1966). *J. Am. Vet. Med. Assoc.* **149**, 400.

Ott, R. L. (1956). *Mich. State Coll. Vet.* **16**, 169 and 195.

Pena, de al A., and Goldzieher, J. W. (1967). *In* "The Baboon in Medical Research" (H. Vagthorg, ed.), Univ. of Texas Press, Austin, Texas. pp. 379 and 383, Vol. 2.

Peredereev, N. I. (1959). *Tru. Mosk. Vet. Akad.* **25**, 98.

Petrovic, M. (1958). *Acta Vet. (Belgrade)* **8**, 101.

Philp, J. R., Grodsky, G. M., and Carbone, J. V. (1961). *Am. J. Physiol.* **200**, 545.

Piccotin, G. (1956). *Clin. Vet.* **79**, 129.

Polson, A., and Malherbe, W. D. (1952). *Onderstepoort J. Vet. Res.* **25**, No. 4, 13.

Powell, W. N. (1944). *Am. J. Clin. Pathol.* **8**, 55.

Pridgen, W. A. (1967). *Lab. Animal Care* **17**, 463.

Prinz, W., and Fiesel, A. (1957). *Z. Tierernaehr. Futtermittelk* **12**, 170.

Quick, A. J. (1938). *J. Am. Med. Assoc.* **110**, 1658.

Rapaport, E., Ketterer, S. G., and Wiegand, B. D. (1959). *Clin. Res.* **7**, 289.

Reichard, H., and Reichard, P. (1958). *J. Lab. Clin. Med.* **52**, 709.

Richards, T. G., Tindall, V. R., and Young, A. (1959). *Clin. Sci.* **18**, 499.

Roberts, H. E. (1968). *Brit. Vet. J.* **124**, 433.

Robertson, W. G., Mixner, J. P., Bailey, W. W., and Lennon, H. D., Jr. (1957). *J. Dairy Sci.* **40**, 977.

Robinson, F. A., and Ziegler, R. F. (1968). *Lab. Animal Care* **18**, 50.

Robinson, S. H., Tsong, M., Brown, B, W., and Schmid, R. (1966). *J. Clin. Invest.* **45**, 1569.

Romagnoli, A. (1954). *Atti Soc. Ital. Sci. Vet.* **8**, 685.

Romagnoli, A. (1958). *Atti Soc. Ital. Sci. Vet.* **12**, 715.

Rosenblum, L. A., and Cooper, R. W. (1968). "The Squirrel Monkey." Academic Press, New York.

Rosenthal, F., and Meier, K. (1921). *Arch. Exptl. Pathol. Pharmakol.* **91**, 246.

Rosenthal, S. M. (1922). *J. Pharmacol. Exptl. Therap.* **19**, 385.

Rosenthal, S. M., and White, E. C. (1925). *J. Am. Med. Assoc.* **84**, 1112.

Rotor, A. B., Manahan, L., and Florentin, A. (1948). *Acta Med. Philippina* **5**, 37.

Roussel, J. D., and Stallcup, O. T. (1966). *Am. J. Vet. Res.* **27**, 1527.

Rowntree, L. G., Hurwitz, S. H., and Bloomfield, A. L. (1913). *Bull. Johns Hopkins Hosp.* **24**, 327.

Royer, M. (1943). "La Urobilina en el Estado Normal y Batologico," 2nd ed. El Ateneo, Buenos Aires, Argentina.

Royer, M., and Biasotti, A. (1932). *Compt. Rend. Soc. Biol.* **111**, 409.

Royer, M., Chiaravalle, A., and Aramburu, H. G. (1941). *Rev. Soc. Arg. Biol.* **17**, 208.

Rudolph, L. A., Schaefer, J. A., Dutton, R. E., Jr., and Lyons, R. N. (1957). *J. Lab. Clin. Med.* **49**, 31.

Rudra, N. B. (1946). *Biochem. J.* **40**, 500.

Sachs, H. (1899). *Z. Klin. Med.* **38**, 87.

Sadun, E. H., Williams, J. S., Martin, L. K. (1966). *Military Med.* **131**, 1094.

Sastry, M. R. S. (1945). *Indian Vet. J.* **21**, 350.

Sborov, V. M., Jay, A. R., and Watson, C. J. (1951). *J. Lab. Clin. Med.* **37**, 52.

Schaffer, J. D. (1949). *Vet. Med.* **44**, 394.

Schaffner, F. (1966). *Recent Advanc. Gastroenterol.* **4**, 69.

Schiff, L., Billing, B. H., and Oikawa, Y. (1959). *New Engl. J. Med.* **260**, 1315.

Schlotthauer, C. F. (1945). *North Am. Vet.* **26**, 349.

Schmid, R. (1956). *Science* **124**, 76.

Schmid, R., Hammaker, L., and Axelrod, J. (1957). *Arch. Biochem. Biophys.* **70**, 285.

Schultz, J. A., Rossow, N., and Urbaneck, D. (1960). *Monatsh. Veterinaermed.* **15**, 257.

Seghetti, L., and Marsh, H. (1953). *Am. J. Vet. Res.* **14**, 9.

Shaw, J. N. (1933). *J. Am. Vet. Med. Assoc.* **82**, 199.

Sherlock, S. (1958). "Diseases of the Liver and Biliary System," 2nd ed. Blackwell, Oxford.

Sherlock, S., Bearn, A. G., Billing, B. H., and Paterson, J. C. S. (1950). *J. Lab. Clin. Med.* **35**, 923.

Shetlar, M. R., Bryan, R. W., Foster, J. V., Shetlar, C. L., and Everett, M. R. (1949). *Proc. Soc. Exptl. Biol. Med.* **72**, 294.

Shibanai, D., Haraga, H., Kikuchi, Y., and Tamai, Y. (1956). *J. Japan. Vet. Med. Assoc.* **9**, 315.

Silen, W., and Eiseman, B. (1960). *Postgrad. Med.* **28**, 445.

Simesen, M. G., and Moller, T. (1959). *Nord. Veterinaermed.* **11**, 787.

Sisk, D. B., Carlton, W. W., and Curtin, T. J. (1968). *Am. J. Vet. Res.* **29**, 1591.

Smith, M. I., Westfall, B. B., and Stohlman, E. F. (1940). *Natl. Inst. Health Bull.* **174**, 21.

Snapp, F. E., Cutmann, M., Li, T. W., and Ivy, A. C. (1947). *J. Lab. Clin. Med.* **32**, 321.

Snell, A. M., Greene, C. H., and Rowntree, L. G. (1925). *A. M. A. Arch. Internal Med.* **36**, 273.

Stary, Z. (1957). *Clin. Chem.* **3**, 557.

Stenius, P. I. (1941). *Skand. Veterinaertidskr.* **31**, 193.

Sterkel, P. L., Spencer, J. A., Wolfson, S. K., Jr., and Williams-Ashman, H. G. (1958). *J. Lab. Clin. Med.* **52**, 176.

Stiebale, H. (1942). Inaugural Dissertation, Tierarztliche Hochschule, Hannover.

Stroebe, F. (1932). *Z. Klin. Med.* **120**, 95.

Svirbely, J. L., Monaco A. R., and Alford, W. C. (1946). *J. Lab. Clin. Med.* **31**, 1133.

Talafont, E. (1956). *Nature* **178**, 312.

Taplin, G. V., Meredith, O. M., Jr., and Kade, H. (1955). *J. Lab. Clin. Med.* **45**, 665.

Tarchanoff, J. F. (1874). *Arch. Ges. Physiol.* **9**, 53.

Thannhauser, S. J., and Schaber, H. (1926). *Klin. Wochschr.* **5**, 252.

Thorpe, E., Gopinath, C., Jones, R. S., and Ford, E. J. H. (1968). *J. Pathol.* **97**, 241.

Tiselius, A. (1930). *Nova Acta Regiae Soc. Sci. Upsaliensis* **7**, No. 4, 107.

Todd, J. C., Sanford, A. H., and Wells, B. B. (1953). "Clinical Diagnosis by Laboratory Methods," 12th ed. Saunders, Philadelphia, Pennsylvania.

Tradati, F., and Abbate, A. (1958). *Arch. Vet. Ital.* **9**, 557.

Udall, R. H., Warner, R. G., and Smith, S. E. (1952). *Cornell Vet.* **42**, 25.

Ugarte, G., Pino, M. E., and Valenzuela, J. (1961). *J. Lab. Clin. Med.* **57**, 359.

van den Bergh, A. A., and Müller, P. (1916). *Biochem. Z.* **77**, 90.

Van Vleet, J. F., and Alberts, J. O. (1968). *Am. J. Vet. Res.* **29**, 2119.

Vardiman, P. H. (1953). *Am. J. Vet. Res.* **51**, 175.

Venturoli, O. M. (1958). *Zooprofilassi* **13**, 603.

Vogin, E. E., Moreno, O. M., Brodie, D. A., and Mattis, P. A. (1966). *J. Appl. Physiol.* **21**, 1880.

Wallace, G. B., and Diamond, J. S. (1925). *A. M. A. Arch. Internal Med.* **35**, 698.

Watson, C. J. (1944). *Am. J. Clin. Pathol.* **14**, 129.

Watson, C. J. (1959). *J. Lab. Clin. Med.* **54**, 1.

Watson, C. J., Schwartz, S., Sborov, V., and Bertie, E. (1944). *Am. J. Clin. Pathol.* **14**, 605.

Webster, L. T., Jr., and Davidson, C. S. (1957). *J. Lab. Clin. Med.* **50**, 1.

Weimer, H. E., and Winzler, R. J. (1955). *Proc. Soc. Exptl. Biol. Med.* **90**, 458.

Werner, A. Y., and Horvath, S. M. (1952). *J. Clin. Invest.* **31**, 433.

Wester, J. J. (1912). *Tijdschr. Veeartsenijk.* **39**, 817.

Wheeler, H. O., Cranston, W. I., and Meltzer, J. I. (1958). *Proc. Soc. Exptl. Biol. Med.* **99**, 11.

Wheeler, H. O., Epstein, R. M., Robinson, R. R., and Snell, E. S. (1960a). *J. Clin. Invest.* **39**, 236.

Wheeler, H. O., Meltzer, J. K., and Bradley, S. E. (1960b). *J. Clin. Invest.* **39**, 1131.

Whitehair, C. C., Peterson, D. R., Van Arsdell, W. J., and Thomas, O. O. (1952). *J. Am. Vet. Med. Assoc.* **121**, 285.

Wilkinson, J. H. (1962). "An Introduction to Diagnostic Enzymology." Arnold, London.

Wirts, C. W., and Cantarow, A. (1942). *Am. J. Digest. Diseases* **9**, 101.

Wisecup, W. G., Hodsen, H. H., Hanley, W. C., and Felts, P. E. (1969). *Am. J. Vet. Res.* **30**, 955.

With, T. K. (1954). "Biology of Bile Pigments." Frost-Hansen, Copenhagen, Denmark.

Wittfogel, H. (1939). *Deut. Tieraerztl. Wochschr.* **47**, 43.

Wolff, W. A., Lumb, W. V., and Ramsay, M. K. (1967). *Am. J. Vet. Res.* **28**, 1363.

Wolfson, S. K., Jr., and Williams-Ashman, H. G. (1957). *Federation Proc.* **16**, 273.

Wolfson, W. G., Cohn, C., Calvary, E., and Ichiba, F. (1948). *Am. J. Clin. Pathol.* **18**, 723.

Woodruff, J. M., and Johnson, D. K. (1968). *Pathol. Vet.* **5**, 327.

Wroblewski, F., and Cabaud, P. (1957). *Am. J. Clin. Pathol.* **27**, 235.

Wroblewski, F., and LaDue, J. S. (1955). *Ann. Internal Med.* [N. S.] **43**, 345.

Wroblewski, F., and LaDue, J. S. (1956a). *Proc. Soc. Exptl. Biol. Med.* **91**, 569.

Wroblewski, F., and LaDue, J. S. (1956b). *Ann. Internal Med.* [N. S.] **45**, 782.

Young, J. E., Younger, R. L., Radcliff, R. D., Hunt, L. M., and McLaran, J. K. (1965). *Am. J. Vet. Res.* **26**, 641.

Zenglein, G. (1930). Theses, Ecole D'Alfort.

Zink, B. (1932). Inaugural Dissertation, Tierarztliche Hochschule, Vienna.

Zinkle, J. G., Bush, R. M., Freedland, R. A., and Cornelius, C. E. (1969). Unpublished, University of California, Davis, California.

6   Pancreatic Function

D. F. Brobst

I. INTRODUCTION

The pancreas is comprised of two unrelated organs within the same stroma. The endocrine function of the pancreatic islets has been discussed in detail in Chapter 1 which dealt with carbohydrate metabolism. The present chapter is concerned with the exocrine functions of the pancreas.

The symptoms of exocrine pancreatic disease are often nonspecific, and physical and roentgen examination are seldom diagnostic in this disease. Since the pancreas is so difficult to evaluate using these approaches the clinician has come to rely on biochemical tests in the diagnosis of pancreatic disease. Certainly, when clinical findings and laboratory results are correlated, the clinical diagnosis can be established with more confidence. Correlation of the clinical and laboratory information and appreciation of pancreatic disease requires a basic understanding of the anatomy and physiology of the pancreas and of the pathological processes which may occur in this organ.

II. PHYSIOLOGY OF THE PANCREAS

Pancreatic juice is composed of a proteinaceous portion which is largely enzyme and a fluid and electrolyte portion. The pancreatic enzymes are synthesized by the acinar cells which are arranged in clusters about the terminal pancreatic ductules. The epithelial cells lining the terminal and interlobular ductules which carry pancreatic juice toward the intestine form the fluid and electrolyte portion of pancreatic juice.

A. PANCREATIC ENZYMES

The enzymes of pancreatic juice are capable of digesting all three types of foods, since the juice contains proteolytic, lipolytic, and amylolytic enzymes. The major proteolytic enzymes, which are secreted as inactive proenzymes, are trypsinogen, chymotrypsinogen, and procarboxypeptidase. Within the intestinal tract trypsinogen is activated by enterokinase, an enzyme secreted by the duodenal mucosa, to trypsin which, in turn, activates chymotrypsinogen and procarboxypeptidase to chymotrypsin and carboxypeptidase, respectively. Trypsin and chymotrypsin split whole and partially digested proteins while carboxypeptidase splits a particular peptide linkage of the peptide chain. Other proteolytic enzymes secreted by the pancreas are ribonuclease, deoxyribonuclease, collagenase, and elastase.

To prevent spontaneous activation of trypsinogen within the pancreas the acinar cells also secrete a trypsin inhibitor. When the pancreas becomes damaged the effects of the trypsin inhibitor may be overcome allowing trypsinogen to be activated causing pancreatic necrosis.

Pancreatic lipase may be secreted in an active form but the activity is enhanced by bile salts. The increased activation by bile salts is due in part to their emulsifying action. As lipase acts only at the oil–water interphase, the finer the emulsion the greater the activity. Pancreatic lipase exhibits its optimum activity under alkaline conditions and hydrolyzes fat to glycerol and fatty acids.

Pancreatic amylase is secreted in an active form and hydrolyzes 1,4-polysaccharides (amylose, amylopectin, and glycogen) to form a mixture of disaccharides and monosaccharides.

In ruminants, where extensive breakdown of food is accomplished by bacterial action in the forestomachs the pancreatic secretions differ from that in monogastric animals. Chromatographic analysis of bovine and porcine pancreatic juice, for example (Neurath, 1962), indicate that digestive processes in the intestine of cattle require less amylase and lipase than do digestive processes in swine (Table I). Taylor (1962) reported that the pancreatic output of fluid, bicarbonate, amylase, protease, and lipase was very low in sheep when compared with the dog. The proportions of amylase and protease in the pancreatic juice of each animal were, however, considered the same. Thus in pancreatitis in ruminants, high elevations of pancreatic serum enzymes would not be expected.

The enzymic composition of pancreatic juice may, in time, adapt to the diet of the animal. A specific adjustment of pancreatic enzymes to the main constituent of the diet has been found for amylase and chymotrypsinogen, which were significantly increased when rats ingested much carbohydrate or much protein (Desnuelle et al.,

1962). Trypsinogen remained nearly constant on all diets. Lipase was not influenced by the lipid content of the diet.

B. Pancreatic Fluid and Electrolytes

Pure pancreatic juice collected from dogs has a pH between 8 and 8.3 and a specific gravity between 1.010 and 1.018 (Hightower, 1966). The volume of fluid secretion by the dog pancreas is approximately 67 ml/kg-24 hours and by the pancreas of the normally fed sheep 9.5 ml/kg-24 hours (Taylor, 1962). The distinguishing chemical characteristic of pancreatic juice is its high bicarbonate (HCO_3^-) content. In the dog, HCO_3^- concentration ranges between 60 and 148 mEq/liter, whereas in sheep the range is 15–30 mEq/liter. Bicarbonate is believed to be secreted by the pancreatic ductule cells under the influence of carbonic anhydrase. The reaction of CO_2 with H_2O is catalyzed by carbonic anhydrase to form H_2CO_3 which dissociates at intracellular pH to $H^+ + HCO_3^-$ (Janowitz and Dreiling, 1962). On the other hand, Rawls *et al.* (1963) suggested that OH^- forming within pancreatic ductule cells from water may combine with metabolic CO_2 to form HCO_3^- which would be secreted into the juice. Carbonic anhydrase does appear to be necessary for maximum secretion of HCO_3^- and the apparent limitation on the maximum rate of HCO_3^- production is the rate of transport of HCO_3^- from cell to duct (Rawls *et al.*, 1963). Alterations in blood pH, plasma HCO_3^-, and CO_2 may bring about certain changes in pancreatic juice. Rawls *et al.* (1963) demonstrated that dogs with metabolic acidosis with decreased total CO_2 secreted pancreatic juice with decreased HCO_3^- concentration. Dogs with metabolic alkalosis with increased total CO_2 had an increased rate of flow of pancreatic juice with increased HCO_3^- concentration.

The concentration of sodium and potassium in pancreatic juice tends to parallel

TABLE I   QUANTITATIVE DISTRIBUTION OF PROTEINS IN BOVINE AND PORCINE PANCREATIC JUICE[a]

Protein[b]	Bovine[c] %	Porcine[d] %
Trypsinogen	14	12
Chymotrypsinogen A	16	5
Chymotrypsinogen B	16	18
Procarboxypeptidase A	19	18
Procarboxypeptidase B + Carboxypeptidase B	7	16
Ribonuclease	2.4	—
Deoxyribonuclease	1.4	5.6
Amylase	< 2	13
Lipase	Trace	6.5
"Esterase"	—	3.8
Unidentified	10	

[a]From Neurath (1962). Courtesy, Little, Brown and Company.
[b]Data given in percent of total proteins, determined chromatographically.
[c]Bovine data by Keller *et al.* (1958).
[d]Porcine data by Marchis-Mouren (1959).

plasma concentrations. Calcium concentration in pancreatic juice of the dog, however, tends to be lower than in the plasma. Zimmerman *et al.* (1967) determined the basal total pancreatic juice calcium of four dogs to range from 3.3 to 4.4 mEq/liter with corresponding serum calcium in the range of 4.0 to 5.5 mEq/liter. The studies of these investigators showed that under conditions in which pancreatic enzymes were being formed in large amounts calcium output was greatest. Their work suggests that calcium was not secreted with the electrolyte components of pancreatic juice but rather with the nonelectrolyte portion and that calcium may be a part of the amylase molecule.

C. Regulation of Pancreatic Secretion

Pancreatic secretion is influenced by both nervous and hormonal mechanisms. Prior to the time food actually enters the stomach, impulses are transmitted along the vagus nerve to the pancreas resulting in the secretion of proenzymes into the pancreatic acini. Most of the proenzymes are stored in the acini until food enters the intestine. At this time the hormones secretin and pancreozymin, which are produced by mucosal cells of the small intestine, are released into the blood, carried to the pancreas and cause release of stored proenzymes. Hydrochloric acid in the chyme is a potent stimulus for release of secretin and peptones and products of protein digestion cause release of pancreozymin.

Secretin stimulates a profuse flow of pancreatic juice high in bicarbonate but low in enzymes. Pancreozymin causes a secretion high in digestive enzymes but with little increase in volume of pancreatic juice. In human medicine, tests based on the ability of the pancreas to secrete enzyme and bicarbonate following the injection of secretin or secretin plus pancreozymin are a useful diagnostic technique in the chronic phase of pancreatitis. In this procedure both the stomach and duodenum are intubated and the secretions are collected separately. In patients with chronic pancreatitis the pancreatic secretion is usually reduced in volume and contains reduced amounts of bicarbonate and enzyme (Marks *et al.*, 1968). The difficulties of intubation and collection of uncontaminated pancreatic secretion has made these procedures of little clinical value in veterinary medicine.

Pancreatic secretion may be modified by antidiuretic hormone (ADH). In dogs in which pancreatic secretion was stimulated by intravenous injection of secretin plus ADH the volume of secretion and bicarbonate concentration were less than if only secretin were administered (Banks *et al.*, 1968). It was theorized that ADH depressed the physiological activity of secreting cells of the pancreatic ducts or that ADH altered the permeability of these cells to various electrolytes, e.g., bicarbonate, in such a way that there would be a net movement of bicarbonate out of the duct system. It therefore appears that ADH acts as a fluid regulator in the pancreas as well as in the kidney.

Glucagon may also be involved in the regulation of pancreatic secretion. Dyck *et al.* (1969) observed that small amounts of glucagon administered intravenously to dogs had no effect upon pancreatic secretion in the resting pancreas but markedly depressed volume flow and enzyme concentration in the gland stimulated with secretin or secretin plus pancreozymin. The mechanism by which glucagon produces this effect is not known, although it is postulated that glucagon may have a protein catabolic effect which would decrease the output of pancreatic enzymes. Glucagon may also reduce the blood flow to the pancreas, as it does to the stomach, and thereby diminish glandular activity.

III. PANCREATIC DISEASE

Pancreatic disease in its various forms is not uncommon in dogs and cats and occurs in other animals as well. The exocrine pancreas may be affected by acute or chronic inflammatory diseases; it may fail to develop to its proper size and thus be hypoplastic or it may undergo atrophic or neoplastic changes.

A. ACUTE PANCREATITIS (ACUTE PANCREATIC NECROSIS)

Acute pancreatitis is more common in dogs than in other animals and is characterized by a sudden onset, acute abdominal pain, digestive disturbance, and sometimes shock. The etiology of acute pancreatitis in dogs is not well understood. Anderson (1968), however, points out that female dogs are more likely to acquire pancreatitis than male dogs and that obesity predisposes to the disease. Lean, active, young dogs are apparently less likely to acquire pancreatitis.

The release of digestive enzymes into the parenchyma and interstitial tissue of the pancreas constitutes the most plausible mechanism in the pathogenesis of pancreatic necrosis and inflammation. The earliest responses to this enzymic activity are edema and vascular engorgement within the pancreas. Progression of edema to hemorrhagic necrosis may be the result of enlargment of the pancreas within its capsule which may lead to ischemia, infarction, and hemorrhage. Geokas *et al.* (1968) have demonstrated in dogs with bile-induced pancreatitis that pancreatic elastase may cause dissolution of elastic fibers in vessel walls causing hemorrhage and thrombosis. Escaped pancreatic lipase may cause necrosis of peripancreatic adipose tissue. After several days of duration, areas of parenchymal necrosis may become infected with enteric organisms and abscesses form.

B. CHRONIC PANCREATITIS

The etiology of chronic pancreatitis is likewise not well established but it is considered that acute necrotizing processes may smolder on asymptomatically as a chronic process. Jubb and Kennedy (1963) have observed that there is little difficulty in finding microscopic areas of acute necrosis in the chronically affected canine pancreas. The end result of the necrotizing process in animals that survive the acute episode is almost complete destruction of the pancreas and replacement by fibrous tissue. With destruction of the acini, deficiencies of digestive enzymes occur. Without trypsin or chymotrypsin in the gut, the stool contains undigested meat fiber (creatorrhea) and there is nitrogen loss (azotorrhea). In the absence of lipase, neutral fat is in the feces (steatorrhea). Without amylase, loss of starch (amylorrhea) occurs, although this is of less importance than the resulting disturbed protein and fat digestion since amylase is found in significant amounts in the succus entericus.

Chronic interstitial pancreatitis may develop in cats and horses (Jubb and Kennedy, 1963) as a result of trematodes or parasite larvae migrating through the interstitial tissue. This type of lesion is seldom of clinical significance but in some cases fibrous tissue may develop to the point where little exocrine parenchyma is present.

C. ATROPHY OF THE PANCREAS

Pancreatic atrophy may exist as primary atrophy of the acinar cells. Anderson and Low (1965) reported several cases of primary atrophy in young dogs (juvenile atrophy). Although the dogs did have signs of digestive failure similar to that seen in chronic pancreatitis, the pancreases of these animals were without signs of inflammation. Also, these animals did not develop diabetes mellitus which often complicates chronic pancreatitis.

Atrophy of the acinar cells may also develop secondary to pancreatic fibrosis and ductal obstruction. A pancreas with secondary atrophy is often misshapen, coarsely nodular, and fibrous. In primary atrophy the pancreas is uniformly involved and is soft, pliable, and thinner than normal.

D. HYPOPLASIA OF THE PANCREAS

Hypoplasia of the acinar tissue of the pancreas has been observed in dogs and calves (Jubb and Kennedy, 1963). These animals develop signs of pancreatic enzyme deficiency, although in dogs this may not occur until the animals are about 1 year of age. This syndrome may thus be clinically indistinguishable from atrophy of the pancreas.

E. NEOPLASIA OF THE PANCREAS

Carcinoma of the pancreas is observed rarely in dogs and cats and implies an origin from exocrine tissues or excretory ducts. Ruwitch *et al.* (1964) reported finding adenocarcinoma of the pancreas of a dog which had occluded the pancreatic ducts producing signs of acute pancreatitis.

IV.   LABORATORY DIAGNOSTIC AIDS

Laboratory procedures used in detecting and measuring pancreatic disease may be considered to be of two types. One type demonstrates the presence or absence of an active pancreatic lesion and is used primarily in detecting the more acute phases of pancreatic disease. The other type is useful when the patient has recovered from the acute phase of the disease and one wishes to determine the degree of damage inflicted upon the pancreas or if pancreatic insufficiency is present. For practical purposes the diagnostic aids can be considered as tests for the acute and chronic phases of pancreatitis.

A. ACUTE PANCREATITIS

1. Serum Amylase

a. SOURCE. The measurement of serum amylase has been the single most important laboratory aid in the diagnosis of acute pancreatitis or acute exacerbations of chronic pancreatitis. In both veterinary and human medicine the pancreas has been considered the primary source of hyperamylasemia. Following ligation of the pancreatic ducts of dogs Hiatt and Warner (1969) observed a marked rise of serum amylase and a subsequent fall to normal in 9 days. The accompanying pathological changes in the pancreas were minimal and they concluded that the pancreas need not be inflamed to be responsible for a marked hyperamylasemia. Similar results were observed by Gibbs and Ivy (1951), however, when the ligated pancreatic ducts were subjected to a pressure of 30 cm water, serum amylase rose twice as fast as in dogs with simple ligation. In those dogs in which the ducts were subjected to pressure the pancreatic changes were of a more severe inflammatory nature than in dogs where the pancreas was simply ligated.

On the other hand, the liver has been considered to be the main source of amylase activity in the blood under normal conditions. Following the injection of puromycin (which inhibits protein synthesis) into rats McGeachin and Johnson (1964) observed liver amylase to fall 50% and that changes in serum amylase levels paralleled those of the liver. Levels of amylase in the salivary glands and pancreas were not significantly affected. The Kupffer cells of the liver may be involved in the transport of amylase in and out of normal liver cells. Hiatt et al. (1968) observed that when Kupffer cells of the rat liver were blockaded by injections of thorium dioxide, liver amylase increased 80% more than controls and serum amylase fell over 45%.

The mucosa of the small intestine of dogs likewise may secrete an amylase. In dogs with strangulated obstructions of the small intestine, Hiatt (1959) observed the serum amylase to be significantly elevated and rises occurred in pancreatectomized dogs with intestinal obstruction as well. Hiatt found little evidence that amylase—producing bacteria were in the intestine. He ascribed the rise of serum amylase to absorption of enzyme seeping through the devitalized gut wall into the peritoneal fluid. Peritoneal fluid often had amylase values higher than the serum.

b. SIGNIFICANCE. Janowitz and Dreiling (1959) were of the opinion that two pathological features within the pancreas influenced the height to which serum amylase elevated in pancreatic disease: (1) continued secretion against obstruction, and (2) disruption of acinar cells and ductular apparatus. Rapid accumulation of inflammatory exudate may increase intraductular pressure and cause sudden elevation of serum amylase. This process may be self-limiting, however, since rapid glandular damage may lead to suppression of secretion. This would be in contrast to gradually increasing ductal obstruction which would maintain elevation of serum enzyme over a longer period of time. Serum amylase values may thus be considered an index of the degree of ductal obstruction of the pancreas. The degree of amylase elevation, however, does not always correlate well with the severity of the pancreatitis.

Egdahl (1958), using dogs with bile-induced pancreatitis, determined that the initial rise of serum enzymes (1–3 hours) after injury was due to absorption of enzymes into the pancreatic venous blood. The later maintenance of rise of enzymes was primarily due to lymphatic absorption of peritoneal fluid of high enzyme content. This fluid resulted from passage of enzyme-containing fluid through the pancreatic capsule.

Amylase levels in acute pancreatitis of man are said to reach a peak within 12–24 hours of the acute attack and gradually subside to normal levels in 2–6 days. This early decrease in amylase levels may not always occur, however. In experimentally induced severe acute pancreatitis in dogs, Zieve et al. (1963) demonstrated serum amylase to remain elevated for as long as 3–5 weeks (Fig. 1).

Stress and certain drugs may also affect serum amylase levels. Hiatt (1959) observed the fasting serum amylase to vary greatly in the same dog from day to day and considered increases in amylase in experimental dogs significant only if they exceeded preoperative levels by 50%. He related serum amylase levels to the dog's age with higher levels in younger dogs. Challis et al. (1957) suggested that since elevations in serum amylase in dogs were extreme following adreno cortical hyperactivity and administration of ACTH the elevations of amylase in pancreatitis might be more correctly attributed to a nonspecific stress reaction.

Serum amylase formerly viewed as a single entity is now considered to be composed of a number of molecular forms termed isoenzymes of amylase (isoamylases). Each of these isoenzymes acts on the same substrate and produces the same end products.

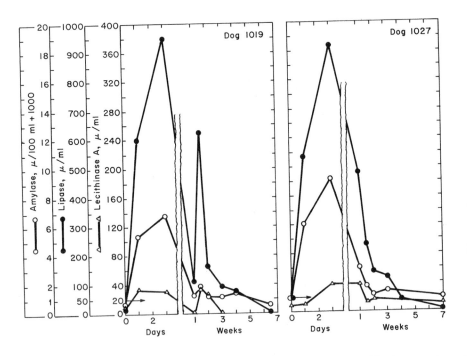

Fig. 1. Serial serum enzyme values in two dogs with severe acute pancreatitis. Arrows represent the upper limit of normal for all enzymes. Reproduced by courtesy of J. Appl. Physiol. 18, 77. Zieve et al. (1963).

Each isoamylase may originate from a different tissue. Berk *et al.* (1965) demonstrated that in the dog the majority of the amylase activity had an electrophoretic mobility similar to that of γ-globulin. A second peak of amylase activity was also in the α- and β-globulin areas. In pancreatectomized dogs the amylase activity in the γ-globulin zones was reduced to a greater degree than that in the α and β zones. This suggests that amylase activity residing in the γ-globulin zone may originate in the pancreas. If it would be possible to determine the tissue source of distinctive isoenzymes of amylase the usefulness of serum amylase in clinical diagnosis would be enhanced.

c. METHODOLOGY.   The principal of serum amylase determination is the enzymic hydrolysis of starch into its constituent maltose and glucose units. The rate of this hydrolysis is measured either by the rate of disappearance (amyloclastic) of starch or by the rate of appearance (saccharogenic) of reducing sugar, i.e., glucose and maltose, in the incubation mixture. A comparison of Somogyi's saccharogenic method and an amyloclastic method of determining serum amylase in dogs has been done by Rapp (1962). He found that the determination of amylase by the saccharogenic method of Somogyi was invalid in the dog due to the presence of maltose in the serum which was additive to amylase activity. Loeb and Edge (1962), using an amyloclastic procedure, suggested the values of 318–1050 Caraway units as normal in healthy dogs.

2. Urine Amylase

In human medicine the determination of the amount of amylase excreted in urine per unit of time has been a valuable test in suspected pancreatitis. In pancreatitis in man it is concluded that urine amylase determination was a more sensitive indication of pancreatitis than serum amylase levels and that it remained elevated for a longer period than serum amylase. Hiatt (1961) concluded that under normal conditions the dog kidney did not appear to clear amylase from the blood. In a case of acute pancreatitis in a dog, Gage and Anderson (1967) demonstrated the presence of amylase in the urine; however, it was not elevated and correlated relatively well with serum values.

3. Serum Lipase

The bulk of the body digestive lipase is produced in the pancreas, although Engstrom *et al.* (1968) have demonstrated evidence of lipase in canine gastric juice. This lipase appeared to be about one-tenth as active as pancreatic lipase. In acute pancreatitis in man serum lipase supposedly becomes elevated several hours after serum amylase and remains elevated for a longer period of time. Zieve (1966) simultaneously determined serum lipase and amylase values in acute pancreatitis in man. He observed lipase values to rise higher than amylase values and concluded that one might therefore expect to record abnormal values for lipase a few days after the amylase has fallen to its normal range. Zieve *et al.* (1963) also observed in dogs with experimentally induced pancreatitis that lipase and amylase values tended to parallel each other and that both were elevated for a period of 3–5 weeks (Fig. 1). It is possible that the diagnostic yield of both serum amylase and lipase taken together is greater than that of each considered separately.

Hyperlipasemia, like hyperamylasemia, may be associated with conditions other than acute pancreatitis. In man, elevations of serum lipase have been reported in intestinal obstruction, peritonitis, and renal insufficiency (Bishop, 1968).

The determination of serum lipase is based on the hydrolysis of an olive oil emulsion into its constituent fatty acids. The fatty acids are titrated with NaOH and the units of lipase are in direct relationship to the number of milliliters of NaOH required to neutralize the fatty acids released per milliliter of serum.

The Sigma-Tietz method requires a 6-hour hydrolysis period and normal values for the dogs are 0.0 to 1.0 units (Small et al., 1964). Brobst and Brester (1967) using a modification of a test (Roe and Byler, 1963) which employed only a 1-hour period of hydrolysis reported normal serum lipase values in the dog of 0.8 to 12.0 Roe-Byler units. The relative ease of tests with short periods of hydrolysis will make serum lipase determination a more acceptable laboratory procedure.

4. Serum Calcium

In acute edematous pancreatitis in man serum calcium may fall to 8–9 mg/100 ml and in severe hemorrhagic pancreatitis hypocalcemia in the range of 5–7 mg/100 ml may be noted with tetany occurring (Marks et al., 1968). In general, hypocalcemia occurs between the second and fifth day of onset of the disease. In a dog with acute pancreatitis a serum calcium of 6.2 mg/100 ml was reported 2 days after admission to the clinic (Gage and Anderson, 1967). With appropriate care the serum calcium was raised to 11 mg/100 ml and the animal recovered. The hypocalcemia has been attributed to the release of pancreatic lipase into the peripancreatic tissue. There the action of lipase upon neutral fats releases fatty acids which in turn form insoluble soaps with calcium ion.

5. Serum Methemalbumin

Serum methemalbumin determinations have been made to differentiate acute hemorrhagic pancreatitis from acute edematous interstitial pancreatitis. Methemalbumin appears to form in acute pancreatitis as the result of the action of pancreatic enzymes on blood which may be present at the lesion. The enzymes digest hemoglobin and break it into two molecules: heme and globin. These same enzymes also oxidize heme to ferric hematin also known as metheme. Metheme is absorbed into the circulation and combines with albumin to form methemalbumin. Joseph et al. (1968) produced experimentally hemorrhagic pancreatitis in dogs and observed that serum amylase became elevated 12 hours postoperatively and returned to normal 36 hours later. Methemalbumin levels began to rise 18 hours after induction of pancreatitis and remained elevated for 3 days. Methemalbumin levels were thus considered a good index for the diagnosis of pancreatitis at a time when serum amylase had returned to normal. In other acute conditions in which hyperamylasemia is observed methemalbumin does not appear to be elevated. The usefulness of this test is evaluating spontaneous pancreatitis in animals is not yet established.

6. *Miscellaneous Procedures*

Deoxyribonuclease activity has been reported to be elevated in the serum during the breakdown of pancreatic tissue. In an experimental study in dogs, Donahue *et al.* (1958) observed serum amylase to be elevated after ligation of the pancreatic ducts but serum deoxyribonuclease had no significant change. However, after experimentally producing pancreatic cell necrosis there was a rise in serum deoxyribonuclease. They concluded that the rise in serum deoxyribonuclease was associated only with cell necrosis.

Hyperlipemia has been observed in some dogs with acute pancreatitis and chronic pancreatitis (Anderson, 1966). When the lipid content of the plasma is above the upper normal limit it appears milky or turbid. In a dog with acute pancreatitis (Gage and Anderson, 1967) hyperlipemia was present during the first 3 days of hospitalization. During this time the serum lipid concentration was as high as 8640 mg %. At the time of discharge on hospital day 11 the serum lipid was 1571 mg % and was considered twice the upper limit of normal. The pathogenesis of hyperlipemia may be related to digestion of fats and release of triglycerides from areas of fat necrosis, an increased release of glycerides from the liver to the plasma, or defective intravascular clearing of glycerides. A "lipemia-clearing" factor in plasma called lipoprotein lipase aids in the release of triglyceride from a lipoprotein complex in the plasma. Kessler *et al.* (1963) demonstrated that lipoprotein lipase activity was present in canine pancreatic juice and postulated that with pancreatic necrosis the source of lipoprotein lipase would be inadequate or that inhibitors of this enzyme would be released thereby interfering with the normal clearing reaction.

B. CHRONIC PANCREATITIS

1. *Serum Enzymes*

Serum amylase and lipase may be elevated if acute exacerbations of pancreatitis occur or if chronic pancreatitis is associated with ductal obstruction. However, with complete destruction of acinar tissue and healing by fibrosis, serum enzyme elevations would not be expected.

2. *Fecal Examination*

When pancreatic insufficiency is under consideration an examination of feces is important as a preliminary screening test. The gross and microscopic findings of a fecal examination may reflect the failure to digest and absorb fats and proteins as a result of pancreatic enzyme deficiencies. Pancreatic enzyme deficiencies can also be detected by the qualitative determination of trypsin in feces. Some of these procedures are not as complicated as the tests used in the diagnosis of acute pancreatitis and thus are presented in greater detail.

a. GROSS AND MICROSCOPIC EXAMINATION.   Grossly the stool is large, of a pale yellow or clay color; it may be glistening with neutral fat, and often has a foul odor. Neutral fat may be detected microscopically by staining a diluted (1:1 with water) sample of feces with Sudan III on a glass slide and observing a large number of orange-reddish staining globules. Muscle fibers stain yellow to brown and undigested muscle fibers can be detected by the presence of cross striations and square-cut ends.

One of the most accurate methods of determining if there is increased fat in the feces is through a quantitative determination of fecal fat residue. Likewise fecal nitrogen determination by the macro-Kheldahl method is one of the more accurate methods of measuring protein digestion. However, these determinations may not differentiate pancreatogenous from intestinal malassimilation and are more suitable for the research laboratory.

b. FECAL TRYPSIN.   There are two tests of fecal enzyme activity which are suited to the veterinary clinical laboratory (Jasper, 1954). The procedures are based on the incubation of gelatin with feces and the subsequent detection of proteolysis.

Tube Test.   This procedure utilizes the digestion of a gelatin solution by the test fecal sample and the detection of proteolysis by the failure of the gelatin solution to gel after incubation.

1. Bring 9 ml of water to 10 ml total volume by adding feces and mix.
2. Warm 2 ml of a 7.5% gelatin solution to 37° C and add 1 ml of 5% sodium bicarbonate and 1 ml of fecal dilution.
3. Incubate at 37°C for 1 hour ($2\frac{1}{2}$ hours at room temperature).
4. Refrigerate for 20 minutes. Failure to gel indicates the presence of trypsin in the sample.

Film Test.   This procedure utilizes digestion of the gelatin of exposed or unexposed X-ray film.

1. Bring 9 ml of 5% sodium bicarbonate solution to 10 ml total volume by adding feces and mix.
2. Immerse a thin strip of X-ray film in the fecal dilution.
3. Incubate at 37°C for 1 hour ($2\frac{1}{2}$ hours at room temperature).
4. Rinse off the film under tap water. A clearing of the submerged portion of the film strip indicates the presence of trypsin in the sample.

Of the two tests, the tube test is recommended as a more accurate procedure for detection of fecal trypsin. The film test is less sensitive with approximately 25% of the results falsely negative. If the film test is used, the tube test should be used for the confirmation of samples negative for trypsin. In either test, control samples using diluent only and a normal fecal sample should be run in conjunction with the suspected sample.

It should be remembered that the gelatin substrate is not specific for trypsin or chymotrypsin and may be hydrolyzed by proteolytic enzymes produced by intestinal bacteria or proteolytic enzymes of the succus entericus. The destruction of enzymes in the feces of constipated animals may also occur, although animals with the pancreatic deficiency are usually not constipated.

3.   Absorption Tests

In veterinary medicine the absorption tests have primarily been concerned with the absorption of fats or vitamins in oil. The tests are based on the principal that dietary fats must be hydrolyzed to fatty acids and glycerol prior to absorption.

It should be remembered that with reduced ability to assimilate fats the defect may lie in a deficiency of pancreatic lipase or an inability of the small bowel to absorb properly digested fats.

a. FAT ABSORPTION. This test is simple to perform, requires a minimum of equipment and involves only visual comparison of the turbidity of the plasma (Anderson and Low, 1965). A heparinized blood sample (5 ml) is drawn from the fasted animal and centrifuged. Then 3 ml/kg of Lipomul* (3 ml/kg of corn oil) are added to a small quantity of food and fed to the dog. A second heparinized blood sample (5 ml) is drawn 2 hours after ingestion of the fat meal and the sample centrifuged. The turbidity of the pre- and postfeeding samples are compared. Normally, the prefeeding sample has clear plasma, while the postfeeding sample has a creamy or turbid appearance (hyperlipemia). If the plasma samples are equally clear, one can assume that either pancreatic exocrine function is absent or that the intestine is incapable of proper absorption. The two conditions can be differentiated by repeating the fat meal at a later date, this time supplemented with pancreatic extract as a source of lipase. If the postfeeding sample is cloudy, this would indicate that absorption from the intestine was normal and that the pancreas was deficient in secretion of lipase. Enteritis may render the test unreliable because of false negative results.

In man a similar fat absorption has been done and the turbidity of the serum was measured with a spectrophotometer at 620 mμ (Brum and Poliner, 1966). Serum turbidity resulting from the fat absorption test was considered here not a test of total fat absorption, and the test was used qualitatively only.

b. LABELED FAT ABSORPTION. Measuring intestinal absorption of radioiodine-labeled triolein, a fat, and radioiodine-labeled oleic acid have proved to be valuable in the differential diagnosis of pancreatic steatorrhea and intestinal malabsorption in dogs. In the absence of pancreatic lipase in the intestine or in the presence of an absorptive failure, the label of orally administered labeled fat (^{131}I-triolein) fails to appear in the blood in a manner characteristic of a normal dog. Whether the failure to appear in the blood is due to pancreatic lipase deficiency or to an intestinal absorptive failure can be determined by feeding a labeled fatty acid, ^{131}I-oleic acid. Since oleic acid is the hydrolysis product of triolein, in pancreatic insufficiency, ^{131}I-oleic acid should be absorbed normally from the gut. Kallfelz et al. (1968) demonstrated that in normal dogs approximately 13% of the oleic acid and 11% of the triolein was absorbed. In a dog with pancreatic fibrosis the absorption of oleic acid was normal but that of triolein was less than 1%, indicating defective hydrolysis.

c. VITAMIN A ABSORPTION. This test is based on the principal that vitamin A in oil can be absorbed from the intestine only in the presence of pancreatic lipase. Thus serum vitamin A in dogs with chronic pancreatitis is often subnormal (Thordal-Christensen and Coffin, 1956). In the test employed by Coffin and Thordal-Christensen (1953) the fasting animal was given a standard dose of oleum percomorphum after a fasting blood sample had been taken. Blood was then assayed for vitamin A at specified times and a significant rise in vitamin A was expected in the normal animal.

*Upjohn Co., Kalamazoo, Michigan.

The absence of an elevation was indicative of absorptive failure. Confirmation that the failure was due to lipase deficiency was obtained by repeating the test with the modification that pancreatic extract was given together with the vitamin A. If the initial absorptive failure was due to lipase deficiency, the second test should result in a normal elevation of serum vitamin A. This is a fairly expensive and difficult procedure, having its use mainly in clinical research.

In summary, the most valuable laboratory means for the recognition of acute pancreatitis has been the determination of serum amylase and lipase. Amylase and lipase values appear to be useful as an index of pancreatic ductal obstruction. Serum lipase levels are believed to remain elevated for a longer period than amylase levels, although experimental investigation indicates that serum amylase and lipase tend to parallel each other. Elevation of serum amylase and lipase may also occur as a result of acute exacerbations of chronic pancreatitis. In chronic pancreatitis, however, as in pancreatic atrophy, insufficiency of the pancreas may develop which can be detected by gross and microscopic examination of the stools, fat absorption tests, and tests for proteolytic enzyme in the stool.

REFERENCES

Anderson, N. V. (1966). *Southwestern Vet.* **19**, 119.
Anderson, N. V. (1968). *In* "Current Veterinary Therapy III: Small Animal Practice" (R. W. Kirk, ed.), p. 526. Saunders Philadelphia, Pennsylvania.
Anderson, N. V., and Low, D. G. (1965). *Animal Hosp.* **1**, 101.
Banks, P. A., Rudick, J., Dreiling, D. A., and Janowitz, H. D. (1968). *Am. J. Physiol.* **215**, 361.
Berk, J. E., Searcy, R. L., Hayashi, S., and Ujihira, I. (1965). *J. Am. Med. Assoc.* **192**, 389.
Bishop, R. P. (1968). *Am. J. Gastroenterol.* **49**, 112.
Brobst, D., and Brester, J. E. (1967). *J. Am. Vet. Med. Assoc.* **150**, 767.
Brum, V. C., and Poliner, I. J. (1966). *Am. J. Gastroenterol.* **45**, 281.
Challis, T. W., Reid, L. C., and Hinton, J. W. (1957). *Gastroenterology* **33**, 818.
Coffin, D. L., and Thordal-Christensen, A. (1953). *Vet. Med.* **48**, 193.
Desnuelle, P., Reboud, J. P., and Abdeljlil, B. (1962). *Ciba Found. Symp. Exocrine Pancreas* pp. 90–107.
Donahue, J. P., Houck, J. C., and Coffey, R. J. (1958). *Surgery* **44**, 1070.
Dyck, W. P., Rudick, J., Hoexter, B., and Janowitz, H. D. (1969). *Gastroenterology* **56**, 531.
Edgahl, R. H. (1958). *Ann. Surg.* **148**, 389.
Engstrom, J. F., Rybak, J. J., Duber, M., and Groenberger, N. J. (1968). *Am. J. Med. Sci.* **256**, 346.
Gage, E. D., and Anderson, N. V. (1967). *Animal Hosp.* **3**, 151.
Gibbs, G. E., and Ivy, A. C. (1951). *Proc. Soc. Exptl. Biol. Med.* **77**, 251.
Geokas, M. C., Murphy, D. R., and McKenna, R. D. (1968). *Arch. Pathol.* **86**, 117.
Hiatt, N. (1959). *Ann. Surg.* **149**, 77.
Hiatt, N. (1961). *Ann. Surg.* **154**, 864.
Hiatt, N., and Warner, N. E. (1969). *Am. Surgeon* **35**, 30.
Hiatt, N., Bonorris, G., and Lanchantin, G. F. (1968). *J. Reticuloendothel. Soc.* **5**, 8.
Hightower, N. C. (1966). *In* "The Physiological Basis of Medical Practice" (C. H. Best and N. B. Taylor, eds.), 8th ed., pp. 1122–1140. Williams & Wilkins, Baltimore, Maryland.
Janowitz, H. D., and Dreiling, D. A. (1959). *Am. J. Med.* **27**, 924.
Janowitz, H. D., and Dreiling, D. A. (1962). *Ciba Found. Symp., Exocrine Pancreas.* pp. 113–133.
Jasper, D. E. (1954). *North Am. Vet.* **35**, 523.
Joseph, W. L., Stevens, G. H., and Longmire, W. P. (1968). *J. Surg. Res.* **8**, 206.
Jubb, K. V. F., and Kennedy, P. C. (1963). "Pathology of Domestic Animals," Vol. 2, pp. 225–238. Academic Press, New York.

Kallfelz, F. A., Norrdin, R. W., and Neal, T. M. (1968). *J. Am. Vet. Med. Assoc.* **153**, 43.

Keller, P. J., Cohen, E., and Neurath, H. (1958). *J. Biol. Chem.* **233**, 344.

Kessler, J. I., Finkel, M., Preiling, D. A., and Janowitz, H. D. (1963). *Proc. Soc. Exptl. Biol. Med.* **113**, 127.

Loeb, W. F., and Edge, L. T. (1962). *Am. J. Vet. Res.* **23**, 1117.

McGeachin, R. L., and Johnson, W. D. (1964). *Arch. Biochem. Biophys.* **107**, 534.

Marchis-Mouren, G. (1959). Thesis, University of Marseille.

Marks, I. N., Bank, S., and Louw, J. H. (1968). *Prog. Gastroenterol.* **1**, 412–472.

Neurath, H. (1962). *Ciba Found. Symp., Exocrine Pancreas* pp. 67–86.

Rapp, J. P. (1962). *Am. J. Vet. Res.* **23**, 343.

Rawls, J. A., Wistraad, P. J., and Maren, T. H. (1963). *Am. J. Physiol.* **205**, 651.

Roe, J. H., and Byler, R. E. (1963). *Anal. Biochem.* **6**, 451.

Ruwitch, J., Bonertz, H. E., and Carlson, R. W. (1964). *J. Am. Vet. Med. Assoc.* **145**, 21.

Small, E., Olsen, R., and Fritz, T. (1964). *Vet. Med.* **59**, 627.

Taylor, R. B. (1962). *Res. Vet. Sci.* **3**, 63.

Thordal-Christensen, A., and Coffin, D. L. (1956). *Nord. Veterinar med.* **8**, 89.

Zieve, L. (1966). *Postgrad. Med.* **40**, A-18.

Zieve, L., Vogel, W. C., and Kelly, W. D. (1963). *J. Appl. Physiol.* **18**, 77.

Zimmerman, M. J., Dreiling, D. A., Rosenberg, I. R., and Janowitz, H. D. (1967). *Gastroenterology* **52**, 865.

The Pituitary and Adrenal Glands: Their Function in Health and Disease

John S. Wilkinson

I. INTRODUCTION

There is no place within the scope of a book of this order to deal *in extenso* with all aspects of pituitary and adrenal function. What is included must then necessarily be what the author considers important and will to some extent reflect his interests and prejudices. Those anxious to read further are referred to Eisenstein (1967), Paschkis *et al.* (1967), Harris and Donovan (1966), and Medway *et al.* (1969).

In this chapter the control and effects of the secretions of the following endocrine glands in health and disease will be discussed: the pituitary–adrenal axis, comprising the adenohypophysis and adrenal cortex; the adrenal medulla; the neurohypophysis; and the pineal gland. In addition, the prostaglandins are briefly mentioned.

A. PITUITARY AND ADRENAL GLANDS

1. *Hormones*

a. ADENOHYPOPHYSIS.   The anterior pituitary produces at least seven well-characterized hormones: growth hormone (GH, somatotropin, STH); adreno-corticotropin (ACTH, corticotropin); thyroid-stimulating hormone (TSH); melanocyte-stimulating hormone (MSH); follicle-stimulating hormone (FSH); interstitial cell-stimulating hormone (ICSH, luteinizing hormone, LH); and prolactin (luteotropic hormone, LTH).

In addition, Levine and Luft (1964) have suggested that the "diabetogenic" effects of GH are due to a contaminant which they have called "adipokinetic"; Louis and Conn (1967) have extracted from bovine adenohypophyses a polypeptide with a prolonged insulin-antagonistic effect, similar to one extracted from the urine of human patients suffering from lipoatropic diabetes; and two lipolytic polypeptides have been characterized by Chrétien and Li (1967). Armstrong *et al.* (1969) have described a polypeptide fraction of ovine GH which may prove valuable in treating human diabetes mellitus.

b. NEUROHYPOPHYSIS.   The pars nervosa produces two hormones: antidiuretic hormone (ADH, vasopressin) and oxytocin.

c. ADRENAL CORTEX.   The hormones of this gland are too numerous to mention individually and additions are constantly being made to those known. The more important are: cortisol (hydrocortisone); corticosterone; aldosterone, and androgens and estrogens.

d. ADRENAL MEDULLA.   Two hormones are produced: epinephrine and nor-epinephrine.

2. *Structure of Pituitary and Adrenal Hormones*

The hormones being discussed are either lipid-soluble steroids (adrenal cortex), or water-soluble polypeptides and glycoproteins (pituitary), and catecholamines (adrenal medulla). The pituitary and medullary hormones are ineffective thera-peutically when given orally because they are digested. The steroids are absorbed unchanged and can therefore be administered by mouth. The anterior pituitary hormones show slight species variations in structure. These differences are sufficient to render them mildly antigenic when used in heterologous species.

a. ADENOHYPOPHYSIS. The hormones of the adenohypophysis are glycoproteins (FSH, TSH, and LH) or peptides (ACTH and GH) of relatively low molecular weight (20,000–24,000 approx.). Species specificity in amino acid content (Wilhelmi, 1968) may account for the variations in response achieved by different workers (Fig. 1).

b. NEUROHYPOPHYSIS. The hormones of the neurohypophysis are polypeptides of about 1100 MW. Their structure is known (Fig. 2) and species differences occur. In the pig and hippopotamus lysine replaces the arginine in position 8.

c. ADRENAL CORTEX. The steroid hormones of the adrenal cortex and gonads are of the same basic structure, the cyclopentanophenanthrene ring (Fig. 3a). Most biologically active steroids are Δ^4,3-one; that is they have a double bond between positions 4 and 5 and oxo-(keto-) group at position 3. Most androgens and estrogens have an oxo-group in the 17 position (17-keto- or 17-oxosteroids, usually abbreviated to 17-KS), although hydroxyl groups may replace the oxo-groups in either of these positions (Fig. 3b). A longer chain at the 17-position, and sometimes a hydroxyl group also, imparts gluco- or mineralocorticoid activity. Cortisol and corticosterone have an hydroxyl group in the 11-position and are sometimes called 11-hydroxy-corticosteroids (11-OHCS) (Fig. 3c).

d. ADRENAL MEDULLA. The medullary hormones (catecholamines) differ from each other only in that epinephrine has a methyl group which norepinephrine lacks (Fig. 4).

3. Mechanisms of Hormone Actions

The mechanisms of many hormonal actions are still unknown. It has been held that they activate enzyme systems; for instance, it was thought that epinephrine and glucagon activated hepatic phosphorylase. This activation has now been shown to be indirect, being mediated through cyclic 3′,5′-adenosine monophosphate (AMP), possibly by activation of the enzyme adenylcyclase.

It has been suggested that some hormones may combine with a cell constituent to actually form an enzyme.

Karlson and Sekeris (1966) have postulated that hormones may function as gene activators, by stimulating synthesis of messenger ribonucleic acid (mRNA) "coded" for specific enzymes. This would account for the well-known effect of cortisol as an enzyme inducer.

B. THE PINEAL GLAND

The pineal gland has received more attention recently and to it have been ascribed a wide variety of functions. These include an antigonadotropic influence on reproduction, control of pigmentation through melatonin, and influences on thyroid, glucosteroid, and aldosterone secretion. It is said to be opposed to the pituitary in many of its functions.

C. THE PROSTAGLANDINS

There has been considerable interest in a newly documented group of biologically active substances: the prostaglandins. These are long-chain fatty acids and are

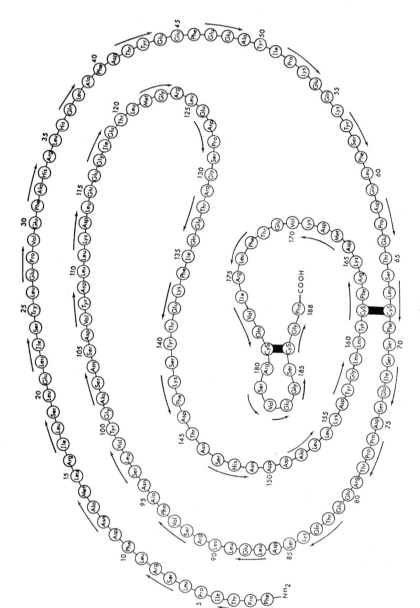

(a)

```
Ser-Tyr-Ser-Met-Glu-His-Phe-Arg-Try-Gly-Lys-Pro-Val-Gly-Lys-Lys-Arg-Arg-Pro-Val-Lys-Val-Tyr-Pro
 1   2   3   4   5   6   7   8   9  10  11  12  13  14  15  16  17  18  19  20  21  22  23  24

                                                              NH₂
                                                               |
Beef:  Asp-Gly-Ala-Glu-Asp-Ser-Ala-Glu-
        25  26  27  28  29  30  31  32  33

                                         NH₂
                                          |
Sheep: Ala-Gly-Glu-Asp-Asp-Glu-Ala-Ser-Glu-      Ala-Phe-Pro-Leu-Glu-Phe
                                                   34  35  36  37  38  39
                            NH₂
                             |
Pig:   Asp-Gly-Ala-Glu-Asp-Glu-Leu-Ala-Glu-
```

(b)

Fig. 1. (a) Structure of human growth hormone. (Li, 1968.) (b) The amino acid sequence of pig, sheep, and beef ACTH. (Li, 1968.)

CyS · Tyr · Phe · Glu(NH₂) · Asp(NH₂) · CyS · Pro · Arg · Gly(NH₂)

Fig. 2.   Structure of arginine vasopressin.

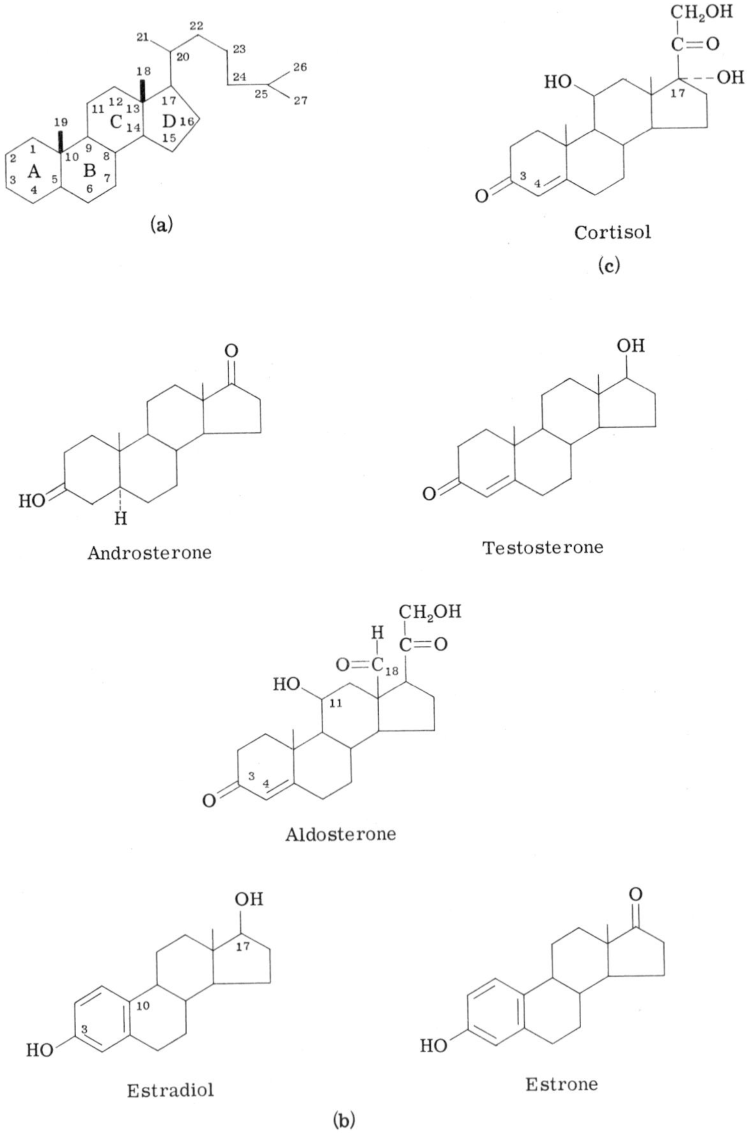

(a)

Cortisol

(c)

Androsterone

Testosterone

Aldosterone

Estradiol

Estrone

(b)

Fig. 3.   (a) The cyclopentanophenanthrene ring. (b) Structure of androgens, estrogens, and aldosterone. (c) Structure of cortisol.

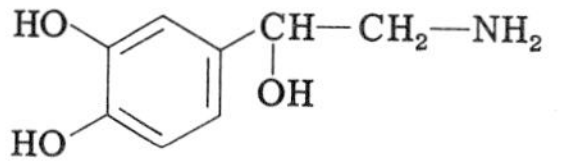

HO—⬡—CH—CH$_2$—NH$_2$
HO   OH

Norepinephrine

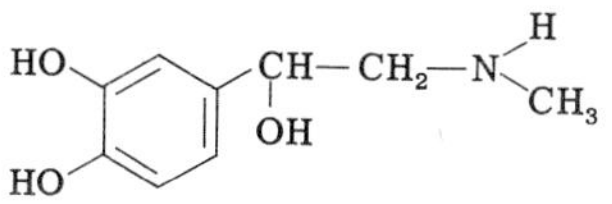

HO—⬡—CH—CH$_2$—N⟨H / CH$_3$
HO   OH

Epinephrine

Fig. 4.   Structure of the catecholamines.

derived from essential fatty acids. They have been isolated from many tissues and are very active in causing smooth muscle contraction or relaxation dependent on the particular substance, dose, and tissue examined (Leading Article, 1968). It has been suggested that their main function is in neurohumoral transmission.

D. CLASSIFICATION OF ENDOCRINE DISEASE

Disease processes in the endocrine system may be classified as hyperfunctional, hypofunctional, nonfunctional, dysfunctional, and ectopic (Wilkinson, 1969). Examples of all these entities may be found in variations of pituitary adrenal function, although dysfunction and ectopic endocrinopathy are not very well documented in veterinary medicine.

1. Hyperfunction

a. ADRENAL CORTEX.   Adrenocortical hyperfunction is the commonest syndrome of excessive endocrine activity. It may be primary, due to adrenocortical neoplasia or secondary, due to excessive ACTH production.

b. ADRENAL MEDULLA.   Medullary hyperfunction due to neoplasia has been suspected but not undeniably established.

2. Hypofunction

a. ADENOHYPOPHYSIS.   Pituitary cachexia may be the end result of almost all pituitary or hypothalamic diseases, whether it is due to neoplasia, ischemia, or inflammation.

In man, individual anterior pituitary hormone deficiencies have been described (Odell, 1966). It is reasonable to assume that similar deficiencies may cause hypothyroidism and adrenal failure in animals. Clarification of this point waits on estimation of peripheral levels of individual tropic hormones (Section II,B,1).

b. ADRENAL CORTEX.   Adrenocortical failure may be due to a number of causes. The gland may be destroyed by nonfunctional neoplastic tissue, inflammation, or infarction.

"The existence of autoimmune disturbances of the thyroid, adrenal and testis is no longer questioned" (Solomon and Blizzard, 1963), and Goudie et al. (1968) have demonstrated that in the human, adrenal antigens are associated with the microsomal fraction of the cell. Autoimmunity has to be considered as a possible cause of primary adrenocortical atrophy in the dog also.

3. Nonfunction

Lesions may be present in endocrine tissue without producing any alteration in function; for example, some adrenal neoplasms, adrenal calcification, and pituitary cysts are without apparent endocrine effect.

4. Dysfunction

In the dysfunctional state there is an excessive liberation of a hormone which is a normal intermediate in biosynthesis but is not usually found in significant concentrations outside the gland. This results from a deficiency of an enzyme whose function is to convert this intermediate hormone to the next compound in the synthetic pathway. Such a situation is induced by the drug mepyrapone (Metopirone*) which selectively blocks 11-hydroxylation.

5. Ectopic Endocrinopathy

This is the result of the production of hormones by nonendocrine tissue, usually neoplastic. It is well documented in man but not as yet described in domestic animals.

Various neoplastic tissues have been shown to cause hypercalcemia due to parathyroid hormone production, hypoglycemia due possibly to the release of an insulin-like substance or an insulin potentiator, polycythemia due to excessive erythropoietin, hyponatremia due to excessive ADH release, and hyperadrenocorticoidism due to excessive amounts of an ACTH-like substance (Lie, 1968). The mechanics of these aberrations are not yet known, but it is becoming clear that tumors may produce almost any hormone. All cells have the same genetic components and therefore the potential to produce any peptide. Specialization of function is achieved by control of some of these processes by "repressors." Malignant cells that produce hormones have possibly lost or escaped from this control (Leading Article, 1967).

E. SPECIES PREVALENCE

Clinical biochemical changes associated with alterations in endocrine function have been studied most widely in the dog and, unless specifically stated otherwise, the discussion following in this chapter refers to dogs.

Table I gives a list of the more important references to abnormalities of function of the pituitary adrenal axis. The list is not exhaustive; for what appears to be a definitive list of pituitary tumors in dogs consult Capen *et al.* (1967). Some of the references list no biochemical findings but are included because they are of importance in other ways.

II. HORMONES OF THE ADENOHYPOPHYSIS

A. SITE OF PRODUCTION

There has been considerable speculation as to the cells responsible for the synthesis of the adenohypophysial hormones. It becomes increasingly likely that individual hormones are synthesized by individual cells and with sufficiently specific

*Burroughs Wellcome.

TABLE I ALTERATIONS IN PITUITARY AND ADRENAL FUNCTION IN DISEASE

Species	Pathological lesions	References
Dog	Pituitary basophil adenomas, 2° adrenocortical hyperplasia	Coffin and Munson (1953)
	Pituitary chromophobe adenomas, 2° adrenocortical hyperplasia	Wilkinson *et al.* (1965) Rijnberk *et al.* (1968b)
	Pituitary chromophobe adenomas and adenomas of pars intermedia, 2° adrenocortical hyperplasia	Capen *et al.* (1967)
	Pituitary chromophobe adenoma, hyperandrogenism	Schwartzman and Fegley (1965)
	Pituitary chromophobe adenoma, adiposogenital syndrome	Hare (1932)
	Pituitary tumors, diabetes insipidus	Brandt (1940)
	Infundibuloma, adiposogenital syndrome, diabetes insipidus	Saunders *et al.* (1951)
	Craniopharyngioma, adiposogenital syndrome, diabetes insipidus	Saunders and Rickard (1952)
	Congenital pituitary deficiency, dwarfism	Baker (1955) Jensen (1959) Hoe (1961)
	Pituitary cachexia	Verstraete and Thoonen (1938; 1939)
	Adrenal neoplasm, 1° adrenocortical hyperfunction	Wilkinson *et al.* (1965) Siegel *et al.* (1967)
	1° adrenocortical failure	Freudiger and Lindt (1958a,b) Annis (1960) Marshak *et al.* (1960) Rothenbacher and Shigley (1966)
	Pheochromocytoma	E.B. Howard and Nielsen (1965)
Horse	Pituitary tumor, hirsutism	Eriksson *et al.* (1956) Backstrom (1963)
	Pituitary tumor, diabetes mellitus	King *et al.* (1962) Loeb *et al.* (1966)
	Pituitary tumor, diabetes insipidus	Brandt (1940)
	Adrenal neoplasm, 1° adrenocortical hyperfunction	Kral (1951)
	Acute adrenocortical failure (Freidrichsen-Waterhouse syndrome)	Jubb and Kennedy (1970)
Cattle	Pituitary and adrenal failure	J.R. Howard *et al.* (1968)
	Adrenal neoplasm, obesity, and sterility	Wright and Conner (1968)
	Pheochromocytoma	Wright and Conner (1968)

techniques it may be possible to demonstrate as many cell types as there are hormones.

The chromophobe cells, because they had no distinctively staining granules, were at first thought to be nonfunctional, either precursor, resting, or exhausted forms of the "functional" cells. Cushing described in man a disease in which a basophil tumor was associated with adrenocortical hyperplasia. Early accounts of a similar condition in dogs also ascribed the condition to basophil neoplasia (Coffin and

Munson, 1953). "Functionally active" chromophobe neoplasms are now commonly reported in man and animals. This more recent histological evaluation has been confirmed by the demonstration of ACTH activity associated with particulate material derived from chromophobe cells (Knutson, 1966).

It has been suggested that specific hormones may originate from specific zones within the adenohypophysis (Section II,B).

B. CONTROL

Regulation of adenohypophysial secretion is mediated neurally through the cerebral cortex and midbrain, chemically through circulating levels of cortisol, thyroxine, glucose, and possibly tropic hormones, and through specific releasing factors. The blood supply to the adenohypophysis is rather unusual and plays a very important role in the regulation of secretion.

1. Blood Supply

In many mammals there are two distinct portal systems supplied from the hypothalamic artery. One has its primary plexus in the hypothalamus (median eminence) and drains by the long portal veins, which mostly lie on the surface of the pituitary stalk, to the secondary plexus in the anterior lobe. The other system has its primary plexus in the region of the lower pituitary stalk and neural lobe of the neurohypophysis and drains via the short portal veins to the sinusoids of the anterior lobe.

These portal systems are the only blood supply to the pituitary in a number of species, there being no arterial supply. The distribution of the individual secondary plexuses within the adenohypophysis is quite discrete, in fact, "the affluent blood of a single portal vessel seems to enter the sinusoids of a rather restricted zone of the pars distalis" (McCann et al., 1968). It is speculated that a given tropic hormone is secreted preferentially by cells receiving blood from a specific portal vessel. If this could be proved it would support the argument that specific zones within the adenohypophysis are responsible for secreting specific hormones and possibly account for the occurrence of individual tropic hormone deficiencies (Section I, D, 2,a).

2. Feedback Mechanisms

Production of tropic hormones is suppressed by elevated levels of target organ hormone and possibly tropic hormone. This may be a direct suppression within the pituitary cell or may be effected at a hypothalamic level through the releasing factors.

3. Releasing Factors

Extracts of different portions of the hypothalamus will specifically stimulate the secretion of individual tropic hormones. These hypothalamic areas are able to "sense" any need for alterations in pituitary secretion. When an increase is necessary, the releasing factor is synthesized in the neurones and passes down the axons to be liberated into one of the pituitary portal systems and carried to the adenohypophysis. Here it promotes either liberation, synthesis, or both, of the corresponding tropic hormone.

Psychic stimuli enhance hypothalamic liberation of releasing factors by pathways from the cerebral cortex.

4.   Adrenocorticotropin Production and Release

ACTH is produced in the pituitary, from whence it is liberated at need in response to corticotropin-releasing factor (CRF). CRF may control the synthesis of mRNA (Kraicer, 1964). ADH has a CRF-like effect and it may increase CRF production. CRF production is controlled by pathways from the cerebral cortex, and perhaps by circulating levels of cortisol and ACTH. Cortisol has been shown to concentrate in the area in the midbrain from whence CRF originates. Emotional stress is mediated through the cerebral cortex. Plasma cortisol levels remain above normal in a proportion of calves for up to 3 weeks after transport (Shaw and Nichols, 1964). A rapid decrease in plasma glucose concentration will enhance ACTH liberation (Matsui and Plager, 1966). Infusion of cortisol into the adenohypophysis will reduce ACTH release. This may be physiologically important. Hypothalamic implantation of thyroxine will stimulate ACTH production in rats but it is doubtful whether a physiological role for thyroxine can be deduced from this experimental observation.

In a series of recent papers Alvarez-Buylla and Alvarez-Buylla (1964, 1967, 1968a,b) have proposed that the pituitary is merely a storage organ whose function can be adequately taken over by a portion of salivary or adrenal gland. They have also demonstrated that a conditioned reflex can be evoked in this system and they postulate that the vagus is involved. These results await clarification and confirmation. If their findings are reproducible, two other explanations may have to be considered: (1) CRF may undergo "condensation" to produce ACTH or (2) it can induce in glandular tissue other than the pituitary the enzyme system necessary for synthesis of ACTH.

5.   Growth Hormone Production and Release

A GH-releasing factor of hypothalamic origin has been demonstrated. There is apparently a feedback mechanism, since peripheral GH-secreting tumors cause a decrease in pituitary eosinophils. MacLeod and Abad (1968) emphasize that the feedback inhibition is on the synthesis of GH rather than on the releasing factor.

The most potent stimulus to GH secretion is hypoglycemia. This is probably due to a lack of carbohydrate substrate for metabolism within the GH-regulating center (Glick, 1968) in the hypothalamus. However, Trenkle (1967) was unable to demonstrate an increase in plasma GH in cattle in response to insulin-induced hypoglycemia. J. Roth et al. (1964) demonstrated that absolute hypoglycemia was not essential but that a rapid fall in plasma glucose levels would stimulate GH release. Both reduction in brain norepinephrine, which probably interferes with neurohumoral transmission, and cortisol reduce GH release.

6. Thyroid-Stimulating Hormone Production and Release

Hypothalamic control of TSH is maintained through TSH-releasing factor (TRF). There is an inverse relationship between ACTH and TSH production, conditions which elevate ACTH secretion suppress TSH, and where TSH is elevated ACTH is depressed. The feedback mechanism is definitely at the pituitary rather than the hypothalamic level. It is likely that thyroxine (T_4) reduces the sensitivity of TSH-producing cells to TRF.

A fall in ambient temperature causes an increase in TSH liberation which is too rapid for any mechanism other than a neural one. However, secretion of TSH declines fairly rapidly if TRF is the only stimulant. The prolonged elevation in TSH production that follows chronic "cold stress" is probably due to increased metabolism and therefore lower plasma levels of T_4. This makes the TSH-producing cells more sensitive to TRF.

7. Melanocyte-Stimulating Hormone Production and Release

The control of MSH has been largely neglected. The factors involved are not mentioned in the major treatise on pituitary function (Harris and Donovan, 1966).

8. Follicle-Stimulating Hormone Production and Release

This hormone is controlled through the hypothalamus. The "higher centers" are involved in the control of all pituitary gonadotropins. FSH production is particularly affected by visual and olfactory stimuli. Secretion of FSH is enhanced by low levels of estrogen but high levels block the releasing factor and stimulate LH production.

9. Interstitial Cell-Stimulating Hormone Production and Release

ICSH, or more conveniently LH-, releasing factor mediates hypothalamic control of this hormone. Androgens, estrogens, and ICSH (LH) inhibit the releasing factor, which is probably why exogenous sex hormones cause tubular degeneration of the testis. Progesterone increases pituitary ICSH levels either by increasing synthesis or by blocking release.

10. Prolactin Production and Release

Hypothalamic control of prolactin secretion departs from the normal in that it is inhibitory not stimulatory. The synthesis and release of prolactin-inhibiting factor (PIF) is blocked by the suckling stimulus, estradiol, epinephrine, perphenazine, and reserpine. It is possible that LHRF is also PIF.

Estradiol, in addition to inhibiting PIF synthesis, in low doses stimulates the release of prolactin from the pituitary. TSH also increases prolactin release. A feedback mechanism is involved but whether this acts through the hypothalamus or directly upon the pituitary is unknown.

C. Actions

1. Adrenocorticotropin

a. Adrenal Cortex. The adrenal cortex responds to ACTH by increasing its output of steroid hormones. This is possibly achieved by enhanced trapping of plasma cholesterol; by specific stimulation of 20-hydroxylation of cholesterol (Hall and Young, 1968) or conversion to Δ^5-pregnenolone (Ney et al., 1967); or possibly by influencing cholesterol synthesis de novo. An increase in adrenal free fatty acids (FFA) parallels the steroid response to ACTH, and there is a similar and perhaps causal increase in lipase and decrease in triglycerides.

Ion flux through the cell and across cell membranes appears to be an important factor in steroidogenesis, and it has been suggested that ACTH may exert an important influence here either directly or through increased levels of 3′,5′ cyclic AMP. Adenylcyclase, an enzyme whose function is to produce 3′,5′ cyclic AMP from adenosine triphosphate (ATP), has been shown in vivo to increase very rapidly following ACTH stimulation. Complicated stimulatory and inhibitory factors have been identified in steroid synthesis and ACTH has been said to act by increasing synthesis of a protein which blocks the inhibitory action of another protein.

Many steps in intermediary metabolism are dependent on sufficient levels of the electron donor nicotinamide adenine dinucleotide (NADH) and it appears that steroid synthesis is no exception. ACTH has been shown to activate glucose-6-phosphate dehydrogenase, an enzyme whose activity determines the levels of available NADH.

The cortical hyperplasia which follows chronic stimulation by ACTH involves frequent mitosis. This requires prolonged high levels of protein and mRNA syntheses. These increases, in response to ACTH, take several hours to reach a peak but are prolonged. The relative insensitivity of the suppressed adrenal cortex to ACTH may be due to the need first to synthesize protein and nucleic acid. Conversely, the gland which has previously been stimulated and then stressed shows an immediate increase in synthesis. However, the hormonal products of this synthesis are not all released immediately; some are temporarily stored and slowly released. This results in a much more prolonged rise in plasma cortisol level, although the levels do not reach the height that would be achieved were all liberated at once (Jones and Stockham, 1966).

The role of ACTH in the regulation of the zona glomerulosa of the adrenal cortex was for a long time uncertain but it has now been established that under certain conditions ACTH causes an increase in aldosterone secretion from this area. While the sodium pool is normal or enlarged, or sodium intake is high, the response of the zona glomerulosa to ACTH is minimal. However, when sodium is depleted cortical sensitivity is much enhanced and ACTH will then cause an increase in aldosterone secretion (Venning et al., 1962). T. C. Lee et al. (1968), however, suggest that in the rat this pituitary glomerulotropic effect is not due to ACTH but to some unidentified substance which stimulates the adrenal cortex indirectly.

b. Extraadrenal Systems. ACTH also acts outside the adrenal, affecting skin pigmentation, peripheral lipolysis, and leukocyte formation.

The main physiological stimulus to the melanocyte is the specific hormone MSH, but ACTH has a minor effect which may lead to increased pigmentation.

The lipolytic effect of ACTH on the adrenal cortex has been mentioned (Section II,C,1,a). It has been shown that this lipolysis is not confined to the adrenal cortex but is also found in the peripheral fat depots where adenylcyclase concentration is increased. The rather specific redistribution of fat which is seen in hyperadrenocorticism in the human may be the result of this lipolysis. It may also contribute to the extremely fatty liver found in the dog.

ACTH has a direct leukocytosis-inducing effect (Massimo et al., 1966), which is distinct from the effect of cortisol upon the bone marrow. It will also reduce capillary permeability in inflammation.

2. Growth Hormone

GH does not have a specific end organ; all tissues are influenced to some extent by its effects upon their metabolism. These effects may be mediated through the adrenal cortex (Campbell et al., 1959).

a. PROTEIN METABOLISM.   This has been reviewed recently by Snipes (1968) who has emphasized once more the interrelated roles of insulin and GH. In the absence of a pituitary gland, growth is retarded or even absent. This can be partially corrected by administration of GH which causes retention of nitrogen, but the full expression of growth occurs only if adequate insulin is also present. It is thought that uptake of amino acids is enhanced by these two hormones in concert but this would not account for all the increase in nitrogen retention, and it is possible that they stimulate other stages in protein synthesis. These may include synthesis of mRNA or enzymic activity of the ribosomes.

Weber et al. (1966) showed that rats carrying transplantable GH-secreting tumors had increased levels of liver glycogen (300%), nitrogen (200%), RNA (200%), and gluconeogenic enzymes.

In sheep GH administration for 4 weeks depressed wool growth, but after treatment was stopped wool growth rose above control values for the following 20 weeks. Possibly the high liver nitrogen that resulted from GH administration was "switched" to wool production (Wheatley et al., 1966).

b. CARBOHYDRATE METABOLISM.   Plasma glucose levels are sometimes elevated by GH. The design of the experiment, the species of test animal and the type of GH used all influence the result of GH administration, and may account for the differences recorded by different authors.

A. Sirek et al. (1964) have shown that GH causes a rise in plasma glucose levels in normal and hypophysectomized but not in Houssay (hypophysectomized–pancreatectomized) dogs, indicating that insulin as well as GH is necessary to produce the rise.

Wallace and Bassett (1966) showed that administration of ovine GH to sheep for 4 weeks caused a rise in plasma insulin levels. They note also that GH will cause an increase in immunoreactive insulin in dogs, and Campbell and Rastogi (1966) state that GH causes a much greater hyperinsulinemia than do glucosteroids.

c. LIPID METABOLISM.   Gans and Butz (1964) demonstrated in dogs that GH was one of the many factors which elevated plasma cholesterol levels. It also increased the plasma-liver cholesterol pool. Cholesterol synthesis per unit weight of liver tissue was not increased but there was an increase in liver size which could have accounted for the increased cholesterol production.

Most workers have found that GH mobilized FFA from peripheral fat depots, and Randle *et al.* (1963) have indicated that the level of plasma FFA may be related to plasma glucose levels. Levine and Luft (1964), however, suggest that there may be a second and heretofore unseparated pituitary hormone which is responsible for the "diabetogenic" effects of GH, including FFA mobilization.

O. Sirek *et al.* (1967), on the other hand, found that bovine GH lowered plasma FFA in normal, hypophysectomized, and Houssay dogs within 30 minutes of injection without any appreciable change in plasma glucose. Bassett and Wallace (1966) also noticed a decline in FFA immediately after administration of ovine GH to sheep but this was followed later by an increase in plasma FFA. Plasma glucose levels also fell in the first hour but rose to hyperglycemic levels during the next 7 hours and blood ketones tended to follow the same pattern.

3. Thyroid-Stimulating Hormone

Hypophysectomy does not produce such a severe hypothyroidism as thyroid-ectomy; the thyroids are able to maintain at least a low level of function following hypophysectomy. TSH only enhances this basic ability. It elevates the metabolic rate of the gland by increasing glucose oxidation and CO_2 production, and it activates the protease which splits T_4 from thyroglobulin. This activation is "immediate," occurring within 30 minutes of the stimulus, and is probably secondary to the increased metabolism. Increased iodine trapping and iodination of tyrosine follows 5–7 hours after the stimulus.

Closely associated with TSH in many pituitary extracts is the exophthalmos-producing substance (EPS). It was originally thought that exophthalmos was produced by TSH but sufficiently purified fractions show high TSH and low EPS, or high EPS and low TSH, activity.

4. Melanocyte-Stimulating Hormone

MSH stimulates tyrosinase activity, probably by increasing synthesis of this enzyme, which is essential to melanin synthesis in mammalian and avian melanocytes. MSH does not influence pigment movement in mammals and birds as it does in the melanophores of cold-blooded animals. The pigment-enhancing effect of ACTH is due to its structure; it has an amino acid chain which has the same sequence as the MSH molecule. The possibility that a deficiency of melatonin, a pineal hormone which decreases skin color, may allow an increase in skin pigmentation in disease has not been investigated.

5. Follicle-Stimulating Hormone

In the male FSH stimulates spermatogenesis. In the female it enhances development of Graafian follicle and estrogen secretion from it.

6. Interstitial Cell-Stimulating Hormone

In the male ICSH stimulates testosterone secretion by the interstitial cells of the testis and so possibly increases plasma and urinary androgen levels.

In birds ICSH, not androgens, is responsible for the development and maintenance of the male nuptial plumage.

In the female LH initiates ovulation and development of the corpus luteum and stimulates the production of progesterone. In man and cattle it is luteotropic, i.e., it maintains the corpus luteum and stimulates progesterone secretion.

At the cellular level it may activate glycogen phosphorylase through 3',5'-AMP. Increased production of NADH, which is essential for steroid synthesis results from glycogenolysis and increased metabolism of glucose-6-phosphate via the pentose phosphate shunt.

7. Prolactin

Prolactin has very different actions in different species. It is luteotropic in sheep but probably not in other species. It also causes mammary alveolar hyperplasia.

D. EXCRETION

Excretory pathways for the anterior pituitary hormones have not been fully elucidated. The gonadotropins are excreted in the urine. It is probable that the other pituitary hormones are also excreted, but investigations have been contradictory. Girard and Greenwood (1968) were unable to find human GH in urine.

E. NORMAL VALUES

Differences in methods of estimation of the adenohypophysial hormones can cause considerable variations in values. Radioimmunoassay is the method of choice for most pituitary hormones, but requires specialized equipment. Bioassays are less specific and less reliable but are the only method available for some hormones in some species.

1. Adrenocorticotropin

This hormone has been measured in pig plasma by Donald and colleagues (1968) who showed the resting level to be less than 40 pg/100 ml. Insulin-induced hypoglycemia caused a rise to 160–174 (mean 392) pg/100 ml and mepyrapone initiated an increase to above 300 pg/100 ml.

2. Growth Hormone

GH concentrations of 41 $\pm$ 19 μg/100 ml were found by Dev (1965) in Hereford cattle and of 4.8 ng/ml in sheep.

F. DISEASE

Hypo-, hyper- and nonfunctional pituitary disease states are recorded. Hypofunctional states commonly arise from pressure changes due to tumors which initially may have produced hyperfunction. Degenerative changes with hemorrhage and necrosis are common (Jubb and Kennedy, 1970). In contrast to man, where infarction is a common cause, pituitary cachexia in domestic animals does not usually follow hypophysial necrosis. The hyperfunctional conditions reported have all resulted from neoplasms. Pituitary cysts are common but rarely affect endocrine function.

1. Peripheral Levels of Tropic Hormones

The author is unaware of any measurement of pituitary hormones in disease states in domestic animals, although Rijnberk et al. (1968a) describe the presence of EPS in sera and one pituitary from cases of adrenal hyperfunction.

It is postulated that in pituitary-induced adrenal hyperfunction there would be elevated levels of ACTH. With the failure of the feedback mechanism in primary adrenocortical failure, high values of ACTH would also be anticipated, but low values would be found in cases with a primary deficit of adenohypophysial ACTH. In man increased ACTH-like activity has been demonstrated in cases of Cushing's syndrome associated with bronchial carcinoma.

Similar assumptions may be made concerning elevation of plasma GH in acromegaly and lowered levels in panhypopituitarism. There is as yet little evidence to support them.

2. Alterations in Peripheral Blood Chemistry

Biochemical alterations in impaired adenohypophysial function are mainly the result of changes in end organ function. There are relatively few changes which are primarily due to the alterations in tropic hormone secretion. Some of the diseases of the anterior pituitary are so rare that no biochemical investigations have been made.

ACTH has a number of extraadrenal effects but it may not be possible to distinguish between these and the results of excessive corticosteroid secretion induced by ACTH. The lipolysis which ACTH is known to cause is probably the origin of the fatty liver but glucosteroids are also involved in fat metabolism and may be responsible. Both steroids and ACTH also induce a neutrophilia.

Panhypopituitarism and pituitary dwarfism are associated with marked biochemical changes which are the results of end organ failure. These are discussed later.

Acromegaly may occur more frequently than it is diagnosed but we know nothing of the chemical changes that occur. One case of acromegaly and diabetes mellitus has been described in a dog but separation of the causes of the biochemical changes is impossible (Groen et al., 1964).

Foley (1956) suggested that variations in pituitary–adrenal function, as indicated by increased insulin sensitivity, occurred in dwarf cattle.

3. Gonadotropins

No biochemical evidence exists of the involvement of pituitary gonadotropins in disease.

Production of the pituitary gonadotropins is more susceptible to surgical trauma and pressure changes than secretion of the other tropic hormones. Gonadotropin secretion is therefore lost early in the natural history of pituitary neoplasia and regression of gonadotropin supported organs results. (The satiety center of the hypothalamus is also affected by the swelling gland early in the disease and hypothalamic overeating and obesity develop.) These two factors cause the signs of the adiposogenital syndrome.

Possibly alterations in gonadotropin metabolism occur in the feminizing syndrome associated with Sertoli cell tumors in dogs. Normal levels of estrogen in testicular venous blood make the syndrome difficult to explain but it is possible that increased metabolism of steroids which influence ICSH secretion or increased metabolism of ICSH itself may occur. Either condition might lead to an eunuchoid state.

III. HORMONES OF THE NEUROHYPOPHYSIS

ADH but not oxytocin has been associated with biochemical changes in disease and the following discussion concerns ADH alone.

A. SITE OF PRODUCTION

ADH is produced in the supraoptic and possibly the paraventricular centers of the hypothalamus. It is probable that individual neurones are specific in their secretion of ADH or oxytocin.

B. CONTROL

The neurohypophysis differs from the adenohypophysis in some of its control mechanisms. There is still neural control via the hypothalamus, although the influence of the cerebral cortex probably is less important. Chemical factors including ethanol, nicotine, and changes in plasma crystalloid osmotic pressure are involved.

1. Blood Supply

Transmission of the neurohumor to the end organ is not dependent on the pituitary portal systems. The hormones are liberated directly from the axons of the hypothalamic neurones into capillaries of the posterior pituitary gland.

2. Feedback Mechanisms

There is no evidence that a feedback mechanism is involved.

3. Releasing Factors

No releasing factor has been demonstrated.

4. Regulation of ADH

The paraventricular and supraoptic nuclei in the hypothalamus are the source of ADH. In this area there are organelles which are responsive to fluctuations of as little as 2% in plasma crystalloid osmotic pressure. ADH is elaborated in the neurones in these centers in response to need. Synthesis is enhanced by chronic dehydration and depressed by overhydration. The initial neurohumor may not be functional; activation may occur further down the axon. The neurosecretory material passes down the axon bound to a protein, neurophysin, and is stored in bulbous expansions of the axon close to the basement membrane of the capillaries of the posterior pituitary. This stored material is liberated in response to an acute stimulus such as acute hemorrhage but after an initial large and rapid response the rate of secretion soon declines.

The mechanism of the dissociation of ADH from the carrier protein and its release into the capillaries is not yet clear. In the plasma the hormone is not protein-bound.

Stimuli for release include alterations in blood volume and increases in intra-thoracic pressure which probably reach the hypothalamus through the baroceptors in the atrium and carotid arteries; pain and emotion also cause an increase in ADH output. Bradykinin, a polypeptide produced by autolytic or bacterial break-down of tissue, causes an antidiuresis possibly by stimulating release of ADH (Silva and Malnic, 1964). Pain itself may also result from the action of a similar polypeptide, pain-producing factor.

C. Actions

1. Vasopressor Action

It is suggested that some of the effect of ADH upon the kidneys is due to its direct vasopressor action upon arterioles. However, at the usual plasma levels there appears to be no effect on the general vasculature. It requires the stimulus of severe acute hemorrhage to elevate plasma ADH levels sufficiently to cause peripheral vasoconstriction.

2. Water Turnover

ADH achieves its results on the renal tubules by influencing the synthesis of $3',5'$-AMP which can be used to replace ADH in some experimental situations. It is uncertain how it increases synthesis. It may stimulate synthesis or activation of adenylcyclase. The increase in $3',5'$-AMP causes an increase in permeability of the tubule to water and, perhaps, to urea also (E. Lee et al., 1967). Both calcium and potassium ion concentrations have been said to influence the sensitivity of the tubule to ADH, a finding which is not universally supported. Ullman and co-workers (1965) showed that tubular sensitivity to ADH was increased during an "acid tide," whereas the need to retain hydrogen ions was associated with reduced sensitivity.

Other factors influencing water transport have been suggested. Fourman and Kennedy (1966), for example, postulate that the vasopressor action of ADH alters the hemodynamics of the renal medulla, thus influencing the countercurrent mechanism. Levels of ADH too low to influence peripheral resistance have been shown to increase renal blood flow. The increase in glomerular filtration rate seen in response to ADH may result from an increase in the number of functional nephrons.

ADH may suppress drinking through the thirst center in the hypothalamus. The reduction in intake in response to ADH injection in some cases of diabetes insipidus is too rapid to have been achieved by other homeostatic mechanisms.

3.   Electrolyte Metabolism

The influence of ADH on sodium, potassium, and chloride excretion appears to be a function of the state of hydration and alimentation of the experimental animal and of the specific response to the type of ADH used. Directly conflicting views have been obtained. For example, Brook and colleagues (1968) found that arginine vasopressin had no effect upon kaliuresis in sheep, whereas Kuhn (1967) found it enhanced potassium excretion. Kuhn (1967) also found that lysine vasopressin was not kaliuretic in sheep but was in dogs. These results, however, may not be directly comparable since there were differences in experimental design.

In the normally hydrated or dehydrated dog ADH had no effect on electrolyte excretion, whereas in the water-loaded dog it causes an increase in sodium, potassium, and chloride loss. In sheep Gans (1964) found that saluresis depended on the dose of arginine vasopressin used.

4.   Steroid Secretion

The increase in secretion of adrenal steroids in response to ADH stimulation is probably not of physiological significance since it appears only at pharmacological levels of the hormone.

D. Excretion

ADH is in part excreted unchanged by both kidneys and liver and in part enzymically degraded by both these organs.

E. Normal Values

Peripheral ADH concentrations of 4 μg/ml plasma, with a half-life ($T_{1/2}$) of 2-7$\frac{1}{2}$ min, and jugular vein levels of 2.0–85 pg/ml (Yoshida *et al.*, 1966) are reported in the dog.

F. Disease

Syndromes of over- and underproduction of ADH are reported in man; in animals only the hypofunctional state is described. The syndrome of inappropriate secretion of ADH has been mentioned (Section 1,C,5). It has been associated with a wide variety of diseases both thoracic and extrathoracic. It has as yet no known counterpart in veterinary medicine.

Diabetes insipidus is due to reduced ADH secretion in the face of chronic dehydration and hyperosmolarity of plasma. The disease may arise from the following:

1. A primary derangement of the sensing elements in the hypothalamus and be associated with no obvious lesions.

2. Destruction of the hypothalamus or neurohypophsis by degenerative processes or pressure atrophy. Koestner and Capen (1967) suggest that the disease in dogs is due to diminished synthesis of the transport protein due to gradually increasing pressure on the supraoptic nucleus by the growing tumor.

3. Insensitivity of the renal tubule to ADH.

Diabetes insipidus arises most commonly from pressure changes due to pituitary tumors or degenerative changes in the hypothalamus. It frequently accompanies adrenocortical hyperplasia of pituitary origin and the adiposogenital syndrome. Renal insensitivity has not been described in dogs.

1. Peripheral Level of ADH

There are no records, of which the author is aware, of levels of ADH in disease. One may anticipate high levels with intrathoracic neoplasms and reduced levels in pituitary or hypothalamic disease.

2. Alterations in Peripheral Blood and Urine Chemistry

a. INAPPROPRIATE SECRETION OF ADH.   There is hyponatremia and hypoosmality of plasma in the presence of hypertonic urine and normal urinary steroid secretion.

b. DIABETES INSIPIDUS.   The cardinal biochemical sign in this disease is a persistently low urinary osmolality or specific gravity. Serum osmolality is elevated but no other serum changes occur.

It should be emphasized here that in some cases of pituitary failure the lack of ADH is masked by the deficiency of cortical steroids secondary to lack of ACTH. In the absence of cortisol, blood volume is so reduced that glomerular filtration reaches levels so low that water reabsorption can occur even in the absence of ADH. The glucosteroids also tend to antagonize the action of ADH and in the absence of this antagonism minimal levels of ADH will maintain water balance.

IV. HORMONES OF THE ADRENAL CORTEX

A. SITE OF PRODUCTION

The adrenal cortex is divided into three distinct zones, the outer zona glomerulosa, the middle zona fasciculata, and the inner zona reticularis.

Aldosterone is secreted by the zona glomerulosa. The other two zones may function as a single entity producing glucosteroids and sex hormones throughout their substance (Cameron and Grant, 1967). If they have separate functions, then the fasciculata produces the glucosteroids and the reticularis the sex hormones.

There is also a fourth, fetal zone, which is of no importance in the normal adult but which may be involved in adrenal hyperplasia (Craig, 1964).

B. CONTROL

Although for convenience the glucosteroids and aldosterone are considered separately, their control is not entirely independent. ACTH stimulates both glucosteroid and, under special conditions, aldosterone secretion also.

1. Glucosteroids

a. ADRENOCORTICOTROPIN.   This, the major controlling factor in steroid synthesis, has been discussed earlier (Section II,C).

b. CORTICOSTEROID FEEDBACK.   Morrow *et al.* (1967) have demonstrated *in vitro* that some adrenal steroids will suppress adrenal protein synthesis. This finding suggests the possibility of a negative feedback control.

2. Aldosterone

a. RENIN–ANGIOTENSIN SYSTEM.   In each nephron there is a group of cells close to the afferent glomerular arteriole. This is the juxtamedullary apparatus which is thought to be sensitive to changes in pressure and pO_2 which are due to alterations in renal perfusion. Hypovolemia and cardiac insufficiency both reduce renal perfusion and stimulate the juxtamedullary apparatus to produce renin. This hormone reacts with or activates a precursor, angiotensinogen (angiotensin I), to liberate the active angiotensin II, which has two functions. First it is a most potent vasoconstrictor and second it stimulates the adrenal to secrete more aldosterone. The importance of this system, at least in the sheep, has been established by Blair-West and colleagues (1968) who demonstrated that a kidney was essential for sustained hypersecretion of aldosterone in hypophysectomized sodium-depleted sheep. It is interesting to note that this system is not important in the cat.

b. ADRENOGLOMERULOTROPIN.   Farrel (1960) extracted from the pineal glands of cattle a substance which increased the output of aldosterone by the zona glomerulosa, and which he called adrenoglomerulotropin. There is also a substance found in pineal tissue which reduces aldosterone release (Wiener 1968a,b).

c. PLASMA ELECTROLYTE LEVELS.   The zona glomerulosa responds to a decrease in plasma sodium and an increase in plasma potassium by increasing aldosterone output. This may be achieved either by increasing the conversion of cholesterol to pregnenolone or corticosterone to aldosterone.

d. ADRENOCORTICOTROPIN.   The zona glomerulosa, normally unresponsive, is rendered sensitive to ACTH by sodium depletion (Section II,C).

C. ACTIONS

Division of adrenal hormones into glucosteroids, which influence carbohydrate metabolism and mineralocorticoids, which, in turn, affect electrolyte metabolism, is artificial and erroneous. All steroids have effects on both metabolic systems, quantitatively considerably different but qualitatively similar. Cortisol is a typical glucosteroid but it has significant effect on salt and water metabolism. The term glucosteroid is itself misleading for both fat and protein metabolism are also subject to steroid influences. It is, however, convenient to separate the different but inter-related metabolic processes of these hormones.

1. Carbohydrate Metabolism

Fundamentally, the glucosteroids are insulin antagonists, although they may increase insulin secretion (Campbell and Rastogi, 1968). There are species variations in the degree of antagonism and in the manner in which it is produced. Impaired peripheral utilization and increased hepatic gluconeogenesis are two of the more important ways in which carbohydrate metabolism is altered.

Hypophysectomy in dogs causes a reduction in body glucose pool, diminished flux of glucose from the liver into the blood, and reduced uptake of glucose by peripheral tissues. Steroid administration increases the glucose pool and hepatic glucose output in these animals. However, glucosteroid excess in both hypophysectomized and normal dogs inhibits peripheral utilization, perhaps by blocking the action of insulin. This inhibition may be immediate in onset, Lecocq *et al.* (1964) found utilization to be reduced by 38% within 30 minutes of the start of a cortisol infusion in normal dogs, or delayed, requiring some time to develop in man (Mills, 1964).

Azuma and Eisenstein (1964) consider that this impairment in peripheral glucose utilization is more important than increased hepatic gluconeogenesis in the development of hyperglycemia in the dog. Basset and colleagues (1966) demonstrated that daily injections of cortisol caused hyperglycemia but no comparable depression of the rate of utilization once higher levels had been reached. Cortisol acts only to reduce utilization at low plasma glucose levels. Pugh (1968) found that the synthetic steroid prednisolone acetate reduced peripheral utilization and raised plasma glucose levels in sheep.

Kitabchi *et al.* (1968) demonstrated in man that physiological levels of glucosteroids increased blood insulin levels in response to an oral glucose load but they were unable to say whether this was a direct effect or was due to an increase in rate of intestinal absorption of glucose.

Hockaday (1965) demonstrated that an increase in blood pyruvate followed glucose and insulin infusions in adrenalectomized but not in entire cats. This can be interpreted as suggesting either that peripheral utilization is impaired after adrenalectomy or that pyruvate production from fatty acid or amino acid metabolism is increased.

The importance of impaired peripheral utilization has been stressed but hepatic gluconeogenesis from amino acids in an important factor in the development of steroid-induced hyperglycemia.

2. Fat Metabolism

Efficient fat absorption requires adrenocortical steroids, but whether or not this is a direct effect on the gut mucosa is not certain.

Glucosteroids are essential for the mobilization of FFA from peripheral tissues by norepinephrine but the mechanism is uncertain. Possibly as a result of this action, the production of ketone bodies is reduced by steroid lack.

3. Protein Metabolism

The glucosteroids are closely involved in protein metabolism. They are both anti-anabolic, i.e., they reduce synthesis, and catabolic, increasing breakdown. The ability of the liver to "trap" amino acids is increased; this reduces the amount available to the peripheral tissues. The liver channels amino acids into urea, glucose, and hepatic protein. The alimentary and urogenital tracts also accumulate nitrogen in this way, whereas the peripheral tissues lose it.

Serum proteins may also reflect the changes in metabolism. Degradation of albumin is increased (Sterling, 1960) and may exceed synthesis which is also elevated. Immune globulin concentrations are initially increased due to lysis of lymphocytes but slowly fall due to suppression of lymphocyte mitosis.

There is a marked increase in hepatic RNA and in some enzyme systems which may be increased up to 1000-fold, whereas other systems are reduced in concentration. Perhaps herein lies the main antagonism between insulin and the glucosteroids. Although insulin tends to reduce the levels of hepatic glucose-6-phosphatase, fructose-1,6-diphosphatase, and other glycogenolytic enzymes, the steroids enhance their activity.

4.   Inflammation and Immune Response

The prime therapeutic importance of the glucosteroids is the suppression of the inflammatory and immune responses.

a. CAPILLARY PERMEABILITY. Loss of fluid from the capillary is reduced by the steroids.

b. VASODILATION.   Glucosteroids prevent vasodilation by reducing histamine liberation, by increasing the vasoconstrictor effect of norepinephrine, and by reducing the liberation of the potent vasodilator kinins (Cline and Helman, 1966). These are polypeptides produced during the inflammatory process from inactive kininogens.

c. PHAGOCYTOSIS. Activity of the reticuloendothelial system is increased by small doses of glucocorticoids, but in excess they suppress phagocytosis (Nicol et al., 1965). Leukocyte diapedesis is reduced.

d. COLLAGEN FORMATION.   This is an important part of the repair process which is suppressed by glucosteroids, which may also cause dissolution of formed fibrous tissue. This may be valuable under some circumstances but it may lead to extension of local infection and prevent wound and fracture repair. Ehrlich and Hunt (1968) state that this suppression can be prevented by vitamin A.

e. ANTIBODY REACTION.   The production of antibody depends on cell division. Mitosis in lymphoid tissue is decreased and immune globulin production is reduced by excessive glucosteroids. There is a more immediate suppression of the cellular response to an antigen antibody reaction.

5.   Calcium and Phosphorus Metabolism

Calcium metabolism shows some quite marked changes in response to glucosteroids. There is a marked depression of uptake from the gut, the result of steroid inhibition of vitamin D. There is evidence also for an inhibition of parathyroid hormone action on bone but this requires further study. There is also some evidence that cortisol may interfere with the hypocalcemic effect of thyrocalcitonin on bone (Thompson et al., 1968). It is claimed that some, at least, of the bone thinning associated with hypercorticoidism arises from interference with protein metabolism, that is, bone matrix production. Cortisol suppresses renal reabsorption of phosphorus and urinary loss increases. Calcium loss is also increased.

6. Salt and Water Metabolism

Aldosterone is the hormone with the greatest effect on sodium metabolism. It stimulates the distal renal tubule to reabsorb Na^+ and to excrete K^+, H^+, NH_4^+, and Mg^{2+}. These results probably originate from an increase in synthesis of RNA and of tubular enzyme function. Cortisol and aldosterone are closely linked in electrolyte balance; for example, cortisol may enhance the kaliuresis produced by aldosterone. It may do this by causing a release of intracellular K^+. Cortisol appears to be responsible for keeping in the exchangeable pool the sodium that is retained by aldosterone activity.

The fluid retention of cardiac failure, cirrhosis, and nephrosis is usually due to secondary hyperaldosteronism together with some other, unidentified factor. It differs from the results of aldosterone administration to subjects not suffering from these conditions, in whom aldosterone has only limited effects. In "normal" subjects given aldosterone, sodium retention occurs to a limited extent only and a natriuresis develops in the face of continued aldosterone administration. This has been called the "escape" phenomenon; its mechanics are uncertain. Hyperaldosteronism is not present in all cases of fluid retention of cardiac, hepatic, or renal origin and a number of other factors have to be elucidated before the full picture is understood.

However, despite their potency, the mineralocorticoids are not always effective in correcting the alteration in the distribution of water within the body that results from overall steroid deficiency. Swingle and Swingle (1967a) showed that, in adrenalectomized dogs maintained on a high salt diet and mineralocorticoids over long periods, plasma volume was reduced to as little as 55% of the initial volume. They ascribe this change to alterations in vasoconstrictive activity of the peripheral circulation. These alterations can be corrected with glucosteroids. This hypovolemia reduces the glomerular filtration rate (GFR). Both are increased very rapidly by cortisol, too rapidly to have been brought about by salt and water retention. Water is mobilized from the intracellular to the intravascular compartment by a route that is still conjectural. Cortisol in pharmacological doses can cause so much loss of potassium in the urine that an alkalosis develops.

The glucosteroids also affect water metabolism. They increase free water clearance, that is, loss of water not associated with electrolyte excretion. They are necessary for maximum tubular impermeability to water in the absence of ADH. The increase in free water clearance has been attributed to an inhibition of ADH activity but this theory does not receive universal support.

7. Lysosomes

At least some of the influence of the glucosteroids on cellular metabolism may be stabilization of lysosomal membrane, although Cline and Helman (1966) maintain this to be pharmacological rather than physiological. The lysosomes are intracellular sacs of autolytic enzymes that escape when the cell is damaged by conditions such as endotoxin shock and ischemia.

8. Vitamin B

An interesting if somewhat unexpected interrelationship is exhibited between nicotinamide and the glucocosteroids. Greengard and colleagues (1966) demonstrated that glucosteroids would prevent the development of signs and cause remission of developed signs in dogs maintained on nictinamide-deficient diets. This may be due to the influence of the steroids on NAD in tissues.

9.   Catecholamines

The interrelationship between the adrenal cortex and medulla is important. There is convincing evidence that the metabolism of catecholamines is dependent on glucosteroids. Coupland (1968) found that corticosterone, in tissue culture, increased methylation of norepinephrine, and Wurtman *et al.* (1968) suggest that this may be achieved by induction of the enzyme which transfers the methyl group.

10.   Bone Marrow and Blood Picture

Clinically, one of the more important effects of the glucosteroids is that on the peripheral blood picture.

a. LEUKOCYTOSIS.   There is an immediate increase in the total white cell count which is more than accounted for by an increase in the neutrophil count. In man this occurs within 5 hours of prednisolone administration (Cream, 1968). The mechanism of this liberation of sequestered or marrow pool leukocytes is not clear.

b. EOSINOPENIA.   The other cell most markedly effected is the eosinophil. There is a reduction in numbers, the mechanism of which is again not fully elucidated. Archer (1963) demonstrated that in the horse there was a very close relationship between the plasma histamine level and the blood eosinophil count and argued that this was cause and effect. However, other workers have been unable to demonstrate such a simple relationship in other species. Blenkinsopp and Blenkinsopp (1967) demonstrated that dexamethasone (a synthetic glucosteroid) caused a migration of eosinophils into the reticuloendothelial system in cats, which accounted for the immediate decline in numbers. Long-term administration caused a suppression of production. Whatever its origin, the change in the eosinophil count tends to reflect, inversely, the circulating cortisol concentration.

c. LYMPHOPENIA.   Immediate lysis of lymphocytes follows an increase in plasma cortisol. This short-term action is further emphasized by the subsequent long-term effect of lymphoid suppression (Section IV,A,3).

d. MONOCYTOSIS AND BASOPHILIA.   The monocytes and basophils do not present such a consistent pattern of change. A monocytosis is the result of high circulating steroids according to Jasper and Jain (1965), while Schalm (1965) describes a basophilia accompanying hypercorticoidism.

e. RED CELL COUNT.   A single injection of a glucosteroid causes a temporary increase in erythropoiesis with an increase in red cell count, and a subsequent fall to below initial levels. Repeated injections cause a persistent elevation of red cell count. Donati and Gallagher (1968) record that a similar affect of ACTH is mediated through the adrenal cortex. The origin of the increase is uncertain. Donati and Gallagher (1968) suggest that this may be due to alterations in metabolism and increased oxygen requirement caused by steroids. If this is the case the increased red cell count may be mediated through erythropoietin. Adrenocortical failure in man causes anemia but hemoconcentration due to contraction of plasma volume in the dog masks any similar change.

11. Parturition

The importance of the intrauterine secretion of adrenocortical steroids by the fetus has been emphasized by Drost and Holm (1968) and Liggins and Kennedy (1968) who have demonstrated its role in the termination of pregnancy.

D. EXCRETION

The glucosteroids and aldosterone, together with their inactive metabolites, are excreted by both the liver and kidneys. In the plasma the active steroids are transported bound to the carrier proteins transcortin and albumin. In the liver a proportion of them is inactivated by conversion to tetrahydro derivatives and thence to 17-KS, cortol or cortolones. Both active and inactive steroids are enzymically conjugated with glucuronic or sulfuric acids. Most of the conjugates are then excreted into the bile but some reflux into the blood to be excreted in the urine. There is some enterohepatic recirculation of the steroids excreted in the bile.

The relative importance of each pathway varies between species and depends on the relative efficiency of hepatic excretion. This influences the amount of conjugate which is refluxed into the plasma, and so determines the relative amounts of protein-bound (unconjugated) and free (conjugated) steroids in the plasma.

Renal clearance is controlled by the degree of protein-binding, protein-bound steroids being retained by the glomerulus. The conjugated steroids pass readily into the glomerular filtrate. Most is excreted in the urine, but a proportion of the filtered load returns to the circulation probably by simple back diffusion in the distal tubule (Beisel et al., 1964). Deck and Siegenthaler (1967) suggest that aldosterone glucuronide is actively excreted by the proximal kidney tubule.

E. NORMAL VALUES

It is perhaps in this field that the most important recent advances have been made. With new techniques more accurate quantitative and qualitative examinations have been made of the steroid constituents of adrenal effluent blood, peripheral blood, and urine. These investigations have also been extended in their scope to include animals which may prove of value as research tools but which have been neglected until the present time. A number of indigenous Australian fauna are included in this group (Weiss and McDonald, 1965, 1966a, b, 1967).

1. Glucosteroids

Unfortunately, it is not possible to compare directly results from different groups working on the same species since different methods give different results. There is no universal agreement on the way in which the results should be presented. However, as the techniques become more specific these variations should become less and eventually be eliminated.

Cortisol and corticosterone are the steroids secreted in the highest concentration in most species. There are specific variations in the cortisol:corticosterone ratio and there may be, as there is in the dog, very marked variations between and in individuals. A circadian rhythm has been well established in some species.

In the plasma much cortisol is normally bound to an α-globulin transcortin for transport, and some may be bound to albumin (Paterson and Harrison, 1968). The remainder is "free," having been conjugated in the liver with glucuronide or sulfate. Both cortisol and aldosterone are adsorbed onto the red cell membrane. The proportion so adsorbed is a function of the hematocrit, transcortin level and steroid concentration. It is decreased in pregnancy (Bartter and Slater, 1966).

a. SHEEP.   The result of steroid assays are shown in Table II. The very high value shown by Vaughan (1965) may have been due to the stress of being handled. The fetal and neonatal lamb adrenal secretes "substantial" quantities of cortisol and corticosterone (Alexander et al., 1968).

Nonspecific chromogens, particularly bionone compounds, have presented problems in urinary steroid assays in cattle and sheep.

b. CATTLE (Table III).   Cupps (1967) was able to recover 32% of radioactivity following intramuscular injection of labeled cortisol into adrenalectomized bulls. Of this 86.3% was in the feces and 14.7% in the urine. Urinary radioactivity reached highest levels within 3–4 hours and had disappeared by 28 hours after injection. Activity appeared in the feces at about 8 hours after injection and reached a maximum by 12–14 hours. It remained steady for about 16–18 hours and then disappeared over the next 40 hours. Unger et al. (1961) emphasized the problems of interfering chromogens in cattle.

c. DOG (Table IV).   The results given by Hechter et al. (1955) represent output of the maximally stimulated gland. The proportion of cortisol bound to protein varies with the concentration, below 2 μg/100 ml, 88% is bound; at 10 μg/100 ml, only 56% is bound (Plager et al., 1963). Rijnberk et al. (1968a) have demonstrated an unequivocal circadian rhythm in six out of eight dogs. Gold (1961) showed that cortisol is excreted as cortone, β-cortolone, tetrahydrocortisol, and tetrahydrocortol in the ratio 1.4:2.0:2.2:1.2. Corticosterone is excreted in urine and feces in the ratio 5:2 (Taylor and Scratcherd, 1963). Urquhart and Li (1968) have examined meticulously the influence of ACTH on adrenocortical secretion.

d. CAT.   Cortisol and corticosterone have both been identified in plasma (Taylor and Scratcherd, 1963). Concentration of steroid metabolites are too low in cat urine to measure by the usual techniques. Those Porter-Silber chromogens present are probably not corticosteroids (Borrel, 1963a,b). At least 50% of corticosterone metabolites are excreted by the liver within 4–5 hours, only 1% may be found in the urine (Taylor and Scratcherd, 1963), about 80% of cortisone is excreted in bile, about 4% in urine (Taylor and Scratcherd, 1967).

e. HORSE.   Zolovick et al. (1966) have shown circadian rhythm in the horse; plasma cortisol and corticosterone were highest at 1000 hours with levels of up to 26.0 and 10.3 μg/100 ml, respectively, but the highest level of cortisone (140 μg/100 ml) was found at 0200 hours. The lowest level for cortisol and corticosterone corresponded with the maximum for cortisone (0200 hours), while cortisone was at low ebb at about 1500 hours. When total combined levels were considered, maximum values (395.3 μg/100 ml) were found at 1000 hours and minimum levels (219 μg/100

TABLE II   NORMAL VALUES OF PLASMA STEROIDS IN SHEEP

Parameter	Values	References
Cortisol secretion rate	1.0 mg/hr ♂ 2.5 mg/hr ♀	Vaughan (1965)
	12 μg/min 132±135 μg/hr 240±135 μg/hr when sodium depleted	Paterson and Harrison (1968) Coghlan *et al.* (1966)
Corticosterone rate	12.7±6.7 μg/hr 20.0±8.5 μg/hr when sodium depleted	Coghlan *et al.* (1966)
Plasma cortisol	18 μg/100 ml (conjugated 4.0 μg, albumin-bound 3.5 μg, transcortin-bound 10.5 μg)	Paterson and Harrison (1968)
Clearance of plasma cortisol	660 ml/min	Paterson (1963)
Body pool of cortisol	130–240 μg	Paterson (1963)

ml) at 2000 hours. Moss and Rylance (1967) did not find free cortisol in horse urine.

f. PIG (Table V).   The very high levels of plasma 17-OHCS found in newborn piglets gradually drops to "adult" levels within 12 months (Dvorak, 1967). Cortisol, cortisone and possibly tetrahydrocorticosterone, tetrahydrocortisol, and aldosterone are present in pig urine (Tegeler and Schulke, 1967). Clark *et al.* (1965) found urinary levels of 17-OHCS too low to measure in the resting animal but concentrations rose to 59 mg/24 hr after ACTH.

TABLE III   NORMAL VALUES OF PLASMA STEROIDS IN CATTLE

Parameter	Values	References
Cortisol: corticosterone ratio		
Adrenal vein	4.4±0.4	Eberhardt (1966)
After ACTH	3.1±0.5	
Jugular vein	0.85–5.94 (mean 2.4)	Estergreen and Venkataseshu (1967)
Cortisol secretion rate		Eberhardt (1966)
Adult: resting	17.0±2.5 μg/kg/hr	
Adult: after ACTH	34.4±2.5 μg/kg/hr	
Calves: resting	44.8±65.5 μg/gm gland/min	Whipp *et al.* (1967a)
Corticosterone secretion rate		
Adult: resting	4.8±1.4 μg/kg/hr	Eberhart (1966)
Adult: after ACTH	12.6±2.3 μg/kg/hr	
Calves: resting	5.6–22.1 μg/gm gland/min	Whipp *et al.* (1967a)
Plasma cortisol	3.2–13.1 μg/100 ml	Estergreen and
Corticosterone	1.5–5.1 μg/100 ml	Venkataseshu (1967)
Cortisol half-life ($T_{\frac{1}{2}}$)	ca. 10 min	Unger *et al.* (1961)

TABLE IV   NORMAL VALUES OF PLASMA AND URINARY STEROIDS IN DOGS

Parameter	Values	References[a]
	Plasma	
Cortisol: corticosterone ratio	20–0.3 (mean 3.39)	Hechter et al. (1955)
Cortisol secretion rate	55–1540 µg/gland-hr.	Hechter et al. (1955)
Coritisol and corticosterone secretion rate	924–1465 µg/gland-hr	Heap et al. (1966)
	30–160 µg/gland-hr 2 hr after hypophysectomy	
Corticosterone secretion rate	0–1130 µg/gland-hr	Hechter et al. (1955)
Cortisol half-life	104 min	Thomasson and Steenburg (1965)
Plasma cortisol (11-OHCS)		
Adrenal vein	86–330 µg/100 ml	Hechter et al. (1955)
Peripheral vein		
Resting	2–10 µg/100 ml	Eik-Nes and Brizzee (1956)
After ACTH IU	25–30 µg/100 ml	
Resting 0800 hr	1.3–9.7 (mean 4.0) µg//100 ml	Rijnberk et al. (1968a)
Resting 1700 hr	0.4–7.0 (mean 3.6) µg/100 ml	
After ACTH		
Resting	< 2.0 µg/100 ml	Plager et al. (1963) .
After ACTH	10 µg/100 ml	
	Urine	
Resting 17-OHCS	2.08 ±0.70 mg/24 hr	Siegel (1968)
Increase after ACTH	0.14–3.97 (mean 1.64) mg/24 hr	
Resting cortisol	861 ±132 µg/24 hr	Wilson et al. (1967)
After ACTH	× 1.6 × 4.0 (mean × 2.7)	
Resting 17-OHCS	0.06–0.32 (mean 0.16) mg/kg-24 hr	Rijnberk et al. (1968a)
After ACTH (50 IU per day for 4 days)	× 4–14	

[a]Earlier references have been omitted since the development of more reliable techniques has made the results no longer applicable.

TABLE V   NORMAL VALUES OF PLASMA STEROIDS IN PIGS

Parameter	Values	References
Plasma 17-OHCS	21.8 ±6.4 µg/100 ml	Topel and Merkel (1967)
Resting		
11-OHCS	6.5–8.6 µg/100 ml	Donald et al. (1968)
1st 24 hr	43.9 ± 9.3 µg/100 ml	Dvorak (1967)
31–45 days	11.5 ± 5.5 µg/100 ml	
12 months	5.1–5.5 µg/100 ml	
Cortisol and corticosterone secretion rates (7—9 weeks old)	945–1270 µg/gm gland-hr	Heap et al. (1966)

2. Oxosteroids (Ketosteroids)

In man the excretion of 17-oxosteroids is used as a measure of androgen secretion since testosterone is excreted in this form. In the dog, some small portion of testosterone may be excreted in this form but the majority is not. We await clarification of significance of these steroids in this species. There is no sex difference. Rijnberk *et al.* (1968a) reported values ranging from 0.02–0.24 (mean 0.06) mg/kg-24 hr and Adlin and Channick (1966) found 0.8–1.2 (mean 1.0) mg/24 hr.

Clark *et al.* (1965) demonstrated marked qualitative and quantitative variations in 17-oxosteroid excretion in entire male and female pigs. Orchidectomized animals of both sexes have similar 17-oxosteroid excretion.

In addition to the major steroids there are numerous others which have been demonstrated in trace concentrations in either peripheral or adrenal vein blood (Oertel and Eik-Nes, 1962). At the moment and with no evidence to the contrary it is assumed that these traces are escaped precursors of the physiologically important end products. This is only an assumption and it may yet be shown that these apparently insignificant compounds have some specific function of their own.

3. Mineralocorticoids

Aldosterone is probably the most potent of all the adrenal steroids. It is present in adrenal effluent blood in all species which have been investigated but there are few data about its concentration.

a. SHEEP. In the resting sodium-replete state sheep secrete aldosterone at 0.71 ± 0.41 μg/min. When sodium-depleted the rate rises to 1.7 ± 0.41 μg/min (Coghlan *et al.*, 1966).

b. CATTLE. Normal calves secrete 0.08 ± 0.03 μg/min-gland. After 14 days of negative sodium balance the rate rises to 1.06 ± 0.90 μg/min-gland (Whipp *et al.*, 1967b).

c. DOGS. Following laparotomy to induce Goldblatt hypertension, dogs excreted 29.1 ± 7.0 μg/24 hr. One week later this figure had declined to 8.6 ± 1.1 μg/24 hr. After hypertension was established, excretion was 14.5 ± 2.7 μg/24 hr.

Hechter *et al.* (1955) demonstrated a very wide range (0–236 μg/hr) in "electrocortin" secretion; adrenal venous blood concentrations ranged from 10–65 μg/100 ml.

F. DISEASE

Aldosterone has not yet been shown to play a major role in disease in domestic animals. In man primary and secondary aldosteronism both exist. The former, due to an aldosterone-secreting tumor, is characterized by fluid retention, hypokalemia, and an increase in exchangeable body sodium. Serum sodium levels may not be altered. Secondary aldosteronism contributes to the fluid retention of congestive heart disease, cirrhosis, and nephrosis. Primary aldosteronism has not been reported in animals. All the syndromes which in man are associated with secondary aldosteronism occur in domestic animals but aldosterone secretion in them has not yet been evaluated. Severe sodium deficiency may develop in cattle grazing in areas of low pasture sodium. This has been demonstrated to occur on the high plains of

Victoria, Australia. Similar but less marked deficiencies may be seen on pastures irrigated with low sodium water (river water). Under these conditions urinary salt loss in minimal and the salivary Na:K drops; both are indications of increased aldosterone secretion. Hypertrophy of the zona glomerulosa has been associated with salt-deficient diets.

Evidence of biochemical changes in endocrine disease is almost entirely confined to the dog and unless specifically stated otherwise all the following comments concern alterations in glucosteroid metabolism in this species.

1. Plasma Cortisol Levels

The wide variations found in normal resting values make it hard to say what plasma cortisol concentrations constitute abnormal levels. There are relatively few assays of plasma cortisol in disease states.

In cases of hyperadrenocorticoidism Wilkinson et al. (1965) found values between 0.8 and 14.2 μg cortisol/100 ml; Capen et al. (1967) between 16.1 and 20.5 (mean 18.8) μg total serum corticosteroids/100 ml; and Rijnberk et al. (1968b) between 4.5 and 22.2 μg 17-β-OHCS/100 ml.

No values have been published for plasma cortisol in adrenal insufficiency.

The levels of plasma cortisol reached in response to ACTH stimulation are perhaps more meaningful. Wilkinson et al. (1965) showed a rise in plasma cortisol from 0.8 to 22 μg/100 ml in a dog with proven adrenocortical hyperplasia following intramuscular ACTH. This increase was as much as that achieved by Eik-Nes and Brizzee (1956) by intravenous injection of ACTH in the normal dog. Rijnberk et al. (1968b) did not report plasma levels following ACTH stimulation in their cases.

2. Urinary Steroids

Values for urinary steroids in disease continue to accumulate, but because of differences in methods and nomenclature, and inadequate series of normal values for the different methods, it is not easy to compare results from case to case.

In most, though not all, cases of adrenocortical hyperfunction, resting values are above the normal range. In one case of adrenocortical hyperfunction Schwartzman and Fegley (1965) found values for 17-KS above 1.0 mg/24 hr in seven out of twelve samples of urine collected, and values for 17-OHCS above 1.0 mg/24 hr in two out of twelve samples. The normal values for their laboratory are 0.01–1.0 mg 17–KS/24 hr and 0.1–1.0 mg 17-OHCS/24 hr. Capen et al. (1967), in a series of cases, found resting urinary steroid values of from 2.8 to 18.2 (mean 10.7) mg 17-OHCS/24 hr, but they reported no comparable normal values.

Again the better test is one which measures the increase in output of steroids following ACTH administration. There is a much greater response from cases of adrenal hyperplasia and from some cases of adrenocortical tumor than there is in the normal dog. After ACTH, urinary steroid excretion in adrenal hyperfunction may increase from normal resting limits by as much as eightfold. Wilson et al. (1967) found an increase in Porter-Silber chromogens from 89 to 740 μg/kg-24 hr. However, neither these authors nor Siegel et al. (1967) were able to demonstrate a satisfactory response to ACTH stimulation in cases with functional adrenocortical carcinoma. In all these cases, however, resting levels of steroid excretion were very high. In such tumors in man normal secretion is usually independent of ACTH control and thus significant urinary steroid increases following ACTH administration are unlikely.

Marshak *et al.* (1960) reported a value of 1.2 mg α-ketolic steroids/24 hr in a case of adrenocortical failure (normal 2.2 mg/24 hr). The diagnosis was confirmed by failure to elicit any increase in secretion with injected ACTH.

To summarize, high resting levels of plasma or urinary 17-OHCS are strongly indicative of adrenal hyperfunction. Resting values for plasma 17-OHCS may be normal in adrenal hyperfunction, but response to ACTH is usually excessive. Resting values for urinary 17-OHCS may be normal or increased, depending partly on the method of estimation used. An excessive response to ACTH is confirmatory. Conversely, low resting values in plasma and urine, and a reduced response to ACTH are found in adrenal hypofunction. The interpretation of dexamethasone suppression and 11-hydroxylation suppression tests, which involve urinary steroid assays are discussed in Section VI,B,C.

3. Salt and Water Metabolism

It is not always possible to differentiate between the effects of the pituitary and the adrenal on water metabolism. A pituitary tumor may interfere with ADH secretion as well as with control of cortisol secretion. This may be demonstrable by the ADH (vasopressin) test (Section VI,D). In primary adrenal hyperfunction the response to exogenous ADH is much less marked. Regardless of origin, however, cases of hypercorticoidism produce urine of low specific gravity, because of the increase in free water clearance which the glucosteroids induce. Some samples may be at the low end of the normal range ($\simeq$ 1018), whereas others are well into the diabetes insipidus range ($<$ 1005). In adrenocortical insufficiency there is a negative water balance with dehydration, hemoconcentration, and a concentrated urine.

Alterations in plasma Na^+ and K^+ levels are of little diagnostic significance in hyperfunctional states, although, terminally, marked alterations may occur (Wilkinson *et al.*, 1965; Rijnberk *et al.*, 1968b). It is worth commenting here that plasma Na^+ levels show a very wide normal range in cattle, and are therefore of little diagnostic value. In adrenal hypofunction plasma Na^+ and K^+ values may not be outside the normal range but the normal Na:K ratio of 30:1 falls terminally to as low as 12:1. Plasma Na^+ levels as low as 100 mEq/liter and plasma K^+ levels up to 8.0 mEq/liter have, however, been found. This level of plasma K^+ is toxic to the myocardium and produces diagnostic alterations in the electrocardiogram. Seiber (1964) described a case of pituitary hypofunction in which a high plasma K^+ reflected the lack of ACTH, but plasma Na^+ was also high.

Low plasma bicarbonate and chloride values are also found since both these are lost in the urine with sodium.

4. Calcium and Magnesium Metabolism

Alterations in calcium metabolism are said to occur in adrenal hyperfunction. The occurrence of calcinosis cutis in dogs with adrenal hyperplasia would support this, although the lesion may be a manifestation of calciphylaxis (Selye, 1962) and not an alteration in overall calcium metabolism. Hypercalcemia is found regularly in experimentally adrenalectomized dogs and cats (Walser *et al.*, 1963) although it is not very prominent in the spontaneous disease.

Wilkinson *et al.* (1965) found two of fifteen samples from eight cases of adrenal hyperfunction to have plasma Ca^{2+} levels above, and four below the normal range. In a cow with suspected adrenal hypofunction secondary to pituitary failure J. R. Howard *et al.* (1968) reported fluctuating plasma Ca^{2+} levels. On 2 days these reached the extraordinarily high levels of 20.8 and 15.5 mg/100 ml. There was also a severe hypoproteinemia at one stage of the disease. Unfortunately no estimations of plasma cortisol, Na^+ or K^+ were made.

Hypomagnesemia is also found in experimentally adrenalectomized dogs (Walser *et al.*, 1963) but the reverse was found in all of twelve samples from eight cases of hyperfunction (Wilkinson *et al.*, 1965).

Osteoporosis is a common finding in Cushing's syndrome in man, but it is only rarely recorded in the dog. Its origin has not been fully elucidated (Riggs *et al.*, 1966) but it may be due to disturbances of calcium balance or alterations in protein metabolism.

5.   Carbohydrate Metabolism

With few exceptions (Jackson, 1960) hyperglycemia is found in all cases of corticoid excess; it may progress to frank diabetes. In the dog primary adrenocortical insufficiency leads to increased insulin sensitivity but hypoglycemia does not always follow. Hypophysectomized dogs succumb to hypoglycemia if not treated (Houssay, 1965); however, in untreated bilaterally adrenalectomized dogs the blood glucose level falls but it does not reach hypoglycemic levels (Swingle and Swingle, 1967b). This suggests that GH is more important than glucosteroids in glucose homeostasis.

The hypoglycemia of newborn piglets cannot be explained in terms of steroid lack since high plasma steroid levels are found immediately after birth. However, these levels may well contribute to the problem by reducing peripheral utilization of glucose and thus exacerbating any existing tissue deficit.

6.   Fat Metabolism

Accumulation of fat in the liver is a frequent if not invariable autopsy finding in adrenal hyperfunction. This may be due to excess ACTH causing an excessive peripheral lipolysis with resynthesis in the liver, or it may be due to excessive glucosteroid depression of lipoprotein synthesis.

Plasma cholesterol values are altered in many endocrine diseases. Adrenal hyperfunction is, with rare exceptions, accompanied by raised plasma levels. This may reflect reduced TSH secretion in a gland compressed by neoplastic tissue.

7.   Protein Metabolism

With the exception of some enzymes there is little biochemical evidence of altered protein metabolism in adrenal hyperfunction, although osteoporosis and muscular weakness is attributed to the marked protein antianabolic or catabolic effect of glucosteroids. In those cases in which they have been assayed serum proteins have shown no significant change.

a. SERUM ALKALINE PHOSPHATASE. This enzyme has been in the author's experience, invariably elevated to quite remarkable levels in adrenal hyperfunction. This may be due either to increased production consequent on enzyme induction, or to failure of excretion by the fatty liver.

b. SERUM GLUTAMIC PYRUVATE TRANSAMINASE (ALANINE AMINOTRANSFERASE). Enzyme induction of glutamic pyruvate transaminase in liver tissue has been shown to result from steroid administration. The raised serum values not infrequently seen in adrenal hyperfunction may arise from this, or from liver damage due to fat accumulation.

c. BLOOD UREA NITROGEN. BUN levels terminally exceed 100 mg/100 ml in most cases of adrenocortical failure, values in other conditions are not altered. This high value is due to decreased renal blood flow resulting from the decrease in plasma volume which, experimentally, may fall to 50% of the normal value.

8. Peripheral Blood Picture

The effect of steroids on the blood picture has been mentioned in Section IV,D, 10. The "hemogram of stress" is quite distinctive. There is a well-developed leukocytosis and the differential count reveals a neutrophilia, a lymphopenia, and usually an eosinopenia. The monocytosis and basophilia noted by Jasper and Jain (1965) and Schalm (1965), respectively, are not commonly reported by other authors.

Changes in the red cell picture do not appear to be of any great significance. The decrease in plasma volume in adrenal failure is due to loss of fluid only, the hematocrit and hemoglobin level are therefore increased. A true polycythemia may or may not occur in adrenal hyperfunction.

9. Reproductive Function

Van Rensburg (1965), in reviewing adrenal function and fertility, mentioned that an enhanced plasma cortisol response to ACTH had been described in habitually aborting Angora goats, and the fetuses showed adrenal hyperplasia. He also commented that in cattle cystic ovaries had been associated with adrenal hyperplasia.

An association between the zona glomerulosa and fertility has been remarked upon (Cupps et al., 1964) in cattle. Testicular degeneration and zona glomerulosa hypertrophy were found in sixteen bulls. It is interesting to speculate that, since the pineal has been associated with gonadotropic and glomerulotropic function there may be a common pineal origin for these two lesions.

Holm et al. (1961) investigated the prolonged gestation syndrome in Friesian cattle and demonstrated adrenal insufficiency.

G. EFFECTS OF PROLONGED GLUCOSTEROID ADMINISTRATION

Glucosteroids are being used therapeutically more frequently and in higher doses. The peripheral blood levels produced are pharmacological and are much higher than any physiological levels. This may have severe effects upon the control of endogenous ACTH and glucosteroids. The production of CRF is depressed and protein synthesis both in the adenohypophysis and adrenal cortex is suppressed. Higher doses and longer therapy increase the degree of suppression. This has been well established in man and is also of importance in domestic animals. It is possible to produce an easily recognizable fully developed adrenocortical hypercorticoidism (Cushing's syndrome) by sufficiently prolonged steroid therapy. An equally serious complication is the likelihood of adrenocortical collapse occurring during or after any "stress" such as surgery in any patient who has received more than minimal steroid therapy (Foord, 1967).

V.   HORMONES OF THE ADRENAL MEDULLA

A. SITE OF PRODUCTION

The adrenal medulla is the main site of production of the catecholamines, although in man at least, there are small extramedullary glands which also produce epinephrine and norepinephrine. It is probable that the two hormones are produced by different cells. In cattle the medulla can be divided into outer epinephrine-rich and inner norepinephrine-rich zones (Zamora et al., 1967).

B. CONTROL

1.   Tropic Hormone

There appears to be no tropic hormone involved.

2.   Neural Control

Control of the adrenal medulla is primarily neural. Like the cortex, however, the medulla is influenced by the hypothalamus which receives stimuli from the cerebral cortex and ascending tracts in the spinal cord. Innervation to the medulla is from spinal nerves $T_{10}-T_{13}$. Acetylcholine from the preganglionic neurones stimulates the cells to liberate epinephrine or norepinephrine. The manner in which one hormone rather than the other is released has not been demonstrated. *In vivo* pain, rage, fear, and cold will all enhance liberation of catecholamines.

3.   Feedback Mechanisms

Norepinephrine synthesis is self-limiting in splenic nerve preparations (Stjärne et al., 1967). This may apply to the adrenal medulla *in vivo*.

C. ACTIONS

The actions of the hormones of the adrenal medulla are aimed at increasing survival at times of stress. They enhance muscular activity both skeletal and myocardial, enabling the animal to either fight or flee. They also mobilize both glucose and fatty acids making both readily available for energy. Basal metabolism is enhanced in a manner which simulates the thyroid hormone. There is an increase in hepatic heat production which is due to the increased metabolism of lactate following glycogenolysis.

Their functions differ only quantitatively. Norepinephrine has a much greater vasoconstricting effect than epinephrine and will thus elevate blood pressure to a greater extent. Increase in cardiac output, elevation of basal metabolic rate, and bronchial dilation are greater following epinephrine.

1. Glycogenolysis

Epinephrine causes hyperglycemia by rapid mobilization of glycogen. One of the enzymes necessary for this process is a phosphorylase which may be present in the inactive form. Epinephrine activates this through 3′,5′-AMP, probably by increasing adenylcyclase activity. Muscle phosphorylase is also activated but muscle glycogenolysis does not contribute directly to the hyperglycemia. The enzyme necessary for the final step in glucose formation is absent and glucose-6-phosphate is metabolized to lactate. This enters the circulation and may be converted to glucose in the liver or used by the heart for energy.

Neural as well as humoral factors may be involved in hepatic glycogenolysis.

2. Lipolysis

Epinephrine and norepinephrine have roughly equivalent lipolytic actions. They cause a considerable increase in plasma FFA. This lipolysis is mediated through increased adenylcyclase levels and therefore elevated 3′,5′-AMP.

3. Electrolytes

Epinephrine causes an increase in plasma Mg^{2+} (Lavor, 1968) but not plasma Ca^{2+} levels (Shim et al., 1968), although plasma phosphorus levels are decreased.

4. Peripheral Blood Picture

a. RED CELLS. Epinephrine causes an immediate increase in red cell count, hematocrit, and hemoglobin concentration. It has been said that this is due to expulsion of the cells from the spleen, but since the plasma protein concentration increases to the same extent as the other factors it is probably due to a shift in water from the intra- to the extravascular compartment.

b. WHITE CELLS. Epinephrine causes a neutropenia which is due to a fall in eosinophils. This eosinopenia does not occur in the absence of glucosteroids.

D. EXCRETION

In man, epinephrine and norepinephrine are degraded to metanephrine and normetanephrine. These may be converted to vanillyl mandelic acid (VMA) which is then excreted in the urine, or conjugated in the liver and excreted in the bile and urine.

E. Normal Values

There is very little information about circulating levels of the medullary hormones in domestic animals or of their excretory products in urine.

Basal epinephrine secretion in the dog averages 7.5 ± 0.01 mg/gland-kg-min and will rise to 31.9 ± 6.1 mg/gland-kg-min following insulin hypoglycemia (Wurtmann et al., 1968).

F. Disease

Excessive production of catecholamines may be due to a pheochromocytoma, a neoplasm which has yet to be diagnosed antemortem in domestic animals. R. H. Roth et al. (1968) suggest that there is a failure in the feedback mechanism in functional tumors of the adrenal medulla.

Retrospective evidence of functional pheochromocytomas is adduced by E. B. Howard and Nielsen (1965) in the dog and Wright and Conner (1968) in cattle. As the condition has not been diagnosed antemortem, no clinical pathology has been described, but the signs to be expected are intermittent hyperglycemia and glycosuria with neutropenia and an increase in plasma FFA.

VI. TESTS OF FUNCTION

A. Thorn Test

The Thorn test has several variations, it is usually based on the eosinopenic response to increased peripheral levels of adrenal glucosteroids but other responses are sometimes used. Administration of ACTH by all routes has been advocated; eosinophil counts are made prior to and at 4 and 7 hours after the dose. The test has been evaluated in dogs (Freudiger, 1958; Martin et al., 1954), cattle (Pehrson and Wallin, 1966; Forenbacher, 1963), horses (Forenbacher, 1963), and pigs (Forenbacher, 1963). A decline in eosinophils of about 70% indicated normal function, a fall of 20% or less is diagnostic of adrenocortical failure. Tests giving intermediate values should be repeated. Occasionally intramuscular ACTH is destroyed and no response is obtained; this can be eliminated by using an intravenous preparation.

The use of eosinopenic response has two drawbacks.

1.   An eosinophilia does not invariably accompany adrenocortical failure and the test may have too low a baseline for a significant fall to be achieved.

2.   The eosinophil count is not related to the plasma cortisol level when this is low.

Hortling et al. (1964) investigated the Thorn test in man and demonstrated that when plasma levels exceeded 25–30 μg/100 ml there was in inverse relationship but when the level of the circulating cortisol was normal or low no such correlation existed. Other responses to ACTH are frequently better. Where they can be estimated, much more satisfactory results can be obtained by using the level of urinary steroid excretion before and after ACTH administration. There is a considerable range over which the urinary steroids may be increased and there may be some overlap between diseased states and normal responses, but it is anticipated that the majority of cases of abnormal function would lie outside the normal range (Section IV,C,D).

1. Cattle

Pehrson and Wallin (1966) concluded that an intravenous infusion of 200 IU of ACTH would produce in normal cattle:

1. a 50% decrease in circulating eosinophils;
2. a 100% increase in neutrophils;
3. an increase of at least 10% in total white cell count; and
4. an increase in blood glucose level of at least 5 mg/100 ml.

They based the preinjection values on the mean of two samples. They bled two or three times over 6–10 hours after the injection. If two criteria are not fulfilled the test should be repeated, if three are missing then adrenocortical failure is likely, although failure of all four is, of course, a better indication. The test may be used to assess the adrenal component of sterility. Sybesma and Van der Veen (1962) used 80 units of a depot preparation and took a 60% decrease in eosinophils to indicate normal function.

2. Dog

In the dog the test is usually confined to an eosinophil count. Two samples are taken at a 30-minute interval to assess resting eosinophil levels. Either 0.1–0.5 IU ACTH/kg or a standard dose of 20 USP units (Siegel and Belshaw, 1968) intramuscularly is then given and blood samples collected for total eosinophil counts at 4 and 7 hours later. In the dog basal levels of plasma cortisol are much lower than those found in man and values as high as 25–30 μg/100 ml may not always be achieved. Plager et al. (1963) showed an increase to only 12 μg/100 ml and Eik-Nes and Brizzee (1956) gave 27 $\pm$ 0.42 μg/100 ml as the value obtained 2 hours following an intravenous injection of ACTH.

Adrenalin is necessary in the dog for the test to function, and although medullary tissue is usually present in the common form of adrenocortical failure, it may also have been destroyed. This presents yet another complicating factor in interpreting the results (Henry et al., 1953).

The Thorn test may be used to differentiate between primary and secondary failure. Where the disease is adrenal in origin there is unlikely to be any response to exogenous ACTH but where the condition arises from a lack of ACTH then the gland will respond to exogenous ACTH. In the dog, however, where adrenocortical atrophy has been induced by prolonged medication with steroids, then cortical response to ACTH may be markedly reduced (Wilson et al., 1967) and in man some cases of panhypopituitarism show a similar refractoriness to ACTH stimulation (Chakmakjian et al., 1968).

B. Mepyrapone Test of Adenohypophysial Function

This test is used to assess anterior pituitary function and depends on normal adrenocortical function. An intrinsic step in the production of glucosteroids is the 11-hydroxylation of cortisone precursors, more specifically 11-deoxycortisol.

Mepyrapone selectively blocks this process and the precursors accumulate and are liberated into the circulation. They do not inhibit ACTH production as cortisol does and this leads to increased production of ACTH. This stimulates more active steroidogenesis up to the stage of 11-hydroxylation with increased excretion of androgens which may be measured as 17-ketosteroids.

One or two 24-hour samples of urine are collected for 24–48 hours prior to administration of 50 mg mepyrapone/lb orally and 24-hour samples of urine collected for 2 days afterward. This usually produces an increase over baseline values of 17-KGS of about 1.6 mg in the first and about 2.3 mg in the second 24-hour period (Siegel and Belshaw, 1968). A poor response, that is little or no increase, usually indicates an inability of the pituitary to produce more ACTH, that is, hypopituitarism. A poor response will also be given by some adrenocortical neoplasms which have escaped from ACTH control (Siegel and Belshaw, 1968).

As with many of these investigations there are indications that all is not as simple as it seems. Adlin and Channick (1966) investigated the result of prolonged mepyrapone administration in dogs and showed that when there was an increase in urinary steroid excretion it was of the order of 100% (from 1.0 to 2.0 mg/24 hr), but that a number of animals showed no response. It must be emphasized, however, that they were using 17-KS estimation not a 17-KGS method.

C. Dexamethasone Suppression Test

The synthetic steroid dexamethasone is a potent suppressor of ACTH release. This action is used to assess the part played by ACTH in cases of adrenal hyperfunction.

In the normal animal dexamethasone administration (0.5 mg/kg, 6-hourly in man) blocks ACTH release and therefore causes a drop in adrenocortical secretion. Suppression also occurs in adrenocortical hyperplasia secondary to adenohypophysial overactivity if sufficiently large doses (2.0 mg/kg every 6 hours) are given. If no suppression occurs it is assumed that the adrenal cortex is not responsive to ACTH. The likeliest cause of such autonomous secretion is neoplasia. Kendall and Sloop (1968), however, have described in man an adrenocortical tumor which was dexamethasone-suppressible.

1. Dog

Baseline urinary 17-OHCS (or 17-KGS) assays are made for 24 or 48 hours before the test; 1–2 mg (depending upon body weight) of dexamethasone is given four times daily for 3 days and urine collected over the three 24-hour periods. Plasma cortisol levels may also be estimated. In most cases of ACTH-dependent adrenal hyperfunction both urinary 17-OHCS and plasma cortisol are reduced by the third day. Autonomous tumors show no such response and occasionally hyperplasia gives inconsistent results (Rijnberk et al., 1968b).

D. Tests of Water Turnover or Posterior Pituitary Function

1. Water Deprivation Test

This test is designed to measure the degree of urinary concentration achieved in response to dehydration and may be carried out in two ways.

a. SET TIME OF DEPRIVATION.   In this test the animal is allowed water and food *ad lib.* for 24 hours. The bladder is then emptied by catheterization if necessary and the specific gravity of the urine noted. All water is withdrawn for the period of the test, usually 12–24 hours. At the end of this period the bladder is again emptied, and finally 1 hour later the patient is once more catheterized. The specific gravity of this last sample is compared with that of the first. A significant increase in concentration suggests the presence of endogenous ADH and the ability of the tubule to react to it; a failure to concentrate argues absence of ADH or failure of the tubules to react.

b. CONTROLLED WEIGHT LOSS.   The previous test takes no account of variations in severity of disease and may subject some patients to little, but others extreme, distress. A test which depends on the loss of a fixed amount of fluid uses as its endpoint a factor which is physiologically related to the disease process.

Barlow and de Wardener (1959) uses a loss of 3% of the body weight as the endpoint in the human and a similar endpoint is advised for use in veterinary medicine. This test has the disadvantage that it requires more frequent catheterization and weighing (usually at hourly intervals, although this depends on the rapidity with which weight is being lost). Failure to concentrate significantly when this amount of dehydration has occurred is interpreted in the same way as in the set time test. An increase in specific gravity of 0.005 or less should be considered an inadequate response.

2.   ADH (Vasopressin) Test

The corollary to the water deprivation test is the ADH test. Failure to concentrate under the stress of water deprivation is due to a lack of endogenous ADH or to an inability of the tubules to respond. In any subject who fails to concentrate, the next step is to administer ADH. This is available in three forms, as aqueous or oily solutions and as a snuff. Either injectable form may be used in this test (dose 1.0 unit/kg body weight). If the aqueous solution is used then urine samples must be taken at hourly intervals for 4 hours after inoculation; if the oily solution is used in this test, samples should be taken at 8, 12, 16, and 24 hours. As vasopressin is a labile drug, if one dose fails to show satisfactory concentration the test should be repeated using a fresh solution or a larger dose. If there is concentration of more than 0.005 then diabetes insipidus has been proven. If there is no response then a tubular defect exists. In man, nephrogenic diabetes insipidus has been described but this has yet to be demonstrated in the dog.

REFERENCES

Adlin, E. V., and Channick, B. J. (1966). *Endocrinology* **78**, 511.
Alexander, D. P., Wintour, E. M., Britton, H. G., James, V. H. I., Nixon, D. A., Parker, R. A., and Wright, R. D. (1968). *J. Endocrinol.* **40**, 1.
Alvarez-Buylla, R., and Alvarez-Buylla, E. R. (1964). *Acta Physiol. Latinoam.* **14**, 245.
Alvarez-Buylla, R., and Alvarez-Buylla, E. R. (1967). *Acta Physiol. Latinoam.* **17**, 253.
Alvarez-Buylla, R., and Alvarez-Buylla, E. R. (1968a). *Acta Physiol. Latinoam.* **18**, 7.

Alvarez-Buylla, R., and Alvarez-Buylla, E. R. (1968b). *Acta Physiol. Latinoam.* **18**, 13.

Annis, J. R. (1960). *Vet. Med.* **55**, 35.

Archer, R. K. (1963). "The Eosinophil Leucocytes," pp. 71–80. Blackwell, Oxford.

Armstrong, J. McD., Bornstein, J., Ng, F. M., and Taft, H. P. (1969). *Brit. Med. J.* **1**, 157.

Azuma, T., and Eisenstein, A. B. (1964). *Endocrinology* **75**, 521.

Backstrom, G. (1963). *Nord. Veterinarmed.* **15**, 778.

Baker, E. (1955). *J. Am. Vet. Med. Assoc.* **126**, 468.

Barlow, E. D., and de Wardener, H. E. (1959). *Quart. J. Med.* **28**, 235.

Bartter, F. C., and Slater, J. D. H. (1966). *J. Physiol. (London)* **184**, 29P.

Bassett, J. M., and Wallace, A. L. C. (1966). *Metab., Clin. Exptl.* **15**, 935.

Bassett, J. M., Mills, S. L., and Reid, R. L. (1966). *Metab., Clin. Exptl.* **15**, 922.

Beisel, W. R., Cos, J. J., Horton, R., Chao, P. Y., and Forsham, P. H. (1964). *J. Clin. Endocrinol. Metab.* **24**, 887.

Blair-West, J. R., Coghlan, J. P., Denton, D. A., Goding, J. R., Wintour, E. M., and Wright, R. D. (1968). *Australian J. Exptl. Biol. Med. Sci.* **46**, 295.

Blenkinsopp, E. C., and Blenkinsopp, W. (1967). *J. Endocrinol.* **37**, 463.

Borrell, S. (1963a). *Biochem. J.* **89**, 51.

Borrell, S. (1963b). *Biochem. J.* **89**, 54.

Brandt, A. J. (1940). *Skand. Veterinartidskr.* **30**, 877.

Brook, A. H., Radford, H. M., and Stacy, B. D. (1968). *J. Physiol. (London)* **197**, 723.

Cameron, E. H. C., and Grant, J. K. (1967). *J. Endocrinol.* **37**, 413.

Campbell, J., and Rastogi, K. S. (1966). *Diabetes* **15**, 30.

Campbell, J., and Rastogi, K. S. (1968). *Can. J. Biochem. Physiol.* **46**, 421.

Campbell, J., Chaikoff, L., Wrenshall, G. A., and Zemel, R. (1959). *Can. J. Biochem. Physiol.* **37**, 1313.

Capen, C. C., Martin, S. L., and Koestner, A. (1967). *Pathol. Vet. (Basel)* **4**, 301.

Chakmakjian, Z. H., Nelson, D. H., and Bethune, J. E. (1968). *J. Clin. Endocrinol. Metab.* **28**, 259.

Chrétien, M., and Li, C. H. (1967). *Can. J. Biochem.* **45**, 1163.

Clark, A. R., Raeside, J. I., and Solomon, S. (1965). *Endocrinology* **76**, 427.

Cline, M. J., and Helman, K. L. (1966). *Science* **153**, 1135.

Coffin, D. L., and Munson, T. D. (1953). *J. Am. Vet. Med. Assoc.* **123**, 402.

Coghlan, J. P., Wintour, M., and Scoggins, B. A. (1966). *Australian J. Exptl. Biol. Med. Sci.* **44**, 639.

Coupland, R. E. (1968). *J. Endocrinol.* **41**, 487.

Craig, P. (1964). Personal communication.

Cream, J. J. (1968). *Brit. J. Haematol.* **15**, 259.

Cupps, P. T. (1967). *J. Dairy Sci.* **50**, 992.

Cupps, P. T., Laben, R. C., Fowler, M. E., and Briggs, J. R. (1964). *J. Dairy Sci.* **47**, 433.

Deck, K. A., and Siegenthaler, W. E. (1967). *Acta Endocrinol.* **55**, 648.

Dev. V. G. (1965). Ph.D. Thesis, University of Missouri.

Donald, R. A., Murphy, S. S., and Nabarro, J. D. N. (1968). *J. Endocrinol.* **41**, 509.

Donati, R. M., and Gallagher, N. I. (1968). *Med. Clin. N. Am.* **52**, 231.

Drost, M., and Holm. L. W. (1968). *J. Endocrinol.* **40**, 293.

Dvorak, M. (1967). *Vet. Med. (Prague)* **12**, 43.

Eberhart, R. J. (1966). Ph.D. Thesis, Pennsylvania State University.

Ehrlich, H. P., and Hunt, T. K. (1968). *Ann. Surg.* **167**, 324.

Eik-Nes, K., and Brizzee, K. R. (1956). *Am. J. Physiol.* **84**, 371.

Eisenstein, A. B. (1967). "The Adrenal Cortex" Churchill, London.

Eriksson, K., Dyrendahl, S., and Grimfelt, D. (1956). *Nord. Veterinarmed.* **8**, 807.

Estergreen, V. L., and Venkataseshu, G. K. (1967). *Steroids* **10**, 83.

Farrel, G. (1960). *Circulation* **21**, 1009.

Foley, C. W. (1956). *J. Animal Sci.* **15**, 1217.

Foord, H. E. (1967). *Vet. Record* **80**, 242.

Forenbacher, S. (1963). *Proc. 17th World Vet. Congr.,* (1963) Vol. 2, p. 1209, Hanover.

Fourman, J., and Kennedy, G. C. (1966). *J. Endocrinol.* **35**, 173.

Freudiger, U. (1958). *Schweiz. Arch. Tierheilk.* **100**, 320.

Freudiger, U., and Lindt, S. (1958a). *Schweiz. Arch. Tierheilk.* **100**, 362.

Freudiger, U., and Lindt, S. (1958b). *Schweiz. Arch. Tierheilk.* **100**, 428.

Gans, J. H. (1964). *Am. J. Vet. Res.* **25**, 918.

Gans, J. H. and Butz, R. L. (1964). *Am. J. Vet. Res.* **25**, 1695.

Girard, J., and Greenwood, F. C. (1968). *J. Endocrinol.* **40**, 493.

Glick, S. M. (1968). *Ann. N. Y. Acad. Sci.* **148**, 471.

Gold, N. I. (1961). *J. Biol. Chem* **236**, 1924.

Goudie, R. B., McDonald, E., Anderson, J. R., and Gray, K. (1968). *Clin. Exptl. Immunol.* **3**, 119.

Greengard, P., Sigg, E. B., Fratta, I., and Zak, S. B. (1966). *J. Pharmacol. Exptl. Therap.* **154**, 624.

Groen, J. J., Frenkel, H. S., and Offerhaus, L. (1964). *Diabetes* **13**, 492.

Hall, P. F., and Young, D. G. (1968). *Endocrinology* **82**, 559.

Hare, T. (1932). *Proc. Roy. Soc. Med.* **25**, 1493.

Harris, G. W., and Donovan, B. T. (1966). "The Pituitary Gland," 3 vols. Butterworth, London and Washington, D.C

Heap, R. B., Holzbauer, M., and Newport, H. M. (1966). *J. Endocrinol.* **36**, 159.

Hechter, O., Macchi, I. A., Korman, H., Frank, E. D., and Frank, H. A. (1955). *Am. J. Physiol.* **182**, 29.

Henry, W. L., Oliver, L., and Rainey, E. R. (1953). *Federation Proc.* **12**, 66.

Hockaday, T. D. R. (1965). *J. Endocrinol.* **65**, 163.

Hoe, C. M. (1961). Thesis, Fellowship of Royal College of Veterinary Surgeons.

Holm, L. W., Parker, H. R., and Galligan, S. J. (1961). *Am. J. Obstet. Gynecol.* **81**, 1000.

Hortling, H., Pekkarinen, A., and Puupponen, E. (1964). *Acta Endocrinol.* **47**, 209.

Houssay, B. A. (1965) Personal communication.

Howard, E. B., and Nielsen, S. W. (1965). *J. Am. Vet. Med. Assoc.* **147**, 245.

Howard, J. R., Adams, W., and Sloss, M. W. (1968). *J. Am. Vet. Med. Assoc.* **152**, 17.

Jackson, R. (1960). *Rocky Mountain Vet.* **8**, 12.

Jasper, D. E., and Jain, N. C. (1965). *Am. J. Vet. Res.* **26**, 844.

Jensen, E. C. (1959). *J. Am. Vet. Med. Assoc.* **135**, 572.

Jones, M. T., and Stockham, M. A. (1966). *J. Physiol. (London)* **184**, 741.

Jubb, K. V. F., and Kennedy, P. C. (1970). *In* "Pathology of Domestic Animals," 2nd ed., 2 vols. Academic Press, New York (in press).

Karlson, P., and Sekeris, C. E. (1966). *Acta Endocrinol.* **53**, 505.

Kendall, J. W., and Sloop, P. R. (1968). *New. Engl. J. Med.* **279**, 532.

King, J. M., Kavanaugh, J. F., and Bentinck-Smith, J. (1962). *Cornell Vet.* **52**, 133.

Kitabchi, A. E., Buchanan, K. D., Vance, J. E., and Williams, R. H. (1968). *J. Clin. Endocrinol. Metab.* **28**, 1479.

Knutson, F. (1966). *Acta Endocrinol.* **52**, 305.

Koestner, A., and Capen, C. C. (1967). *Pathol. Vet. (Basel)* **4**, 513.

Kraicer, J. (1964). *Biochim. Biophys. Acta* **87**, 703.

Kral, C. F. (1951). *J. Am. Vet. Med. Assoc.* **118**, 235.

Kuhn, E. (1967). *Arch. Intern. Pharmacodyn.* **168**, 417.

Lavor, P. (1968). *Ann. Biol. Animale, Biochim., Biophys.* **8**, 461.

Leading Article. (1967). *Lancet* **I**, 86.

Leading Article. (1968). *Lancet* **I**, 30.

Lecocq, F. R., Mebane, D., and Madison, L. L. (1964). *J. Clin. Invest.* **43**, 237.

Lee, E., Cross, R. B., and Thornton, W. (1967). *Australian J. Exptl. Biol. Med. Sci.* **45**, 6.

Lee, T. C., van der Wal, B., and de Wied, D. (1968). *J. Endocrinol.* **42**, 465.

Levine, R., and Luft, R. (1964). *Diabetes* **13**, 651.

Li, C. H. (1968). *Perspectives Biol. Med.* **11**, 498.

Lie, J. T. (1968). *Med. J. Australia* **2**, 508.

Liggins, G. C., and Kennedy, P. C. (1968). *J. Endocrinol.* **40**, 371.

Loeb, W. R., Capen, C. C., and Johnson, L. E. (1966). *Cornell Vet.* **46**, 623.

Louis, L. H., and Conn, J. W. (1967). *J. Lab. Clin. Med.* **70**, 1016.

McCann, S. M., Dhariwhal, A. P. S., and Porter, J. C. (1968). *Ann. Rev. Physiol.* **30**, 589.

MacLeod, R. M., and Abad, A. (1968). *Endocrinology* **83**, 799.

Marshak, R. R., Webster, G. G., and Skelley, J. F. (1960). *J. Am. Vet. Med. Assoc.* **136**, 274.

Martin. J. E., Skillen, R. G., and Deubler, J. (1954). *Am. J. Vet. Res.* **15**, 489.

Massimo. L., Gaiero, G., and Braito. A. (1966). *Minerva Med.* **6**, 22.

Matsui, N., and Plager. J. E. (1966). *Endocrinology* **79**, 737.

Medway, W., Prier, J. E., and Wilkinson, J. S. (1969). "Textbook of Veterinary Clinical Pathology." Williams & Wilkins, Baltimore, Maryland.

Mills, I. H. (1964). "Clinical Aspects of Adrenal Function," p. 49. Blackwell, Oxford.

Morrow, L. B., Burrow, G. N., and Mulrow, P. J. (1967) *Endocrinology* **80**, 883.

Moss, M. S., and Rylance, H. J. (1967). *J. Endocrinol.* **37**, 129.

Ney, R. L., Dexter, R. L., Davis, W. W., and Garren, L. D. (1967). *J. Clin. Invest.* **46**, 1916.

Nicol, T., Vernon-Roberts, B., and Quantock, D. C. (1965). *J. Endocrinol.* **33**, 365.

Odell, W. D. (1966). *J. Am. Med. Assoc.* **197**, 1006.

Oertel, G. W., and Eik-Nes, K. B. (1962). *Endocrinology* **70**, 39.

Paschkis, K. E., Rakoff, A. E., Cantarow, A., and Rupp, J. J. (1967). "Clinical Endocrinology," 3rd ed. Harper (Hoeber), New York.

Paterson, J. Y. F. (1963). *Biochem. J.* **86**, 1P.

Paterson, J. Y. F., and Harrison, F. A. (1968). *J. Endocrinol.* **40**, 37.

Pehrson, B., and Wallin, O. (1966). *Acta Vet. Scand.* **7**, 35.

Plager, J. E., Knopp, R., Slaunwhite, R., and Sandberg, A. A. (1963). *Endocrinology* **73**, 353.

Pugh, D. M. (1968). *Brit. Vet. J.* **124**, 259.

Randle, P. J., Garland, P. B., Hales, C. N., and Newsholme, E. A. (1963). *Lancet* **1**, 785.

Riggs, B. L., Jowsey, J., and Kelley, P. J. (1966). *Metab., Clin, Exptl.* **15**, 773.

Rijnberk, A., der Kinderen, P. J., and Thijssen, J. H. H. (1968a). *J. Endocrinol.* **41**, 387.

Rijnberk, A., der Kinderen, P. J., and Thijssen, J. H. H. (1968b). *J. Endocrinol.* **41**, 397.

Roth, J., Glick, S. M., Yalow, R. S., and Berson, S. A. (1964), *Diabetes* **13**, 355.

Roth, R. H., Stjärne, L., Levine, R. J., and Giarman N. J. (1968). *J. Lab. Clin. Med.* **72**, 397.

Rothenbacker, H., and Shigley, R. F. (1966). *J. Am. Vet. Med. Assoc.* **149**, 406.

Saunders, L. Z., and Rickard, C. G. (1952). *Cornell Vet.* **42**, 490.

Saunders, L. Z., Stephenson, H. G., and McEntee, K. (1951). *Cornell Vet.* **41**, 445.

Schalm, O. (1965). "Veterinary Hematology," 2nd ed., p. 440. Lea & Febiger, Philadelphia, Pennsylvania.

Schwartzman, R. M., and Fegley, H. (1965). *J. Am. Vet. Med. Assoc.* **147**, 642.

Seiber, S. E. (1964). Personal communication.

Selye, H. (1962). "Calciphylaxis," Univ. of Chicago Press, Chicago, Illinois.

Shaw, K. E., and Nichols, R. E. (1964). *Am. J. Vet. Res.* **25**, 252.

Shim, S. S., Copp, D. H., and Patterson, F. P. (1968). *Can. J. Physiol. Pharmacol.* **46**, 43.

Siegel, E. T. (1968). *Am. J. Vet. Res.* **29**, 173.

Siegel, E. T., O'Brien, J. B., Pyle, L., and Schryver, H. (1967). *J. Am. Vet. Med. Assoc.* **150**, 760.

Siegel, E. T., and Belshaw, B. E. (1968). *Current Vet. Therapy* **3**, 545.

Silva, M., and Malnic, G. (1964). *J. Pharmacol. Exptl. Therap.* **146**, 23.

Sirek, A., Schoeffling, K., Webster, M., and Sirek, O. V. (1964). *Can. J. Physiol. Pharmacol.* **42**, 299.

Sirek, O., Sirek, A., Przybylska, K., Doolan, H., and Niki, A. (1967). *Endocrinology* **81**, 395.

Snipes, C. A. (1968). *Quart. Rev. Biol.* **43**, 127.

Solomon, I. L., and Blizzard, R. M. (1963). *J. Pediat.* **63**, 1021.

Sterling, K. (1960). *J. Clin. Invest.* **39**, 1900.

Stjärne, L., Lishajko, F., and Roth, R. H. (1967). *Nature* **215**, 770.

Swingle, W. W., and Swingle, A. J. (1967a). *Proc. Soc. Exptl. Biol. Med.* **125**, 811.

Swingle, W. W., and Swingle, A. J. (1967b). *Endocrinology* **81**, 406.

Sybesma, W., and Van der Veen, H. E. (1962). *Tijdschr. Diergeneesk.* **87**, 691.

Taylor, W., and Scratcherd, T. (1963). *Biochem. J.* **86**, 114.

Taylor, W., and Scratcherd, T. (1967). *Acta Endocrinol.* **56**, Suppl. 119, 139.

Tegeler, G., and Schulke, B. (1967). *Arch. Exptl. Veterinaermed.* **21**, 777.

Thomasson, B., and Steenburg, R. W. (1965). *Am. J. Physiol.* **208**, 84.

Thompson, J. S., Palmieri, G. M. A., Eliel, L. P., and Butler, G. A. (1968). *Endocrinology*, **83**, 470.

Topel, D. G., and Merkel, R. A. (1967). *J. Animal Sci.* **26**, 1017.

Trenkle, A. (1967). *J. Animal Sci.* **26**, 1497.

Ullman, T. D., Czaczkes, W. J., and Menczel, J. (1965). *J. Clin. Invest.* **44**, 746.

Unger, F., Rosenfeld, G., and Dorfman, R. I. (1961). *Am. J. Vet. Res.* **22**, 313.

Urquhart, J., and Li, C. C. (1968). *Am. J. Physiol.* **214**, 73.

van Rensburg, S. J. (1965). *J. S. African Vet. Med. Assoc.* **36**, 491.

Vaughan, L. P. V. (1965). *J. Endocrinol.* **33**, iii.

Venning, E. H., Dyrenfurth, T., Dosseter, J. B., and Beck, J. C. (1962). *Metab., Clin. Exptl.* **11**, 254.

Verstraete, A., and Thoonen, J. (1938). *Vlaams Diergeneesk. Tijdschr.* **7**, 186.

Verstraete, A., and Thoonen, J. (1939). *Vlaams Diergeneesk. Tijdschr.* **8**, 304.

Wallace, A. L. C., and Bassett, J. M. (1966). *Metab., Clin. Exptl.* **15**, 95.

Walser, M., Robins, B. H., and Buckett, J. W. (1963). *J. Clin. Invest.* **42**, 456.

Weber, G., Singhal, R. L., Hird, H. J., and Furth, J. (1966). *Endocrinology* **79**, 865.

Weiss, M., and McDonald, I. R. (1965). *J. Endocrinol.* **33**, 202.

Weiss, M., and McDonald, I. R. (1966a). *J. Endocrinol.* **35**, 207.

Weiss, M., and McDonald, I. R. (1966b). *Gen. Comp. Endocrinol.* **7**, 345.

Weiss, M., and McDonald, I. R. (1967). *J. Endocrinol.* **39**, 251.

Wheatley, I. S., Wallace, A. L. C., and Bassett, J. M. (1966). *J. Endocrinol.* **35**, 341.

Whipp, S. C., Weber, A. P., Usenik, E. A., and Good, A. L. (1967a). *Am. J. Vet. Res.* **28**, 671.

Whipp, S. C., Beary, M. E., Usenik, E. A., Weber, A. F., and Good, A. L. (1967b). *Am. J. Vet. Res.* **28**, 1343.

Wiener, H. (1968a). *N. Y. State J. Med.* **68**, 912.

Wiener, H. (1968b). *N. Y. State J. Med.* **68**, 1019.

Wilhelmi, A. E. (1968). *Yale J. Biol. Med.* **41**, 199.

Wilkinson, J. S. (1969). *In* "Textbook of Veterinary Clinical Pathology" (W. Medway, J. E. Prier, and J. S. Wilkinson, eds.), p. 181. Williams & Wilkins, Baltimore, Maryland.

Wilkinson, J. S., Medway, W., Siegel, E. T., Schwartzman, R., and Craig, P. (1965). *J. Am. Vet. Med. Assoc.* **147**, 1650.

Wilson, R. B., Kline, L. J., Clark, T. J., Hendricks, E. C., and Grossman, M. S. (1967). *Am. J. Vet. Res.* **28**, 313.

Wright, B. J., and Conner, G. H. (1968). *Cancer Res.* **28**, 251.

Wurtman, R. J., Casper, A., Pohorecky, L. A., and Bartter, F. C. (1968). *Proc. Natl. Acad. Sci. U.S.* **61**, 522.

Yoshida, S., Ibayoshi, H., Murakawa, S., and Nakao, K. (1966). *Endocrinology* **79**, 871.

Zamora, C. S., Weber, A. F., and Whipp, S. C. (1967). *Am. J. Vet. Res.* **28**, 1351.

Zolovick, A., Upson, D. W., and Eleftheriou, B. E. (1966). *J. Endocrinol.* **35**, 249.

8 Thyroid Function

J. J. Kaneko

I. INTRODUCTION

Disorders of the thyroid gland are the most common endocrine disorders in man and an extensive historical and scientific literature is available. In domestic animals, however, thyroid function and its disorders are less well known and documented. The importance of thyroid function and its diseases will become even more important as longevity of some domestic species increases. This is already evidenced by the rapidly growing literature concerning thyroid function in the dog.

Recent advances in the understanding of thyroid physiology and in the development and refinement of methods of testing thyroid function will certainly add impetus to the study of thyroid disease. In this chapter, the anatomy, physiology, and diseases of the thyroid will be briefly reviewed as a corollary to the understanding of thyroid function. Emphasis is placed on an understanding of the physiological bases of a variety of thyroid function tests, most of which are now readily available to the veterinary clinician.

II. ANATOMICAL CONSIDERATIONS

The thyroid gland of animals is a bilobed structure which overlays the trachea and is located just below the larynx. Anatomical variation of the gland is quite marked between species and, to a lesser extent, within a given species. The isthmus connecting the two lobes of the thyroid varies most markedly between the species. Man and the pig have a large discrete isthmus which forms a pyramidal lobe connecting the two lateral lobes. The cow has a fairly wide band of glandular tissue which forms the connecting isthmus. In the horse, sheep, goat, cat, and dog, the isthmus is a narrow remnant and may even be nonexistent. The size of the lobes is increased and the isthmus may be present in these animals under conditions of increased thyroid stimulation.

The thyroid gland is a highly vascularized tissue with a rapid blood flow. The glandular tissue of the thyroid is composed of follicles whose lumens contain a thick clear fluid, the colloid. The size of the follicles and their cells vary according to the functional state of the gland. The cells can vary from the less active squamous type to the highly active tall columnar cells.

III. PHYSIOLOGY

The thyroid gland is unique among the endocrine glands in that an integral part of its hormone, L-thyroxine (T_4), is a micronutrient, iodine, which is available to the animal in only limited amounts. This is compensated for by the presence of a very efficient trapping mechanism. Also, while most endocrine glands store little of their hormones, the thyroid manages to store quantities of its hormone sufficient for from one to several weeks (biological half-time) depending upon the species. The thyroid gland is also one of the larger of the endocrine glands and contains about 20% of the total body iodine. Its iodine content and size varies with iodine intake and the state of thyroid function but it usually contains 10–40 mg iodine/100 gm tissue.

A. Iodine Metabolism

1. Absorption and Excretion

Iodine may be absorbed into the body in a wide variety of soluble chemical forms but usually as iodides (I^-), iodates (IO_4^-), and as the hormonal forms. Iodide may be absorbed from any moist body surface but its chief route of entry into the general circulation is by absorption through the small intestine. The I^- in the circulation is trapped principally by the thyroid gland, with some trapping by the salivary gland and a minimal amount by the gastric mucosa, placenta, and mammary gland. In the ruminant, 70–80% of an oral dose is absorbed in the rumen and 10% in the omasum (Barua *et al.*, 1964).

The main route of excretion of I^- is by the kidneys through which almost all the I^- that was not trapped by the tyroid is lost in the urine. A small but significant amount is lost in the saliva and minimal amounts are lost in the feces, sweat, and milk. In ruminants, a significant amount may be lost in the feces as well (Bustad *et al.*, 1957, 1962)

2.   Functions of the Gland

The role of the thyroid in the synthesis and release of thyroid hormones is shown in Fig. 1 and the structures of the important thyroid hormones are shown in Fig. 2. Initially, the I^- that is absorbed into the general circulation is taken up by the thyroid follicular cells by a highly efficient trapping and concentrating mechanism. It does this against a concentration gradient which can be from 1:20- to 1:500-fold across the thyroid cell membrane. It is an active transport process, thought to be enzymic in nature, requires oxygen, and can be assumed to utilize high-energy phosphate bonds in the form of ATP (Freinkel and Ingbar, 1955; Slingerland, 1955). Although I^- may enter the thyroid cell by diffusion or by deiodination of preexisting iodinated compounds within the gland, active transport is the most important concentrating mechanism. This trapping of I^- is also the basis for use of the uptake of radioactive iodine (^{131}I) as a test of thyroid function which is described in Section IV,I. The uptake of I^- is stimulated by the thyroid-stimulating hormone (TSH) and blocked by thyrotoxic agents such as thiocyanate (SCN^-), perchlorate (ClO_4^-), and by large amounts of I^- itself. The sites of these and other blocks in the thyroxine biosynthetic pathway are also shown in Fig. 1.

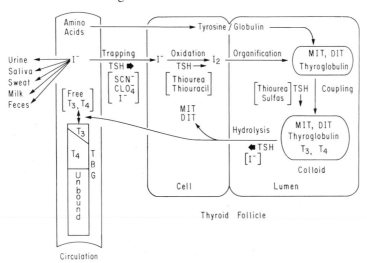

Fig. 1.   Pathways of iodine metabolism and thyroid hormone synthesis. Sites, direction, and relative degree of thyroid-stimulating hormone action are shown by arrows. Goitrogenic blocking agents and their sites are shown in brackets.

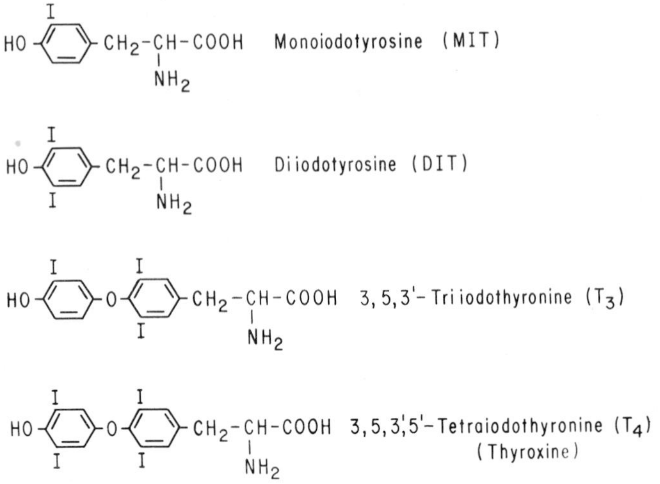

Fig. 2.   Chemical structures of the major iodinated compounds of the thyroid gland.

As shown in Fig. 1, the first step after trapping involves an oxidation of iodide (I^-) to iodine (I_2) by a peroxidase. This reaction is inhibited by the thyrotoxic agents such as thiouracil and thiourea. The I_2 next conjugates with the tyrosine moiety of thyroglobulin to form the mono- (MIT) and diiodotyrosines (DIT) (Fig. 2). This reaction is sensitive to blocking by sulfa drugs and p-aminobenzoic acid (PABA). The iodinated tyrosines are next coupled to form either the L-3,5,3'-triiodo-thyronine (T_3) or L-3,5,3',5'-tetraiodothyronine (T_4), the principal thyroid hormones. These latter reactions appear to occur in the follicular lumen where thyroglobulin acts as the acceptor protein upon which T_3 and T_4 are synthesized. Thyroglobulin is a glycoprotein which, under normal conditions, is found only in the thyroid follicle. The thyroid hormones bound to the thyroglobulin are stored in the follicular lumen as colloid.

A second major site of action of TSH is to stimulate the release of thyroid hormones from the gland. TSH appears to activate the enzymic hydrolysis of colloid to release its T_4, T_3, MIT, DIT, and other iodinated compounds. T_4 and T_3 are released into the circulation while MIT and DIT are metabolized and their iodine is recycled within the gland. About 90% of the hormone released into the circulation is T_4 and 10% is T_3. The oxidation and coupling are two additional sites of TSH action (Fig. 1).

T_4 is mainly transported in the plasma bound to a specific plasma protein, thyroxine-binding globulin (TBG). A small amount is bound to thyroxine-binding prealbumin (TBPA) and to albumin. T_3, on the other hand, is bound only to TBG (Klebanoff, 1965) and less tightly than T_4. About 99.95% of the T_4 in plasma is bound to the protein and only a small fraction, 0.05%, is present in the free or unbound state (T_f). These fractions are diagrammatically shown in Fig. 1. This free L-thyroxine (T_f) is thought to be the metabolically active form of the thyroid hormone. This is the active hormone thought to function in cell metabolism and in TSH feedback control. Measurements of T_f would therefore seem to be the most definitive test of thyroid function.

There are two principal factors of importance in the regulation of the amount of T_f. These are the total amount of T_4 in the plasma and the amount of the binding protein, TBG. The T_f level in plasma is usually maintained by a balance of these two factors and, in general, when T_4 increases, T_f increases, and when TBG increases, T_f decreases:

$$T_f = k\frac{T_4}{TBG}$$

Only about one-third of the binding sites for T_4 on the TBG molecule are occupied but this ratio is usually constant enough so that T_4 can be considered proportional to TBG. Thus, T_4 is also, in most instances, directly proportional to the amount of T_f and, therefore, T_4 or PBI also become direct measures of thyroidal activity.

B. MECHANISM OF THYROXINE ACTION

After the administration of T_4, its first effects are noted in 24–48 hours and its maximal effects are noted in 7–10 days. T_3 takes a shorter time and is more active, perhaps due to its low affinity for TBG. T_3 was therefore thought for some time to be the active form of the thyroid hormone. The "free" thyroxine (T_f) is now considered to be the most likely active form of the thyroid hormone. Certain of the effects of T_4 are consistent and these are noted in Table I. The requirements for T_4 for these activities vary and increased amounts are required for growth, pregnancy, and lactation.

The exact mechanism of T_4 action at the cellular level is poorly understood. While the overall effects of T_4 on the animal have been well documented, the definitive evidence for a unified concept of T_4 action (or actions) cannot yet be stated. The view that T_4 acts by a direct effect on oxidative enzymes has been attractive but there is no firm evidence that T_4 in any way alters the activity of various enzymes. A similar uncertainty is present regarding the concept that T_4 might alter the structure or properties of the mitochondrial membrane to promote increased metabolism. T_4 is also known to increase protein synthesis (Tata et al., 1963; Tapley, 1964) and these effects occur within the latent period for the calorigenic action of T_4. Thus, the anabolic effects of T_4 may be the result of general stimulation of protein synthetic activity (which would also require large amounts of energy).

A most attractive hypothesis which has remained prevalent in spite of valid criticism is the uncoupling of oxidative phosphorylation (Ox-Phos) by T_4. Under

TABLE I   EFFECTS OF THYROXINE

Physiological	Temperature increase
Calorigenic	BMR (O_2 consumption) increase
Carbohydrate metabolism	Increased glucose turnover; absorption
Protein metabolism	Anabolic; positive N balance
Lipid metabolism	Decrease blood cholesterol
Development	Stimulus growth and maturation
Reproductive	Fertility, pregnancy, ovulation
Hematological	Tendency for polycythemia; anemia in absence

normal conditions, 3 moles of ATP(P) are synthesized per atom of oxygen ($\frac{1}{2}O_2 = O$) utilized in the cytochrome oxidative system; hence P:O ratio = 3. If less ATP is formed for the same or even greater use of O, the system is said to be uncoupled; P:O ratio is less than 3. Thyroxine has been repeatedly shown to uncouple Ox-Phos so that O_2 consumption must be increased to maintain the same amounts of needed ATP and the large amount of energy not incorporated into ATP is dissipated away as heat. This mechanism indicates that T_4 does have an effect on an enzymic process but it cannot be stated whether it is a direct one or an indirect membrane effect. Furthermore, demonstration of this effect does require considerably more than physiologic amounts of T_4. Thus, it is possible that the action of T_4 represents a combination of actions where its anabolic effects are the result of protein synthetic activities and its catabolic effects are the result of uncoupling of Ox-Phos.

C. REGULATION OF THE THYROID

1. Thyroid-Stimulating Hormone

The principal control of the thyroid gland is dependent upon thyroid-stimulating hormone (TSH) secreted by the anterior pituitary gland, which in turn is mediated through the hypothalamus. Control of TSH secretion is in turn by a system of feedback control based on the product of the target gland, thyroxine. The iodine levels in the blood and thyroid also affect the control mechanism. The secretion of TSH by the pituitary is dependent upon the levels of unbound or "free" thyroxine (T_f) in the blood. By negative feedback inhibition high levels of the T_f depress TSH and vice versa. Although the iodine-containing thyroid hormones may act directly on the thyroid gland, their principal regulatory effect is on the pituitary and certain regions of the hypothalamus. Both structures respond to increased thyroxine levels by depressing TSH release but the pituitary response may be the faster acting. A transmitting agent from the hypothalamus, the thyrotropin-releasing factor (TRF), stimulates the pituitary to release TSH when levels of T_f are low.

The pituitary TSH has a number of effects on the thyroid gland. The gland increases in size, the follicular cell height increases, and there is a loss of colloid. The response of the thyroid gland to TSH is also affected by the level of stable iodine intake. When the level of stable iodine intake is high, the action of TSH is suppressed and the size and activity of the follicular cells is decreased. When the level of stable iodine intake is low, there is an increase in the number and size of cells and in uptake and release of iodine, which is most likely the result of the increase in TSH secretion.

2. Long-Acting Thyroid Stimulator

In recent years, a second thyroid stimulatory factor has been discovered in the serum which appears to be closely involved in the mechanism of thyrotoxicosis (Adams, 1958; McKenzie, 1958). It differs from TSH in that it is cleared from the blood more slowly and produces its thyroid-stimulating effects many hours (8–24) after that observed for TSH. It is therefore referred to as long-acting thyroid stimulator or LATS. Studies of LATS have been largely confined to man where it has been closely correlated with hyperthyroidism (Lipman, 1967). Little is yet known of this factor with regard to its origin, nature, and role in thyroid function.

IV. THYROID FUNCTION TESTS

The diagnosis of diseases of the thyroid gland in animals is very often obscured by the nonspecific nature and variety of clinical signs. Routine rapid laboratory aids to diagnosis, such as urinalysis, are of little value to the physical examination. As such, the laboratory tests of thyroid function become of great importance in the diagnosis of thyroid disease. In recent years, improvements and refinements of standard tests and the development of new tests have progressed to the point where a variety of tests are now available to the veterinary clinician. A select few show promise of becoming the most definitive measures of circulating thyroid hormone levels or thyroid function and these can and should become an integral part of the diagnostic armamentaria for thyroid disease in animals.

A. HEMATOLOGY

A moderate normocytic normochromic anemia is sometimes associated with clinical hypothyroidism in the dog. This anemia has also been observed in man and in experimental animals and is known to be of a depression type (Cline and Berlin, 1963). The stained blood smear characteristically shows little or no evidence of active erythrogenesis such as anisocytosis, polychromasia, or nucleated red cells. Leptocytosis may be especially prominent. The hemogram is characteristic of the depression type of anemia associated with a variety of diseases such as neoplasia, chronic infection, etc. This anemia is therefore not diagnostic for hypothyroidism but, conversely, in cases of unexplained hypoplastic or depression anemia, hypothyroidism should be considered.

B. BASAL METABOLIC RATE (BMR)

This test measures the O_2 consumption of the animal under rigidly standardized conditions, and has been a classical test of thyroid function in man. It has found little application in veterinary medicine due to the difficulty of maintaining animals under basal conditions. Even under anesthesia, basal conditions are not necessarily maintained.

C. SERUM CHOLESTEROL

The level of plasma or serum cholesterol is affected by the status of thyroid activity and, in general, it varies inversely with the degree of activity. In the past, considerable reliance has been placed upon the use of serum cholesterol levels as an index of thyroid function. Hypothyroidism is generally associated with an elevation in serum cholesterol. The normal range for serum cholesterol, however, is wide and elevations are frequently seen in a variety of conditions unrelated to thyroid activity. These include the nature of the diet, hepatic function, bile duct obstruction, and diabetes mellitus. The wide normal range and variety of factors influencing the cholesterol level limits its usefulness as a test of thyroid function. The diagnostic accuracy of serum cholesterol for hypothyroidism in the dog is about 60%. However, when the levels are very high, greater than 500 mg/100 ml, and diabetes mellitus is eliminated, its diagnostic accuracy is greatly increased and this test can be of great value. To be of greatest diagnostic significance, this test should be employed in combination with other tests of thyroid function.

Conversely, it would seem reasonable that lowered serum cholesterol levels might be similarly employed for hyperthyroid states but the inconsistencies are such that this test is useless for this purpose. On the other hand, cholesterol level responds quickly and consistently to thyroid therapy and can be employed as a guide to proper dosage.

A detailed discussion of cholesterol metabolism and its association in various diseases are given in Chapter 2. Table II gives the normal cholesterol values of a number of domestic animals. For the dog, 125–250 mg/100 ml of serum is considered normal (Kaneko, 1963).

D. Serum Protein-Bound Iodine (PBI)

A more direct test of thyroid function would be the measurement of the amount of thyroid hormone in the blood. As already described, almost all the T_4 in plasma is bound to plasma proteins (TBG). Also, about 90% of the iodine in plasma protein is that of T_4 with the remainder being T_3 and other iodine derivatives. Since this percentage is usually quite constant, a measure of the amount of iodine bound to the protein (PBI) in plasma is a reflection of the amount of circulating thyroid hormone. The PBI would vary directly with the degree of thyroid activity and be low in the hypothyroid and high in the hyperthyroid. It has been and continues to be a useful index of thyroid function. A more precise, though less commonly employed, reflection of T_4 is the butanol extractable iodine (BEI). The BEI is the organic iodine which is soluble in butanol, is predominantly thyroxine and has been found to be a reliable index of thyroid function in man (Schultz et al., 1954).

Methods for the determination of PBI are beyond the scope of this section even though the procedure has been somewhat simplified. The automated chemical analysis of PBI has made this a fairly common test and is likely to continue to be widely used. Many commercial laboratories can furnish accurate results quickly by this method and is to be recommended. The determination of PBI still remains as one of the most rigorous of quantitative determinations, yet the results, particularly in animals, are often equivocal and sometimes valueless. In each step of the procedure, from the initial venipuncture to its final determination, precautions must be taken to avoid contamination with any iodine-containing compounds and resultant errors. Contamination can be checked by measuring total serum iodine (SI) and if it is greater than 25 μg/100 ml, the PBI should be considered unsatisfactory. A normal range for SI of 14–52 μg/100 ml (Taurog and Chaikoff, 1946) and 5–20 μg/100 ml (Siegel and Belshaw, 1968) has been reported. Prior to sampling, the history of previous medication should be ascertained so that errors from this source may be avoided. The automated analyzers have largely reduced the human error in the laboratory but cannot reduce the prior contamination. The iodine-containing compounds of sodium or potassium iodide increase the PBI, require about 10–14 days for disappearance from the blood and are the chief sources of error in PBI data. The iodinated dye, diodrast, used to visualize the urinary tract, persists for 10–20 hours; while desiccated thyroid or thyroxine given as medication requires 1 to 2

TABLE II PLASMA CHOLESTEROL CONCENTRATION IN VARIOUS SPECIES[a]

Species	Total (mg%)	Free (mg%)	Ester (mg%)	Reference
Cat	95–130			Kritchevsky (1958)
	93±24	30±10	63±23	E. M. Boyd (1942)
	98±7.3			Morris and Courtice (1955)
Cow	80–120			Kritchevsky (1958)
	110–32	37±15	73±15	E. M. Boyd (1942)
Pregnant, nonlactating	241.9			Lennon and Mixner (1957)
Lactating, nonpregnant	96.1			Lennon and Mixner (1957)
Heifers, 15–18 months	105.6			Lennon and Mixner (1957)
Calves	123			Lennon and Mixner (1957)
Dog	125–250			Kaneko (1969)
	110–135			Kritchevsky (1958)
	110±28	51±20	59±19	E. M. Boyd (1944)
	194±35			Morris and Courtice (1955)
Low-fat diet	140			G. S. Boyd and Oliver (1958)
High-fat diet	280			G. S. Boyd and Oliver (1958)
Fowl (chicken, ducks, geese)	100–200			Kritchevsky (1958)
Cockeral	100±23	34±9	66±19	E. M. Boyd (1942)
Nonlaying hens.	116±2 to 152±2			Leveille et al. (1957)
Laying hens	208±15 to 285±24			Leveille et al. (1957)
Goat	80–130			Kritchevsky (1958)
Horse	83–140			Kritchevsky (1958)
	96.8±2.8	15.7	81.1	Norcia and Furman (1959)
	128±12			Morris and Courtice (1955)
Rabbit	30–70			Kritchevsky (1958)
	45±18	22±13	23±12	E. M. Boyd (1942)
Sheep	70			G. S. Boyd and Oliver (1958)
	64±12			Morris and Courtice (1955)
Swine (low-fat diet)	35.6–53.7	5.7–10.9	28–48	Reiser et al. (1959)

[a]Modified from Carroll (1963).

TABLE III SOME DRUGS WHICH AFFECT THYROID FUNCTION TESTS

Compounds	Effect on ^{131}I uptake	Effect on PBI	Effect on T_3 uptake	Duration of effect (average period)
Iodides				
Lugol's, cough syrup, vitamin preparations	Decr	Incr	None	10–30 days
Iodine antiseptics	Decr	Incr	None	10–30 days
Iodine-containing drugs	Decr	Incr	None	10–30 days
X-rays contrast media				
Iodoalphionic acid (Pheniodal)	Decr	Incr	None	3–12 months
Iodopyracet (Diodrast)	Decr	Incr	None	2–7 days
Iodized oil (Oleum Iodatum)	Decr	Incr	None	½–3 years
Most IV contrast media	Decr	Incr	None	2–6 weeks
Most gallbladder media	Decr	Incr	None	3 weeks–3 months
Hormones				
Thyroid Extract	Decr	Incr	Incr	4–6 weeks
Triiodothyronine	Decr	Decr	Decr	2–4 weeks
ACTH	Decr	None	Incr	2 weeks
Estrogens	None	Incr	None	—
Oral contraceptions	None	Incr	None	—
Androgens	None	None	Incr	—
Thiocarbamide compounds				
Thiouracil	Decr	Decr	None	5–7 days
Propylthiouracil	Decr	Decr	None	5–7 days
Thiocyanate	Decr	Decr	None	14–21 days
Phenylbutazone	Decr	None	Incr	14 days
Bromides	Decr	None	—	10–30 days
Antihistamines	Decr	None	—	7 days
Diphenylhydantoin (Dilantin)	None	Decr	Incr	7–10 days
Others				
Salicylates	None	None	Incr[a]	—

[a]Effect depends on the method.

weeks to disappear. Some of these compounds are listed in Table III. It should also be noted that many cough syrups and some vitamin preparations contain iodine in one form or another and will also cause an increase in PBI. Care should also be taken that the area selected for venipuncture is not cleansed with an iodine-containing antiseptic. All glassware with which the blood sample will come in contact should be specially cleaned and used only for PBI sampling. Disposable syringes and needles are excellent for this purpose and may be used without further cleaning. In routine practice, the use of disposable equipment and special tubes which can be obtained from the clinical laboratory performing the test are to be recommended.

The determination of PBI has been of considerable value and is widely employed as an aid to diagnosis of thyroid disease. The normal range for man is 4.0–8.0 μg/100 ml serum as compared to 1.8–4.5 μg/100 ml for the dog. Values below the range are considered indicative of hypothyroidism and those above as hyperthyroid. This and other measures of T_4 levels and the radioiodine tests *in vitro* and *in vivo* are presently the most widely used tests of thyroid function. The range of PBI in animals as shown in Table IV is, in general, considerably lower than in man. The apparent decreased dependence of the dog upon thyroid hormone has been observed by a number of authors (Danowski *et al.*, 1946; Mayer, 1947; Glock, 1949). The usefulness of the PBI determination in dogs is somewhat obscured by these low normal levels and the normal levels found in patients in which other parameters of thyroid function (including biopsy) indicated a definite hypofunction of the thyroid (Kaneko *et al.*, 1959). Extrathyroidal synthesis of iodine-containing compounds by the dog is a possible explanation for this phenomenon. As such, PBI values in dogs should be interpreted with care, even when they fall within the normal range.

E. THYROXINE DETERMINATION BY COLUMN CHROMATOGRAPHY (T₄-COL)

A more specific approach to the determination of total circulating T_4 is the column chromatographic procedure for extracting T_4 from the serum (Pilleggi *et al.*, 1961; Fisher *et al.*, 1965). This procedure uses an anion exchange resin to remove T_4, T_3, other iodoamino acids, and iodides from the serum. These compounds are then eluted off the resin and only the fractions containing T_4 and T_3 are collected. Iodine is measured in these fractions and the thyroxine iodine by column is reported as μg I/100 ml (T₄-Col).

This test is superior to the PBI because of very much less interference by inorganic iodine or iodine-containing compounds. However, iodine containing radiographic contrast media will interfere with the test (Kaihara *et al.*, 1969).

TABLE IV   SERUM PROTEIN-BOUND IODINE (PBI) IN DOMESTIC ANIMALS

Species	PBI[a]	Reference
Dog	2.3 (1.5–3.5)	Siegel and Belshaw (1968)
	3.4 ±1.0 (1.5–5.1)	Mallo and Harris (1967)
	2.3 ±0.8 (1.1–4.3)	Quinlan and Michaelson (1967)
	1.99 ±0.24	Theran and Thornton (1966)
	2.6 ±0.18	O'Neal and Heinbecker (1953)
	2.7 (1.8–4.5)	Kaneko (1969)
Cat	3.5 (2.5–6.0)	Kaneko (1969)
Horse, thoroughbred	1.86 ±0.29 (1.2–2.5)	C. H. G. Irvine (1967b)
	2.2 ±0.6 (1.5–3.5)	Kaneko (1964)
	1.6–2.7	Trum and Wasserman (1956)
Pig, Landrace	2.7 ±0.1	Sorenson (1962)
Large white	4.4 ±0.2	Sorenson (1962)
Dairy cattle	2.73–4.11	Long *et al.* (1951)
Lactating	3.7 ±0.3	Sorenson (1962)
Pregnant heifers	5.0 ±0.7	Sorenson (1962)
Nonpregnant heifers	3.3 ±0.1	Sorenson (1962)
Beef cattle	2.19	Long *et al.* (1951)
Steers	2.5 ±0.3	Sorenson (1962)
Sheep	3.8 ±1.0 (3.6–4.0)	Hackett *et al.* (1957)
Goats, miniature	4 (2–5)	Ragan *et al.* (1966)

[a]μg/100 ml serum. Values are means with their standard deviations where available. The ranges are given in parentheses.

Only a limited amount of data is presently available by this method. The normal range in dogs for T_4-Col is about 1.1–2.3 μg I/100 ml serum ($\bar{x} = 1.5$) (Kaneko, 1969) and is understandably lower than the PBI. At present, this value can be considered tentative.

F. Thyroxine Determination by Competitive Protein Binding (T_4-CPB)

A new procedure for T_4 determination has recently been developed (Murphy and Pattee, 1964) which does not depend in the colorimetric measurement of iodine and is gaining wide acceptance. It is based on the T_4-binding properties of thyroxine-binding globulin (TBG) and is not interfered with by exogeneous iodine contaminants such as contrast media. The procedure involves the extraction of T_4 from the patient serum and the T_4 is incubated with human TBG which has been saturated with ^{125}I-T_4. The ^{125}I-T_4 on the TBG is displaced from the TBG by the patient T_4 in an amount proportional to the amount of patient T_4. The displaced TBG is counted for radioactivity and from a standard curve, the amount of thyroxine or thyroxine iodine is read directly in μg/100 ml.

The advantage of the T_4-CPB is that iodine compounds or iodides do not interfere. Interference is caused only by compounds which compete with T_4 for the binding sites. Only Dilantin and salicylates in large amounts compete and interfere to any extent but in small amounts, their interference is negligible (Sparagana et al., 1969). These and other recent comparative studies (Lucis et al., 1969) indicate that the T_4-CPB is likely to become a widely used measure of serum thyroxine.

Since the method is a measure of T_4, the results theoretically should be identical to T_4-Col. Limited data, however, indicate that the normal range in dogs for T_4-CPB is about 1.4–2.7 μg I/100 ml serum ($\bar{x} = 1.9$) (Kaneko, 1969). Kallfelz (1969) reported a slightly wider range (1.7–4.4 μg I/100 ml) for T_4-CPB with a mean of 2.83 ± 0.94. These values were calculated from a range of total T_4 values of 2.6–6.1 μg/100 ml (4.34 ± 1.44) in six dogs. The clinical significance of PBI, T_4-Col, or T_4-CPB is the same since all are measurements of total T_4.

G. "Free" Thyroxine (T_f)

The "free" thyroxine (T_f) is thought to be the metabolically active fraction of the total circulating thyroxine. As previously described (Section III,B), the amount of T_f is governed by the equilibrium between T_f, TBG, and T_4.

$$T_f = k\frac{T_4}{TBG}$$

The determination of T_f would also be the most accurate parameter of thyro-metabolic status.

The concentration of T_f, however, is extremely low and difficult to determine; its determination is based, in part, upon analysis of T_4-I, either by column or CPB. Therefore, interferences can occur. The T_f levels for the beagle is 3.53 ± 0.34 mμg/100 ml serum (Michaelson, 1969).

H. *In Vitro* ^{131}I-Triiodothyronine Uptake (T$_3$ Uptake)

The uptake of ^{131}I-triiodothyronine by red cells (T$_3$ uptake) was observed and proposed by Hamolsky *et al.* (1957, 1959) as an *in vitro* test of thyroid function. This test measured the *in vitro* partition of ^{131}I-labeled T$_3$ between the TBG of serum and a secondary binding agent, in this case, red cells. Serum TBG is the primary binding agent and it binds T$_4$ more firmly than it does T$_3$. Therefore, added ^{131}I-T$_3$ is bound to added red cells or other added agents, such as resins. A radioactive count of the red cell (or resin) will thus be a measure of the unbound TBG which, in turn, depends upon the amount of T$_4$ bound to TBG. The uptake would be low in hypo- and high in hyperthyroidism.

There is a large group of modifications to the basic test which utilizes different binding techniques or agents and many are available in kit form. Recently, Pain and Oldfield (1969) surveyed six T$_3$ methods including the red cell uptake, resin uptake, resin sponge uptake, Sephadex, T$_3$-charcoal-hemoglobin and the thyroid-binding index. They concluded that the original red cell T$_3$ uptake gave overall satisfactory results but only two of the newer methods, Sephadex and charcoal, gave satisfactory results for both hyper- and hypothyroidism. On the basis of ease of performance, the T$_3$-charcoal-hemoglobin test (W. J. Irvine and Standeven, 1968) would appear to be the test of choice.

The T$_3$ tests have found widespread use as a thyroid function test because of its ease and *in vitro* nature. It is useful with contaminated sera, during pregnancy, and as an adjunct to other tests. The ranges, however, usually overlap and the results are poorly correlated with thyroid activity. By the T$_3$-resin sponge method, Kallfelz (1969) reports an uptake of 40–56% (49.75 ± 5.51%) for dogs. Wilson *et al.* (1961) reported T$_3$ uptake by the red cell to be about 10–30% for dogs. For horses, the T$_3$-resin sponge method was 46–57% (51.5 ± 2.9%) in nonpregnant mares but was not evaluated for thyroid function (Kuhns *et al.*, 1969). The thyroid-binding index in horses was 0.80–1.20 (1.03 ± 0.14) (Kaneko, 1964). In contrast to the uptake, this index is high in hypo- and low in hyperthyroidism.

I. Thyroidal Radioiodine Uptake

The uptake of radioiodine (^{131}I or ^{125}I) as a tracer for thyroid function is based upon the principle that the metabolic behavior of ^{131}I is inseparable from the behavior of the nonradioactive stable isotope of iodine, ^{127}I. As such, injected or ingested tracer amounts of ^{131}I follows the same metabolic pathway in the animal as stable iodine as shown in Fig. I. The radioiodine uptake test has been used for more than three decades (Hamilton and Soley, 1939) and remains as one of the most definitive tests for thyroid function.

The use of tracer doses of ^{131}I adds no significant amount of iodine to the system (1 μCi ^{131}I = 8 × 10^{-6} μg iodine) and only minimal exposure of the subject to radiation. The amount of ^{131}I used as tracer depends on a variety of factors such as size, age, thyroid gland size, dietary iodine, and the instrumentation used for detection. The fundamentals of isotopology are discussed further in Chap. 9, Vol. II on Radioisotopes. Metz (1969) has developed a mathematical formulation for calculation of the minimal dose of ^{131}I which can be as little as 1 μCi for a man. Since high doses can cause functional impairment to the thyroid gland, it is important that only a minimal dose be used. For practical clinical purposes, this minimum should be established; in our system, 10–30 μCi is used for the dog. The dose is given intravenously, although the oral route would also suffice.

The high energy γ-radiation of ^{131}I also permits ease of counting radioactivity *in vitro* and *in vivo* and by appropriate procedures, various parameters of thyroid function can be assessed. A number of procedures have been used to study thyroid physiology in goats and cattle (Pipes and Turner, 1956), sheep (Bustad *et al.*, 1958), swine (Seigneur *et al.*, 1959), and horses (Trum and Wasserman, 1956).

A standard technique is to monitor the amount of ^{131}I taken up by the gland using an external scintillation detector placed over the thyroid region of the neck (see Fig. 1, Chap. 9, Vol. II). The uptake is expressed as the percent of the injected dose. Ideally, the uptake should be measured frequently after injection and a time-uptake curve should be constructed for 3–4 days. For clinical purposes in the dog, a single measurement at 72 hours is usually satisfactory for the hypothyroid but the time-uptake curve is required for the differential diagnosis of hyperthyroidism.

The correlation of the 72-hour thyroidal-^{131}I uptake with the degree of thyroid function and its use as a reliable diagnostic test of thyroid disease in dogs has been shown (Kaneko *et al.*, 1959; Lombardi *et al.*, 1962). The time interval employed is the time at which the normal dog accumulates a maximal amount of administered isotope. The results are then reported as a percentage of the administered dose which was taken up by the thyroid gland.

The procedure in the dog has been to measure the thyroidal uptake of ^{131}I at 72 hours after injection. The percent uptake is calculated from the following:

$$\frac{\text{Neck count} - (\text{stifle count} \times 1.1)}{\text{Standard count}} \times 100 = \% \text{ uptake}$$

The standard count represents the injected dose of ^{131}I as counted in a thyroid neck phantom. The factor, 1.1, is used to correct the stifle count to obtain the body background. The body background can also be obtained by shielding the thyroid region of the neck and counting. Using this method, an uptake of 10–40% is considered to be within the normal (euthyroid) range for the dog. Values below 10% are considered indicative of hypofunction of the thyroid and those above 40% as indicative of hyperfunction. A slightly lower euthyroid range (7–37%) has recently been reported by Lombardi *et al.* (1962).

It is well known that a large number of iodine-containing compounds, in addition to exogenous thyroid hormone, may interfere with thyroid function tests (Table III). Most of these compounds depress the ^{131}I uptake. These include various forms of iodine compounds as used in diagnostic radiology, expectorants, vitamin preparations, and topical tinctures of iodine. The length of time that the uptake studies may be affected varies with the agent from a few hours to as long as several years. In general, it is well to defer the uptake test for at least 3 weeks if iodine compounds have been administered.

J. Protein-Bound ^{131}I (PB ^{131}I) and the Conversion Ratio (PB ^{131}I-CR)

These tests may be carried in conjunction with the ^{131}I uptake test. Following the accumulation of ^{131}I by the thyroid gland, thyroid hormone containing ^{131}I is synthesized and released into the circulation. The amount of ^{131}I bound to plasma protein (PB ^{131}I) should reflect the status of thyroid activity in the same manner as the amount of nonradioactive iodine (^{127}I) bound to plasma protein, i.e., the PBI. PB ^{131}I and PBI differ, however, in the techniques employed for their measurement and expression of the results. Injected ^{131}I is taken up by the thyroid and released into the circulation as thyroxine-^{131}I which is then bound to plasma protein. The plasma protein-bound ^{131}I (PB ^{131}I) is conveniently separated from the ^{131}I iodide ion of the circulation by the newly developed resin techniques (Scott and Reilly, 1954; Zieve et al., 1956). This test usually requires a higher dose (50 μCi) of ^{131}I than used in the standard uptake test in order to obtain satisfactory count rates of the serum. An accurate measure of the injected dose is also required because the PB ^{131}I is expressed as the percent of the injected dose per liter of serum. A modification of the PB ^{131}I is to measure the radioactivity of the isolated plasma proteins and of the whole plasma and the result expressed as the conversion ratio (PBI^{131}-CR):

$$\frac{\text{Plasma protein radioactivity}}{\text{Total plasma radioactivity}} \times 100 = \frac{\text{PB }^{131}\text{I}}{\text{PB }^{131}\text{I} + {}^{131}\text{I}} \times 100 = \text{CR (\%)}$$

The CR describes the percentage of the total ^{131}I in the plasma which is accounted for by ^{131}I bound to protein. As such, it reflects the amount of labeled thyroid hormone formed by the gland and becomes a measure of thyroid function. A CR of 2–6% has been reported (Lombardi et al., 1962) for normal dogs. This test is useful in the diagnosis of hyperthyroidism in man but its diagnostic value in thyroid disease of animals awaits further confirmation.

K. Thyroxine Secretion Rates (TSR)

The output of thyroxine by the thyroid gland should be a direct indicator of thyroid function and can be indirectly determined by several methods. Most data on thyroxine secretion rates (TSR) in domestic species have been obtained by a technique based on the amount of exogenous L-thyroxine necessary to inhibit the release of ^{131}I by the thyroid, i.e., by thyroxine substitution. An alternate method has been to calculate the TSR from the fractional turnover rate of injected ^{131}I-thyroxine and the T_4 or PBI. The TSR has been determined in most domestic species including the cow (Pipes et al., 1963), sheep (Henneman et al., 1955), goat (Flamboe and Reineke, 1959), pig (Sorenson, 1962), and horse (C. H. G. Irvine, 1967a). There is a fairly wide variation in the reported values which is probably the result of the differences in technique and conditions of the study. The TSR is also affected by age, lactation, diet, season, and training in the case of horses. In animals, the TSR appears to vary from a low of about 0.108 mg/100 kg/day in the horse (C. H. G. Irvine, 1967a) to a high of about 0.46 mg/100 kg/day in the cow (Sorenson, 1962).

L. Response to Thyroid-Stimulating Hormone (TSH)

The response of an animal to TSH injection is also a means to differentiate hypothyroidism which is primarily due to thyroid pathology from a hypothyroid state which is secondary to pituitary hypofunction. The response can be followed by the ^{131}I uptake, PBI, or other test of thyroid function. In pituitary hypofunction, the absence of a stimulus (TSH) for normal thyroid hormone metabolism would account for the manifestations of hypothyroidism. If the thyroid gland has remained functional, administration of TSH should result in subsequent ^{131}I uptakes increasing to within the normal range. This technique has been applied in the dog by the IM injection of 10 units of TSH prior to performance of the standard 72-hour ^{131}I uptake test (Kaneko *et al.*, 1959). This test has been extended (Siegel and Belshaw, 1968) so that an ^{131}I uptake curve is first determined for 72 hours, 3 μ of TSH are then injected b.i.d. for 3 days and followed by 10 units of TSH just prior to conducting a second 72-hour ^{131}I uptake curve.

The PBI determination has also been used as a measure of TSH response (Siegel and Belshaw, 1968). This is a simpler and more rapid test. A control serum sample for PBI is obtained, 10 μ of TSH injected and after 24 hours, a second serum sample for PBI is obtained. The normal dog responds with a mean increase of 3 μg/100 ml. In secondary hypothyroidism with functional thyroid tissue, an increase of at least 1 μg/100 ml is seen, while in primary hypothyroidism, there is less than 0.5 μg/100 ml increase in the PBI.

V.   DISORDERS OF IODINE METABOLISM

Goiter may be defined as any enlargement of the thyroid gland which is not due to inflammation or malignancy. There are two general types of goiters: (1) nontoxic goiters, which produce normal amounts of hormone (simple goiter) or less than normal amounts of hormone (hypothyroid), and (2) toxic goiters, which are characterized by excessive production of hormone (hyperthyroid). The complex steps in the synthesis of thyroxine have been described in the preceding sections. Almost all steps involve either hormonal or enzymic action and it is apparent that a defect at any step or a deficiency can result in thyroid disease.

The simple form of nontoxic goiter is said to be "compensated" because there has been a compensatory increase in thyroid activity and mass (hyperplasia and hypertrophy) such that the tissue secretes as much T_4 as does a normal gland. When the secretion of T_4 is less than that of the normal, hypothyroidism occurs.

Hypothyroidism may be the result of a variety of causative factors. Iodine deficiency (endemic goiter) is a well-known cause of goiter. Goitrogenic materials, either natural or as drugs induce goiters by their blocking effects on steps in the iodine metabolic pathways (Section III,A). Thyroiditis with similarities to Hashimoto's thyroiditis in man has been reported in about 12% of beagles (Beierwaltes and Nishiyama, 1968). Antithyroglobulin antibodies were reported in these dogs. In the adult dog, follicular atrophy is probably the most common cause of hypothyroidism (Clark and Meier, 1958; Siegel and Belshaw, 1968). There are also a number of rare types of familial goiter associated with defects in hormone synthesis (dyshormonogenesis) in man (Stanbury, 1966), which may find their counterpart in sheep (Rac *et al.*, 1968) and cattle (Van Zyl *et al.*, 1965). Finally, hypothyroidism may be secondary to a pituitary insufficiency as described earlier. Hypothyroidism, particularly in the dog, is an important differential diagnosis. The hypothyroid dog is typically obese and lethargic with dry skin, myxedema, and a sparse hair coat. It is therefore an important consideration in the differential diagnoses of the dermatoses. The requirement of T_4 for normal reproduction, growth, and development is well known and also makes thyroid disease an important consideration in reproduction and its disorders.

Hyperthyroidism or toxic goiter is characterized by increased T_4. It has been reported to occur in dogs but is apparently quite a rare condition (Meier and Clark, 1958). These dogs usually exhibit symptoms of hypermetabolism as a result of the excess T_4 such as hyperexcitability and hyperactivity. The most common form of hyperthyroidism is a toxic diffuse hyperplasia of the thyroid (Graves disease in man). Less commonly, a multinodular form or a single adenoma occurs and, in animals, they may all be collectively described as adenomas (Smith and Jones, 1966). In recent years, there has been evidence that the thyroid in Graves disease is responding to a substance other than TSH. This substance is long-acting thyroid stimulator (LATS) which is present only in serum or Graves disease patients and has already been discussed.

Tumors of the thyroid, on the other hand, appear to be of relatively frequent occurrence (Lucke, 1964). Almost all, however, are benign and their significance as a clinical disease entity remains unclear since Brodey and Kelly (1968) found no evidence of clinical thyroid disease in their study of thyroid tumors.

REFERENCES

Adams, D. D. (1958). *J. Clin. Endocrinol. Metab.* **18**, 699.
Barua, J., Cragle, R. G., and Miller, J. K. (1964). *J. Dairy Sci.* **47**, 539.
Beierwaltes, W. H., and Nishiyama, R. H. (1968). *Endocrinology* **83**, 501.
Boyd, E. M. (1942). *J. Biol. Chem.* **143**, 131.
Boyd, E. M. (1944). *Can. J. Res.* **22E**, 39.
Boyd, G. S., and Oliver, M. F. (1958). *In* "Cholesterol" (R. P. Cook, ed.), p. 187. Academic Press, New York.
Brodey, R. S., and Kelly, D. (1968). *Cancer* **22**, 406.
Bustad, L. K., George, L. A., Jr., Marks, S., Warner, D. E., Barnes, C. M., Herde, K. E., and Kornberg, H. A. (1957). *Radiation Res.* **6**, 380.
Bustad, L. K., Warner, D. E., and Kornberg, H. A. (1958). *Am. J. Vet. Res.* **18**, 893.
Bustad, L. K., Barnes, C. M., George, L. A., Jr., Herde, K. E., Horstman, V. G., Kornberg, H. A., McKenney, J. R., Persing, R. L., Marks, S., Seigneur, L. J., and Warner, D. E. (1962). *In* "Use of Radioisotopes in Animal Biology and the Medical Sciences" (M. Fried, ed.), Vol. 1, p. 401. Academic Press, New York.
Carroll, E. J. (1963). *In* "Clinical Biochemistry of Domestic Animals" (C. E. Cornelius and J. J. Kaneko, eds.), p. 58. Academic Press, New York.
Clark, S. T., and Meier, H. (1958). *Zentr. Veterinaermed.* **5**, 17.
Cline, M. J., and Berlin, N. I. (1963). *Am. J. Physiol.* **204**, 415.
Danowski, T. S., Man, E. B., and Winkler, A. W. (1946). *Endocrinology* **38**, 230.
Fisher, D. A., Oddie, T. H., and Epperson, J. (1965). *J. Clin. Endocrinol. Metab.* **25**, 1580.
Flamboe, E. E., and Reineke, E. P. (1959). *J. Animal Sci.* **18**, 1135.
Freinkel, N., and Ingbar, S. H. (1955). *J. Clin. Endocrinol. Metab.* **15**, 598.
Glock, G. E. (1949). *J. Endocrinol.* **6**, 6.
Hackett, P. L., Gaylor, D. W., and Bustad, L. K. (1957). *Am. J. Vet. Res.* **18**, 338.
Hamilton, J. G., and Soley, M. H. (1939). *Am. J. Physiol.* **127**, 557.
Hamolsky, M. W., Stein, M., and Freedberg, A. S. (1957). *J. Clin. Endocrinol. Metab.* **17**, 33.

Hamolsky, M. W., Golodetz, A., and Freedberg, A. S. (1959). *J. Clin. Endocrinol. Metab.* **19**, 103.

Henneman, H. A., Reineke, E. P., and Griffin, S. A. (1955). *J. Animal Sci.* **14**, 419.

Irvine, C. H. G. (1967a). *J. Endocrinol.* **39**, 313.

Irvine, C. H. G. (1967b). *Am. J. Vet. Res.* **28**, 1687.

Irvine, W. J., and Standeven, R. M. (1968). *J. Endocrinol.* **41**, 31.

Kaihara, S., Carullit, N., and Wagner, H. N., Jr. (1969). *J. Nucl. Med.* **10**, 281.

Kallfelz, F. A. (1969). *J. Am. Vet. Med. Assoc.* **152**, 1647.

Kaneko, J. J. (1963). *In* "Clinical Biochemistry of Domestic Animals" (C. E. Cornelius and J. J. Kaneko, eds.), p. 310. Academic Press, New York.

Kaneko, J . J. (1964). *Proc. 10th Ann. Conv. Am. Assoc. Equine Practitioners.* p. 125. Denver, Colo.

Kaneko, J. J. (1969). Unpublished data.

Kaneko, J. J., Tyler, W. S., Wind, A. P., and Cornelius, C. E. (1959). *J. Am. Vet. Med. Assoc.* **135**, 10.

Klebanoff, S. J. (1965). *In* "Physiology and Biophysics" (T. C. Ruch and H. D. Patton, eds.), 19th ed., p. 1147. Saunders, Philadelphia, Pennsylvania.

Kritchevsky, D. (1958). "Cholesterol," p. 279. Wiley, New York.

Kuhns, L. J., Tallman, D. F., and Sippel, W. L. (1969). *J. Comp. Lab. Med.* **3**, 27.

Lennon, H. D., and Mixner, J. P. (1957). *J. Dairy Sci.* **40**, 1424.

Leveille, G., Fisher, H., and Weiss, H. S. (1957). *Proc. Soc. Exptl. Biol. Med.* **94**, 383.

Lipman, L. M. (1967). *Am. J. Med.* **43**, 486.

Lombardi, M. H., Comar, C. L., and Kirk, R. W. (1962). *Am. J. Vet. Res.* **23**, 412.

Long, J. F., Gilmore, L. O., Curtis, G. M., and Rife, D. C. (1951). *J. Animal Sic.* **10**, 1027.

Lucis, O. J., Cummings, G. T., Matthews, S., and Burry, C. (1969). *J. Nucl. Med.* **10**, 160.

Lucke, V. M. (1964). *J. Small Animal Pract.* **5**, 351.

McKenzie, J. M. (1958). *Endocrinology* **63**, 372.

Mallo, G. L., and Harris, A. L. (1967). *Vet. Med./Small Animal Clinician* **62**, 533.

Mayer, E. (1947). *Endocrinology* **40**, 165.

Meier, H., and Clark, S. T. (1958). *Zentr. Veterinaermed.* **5**, 120.

Metz, C. E. (1969). *J. Nucl. Med.* **10**, 475.

Michaelson, S. M. (1969). *Mod. Vet. Pract.* **50**, 43.

Morris, B., and Courtice, F. C. (1955). *Quart. J. Exptl. Physiol.* **40**, 127.

Murphy, B. E. P., and Pattee, C. J. (1964). *J. Clin. Endocrinol. Metab.* **24**, 187.

Norcia, L. M., and Furman, R. H. (1959). *Proc. Soc. Exptl. Biol. Med.* **100**, 759.

O'Neal, L. W., and Heinbecker, P. (1953). *Endocrinology* **53**, 60.

Pain, R. W., and Oldfield, R. K. (1969). *Tech. Bull. Regist. Med. Technol.* **39**, 139.

Pilleggi, V. J., Lee, N. D., Golub, O. J., and Henry, R. J. (1961). *J. Clin. Endocrinol. Metab.* **21**, 1272.

Pipes, G. W., and Turner, C. W. (1956). *Missouri, Univ., Agr. Expt. Sta., Res. Bull.* **617**, 1.

Pipes, G. W., Bauman, T. R., Brooks, J. R., Comfort, J. E., and Turner, C. W. (1963). *J. Animal Sci.* **22**, 476.

Quinlan, W., and Michaelson, S. M. (1967). *Am. J. Vet. Res.* **28**, 179.

Rac, R., Hill, G. N., and Pain, R. W. (1968). *Res. Vet. Sci.* **9**, 209.

Ragan, H. A., Horstman, V. G., McClellan, R. D., and Bustad, L. K. (1966). *Am. J. Vet. Res.* **116**, 161.

Reiser, R., Sorrels, M. F., and Williams, M. C. (1959). *Circulation Res.* **7**, 833.

Schultz, A. L., Sandhaus, S., Demorest, H. L., and Zieve, L. (1954). *J. Clin. Endocrinol. Metab.* **14**, 1062.

Scott, K. G., and Reilly, W. A. (1954). *Metab., Clin. Exptl.* **3**, 506.

Seigneur, L. J., Test, L. D., Bustad, L. K. (1959). *Am. J. Vet. Res.* **20**, 14.

Siegel, E. T., and Belshaw, B. E. (1968). *In* "Current Veterinary Therapy" (R. W. Kirks, ed.), 3rd ed., p. 545. Saunders, Philadelphia, Pennsylvania.

Slingerland, D. W. (1955). *J. Clin, Endocrinol. Metab.* **15**, 131.

Smith, H. A., and Jones, T. C. (1966). "Veterinary Pathology," p. 1073. Lea & Febiger, Philadelphia, Pennsylvania.

Sorensen, P. H. (1962). *In* "Use of Radioisotopes in Animal Biology and the Medical Sciences" (M. Fried, ed.), Vol. 1, p. 455. Academic Press, New York.

Sparagana, M., Phillips, G., and Kucera, L. (1969). *J. Clin. Endocrinol Metab.* **29**, 191.

Stanbury, J. B. (1966). *In* "The Metabolic Basis of Inherited Disease" (J. B. Stanbury, J. B. Wyngaarden, and O. S. Fredrickson, eds.), p. 215. McGraw-Hill, New York.

Tapley, D. F. (1964). *Mayo Clinic Proc.* **39**, 626.

Tata, J. R., Ernster, L., Lindberg, O., Arrhenius, E., Pederson, S., and Redman, R. (1963). *Biochem. J.* **86**, 408.

Taurog, A., and Chaikoff, I. L. (1946). *J. Biol. Chem.* **163**, 313.

Theran, P., and Thornton, G. W. (1966). *J. Am. Vet. Med. Assoc.* **148**, 562.

Trum, B. F., and Wasserman, R. H. (1956). *Am. J. Vet. Res.* **17**, 271.

Van Zyl, A., Schulz, K., Wilson, B., and Pansegrouw, D. (1965). *Endocrinology* **76**, 353.

Wilson, R. B., Dickson, W. M., and Dost, F. N. (1961). *Vet. Med.* **46**, 285.

Zieve, L., Vogel, W. C., and Schultz, A. L. (1956). *J. Lab. Clin. Med.* **47**, 663.

Calcium, Inorganic Phosphorus, and Magnesium Metabolism in Health and Disease

Mogens G. Simesen

I. CALCIUM AND INORGANIC PHOSPHORUS METABOLISM

Over 70% of the ash of the body consists of calcium and phosphorus. More than 99% of the total calcium and 80–85% of the phosphorus are contained in the skeleton and in the teeth. The minor portions present in the body fluids, though negligible in size, play an extremely important role in the maintenance of normal body functions. The calcium in the extracellular fluids is critical for (1) normal neuro-muscular excitability; (2) capillary and cell membrane permeability; (3) normal muscle contraction; (4) normal transmission of nerve impulses; and (5) normal blood coagulation.

Phosphorus outside the skeleton plays an even more fascinating part. It is in-volved in vital cellular structures and serves in degradation and synthesis of numerous carbon compounds. High-energy phosphate bonds play a fundamental role in storage, liberation, and transfer of energy. Finally, the ability of phosphorus to be excreted either as $H_2PO_4^-$ or HPO_4^{2-} gives a broad margin for the acid–base metabolism in the body.

A. Calcium and Phosphorus in Composition and Formation of Bone

Normal adult bone is composed of approximately 45% water, 25% ash, 20% protein, and 10% fat. In mammals the ash is made up of 36% calcium, 17% phos-phorus, and 0.8% magnesium.

Calcium is found in the bones partly as tricalcium phosphate and partly as calcium carbonate, probably related in a complex apatite structure, whose formula may be written as $CaCO_3 \times nCa_3(PO_4)_2$. However, bone does not seem to have a constant composition. The crystals apparently admit and absorb various ionic groups without change in the geometry of the crystal lattice; hence bone contains, besides calcium and phosphorus, variable proportions of carbonate, fluoride, citrate, sodium, potassium, and magnesium. There appears to be a clear difference between young and adult bone: the salt determining solubility in young bone is octocalcium phosphate and that in adult bone is hydroxyapatite. This difference offers an explanation for the higher incidence of serum inorganic P in young animals (Mac-Gregor and Brown, 1965).

Calcium and phosphorus always occur in approximately 2:1 ratio, and this is not altered even in conditions of partial demineralization of the bones. The percentage of calcium and phosphorus or of ash in bone, without ash weight, therefore, is a poor indication of an animal's mineral reserve (D. L. Duncan, 1958). Cancellous bone is more readily resorbed than compact bone and, accordingly, changes are best demonstrated in vertebrae or ribs.

Bone mineral is readily mobilized to maintain the level of serum calcium, but less readily to maintain that of phosphorus, so that a low serum inorganic phosphate level is the first sign of deficiency of phosphorus.

All bone formation involves (1) the production of a suitable matrix of organic material consisting of collagenous fibrils and a binding substance of mucoproteins, and (2) the precipitation of bone salts in the binding substance. Osteoblasts bring about both processes.

The precipitation of insoluble calcium salts at the site of bone formation is favored by secretion of a phosphatase, which, in alkaline solution, converts organic esters of phosphoric acid into inorganic phosphate. The phosphatase is formed by osteoblasts (Robison, 1923). Some phosphatase reaches the blood stream and is found in the circulating blood.

The possibility and extent of deposition depend on the concentration of calcium and phosphorus in the serum and interstitial fluid. If calcium and/or phosphate concentrations are too low, even the phosphatase activity may not be effective enough to induce calcification. In rickets, the undersaturation of body fluids with calcium and phosphate retards new bone formation in the epiphysis and also causes excessive resorption of bone from the diaphysis.

It is in cancellous bone with its extensive surface exposed to interstitial fluid that most of the bone turnover of calcium and phosphate takes place. Mobilization and deposition of calcium is controlled by the output of parathyroid hormone and thyrocalcitonin.

Although the action of vitamin D is predominantly an enhancement of calcium absorption from the intestine, it is also essential for the normal growth of bones, exerting a specific effect at the site of calcification. Defects in this mechanism result in rickets.

B. CALCIUM AND PHOSPHORUS ABSORPTION

Ultimately, the calcium contained in the diet per se will determine the amounts of calcium absorbed from the gastrointestinal tract, and in most species the blood calcium level tends to rise or fall with the dietary calcium level. This seems to be true in sheep (Franklin et al., 1948). In cattle, however, it seems difficult to provoke a decrease of the serum calcium level by feeding a calcium-deficient diet (Groenewald, 1935). Diets rich in calcium or diets with high Ca:P ratios may cause a slight increase of the blood calcium level of cattle (Saarinen, 1950).

The efficiency of calcium absorption may increase in conditions causing increasing demands, for instance, during pregnancy or lactation. The same effect may be brought about during deficient dietary intake of calcium. Studies with ^{45}Ca in cattle and goats have revealed that "true digestibility" is at its greatest level during the peak of the lactation period (Visek et al., 1952, 1953b). Calcium absorption decreases with increasing age.

The formation of rather insoluble calcium compounds in the intestine may reduce calcium absorption. Thus it has been shown that oxalate may reduce calcium absorption in rats due to formation of insoluble calcium oxalate, which is lost in the feces (Talapatra et al., 1948). In ruminants microbial decomposition of oxalates in the rumen has been demonstrated (Oslage et al., 1960). The degradation of oxalates may result, however, in alkalosis, thus upsetting mineral equilibrium and affecting calcium metabolism indirectly (Watts, 1959). Large quantities of oxalates (fresh leaves of sugar beets may contain as much as 7% of potassium oxalate) may, however, overload the ruminal capacity of metabolizing the oxalate, immobilize the calcium in the alimentary tract, and thus contribute significantly in the development of hypocalcemia.

Phytates, present in rather high levels in cereals, are of considerable importance in calcium and phosphorus metabolism in monogastric animals (Hoff-Jørgensen, 1946; Mellanby, 1949). Phosphorus bound in this manner is not utilized by monogastric animals unless it is decomposed (hydrolyzed) by the enzyme phytase. If this does not occur, the body is deprived, not only of phosphorus, but of calcium as well. This is due to the fact that this substance, inositol hexaphosphoric acid, at a pH of 5–7, will form a very insoluble calcium salt in the intestine. In ruminants phytin is completely hydrolyzed in the rumen (Reid *et al.*, 1947).

It has been shown (Storry, 1961a,b) that abomasal digesta of sheep may contain materials which bind Ca above pH 5. Nucleic acids which are formed in the rumen and pass largely unchanged to the duodenum are potent Ca-binding agents (Chang and Carr, 1968) and are presumably in part responsible for this binding (R.H. Smith *et al.*, 1968).

The chelating agent, ethylenediaminetetraacetic acid (EDTA) has also been shown to inhibit the absorption of calcium from the small intestine of sheep (Van'T Klooster and Care, 1966).

Calcium is apparently absorbed primarily from the oral portion of the small intestine, and most of the evidence indicates that increased acidity of the gastro-intestinal fluid favors calcium absorption (Granström, 1908; Hart *et al.*, 1931). Oral administration of acid increases intestinal absorption, at the same time leading to increased urinary excretion of calcium.

The Ca:P ratio of the diet greatly influences the absorption of calcium and phosphorus. The dietary level of calcium or phosphorus tends to limit the absorption of the remaining element. As the Ca:P ratio becomes wider the requirement for vitamin D increases (see Section IV). In the nonruminant a Ca:P ratio wider than 3:1 results in undesirable effects, whereas Ca:P ratio less than 1:1 is tolerated. Ruminants, on the other hand, will tolerate Ca:P ratios of 7:1 without undesirable effects, but with Ca:P ratios lower than 1:1 decreased performance is observed (Wise *et al.*, 1963; Young *et al.*, 1966).

Evidence in the sites of absorption of calcium and phosphorus from the gastro-intestinal tract has been obtained from studies using radioactive isotopes. Oral administration of [^{32}P] phosphate to dairy cows (Saarinen *et al.*, 1950) or [^{32}P] casein to young calves (Lofgreen *et al.*, 1951) was followed by two maxima for specific activity of blood phosphorus. The maxima occurred at approximately 4 and 15 hours in calves and 6 and 30 hours in cows. These results would seem to indicate absorption of phosphorus at two sites, the rumen and the small intestine. Available evidence now suggests that the rumen epithelium is relatively impermeable to the phosphate ion as it is to Ca and Mg (Phillipson and Storry, 1965).

The delay between oral administration of ^{45}Ca and time of maximum specific activity in blood calcium was 30 hours in the cow (Visek *et al.*, 1953b) and 12–18 hours in the goat (Visek *et al.*, 1952), indicating that calcium absorption occurred mainly in the intestine, whereas the absorption from the forestomachs was negligible.

C. Vitamin D

Apart from dietary intake of calcium, vitamin D is a most important factor in regulating the absorption of calcium. Vitamin D has a direct effect on the mineralization of bone, as well as on the intestinal absorption of calcium (Greenberg, 1945).

Vitamin D is involved in the mechanism that balances skeletal and blood calcium. Injection of vitamin D in dogs fed a low calcium or calcium-free diet will thus induce bone resorption and hypercalcemia (Hess *et al.*, 1931). Also, in cattle (Hibbs and Pounden, 1955) and swine (Pedersen, 1945) massive doses of vitamin

D have been reported to cause increased blood calcium levels. In these cases increased intestinal absorption of calcium as well as mobilization from bone would account for the increase.

Vitamin D facilitates intestinal absorption of calcium and, at the same time, lowers the intestinal pH. Apparently intestinal absorption of phosphate is also somewhat increased. Calcium salts, particularly phosphate and carbonates, are easily soluble in acid solutions and relatively insoluble in alkaline solutions. Accordingly factors increasing intestinal acidity will favor absorption of calcium and vice versa.

Vitamin D, especially dihydrotachysterol, has been successfully used in the treatment of parathyroid insufficiency in humans (E. Rose and Sunderman, 1939). Most of the compounds with vitamin D activity are more effective in the treatment of parathyroid insufficiency than is parathyroid extract itself (McChesney and Giacomino, 1945).

D. Calcium and Phosphorus Excretion

The fecal calcium, mainly dietary in origin, may be partitioned into exogenous and endogenous calcium. The exogenous fecal calcium is undigested calcium from the food. The endogenous fecal calcium is the fraction of fecal calcium derived from secretions of calcium into the digestive tract, mainly in the small intestine. Calcium-45 studies have indicated that the small intestine is by far the most important.

Knowledge of endogenous fecal calcium and phosphorus is important for determination of the "true" digestibility of food calcium and phosphorus. The apparent digestibility: (food Ca-fecal Ca)/food Ca is a valid basis for estimating the "true" digestibility, only when the endogenous calcium or phosphorus is a small part of the total fecal calcium or phosphorus.

In cattle the endogenous calcium has been estimated to be 4–7 gm daily (Visek et al., 1953a; Comar et al., 1953) and it has been shown that the amount of endogenous fecal calcium is directly proportional to body weight and is little influenced by short-term dietary changes. Hansard et al. (1954) have shown that the level of endogenous calcium in feces changes appreciably with age, becoming progressively greater in old animals.

In rats there is evidence that the amount of endogenous fecal calcium is influenced by vitamin D. Thus, Nicolaysen (1937) showed an increased excretion of metabolic fecal calcium in vitamin D-deficient rats on a calcium- and phosphorus-free diet.

Inorganic phosphorus, too, is excreted in the urine and digestive secretions. The endogenous fecal phosphorus was estimated by Kleiber et al. (1951), Lofgreen and Kleiber (1953), and Luick and Lofgreen (1957). In lactating cows the value was found to be 10–14 gm phosphorus daily, or about twice the amount of endogenous calcium. The site of transfer of endogenous phosphorus into the gastrointestinal tract was studied by A. H. Smith and co-workers 1955a,b, 1956; Lofgreen et al., 1952). The animals were given injections of ^{32}P and sacrificed at intervals following injection. The specific activity of phosphorus was determined in plasma and in various segments of the gastrointestinal tract and their corresponding contents. In swine (A. H. Smith et al., 1955a) most of the endogenous phosphorus appeared to enter the small intestine, and endogenous phosphorus was reabsorbed to a greater extent than dietary phosphorus in the posterior portion of the digestive tract. In dairy cows (A. H. Smith *et al.*, 1956) and sheep (A. H. Smith *et al.*, 1955b) the main site of phosphorus excretion was the rumen (saliva).

1.   Urinary Excretion

The urinary excretion of calcium and phosphorus is regulated. Part of the filtrated calcium and phosphorus is reabsorbed in the renal tubules. Reabsorption of phosphorus takes place in the proximal end of the tubules and is probably brought about by enzymic activity.

The renal threshold for calcium excretion is between 6.5 and 8.0 mg/100 ml, little being eliminated at lower concentrations.

Mineral acids fed to cows increase the urinary calcium excretion (Hart *et al.*, 1931). The same is true of nonionized Ca complexes such as citrate and EDTA. They are not subject to tubular reabsorption in the kidney, and therefore renal calcium excretion is enhanced.

As a rapid method for estimation of urinary calcium the so-called Sulkowitch test has been considered as a valuable clinical tool for serum calcium on the spot in cases of parturient paresis. Examinations of the reliability of the test (Detweiler and Martin, 1949; Roberts *et al.*, 1951; Hallgren, 1955) have shown it to be of little value or even misleading (1) because of poor correlation between serum calcium and urine calcium and (2) because of the difficulty of achieving safe estimation of the urinary level of calcium by means of the test. A reliable, 15-minute semi-quantitative test for serum calcium has recently been proposed (Mayer *et al.*, 1965).

In cattle the rate of urinary phosphorus excretion amounts to only a fraction of 1% of the rate of phosphorus excretion in the feces (Kleiber *et al.*, 1951). In contrast, urinary phosphorus excretion in man may exceed the excretion of fecal phosphorus (Clark, 1925). This characteristic difference apparently is attributable to the alkaline urine herbivora normally excrete. An alkaline pH seriously limits the possibilities for simultaneous excretion of calcium and phosphate.

2.   Mammary Secretion

In lactating animals considerable amounts of calcium and phosphorus are secreted in the milk, and several of the constituents are found in concentrations higher than that of the blood. Thus, the concentration of calcium is increased by a factor of 12–13, that of phosphorus about 7, and that of magnesium about 6.

Blood samples drawn from mammary veins may have an inorganic phosphorus level of about 1 mg/100 ml higher than that of blood from the jugular vein (Meigs *et al.*, 1919). The level of serum calcium is, on the other hand, usually lower in the mammary vein than in the jugular vein (Hallgren, 1940).

II.   SERUM CALCIUM AND PHOSPHORUS LEVELS

The serum concentration of calcium in normal adult animals averages 10 mg/100 ml (5 mEq/liter, or 2.5 mmoles/liter). The normal range is usually stated to be

9–12 mg/100 ml (details in Table I). The serum calcium concentration of normal young animals is of the same order as that of adults. The quantity of calcium contained in red blood cells is negligible.

Ultrafiltrable serum calcium in cattle has been found to constitute from 40 to about 60% of total serum calcium (Boogaerdt, 1954; R. H. Smith, 1957; Hallgren et al., 1959).

Most of the phosphorus of blood is present as organic esters of phosphorus within the red cells; these contain small amounts of inorganic phosphorus at any given moment. Serum contains about 14–15 mg total phosphorus/100 ml, but of this 5–8 mg is lipid phosphorus. A trace of the rest is ester phosphorus, the most significant portion of the remainder being inorganic phosphate. The main difficulty in determining serum inorganic phosphate arises from the fact that if a portion of the red cells undergoes hemolysis, the phosphoric esters present in these cells may undergo hydrolysis with consequent liberation of phosphate. Serum inorganic phosphate concentration in normal adult animals is 4–7 mg/100 ml, horses and dogs being the exceptions (see Table II). Young animals usually have a higher and more variable concentration (5–9 mg/100 ml). The inorganic phosphate level appears to be intimately related to carbohydrate metabolism. During increased carbohydrate utilization the level tends to decrease, and during fasting an increase usually is observed (1–2 mg/100 ml). A principal rule—to which, however, there are many exceptions—says that increasing serum phosphorus is accompanied by decreasing serum calcium. Principally, the actual concentrations will depend upon the following conditions: (1) intestinal absorption, (2) uptake from the skeleton,

TABLE I   CONCENTRATION OF CALCIUM IN BLOOD OF NORMAL ANIMALS

| Species | Blood fraction[a] | Value (mg/100 ml) | | | Reference |
		No. of animals sampled.	Mean	Standard deviation	
Shetlands pony	S	8	10.2	±1.0	Eriksen and Simesen (1970)
Horse	S	30	12.4	±0.58	Jennings and Mulligan (1953)
Cattle	S	185	11.08	±0.67	Crookshank and Sims (1955)
Cattle	S	90	10.2	±0.28	Mylrea and Bayfield (1968)
Cattle	B	833	7.4	±0.8	Lane et al. (1968)
Cattle at parturition	S	31	8.07		Blosser and Smith (1950b)
Sheep	S	722	12.16	±0.28	Hackett et al. (1957)
Sheep	P	517	9.2	±1.0	Marsh and Swingle (1955)
Pig (6 months old)	S	50	9.65	±0.99	Simesen (1963a)
Pregnant sow	S	14	10.11	±1.08	Simesen (1963a)
Goat	S	30	10.3	±0.7	Murty and Kehar (1951)
Cat	S	10	8.22	±0.97[b]	Bloom (1957)
Dog	S	9	10.16	±2.04	Eichelberger et al. (1948)

[a] S = serum; P = plasma; B = whole blood.
[b] Standard deviation was estimated from range and number of observations.

TABLE II   CONCENTRATION OF PHOSPHORUS (INORGANIC) IN BLOOD OF NORMAL ANIMALS

Species	Blood fraction[a]	No. of animals sampled	Mean	Standard deviation	Reference
			Values (mg/100 ml)		
Shetlands pony	S	8	4.9	±1.1	Eriksen and Simesen (1970)
Horse	B	2	2.1	±2.2	Rapoport and Guest (1941)
Cattle	S	25	5.5	±0.8	Mylrea and Bayfield (1968)
Heifers	S	25	6.2	±0.6	Mylrea and Bayfield (1968)
Calves	S	20	8.9	±0.6	Mylrea and Bayfield (1968)
Cattle	B*	838	6.1	±0.8	Lane et al. (1968)
Cattle	S	185	5.56	±1.56	Crookshank and Sims (1955)
Goat	B	2	6.8–8.4 (range)		Rapoport and Guest (1941)
Sheep	P	517	4.3	±0.9	Marsh and Swingle (1955)
Sheep	S	919	5.21	±0.11	Hackett et al. (1957)
Pig (6 months old)	S	43	10.94	±0.98	Simesen (1963a)
Pregnant sow	S	12	7.87	±1.42	Simesen (1963a)
Cat	S	10	6.40	±1.17[b]	Bloom (1957)
Dog	B	13	3.2		Rapoport and Guest (1941)
	P	20	4.3		Baer et al. (1957)

[a]S = serum; P = plasma; B = whole blood; B* = whole blood in trichloracetic acid.
[b]Standard deviation was estimated from range and number of observations.

(3) amounts of parathyroid hormone and thyrocalcitonin, and (4) urinary excretion.

W. M. Allcroft and Godden (1934) have shown that calves at birth and for the first 8 weeks of life show rather high levels of serum calcium and inorganic phosphorus. In the adult stage increasing age has been reported to be associated with a slight decline in serum calcium and a marked decline in inorganic phosphorus (Payne and Leech, 1964).

A. Parathyroid Hormone

In conditions with poor absorption of calcium from the intestinal tract the plasma calcium level is maintained primarily by its mobilization from the bones through the action of the parathyroid hormone (PTH). Its physiological actions, which are exerted in the metabolism of both calcium and phosphorus, may be illustrated by outlining the consequences of (1) removal of the parathyroid glands and (2) injection of PTH.

Effect of parathyroidectomy: Decreased urinary output of phosphate; increased serum phosphate level; decreased urinary calcium output; and decreased serum calcium level.

Effect of injection of PTH: Increased urinary phosphate excretion; decreased serum phosphate level; increased urinary calcium excretion; and increased serum calcium concentration.

Early studies on the physiology of the parathyroids led to two conflicting opinions concerning the actual mechanism. One school of thought (Albright et al., 1929; Albright and Reifenstein, 1948) felt that the primary effect of PTH was to increase renal excretion of phosphorus by diminishing tubular absorption of the phosphorus filtered by the glomeruli. In other words, the hormone increased the ratio of phosphorus clearance to inulin clearance. As a result, the serum phosphorus level rapidly declines, and the serum body fluids become unsaturated with respect to calcium phosphate. Calcium phosphate is therefore liberated from the bones. Since phosphorus is still being rapidly excreted, only serum calcium rises. When serum calcium has increased above the threshold value for renal excretion, more calcium is excreted in the urine. Thomson and Collip (1932), on the other hand, proposed that the primary action of the hormone was to induce dissolution of bone, possibly by increasing the numbers and activity of osteoclasts. The increased excretion of phosphate followed as a secondary effect.

According to the present view (McLean and Urist, 1955) the skeleton is the chief factor in stabilizing the calcium concentrations of the extracellular fluids. A dual mechanism exists for the PTH control of plasma calcium level. One mechanism involves a simple chemical equilibrium between labile fractions of the bone mineral and plasma. This dynamic equilibrium is adequate to maintain serum calcium at approximately 7 mg/100 ml. The mechanism is independent of the PTH.

The second part of the regulatory mechanism depends on the parathyroid gland. The hormone regulates resorption of calcium and phosphate from cancellous bone as well as the excretory mechanism of phosphate and is thus able to increase serum calcium to the normal level of 9–12 mg per 100 ml.

The primary stimulus to secretion of PTH is the calcium level itself. A decrease in serum calcium stimulates the production of PTH and an increase in the serum calcium depresses the excretion (McLean's negative feedback mechanism). Hypermagnesemia also appears to have an inhibitory effect on the rate of excretion (Care et al., 1966). It has been difficult to assess the importance of the parathyroids in ruminants (Boda and Cole, 1956), even though considerable interest is attached to this problem because of the great frequency of parturient paresis in dairy cattle.

B. Thyrocalcitonin

In 1962 Copp et al. were able to show that perfusion of the thyroid-parathyroid gland complex with blood of high calcium concentration resulted in liberation of a previously unrecognized hormone, a fast-acting hypocalcemic factor, which they named calcitonin. Since then, evidence has steadily been accumulating confirming the existence of such a calcium-lowering hormone.

Hirsch et al. (1963) introduced the name thyrocalcitonin, because they found that the hormone could be extracted from rat thyroid. The hormone is only found in the scattered parafollicular "C" cells (Bussolati and Pearse, 1967) which arise embryologically from the ultimobranchial body (Pearse and Calvalheira, 1967). In mammals these cells occur imbedded in the thyroid and parathyroid. The regular follicular cells of the thyroid are not involved in thyrocalcitonin production.

Tenenhouse et al. (1965) have reported a procedure capable of yielding thyrocalcitonin of high purity, and have shown thyrocalcitonin to be a polypeptide with a molecular weight of approximately 8700.

Mode of Action

Following injection of thyrocalcitonin, hypocalcemia accompanied by hypophosphatemia and phosphaturia have been demonstrated (Kenny and Heiskell, 1965). A hypocalcemic and hypophosphatemic response to exogenously administered thyrocalcitonin has now been demonstrated in the rat, guinea pig, goat, man, and dog (Stahl and Kenny, 1967; Cramer *et al.*, 1969).

The sensitivity to thyrocalcitonin has been found to decrease with increasing age (Copp and Kuczerpa, 1967; Care and Duncan, 1967).

The most probable explanation for the action of thyrocalcitonin is that it causes a net transfer of calcium from blood into bone (MacIntyre *et al.*, 1967). This is supported by the negative evidence that the rapid loss of calcium from plasma following intravenous injection of the hormone is neither prevented by previous nephrectomy or removal of the gastrointestinal tract, nor accompanied by a rise in the calcium content of cardiac or skeletal muscle (Aliapoulios *et al.*, 1965; Gudmundsson *et al.*, 1966).

Hirsch *et al.* (1963) found that thyrocalcitonin does not act by neutralizing PTH. Friedman and Raisz (1965) pointed out that the relative changes in plasma calcium, inorganic phosphate, and magnesium concentrations after injection of thyrocalcitonin are consistent with the suggestion that bone is the principal target organ. Milhaud *et al.* (1965) and Martin *et al.* (1966) finally presented evidence indicating that the shift in blood–bone calcium equilibrium caused by thyrocalcitonin is due to inhibition of bone resorption.

Besides the effect on bone, Robinson *et al.* (1966) have demonstrated a phosphaturic effect of thyrocalcitonin.

Care *et al.* (1967) have recently suggested that the secretion of thyrocalcitonin is controlled by a negative feedback mechanism operating through the plasma concentration. Because of the rapidity of its release, action, and elimination, relative to PTH, thyrocalcitonin is thought to act as a fine regulator of calcium homeostasis. It is, however, difficult to assess the physiological role of thyrocalcitonin, if it is secreted only when blood calcium levels rise above normal, since, in most mammals studied, hypercalcemia rarely exists in the normally functioning animal. Klein and Talmage (1968) have recently presented evidence for the secretion of thyrocalcitonin also at normal and subnormal plasma calcium levels, and thus suggested that thyrocalcitonin not only plays a role in preventing hypercalcemia, but that it might also contribute to the maintenance of normal calcium homeostasis and bone metabolism.

C. Miscellaneous Factors

Thyroid hormone has been reported to increase the fecal excretion of calcium in dogs (Logan *et al.*, 1942) and lactating dairy cattle (E. C. Owen, 1948), but no effect upon serum calcium and phosphate concentrations has been demonstrated.

Estrogens have been found to depress the serum calcium level, simultaneously elevating the level of inorganic phosphate (Folley, 1936; G. Horvath and Kutas, 1959) in sows, mares, and cows. In bitches, on the contrary, the changes were erratic.

III. ABNORMAL CALCIUM AND PHOSPHORUS METABOLISM

A. HYPERCALCEMIA

Increase in the serum calcium concentrations is found during hyperparathyroidism or induced from administration of excessive amounts of vitamin D.

B. HYPOCALCEMIA

Hypocalcemia is one of the most constant and characteristic features of diminished parathyroid function. The clinical and metabolic aspects of hypoparathyroidism are discussed in connection with parturient paresis.

Deficiency of vitamin D often causes pronounced hypophosphatemia in early stages followed later by a fall in serum calcium.

In sheep, sudden deprivation of feed or forced excercise may cause marked depression of serum calcium levels. Hypocalcemia also occurs in lactating cows after periods of starvation and during bovine ketosis (W. M. Allcroft, 1947a; Simesen, 1958). During bovine ketosis there is a simultaneous increase in urinary calcium excretion (Sjollema, 1932a).

Moderate hypocalcemia is a common finding during diseases with protein-losing gastroenteropathies, where it has been shown that the hypocalcemia is due to gastrointestinal loss of calcium bound to albumin (Nielsen, 1966).

Hypocalcemia is observed in cases of acute pancreatitis. In these cases the hypocalcemia has been attributed to sudden removal of large amounts of calcium from the blood plasma as a result of its fixation as insoluble calcium soaps by fatty acids in areas of fat necrosis.

C. PARTURIENT PARESIS (MILK FEVER)

Milk fever is an afebrile disease, which is typically associated with parturition and the very beginning of lactation. It is characterized by a sudden progressive paresis, paralysis, or coma, and, if untreated, usually terminates in death. The main chemical changes in blood serum are a marked decrease in total as well as ionized calcium and of total as well as inorganic phosphorus and an increase in magnesium. An excellent review on parturient paresis in dairy cattle was published by Hibbs (1950).

The first epoch in the history of milk fever was initiated when a Danish veterinarian by the name of J. Schmidt (1897) discovered that udder insufflation resulted in recovery. This treatment reduced the mortality hazard of milk fever from 60–70% to about 15%. Since then students of milk fever have been probing this phenomenon (Fish, 1928, 1929a; Niedermeier and Smith, 1950; Marshak, 1956), and even today udder insufflation is, under certain conditions, the therapy of choice (Marshak, 1956).

1. Clinical Biochemical Manifestations

Since Little and Wright (1925) published their first results proving that milk fever in cattle was associated with hypocalcemia, there has been a tendency to

TABLE III   BIOCHEMICAL FINDINGS IN CATTLE WITH MILK FEVER, WITH GRASS TETANY AND IN NORMAL CATTLE[a]

Condition	Calcium ion (mg/100 ml)	Total calcium (mg/100 ml)	Inorganic phosphorus (mg/100 ml)	Magnesium (mg/100 ml)
Milk fever	0.44	4.35	2.16	2.19
Grass tetany	1.18	6.65	4.33	0.46
Normal cattle	1.65	9.35	4.57	1.66

[a]From Sjollema and Seekles (1932).

regard these two conditions as synonymous. Numerous reports subsequent to the originals have been made by Dryerre and Greig (1925, 1928), Little and Wright (1925, 1926), and others. Greig (1930) reported minimum, maximum, and average serum calcium values of 3.00, 7.76, and 5.16 mg, respectively, per 100 ml in 82 cases of milk fever. No hypocalcemia was found in diseased animals which did not have milk fever.

Fish (1929b) reported average blood plasma values of 3.31 mg/100 ml for calcium and 2.39 mg/100 ml for inorganic phosphate, and Sjollema and Seekles (1932) (see Table III) drew attention to the difference between the biochemical findings in milk fever, grass tetany, and normal cows.

Previously, Palmer and co-workers (Palmer and Eckles, 1930; Palmer et al., 1930) had reported decreased blood levels of both calcium and phosphate in normal cattle at parturition. Wilson and Hart (1932) demonstrated that this decrease was more pronounced in older cattle than in first-calf heifers, and they presented additional evidence to show hypocalcemia to be an essential factor in milk fever. These findings were confirmed (W. M. Allcroft and Green, 1934; W. M. Allcroft and Godden, 1934), and an increase in serum magnesium was reported to take place in normal cattle at parturition (Table IV).

Barker (1939) recognized three types of hypocalcemia. The clinical symptoms depended on the level of serum magnesium varying from extreme nervousness and tetany, when magnesium was low, to a comatose condition, when magnesium was high. Robertson (1949), however, was unable to confirm this classification of types of milk fever.

TABLE IV   BLOOD CHANGES AT NORMAL PARTURITION (PERCENTAGE CHANGE FROM 2 DAYS PREPARTUM)[a]

Group	Number of animals	Serum calcium (% fall)	Inorganic phosphorus (% fall)	Serum magnesium (% rise)
First calvers	7	11.7	33.8	7.7
Second calvers	8	17.6	38.4	24.1
Third calvers	9	22.9	46.4	34.4
Fourth and subsequent calving	8	30.6	48.1	35.9

[a]Robertson et al. (1956).

Blood calcium exists principally in two fractions: a diffusible ionized form, which accounts for 3.6 to 7.7 mg/100 ml (Hallgren *et al.*, 1959), and a nondiffusible protein-bound fraction. The combination of calcium with serum protein can be split readily when serum calcium is removed by dialysis or oxalate precipitation. The ratio between the different calcium fractions in the blood is determined by the law of mass action.

The decrease in total calcium content at normal parturition relates almost entirely to the bound calcium fraction. During milk fever a reduction is found in both calcium ion concentration and bound calcium (Hallgren *et al.*, 1959) as well as in the total and ultrafiltrable fraction (Straub *et al.*, 1959).

In normal calving cows a reduction is found in organically bound phosphorus as well as in inorganic phosphorus. During milk fever the values for inorganic phosphorus is still lower, while the content of organically bound phosphorus is of the same order as in normal cows after calving (G. Carlström, 1969).

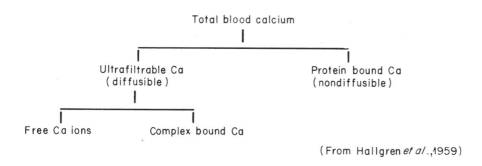

(From Hallgren *et al.*,1959)

Calcium is transported by the blood and is constantly being exchanged. According to Moodie (1960) the total amount of circulating calcium is approximately 1.5–2.0 gm, and the daily turnover of calcium within the body may vary from about 10 gm in the nonproductive cow up to more than 35 gm in the lactating cow (Fig. 1). Thus, a quantity of calcium equal to the total amount in circulation may be removed every 1 to 5 hours depending on the physiological state of the animal.

2. Other Findings

A decrease in blood citric acid (Blosser and Smith, 1950a) has been reported in milk fever cows as compared with healthy cows at parturition. The levels of citric acid seem to reflect those of calcium. Calcium and citrate metabolism, however, are known to be closely related (Lichtwitz *et al.*, 1961). Both calcium and citrate are present in bone salts, and they form a soluble poorly ionized complex. Therefore, even if citrate concentration may influence the disposition and resorption of bone salts, it seems impossible to decide whether the changed citric acid levels in parturient paresis only mirror the calcium citrate reciprocity, or if they indicate a decreased mobilization from the skeleton (Jönsson, 1960).

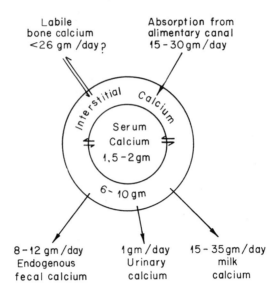

Fig. 1.   The exchange of calcium between serum and tissue in lactating cows (from Moodie, 1960).

A marked increase of blood glucose and pyruvic acid in both normally calving cows and cows developing milk fever has been found, the levels being considerably higher in the latter group (Van Soest and Blosser, 1954; Ward *et al.*, 1953). A statistical significant negative correlation between blood glucose and plasma inorganic phosphate, and between blood pyruvate and inorganic phosphate was demonstrated.

A number of reports indicating a connection between the activity of the adrenal cortex and milk fever have appeared.

Garm (1950) has reported marked lymphopenia and eosinopenia as well as adrenocortical hypertrophy in cows with milk fever. Holcombe (1953) found a low urinary excretion of reducing corticoids and neutral steroids, thus indicating adrenocortical exhaustion. But since a decrease of the circulating lymphocytes and eosinophils and an increase of neutrophils and blood glucose occur normally at parturition, and since ACTH has a similar effect to that of parturition on these blood constituents, Merrild and Smith (1954) suggest that an increased excretion of adrenocortical hormones occurs in response to the stress of parturition. Later on these workers found that milk fever may produce a stress sufficient to increase adrenocortical activity, as measured by the leukocyte response, but they could not support the findings of adrenocortical exhaustion, since they demonstrated that ACTH administration to milk-fever cows resulted in the usual response (V. R. Smith and Merrild, 1954). Neither could Ward (1956), in the study of the changes in the blood and urinary levels of sodium and potassium in normal cows and in cows with milk fever, find any indication of adrenal involvement to a greater extent than that associated with the act of parturition. Recently, Jonsgård (1963) reviewed a series of experiments on the prophylactic effect of glucocorticoids and ACTH and concluded that there is no convincing evidence that adrenal hypofunction is the cause of the disease, and administration of adrenal corticoids appears to have no prophylactic effect.

The data of Ward (1956) indicate that hematocrit values are higher in milk fever cows prior to treatment than in healthy cows at parturition. Van Soest and Blosser (1954), however, found that higher hematocrit values were typical for all cows at the time of parturition. As early as 1932 evidence was given that anhydremia (dehydration) was not an important factor in milk fever (L. T. Wilson and Hart, 1932).

Larson and Kendall (1957) have recorded a lowering of serum protein at calving time compared with 4 weeks precalving, and Vigue (1952) reported low total serum protein levels in cases of milk fever. Hallgren *et al.* (1959) and Marshak (1956), however, were unable to demonstrate any decrease in the serum proteins of cows with hypocalcemia.

Minor changes in blood pH during milk fever have occasionally been reported (Hallgren *et al.*, 1959; Aalund and Nielsen, 1960). In studies on milk fever, Hallgren (1940) demonstrated a hypotension, the degree of which, however, was minimal and not associated with vasomotor collapse. In 140 healthy cows the systolic blood pressure was 110–185 mmHg as compared with a range of 80–150 mmHg in 44 cases of milk fever. In the majority of those with milk fever (39 cases) the pressure was found to be between 105 and 140 mmHg.

Cholinesterase activity has been studied during milk fever (Seekles and Van Asperen, 1949). No alterations could be demonstrated.

3. Experimental "Milk Fever"

In an attempt to produce an experimental condition similar to milk fever, several investigators (Seekles *et al.*, 1931; Petersen *et al.*, 1931; B. Carlström, 1933; Hallgren *et al.*, 1959; Moodie, 1960; and others) have injected sodium oxalate into cows and observed the symptoms. Following slow intravenous injection of 20–40 gm oxalate the serum calcium is greatly reduced. Clinical symptoms terminating in clonic convulsions and death occur when serum calcium levels lower than 4 mg/100 ml are reached. The hypocalcemia thus produced is largely due to a lowering of the amount of calcium ions (Hallgren *et al.*, 1959).

The decreased ratio Ca:Mg in milk fever caused Klobouk (1932), Pribyl (1933), and Schulhof (1933) to assume magnesium narcosis to be the cause of milk fever, and subsequently magnesium sulfate was injected into calves until a Ca:Mg ratio similar to that found in milk fever was reached. In such cases injections of $CaCl_2$ were demonstrated to be curative.

Hibbs *et al.* (1945, 1946) showed that the anesthetic effect of magnesium is due to the ratio Ca:Mg regardless of whether the serum calcium comes down to meet the serum magnesium, as in milk fever or when oxalate is injected, or the serum magnesium goes up to meet the serum calcium, as when magnesium salts are injected. Hibbs therefore concluded (1950) that the relatively high serum magnesium accounts for the lack of tetanic symptoms in typical milk fever and for the comatose condition, which is usually seen in spite of the low blood calcium level.

4. Etiological Considerations

To illustrate our present concept of milk fever, only two sets of theories need to be mentioned: (1) the hypoglycemia theory and (2) the parathyroid (hypocalcemia) theory.

Until about 1925 little experimental work was done concerning the etiology of milk fever. In 1885 Nocard had noticed "sugar" in the urine of milk-fever cows (at that time it was not possible to distinguish between glucose and lactose).

Then in 1925 suddenly two sets of theories were advanced. Widmark and Carlens (1925a,b,c,) attributed the disease to glucose deficiency (a hypoglycemic coma) brought on by the intensity of mammary secretion. At the same time, in a working hypothesis, without experimental evidence to support it, Dryerre and Greig (1925) in Scotland claimed that "the nature of milk fever may be understood as a parathyroid deficiency resulting in the accumulation of toxic substances such as guanidine, and a fall in blood calcium, the fall in calcium being further accentuated by lactation."

These two new theories caused an increasing interest in chemical blood analysis, and in the next few years both theories were subjected to intensive scientific investigation.

a. THE HYPOGLYCEMIA THEORY.   It was soon shown that a hyperglycemia rather than a hypoglycemia was characteristic of milk fever (Hayden, 1924–1925; Fish, 1927, 1928; Greig, 1926). But then supporters of the hypoglycemia theory (Auger, 1926, 1927) replied that the high blood "sugar" demonstrated was due to lactose not available to the tissues. Thus, although an increase occurred in total "sugar," the actual available sugar (i.e., glucose) was still deficient during milk fever. The matter was conclusively cleared up, when Hayden (1927), by means of the new Folin-Svedberg fermentation method (Folin and Svedberg, 1926), was able to demonstrate a hyperglycemia during milk fever.

b. THE PARATHYROID (HYPOCALCEMIA) THEORY.   As early as May, 1925, Little and Wright reported their first results showing milk fever in cattle to be associated with a hypocalcemia. Since then this finding has been repeatedly confirmed, and the research almost exclusively directed toward the cause of this phenomenon.

The assumption of a guanidine toxemia due to parathyroid deficiency was soon refuted (Hayden, 1929), and PTH was reported to be of dubious value in preventing or curing milk fever (Little and Mattick, 1933). Jackson *et al.* (1962) have recently confirmed this finding. They concluded that parturient cows were not responsive to PTH extract, and its administration just after calving had no apparent effect on the occurrence or severity of milk fever.

Greig (1930) demonstrated that the blood calcium rose rapidly to normal in milk-fever cases treated with udder inflation. The recovery followed, when a blood serum calcium concentration of about 7 mg/100 ml was reached. Later Niedermeier and Smith (1950) demonstrated that different cows recover at different serum calcium levels, and they have suggested that the relative levels of calcium, phosphate, and magnesium may be important in the symptomatology of milk fever.

The question whether the sudden demand for calcium and phosphorus at the onset of lactation might be responsible for the drop in serum calcium and phosphorus found in parturient paresis, has been subject to considerable interest (B. Carlström, 1933). However, studies reported by V. R. Smith and Blosser (1947), and Jonsgård (1965) showed that prepartum milking had little or no effect on reducing the incidence of parturient paresis. Nor did complete milking of cows immediately following parturition increase the incidence (V. R. Smith *et al.*, 1948; J. R. Owen, 1954). Furthermore, Hibbs (1947) showed that cows with milk fever produced no more colostrum than normal cows during the postparturient period. Ash and calcium content of the colostrum from cows with milk fever were no higher than that of normal postparturient cows. Finally it was shown that mastectomy in susceptible cows eliminates parturient paresis as well as the usual alterations in blood constituents during parturition (Niedermeier et al., 1949; Robertson et al., 1956). The mammary drain of calcium has recently been reconsidered (Kronfeld, 1970).

From these experiments it appears that although the udder is essential in the pathogenesis of parturient paresis, the aberrations responsible for the temporary failure of the mechanisms of calcium homeostasis have to be found somewhere other than the udder. Consideration of these matters led to the conclusion that hypocalcemia in the recently calved cow is essentially a failure to obtain sufficient calcium from the gut and/or bone. From Fig. 1 it will be seen that a cow secreting colostrum at 3–4 gallons a day could not provide the calcium needed for this plus that for endogenous fecal calcium from either the skeleton or the digestive system alone.

As mentioned above, the calcium equilibrium between skeleton and blood is maintained by a dual mechanism. One part is the action of PTH on the skeletal calcium; the other is a chemical equilibrium between bone calcium and blood. Until recently the pros and cons of PTH insufficiency as an etiological feature in milk fever have been almost exclusively based on indirect evidence, and therefore Hibbs (1950) stated: "In weighing all the experimental evidence that has been reported on the various phases of the milk fever problem, the theory of Dryerre and Greig seems to come the nearest of all theories to explaining the cause of the disease."
i. *Renewed examination of parathyroid function.*   Garm (1951) reported significantly higher absolute and relative parathyroid weights in cows with parturient paresis than in normal nonpregnant cows. Blosser and Albright (1956) stated that the blood and urine excretion picture during parturient paresis did not conform to that of hypoparathyroidism in man and laboratory animals, and later Marshak (1957), and more extensively Jönsson (1960), in histological studies evaluated the parathyroid function in normal cows and in cows with parturient paresis. Both concluded that there was no indication of parathyroid insufficiency in cows with parturient paresis.

In the last few years several studies of the response to experimental hypocalcemia have been made (Payne et al., 1963; V. R. Smith and Brown, 1963; Payne, 1964; Mayer et al., 1966). The idea behind some of these experiments was the observation that recovery from EDTA-induced hypocalcemia was found to be prolonged in parathyroidectomized dogs (Payne et al., 1963; Payne, 1964). If a parathyroid insufficiency was involved in parturient paresis a response similar to this would be expected. The experiments showed, however, that milk fever-prone cows were not more than normally prone to experimental hypocalcemia. When symptoms occurred, they appeared during the period when plasma Ca was returning to normal and not, as might have been expected, immediately after injection, when the plasma Ca was at its lowest concentration. During the EDTA-induced hypocalcemia a consistent fall was observed in inorganic phosphate; no changes were seen in plasma Mg.

Mayer et al. (1966) studied hypocalcemia spontaneously occurring as well as experimentally induced. From these observations it was deduced that the degree of hypocalcemia seemed to be more crucial to the development of paresis than duration. Their results are consistent with the above-mentioned finding (Payne, 1963) that hypocalcemia may exist for hours before symptoms develop.

Nelson *et al.* (1963) studied the effect of age and calcium-free diet on thyroparathyroidectomized sheep and showed that adult sheep were more tolerant to thyroparathyroidectomy than young animals. Adult animals were capable of correcting the hypocalcemia and maintain serum calcium above symptomatic levels, whereas serum calcium declined rapidly in young thyroparathyroidectomized sheep and fatal tetany often followed. Serum magnesium was only affected when feed intake decreased.

Ramberg *et al.* (1967) made slow, continuous EDTA infusions in parathyroidectomized as well as normal cows. In the intact cows it was demonstrated (with radioimmunoassays) that plasma PTH and plasma calcium concentration was inversely proportional regardless of whether plasma calcium was falling or rising. In the parathyroidectomized cows no detectable response in plasma PTH could be demonstrated and plasma calcium fell at a constant rate for 13 hours.

ii. Parathyroidectomy. Stott and Smith (1957) reported results of parathyroidectomy in cattle. Following radical thyroparathyroidectomy in five pregnant nonlactating cows and in one nonpregnant lactating cow, the serum calcium dropped from an average of 10.3 mg/100 ml to an average of 7.2 mg/100 ml on the second day after operation. The inorganic phosphate decreased to a lesser extent. The subnormal values persisted for 2–3 weeks; serum calcium then returned to normal, whereas inorganic phosphate usually increased above preoperative levels. The cows did not exhibit signs of milk fever, and the absence of the parathyroids did not have any adverse effect on pregnancy or parturition and did not cause any cessation of lactation. The cows were kept on a normal diet with high Ca:P ratio.

iii. Balance studies. Usually the dry cow is in positive calcium and phosphorus balance, whereas lactating cows during the first month of lactation are in negative balance (D. L. Duncan, 1958). The change from positive to negative balance occurs over a period of a very few days at the time of parturition. In contrast to this, Ward *et al.* (1952) found that cows developing milk fever had a severe negative calcium balance during the last 15 days of pregnancy. These findings contrast sharply with the findings of Boda and Cole (1956) indicating that a negative calcium balance before parturition has a prophylactic influence on milk fever.

iv. Absorption from the alimentary tract. About the time of calving the variable nature of the animal's appetite precludes use of conventional balance experiments as a means of determining the quantities of calcium absorbed on an hourly or daily basis. Robertson *et al.* (1960) and Moodie and Robertson (1961, 1962) therefore produced indirect evidence in support of their suggestion that the cow around the calving time is dependent not only on release of calcium from bone but also on a continuous uptake of calcium from the alimentary tract. Loss of appetite, reduced fecal excretion, and reduction in alimentary activity were changes reported to take place at parturition in normal calving cows. To stress the importance of uninterrupted absorption of calcium from the alimentary tract in heavy milking cows and cows at time of parturition Moodie (1960) had previously introduced hypocalcemia and milk-feverlike symptoms in lactating cows by injection of hyoscine hydrobromide, an alkaloid paralyzing the cholinergic nerve fibers, thus antogonizing acetylcholine. The mechanism responsible for the milk-feverlike syndrome was held to be the impaired absorption of calcium brought about through the bowel stasis.

A similar, milk-feverlike picture has been induced by fasting lactating cows (Halse, 1958a; Robertson et al., 1960). In both cases it appears that a loss of calcium through the milk is a necessary prerequisite.

5. Methods of Prevention of Milk Fever

a. VITAMIN D. The use of vitamin D_2 as a preventive was first tried by Greig (1930), but it was not until 1955 that Hibbs and Pounden demonstrated the possibilities of this method of prevention. The administration of 30 million IU of vitamin D_2 fed daily for at least 4 or 5 days, but no longer than 7 days, prepartum prevented milk fever in mature cows with previous milk-fever histories. Later on they reported that approximately the same protection could be obtained with a dosage level of 20 million IU, whereas 15 million IU daily yielded a lower protection (Hibbs and Conrad, 1960). The protection increased during the first 3 days of vitamin D_2 feeding, remained at a high level the third through the seventh day, and dropped precipitously after 1 day had elapsed following cessation of vitamin D_2 feeding. Dell and Poulton (1958) have confirmed the reports on the value of vitamin D_2 as a milk-fever preventive. In studies with more than 400 cows, the addition of 30 million IU of vitamin D_2 daily to the grain during the time from approximately 72 hours prepartum until 48 hours postpartum decreased the incidence of milk fever by approximately 70% below that of the controls.

The protection afforded by vitamin D_2 has been attributed to its calcemic effect, indicated by the relatively high serum calcium level maintained during the critical postpartum period. This is apparently not due to parathyroid stimulation, but to increased absorption of calcium and phosphorus from the digestive tract (Conrad et al., 1956; Capen et al., 1966b; Muir et al., 1968). Harmful effects due to prolonged feeding of vitamin D_2 have been reported (Cole et al., 1957; Payne, 1963).

In order to minimize the risks of harmful effects due to prolonged feeding of vitamin D_2, the use of vitamin D_3 as injection was introduced (Seekles et al., 1958). It is claimed that 10 million IU of vitamin D_3 given 2 to 8 days before calving will prevent the disease in 84% of the animals, compared with 82% when vitamin D_2 is given orally (Seekles et al., 1964). The danger of causing metastatic calcifications and other harmful effects exists also when vitamin D_3 is used (Manston and Payne, 1964). Pregnant cows are more susceptible to calcifications than nonpregnant cows (Capen et al., 1966a). Thyroxine administered with the vitamin D_3 as well as adjustment of the dietary Ca:P ratio prior to treatment are reported to be of value in reducing calcifications (Payne and Manston, 1967). The intramuscular route of vitamin D_3 injection is recommended (Seekles et al., 1964).

A serious disadvantage of both vitamin D methods is the necessity of accurately estimating the calving date.

b. DIETARY ADJUSTMENT OF Ca:P RATIO. The use of low-calcium, high-phosphorus, prepartal diet was suggested by Boda and Cole (1954, 1956). The purpose of this diet was to stimulate the production of endogenous PTH by causing stimulation of these glands before the initiation of lactation and the increased demand for calcium mobilization occurs. They divided 69 aged Jersey cows into groups of 4 cows each and fed them on diets containing various Ca:P ratios for varying periods of time prepartum. Clinical signs of milk fever were evident in 30% of the cows receiving diets with a Ca:P ratio of 6:1, in 15% of those receiving diets with a Ca:P ratio of 1:1, and in none of those receiving diets with a Ca:P ratio of 1:3.3. In agreement with these figures Ender *et al.* (1956, 1962) found increased incidence of milk fever in cows on an experimental high-calcium diet (Ca:P ratio between 5:1 and 10:1). These investigators further point out that the milk fever-inducing effect of a given fodder also is strongly influenced by its alkali alkalinity. Fodder containing large quantities of acid (AIV ensilage), i.e., low alkali alkalinity, resulted in practically no cases of milk fever, and vice versa.

In a study to determine how cows, which have been prefed a diet as recommended by Boda and Cole, are better able to maintain normal serum calcium levels, Luick *et al.* (1957a,b) estimated the reservoirs of mobilizable skeletal calcium. Their results indicated larger calcium reservoirs and a slower turnover in treated cows. Since such cows are in negative calcium balance, the increasing reservoirs (pool size) can only be due to adjustment in the bone itself, i.e., an increase in the mobilizable calcium at the expense of stable calcium. Stable bone thus became vascularized and therefore identified as part of the mobilizable calcium pool.

A major disadvantage in this method of prevention is the difficulty in producing a palatable diet with a Ca:P ratio of 1:3.

c. DRENCHING WITH CALCIUM CHLORIDE. A third method of milk-fever prevention appeared when Glawischnig (1962) reported that oral drenching with calcium chloride had a beneficial effect on the initial milk-fever attack as well as on relapses. A calcium chloride gel in which changes in viscosity and other properties disguised its salty chloride taste was formulated and its preventive effect investigated (Ringarp *et al.*, 1967). A statistical significant beneficial effect was demonstrated. The milk-fever incidence declined in one series of experiments from 57% in the controls to 7.6% in the dosed animals.

It is recommended that calcium chloride be given daily from several days before calving until 2 days after calving. As with the vitamin D method the greatest difficulty is to determine the exact time of calving. The treatment can, however, be extended up to 3 weeks if necessary.

D. CONDITIONS SIMILAR TO PARTURIENT PARESIS IN OTHER ANIMALS

A condition similar to parturient paresis occurs in many animals. Thus Greig (1929) and later Leslie (1931) showed that serum calcium is subnormal in lambing sickness of ewes. Hypocalcemia has also been reported from Australia (McClymont, 1947; Franklin *et al.*, 1948) and the United States (Asbury, 1962). Recently a presumed hypocalcemia of hill ewes in the North of England, the so-called "Moss-ill" has been described (Littlejohn and Hebert, 1969).

In mares, lactation tetany or transit tetany have been found associated with acute hypocalcemia (Montgomery *et al.*, 1929). Others have reported hypocalcemia in the sow (Kjeldberg, 1940; Craige and Beck, 1941), the goat (Van Maltits, 1945), the bitch (Barto, 1932; Crosfield, 1941), and the rabbit (Wenger, 1945).

E. HYPERPHOSPHATEMIA

High values of serum inorganic phosphate are observed in renal failure (8 to 25 mg/100 ml). A rise also may occur during the period of healing of fractures.

F. HYPOPHOSPHATEMIA

Serum inorganic phosphate is markedly influenced during periods of inadequate phosphorus intake. This condition is described in Section IV,B,4.

G. POSTPARTURIENT HEMOGLOBINEMIA

The relation of postparturient hemoglobinemia and aphosphorosis has not been clearly established. It is a disease mainly affecting heavy-producing cows. Recently calved cows are most susceptible. The hemoglobinuria appears suddenly and in the next 24 to 48 hours further symptoms occur. These include anemia, rapid loss of condition, listlessness, inappetence, slight icterus, and increased heart rate with a shallow, rapid respiration. Often milk yield is only little disturbed. On autopsy the main findings are anemia, icterus, and central lobular necrosis of the liver (Hjärre, 1930).

The disease was first recognized by Cumming (1853). It occurred on old farms with poor soil especially following periods of drought. In the United States it is frequently associated with the feeding of beet by-products and alfalfa hay (Madsen and Nielsen, 1940). In Australia the occurrence has been observed in herds grazing on winter oats (Parkinson and Sutherland, 1954).

Madsen and Nielsen (1940) first reported the disease to be associated with hypophosphatemia. They reproduced the disease by feeding a high-producing dairy cow a low phosphorus ration consisting of alfalfa and dried beet pulp (Madsen and Nielsen, 1944). The main biochemical findings are those of hypophosphatemia (in spite of the hemoglobinemia), pronounced anemia, and icterus. Thus, out of 67 blood samples from cattle, on farms where postparturient hemoglobinemia occurred, 23 showed blood inorganic phosphate levels below 1 mg/100 ml (Mullins and Ramsay, 1959). In the same study the osmotic fragility of the red blood cells was reported to be within normal range. Otherwise, no consistent alterations have been shown.

The centrilobular necroses of the liver have been shown to be secondary to the hemoglobinemia (Hjärre, 1930), and subsequent studies have shown the necroses to disappear rapidly during recovery (Møller and Simesen, 1959).

A very consistent finding in herds affected with postparturient hemoglobinemia has been the hypophosphatemia. However, herds with extremely low blood phosphate levels where neither anemia nor postparturient hemoglobinemia exists, are well known. Therefore the existence of a factor able to produce hemoglobinemia in hypophosphatemic animals has been suggested. Freudenberg (1955) reproduced the disease in three of four dairy cows fed a diet of fresh and ensiled sugar beet leaves and alfalfa hay. The diet had a Ca:P ratio of 4:1. In two herds fed the same forage supplemented with concentrates and minerals, no sign of disease occurred. It is concluded that two factors are necessary for the development of postparturient hemoglobinemia: a hypophosphatemia and on top of this a hemolytic effect of saponins, present in sugar beet leaves as well as in alfalfa hay.

IV. BONE DISORDERS

Failure to assimilate calcium and phosphorus normally may be due to a limited supply of these elements or to factors concerned in their assimilation, notably vitamin D. Such a failure will be reflected differently by immature and adult individuals according to the stage of bone development. Various terms have been used to designate the different conditions. The term *osteoporosis* is used when the abnormalities occur in the formation of the osteoid matrix and are not due to any disturbance in calcium and phosphorus metabolism. If the fundamental defect is in the metabolism of calcium and phosphorus the conditions are included under the designations *rickets* and *osteomalacia*.

A. ALKALINE PHOSPHATASE

Phosphatases are enzymes capable of hydrolyzing monophosphoric esters with the liberation of inorganic phosphate. Alkaline phosphatases have their maximal activity at pH 8.5–9.5, and they are activated by Mg ions (Erdtman, 1928). They are present in practically all tissues (intestinal mucosa, renal tubule cells, and bile), but apparently only the alkaline phosphatase of the osteoblasts has its site of function outside the cells. Therefore, some of the osteoblastic phosphatase continuously reaches the plasma and circulates in the blood stream.

The concentration of serum alkaline phosphatase tends to remain constant. Alkaline phosphatase is found normally in the bile and the level is increased in obstructive jaundice. In human rickets there is a marked increase in serum alkaline phosphatase activity. This is the first apparent evidence of the disease and the last finding to disappear after recovery. In osteomalacia an increase in serum alkaline phosphatase level occurs, whereas no increase is found during osteoporosis.

Alkaline phosphatase activity in domestic animals has been reported as Bodansky, King Armstrong, or Bessey-Lowrey units (see Chapter 5, Section VII).

W. M. Allcroft and Folley (1941) found the variation in serum alkaline phosphate activity 0.3–114.3 and 3.0–166.1 units/100 ml in apparently normal cows and ewes, respectively (King Armstrong units/100 ml). In the single individual, however, the level remains within a fairly narrow range. In both cattle and sheep serum phosphatase activity progressively decreased with advancing age until maturity was reached. During pregnancy a slight increase was observed, although changes in the level during pregnancy did not appear to be correlated with any stage of pregnancy. A marked increase in activity has been reported associated with the approach of parturition (Wilson, 1955; Ford, 1958). Serum alkaline phosphatase activity has been found to be low during hypomagnesemic tetany (Halse, 1948).

Wise *et al.* (1958) have reported that increased phosphatase activity accompanied decreased serum inorganic phosphate levels in 3- to 6-month-old calves fed different levels of dietary phosphorus. The phosphatase level responded rapidly to a change in the blood level of phosphorus, but after an initial change the phosphatase level returned to its "normal" level.

Reports have appeared describing alkaline phosphatase activity in swine (Luecke *et al.*, 1958; Brown *et al.*, 1966; Baustad *et al.*, 1967), horse (Earle and Cabell, 1952; Jennings and Mulligan, 1953; Krook and Lowe, 1964) and dogs (Campbell, 1960; Campbell and Douglas, 1965). In cats alkaline phosphatase has been reported to be excreted through the kidney. Even ligation of the bile duct does not increase the level (Bloom, 1960). In the diagnostic biochemistry of domestic animals, however, the estimation of alkaline phosphatase activity has never achieved a position comparable to that in human medicine. Isoenzymes of alkaline phosphatase are known to exist and would seem to warrant further examination.

B. Rickets and Osteomalacia

1. Rickets

Rickets is a disease which particularly affects growing animals. It is a disorder in which the main feature is a failure of calcium salts to be deposited promptly in the newly formed bone matrix. The typical lesion of rickets is defective endochondral mineralization of the "zone of provisional calcification" of the long bones. The cause may be an inadequate supply of calcium and/or phosphorus and/or vitamin D. In the mature animal a similar lack of calcium, phosphorus, and/or vitamin D leads to osteomalacia. Absorption of calcium may be low in spite of a high-calcium intake if the body does not contain vitamin D. The vitamin D requirement, on the other hand, is markedly influenced by the Ca:P ratio of the diet. An optimal Ca:P ratio calls for minimal vitamin D and vice versa.

Rickets has been described in a number of different animals. Some authors have used such terms as "low-phosphorus rickets" and "low-calcium rickets." In both cases the normal bone mineralization is impeded, causing structural bone abnormalities of similar nature. Blood analysis has been used extensively in the study of these deficiencies. In general, a decrease in the blood level of inorganic phosphate or calcium or both is found. In the diagnosis of severe phosphorus deficiency, blood inorganic phosphate analysis has proved extremely useful (Theiler and Green, 1932). Sometimes, however, the results of blood analysis are difficult to interpret. This applies particularly to data on calcium levels and is due to the hormonal control of the serum calcium concentration. In rickets, therefore, analysis of blood and bone may often provide evidence, but a final diagnosis is best obtained by histopathological examination of epiphyseal cartilage.

In sheep, deficiencies of vitamin D, calcium and/or phosphorus, or combinations of phosphorus and vitamin D have been described.

a. Vitamin D Deficiency. Franklin et al. (1948) reported that inadequate dietary vitamin D or lack of ultraviolet irradiation results in a drop in serum calcium and inorganic phosphorus levels in the growing sheep in spite of a high dietary intake of calcium and phosphorus. Benzie et al. (1959) confirmed this observation and showed that the drop in serum calcium was accompanied by skeletal resorption. Quaterman et al. (1964) was able to estimate the vitamin D activity directly in the blood of sheep. They showed that the vitamin D activity in the blood was reduced to very low levels in sheep kept indoors during the summer. The normal summer rise was also found much reduced if the sheep were not clipped in the spring. Quaterman et al. (1964) showed that an intramuscular injection of 1 million IU vitamin D raised the blood to over normal and maintained normal levels for over 4 months.

In lambs kept indoors for more than 3 weeks after birth, hypocalcemia has been observed, and lack of vitamin D is suggested as being the main cause (Lode and Øverås, 1968). About 20% revealed clinical symptoms, viz, tetany. The relation between rickets in lambs deficient in vitamin D and rates of growth has been elucidated by Duckworth et al. (1943).

b. CALCIUM AND/OR PHOSPHORUS DEFICIENCY. Rations deficient in calcium or with a wide Ca:P ratio will readily induce a severe fall in the serum calcium level when fed to sheep. The hypocalcemia can be induced with decreasing readiness in lactating ewes, sucking lambs, 3- to 6-month-old weaners, in-lamb ewes, and full-mouthed dry ewes (Franklin et al., 1948).

Moderately large depression in serum calcium levels was found by McRoberts et al. (1965a,b) in young sheep fed a diet of low calcium content for several months. Reduced ash content of the bone and retarded eruption of teeth with slight hypoplasia of the enamel were observed. During the repair period a tendency to prognathism was seen.

c. PHOSPHORUS AND VITAMIN D DEFICIENCY. Diets low in phosphorus or low in phosphorus and vitamin D have been found to cause a marked depression of blood inorganic phosphate, bone of extremely poor quality (ash analysis and radiographically), and severe clinical signs of rickets with bent fore and hind legs, swollen joints and collapse of the digits resulting in plantigrade instead of digitigrade gait (McRoberts et al., 1965a; Miller, 1946). After about 12 months on this diet low in phosphorus and vitamin D the clinical condition "open mouth" or "gagged bite" developed. In similar animals fed a control diet or a diet low in calcium these defects were not observed (McRoberts et al., 1965b). Nisbet et al. (1966, 1968) have also reported rickets and dental malocclusion in young sheep (hoggs) caused by deficiency of phosphorus and vitamin D. Blood values were reported and compared with normal values provided from sheep with uncomplicated osteoporosis (cappi).

Studies of rickets in goats have been made by Wieland (1940).

d. RICKETS IN CALVES (Hibbs et al., 1945; Colovos et al., 1951). One of the first symptoms of low vitamin D rickets in calves is a decrease in the serum calcium and/or inorganic phosphorus values. Usually the clinical symptoms, difficulty in locomotion, stiffness in gait with swollen and stiff joints, straight pastern, irritability, tetany, and convulsions are preceded by the decrease in serum calcium and inorganic phosphorus.

In young calves a calcium-deficient diet results in failure of normal bone growth. The bones have a low content of calcium and phosphorus. The serum calcium levels, however, usually remain normal even in severe deficiency (Wentworth and Smith, 1961).

A mild rickets caused by low phosphorus intake may be seen in calves housed for long periods of the year. The calves seem not to be as sensitive as adults. In herds where cows are found severely affected by phosphorus deficiency the calves are often found normal. A fall in serum inorganic phosphate values is the first evidence of a phosphorus deficiency.

e. RICKETS IN HORSES. There exist few reports describing rickets in foals (Åkerblom, 1952). Rachitic changes may be seen in ribs from young animals fed diets able to induce osteodystrophia fibrosa. Groenewald (1949) thus reported histological evidence of rickets in one out of four fillies fed an experimental diet with a Ca:P ratio of 1:5 for 10 months. Since rickets is a disease in which the bones are still growing, and osteomalacia is the disease in bones which have ceased to grow, and since all bones do not cease growth at the same time, it is evident that the two diseases may coexist in the one skeleton.

f. RICKETS IN PIGS. Special interest was taken by Pedersen (1940) in studying the role of phytin and phytase in the production of rickets in pigs. It was found that 20% of the phytic acid in cereals that contain phytase is split during digestion. The amount of phytic acid which is not split combines with calcium in the proportion of 1 part calcium to 1.1 to 1.6 parts phytic acid, thus reducing the amount of utilizable calcium. These findings indicate that the requirement for calcium and phosphorus in the pig's diet varies with the type of cereal used. In experiments with dogs, Mellanby (1949) subsequently found that phytate, in the presence of vitamin D either in the food or stored in the body, consistently reduced calcium absorption to a greater extent than an equal amount of phosphorus given as phosphate. In the absence of vitamin D, on the other hand, phosphate was as effective as phytate in inhibiting the absorption of calcium. The concentration of sulfur ions affects absorption of calcium, phosphorus, and magnesium. Møllgaard (1943) reported that in balance experiments with pigs as little as 0.5 gm of sulfur (S^{2-}) fed per day reduced the absorption of calcium and phosphorus greatly. In a few months, serum calcium and inorganic phosphate decreased to low levels. If vitamin D was deficient, simultaneously severe rachitic changes occurred. Calcium and phosphorus requirements of animals are presented in Table V. Rickets caused by vitamin D deficiency in pigs fed diets with various calcium and phosphorus contents was found to be accompanied by a fall in serum calcium levels. This drop was rapidly followed by a 100–200% rise in the levels of alkaline phosphatase (Baustad et al., 1967).

g. RICKETS IN DOGS AND CATS. Vitamin D, phosphorus, and calcium all play a role in prevention of rickets in dogs (Campbell and Douglas, 1965). In young, rapidly growing puppies a deficiency of vitamin D is a common cause of rickets.

TABLE V   CALCIUM AND PHOSPHORUS REQUIREMENTS OF ANIMALS[a]

	Horse[b] mature weight		Dairy cow[c]		Sheep[d]	
	(270 kg)	(635 kg)	Growing (50 kg)	Lactating (550 kg)	Growing (27 kg)	Lactating (54 kg)
Calcium	0.41	0.40	0.40	0.20	0.21	0.28
Phosphorus	0.41	0.32	0.30	0.20	0.19	0.21

	Pig[e]			Mink[g]	
	Growing (10 kg)	Lactating (170 kg)	Dog[f]	Growing	For maintenance
Calcium	0.8	0.6	1.0	0.4	0.3
Phosphorus	0.6	0.4	0.8	0.4	0.3

[a]Values are percent of diet. Data are from the following titles published by National Academy of Sciences, National Research Council, Committee on Animal Nutrition.
[b]"Nutrition Requirements of Horses." 2nd rev. ed., 1966, No. 6.
[c]"Nutrition Requirements of Dairy Cattle." 3rd rev. ed., 1966, No. 3.
[d]"Nutrition Requirements of Sheep." 4th rev. ed., 1968, No. 5.
[e]"Nutrition Requirements of Swine." 6th rev. ed., 1968, No. 2.
[f]"Nutrition Requirements of Dogs." Revised, 1962, No. 8.
[g]"Nutrition Requirements of Mink and Foxes." 1st rev. ed., 1968, No. 7.

Indian workers (Raghavachari, 1943; Patwardhan *et al.*, 1945) have found the serum calcium level to decrease progressively during the development of rickets in dogs fed a normal diet devoid of vitamin D. The inorganic phosphate values decreased slightly. When vitamin D was given, the serum calcium level rose before that of inorganic phosphate. When a diet low in phosphate was given, the serum calcium level increased and the inorganic phosphate level decreased. Also in dogs diets high in phytates adversely influence the absorption of calcium (Hoff-Jørgensen, 1946).

In cats similar results have been reported (Gershoff *et al.*, 1957).

h. Rickets in the Silver Fox. In the silver fox, the serum calcium and phosphorus levels have been found to be normal when rickets were caused by a diet with a Ca:P ratio of 7:1 and a very low vitamin D content (Ott and Coombes, 1941). In fox puppies on a similar diet, but low in phosphorus, normal serum calcium values were found. Serum inorganic phosphate, however, decreased to 2 to 4 mg/100 ml (Ender *et al.*, 1949a). On a low-calcium diet, on the other hand, with a Ca:P ratio below 0.85, the serum calcium decreased to 6–7 mg/100 ml. Coincidentally increased muscle tonus and tetany were observed in this group.

i. Rickets in Mink. When mink are fed a diet low in vitamin D and/or with abnormally low Ca:P ratio (below 1:1), they develop rickets (S. E. Smith and Barnes, 1941; Bassett *et al.*, 1951). When the diet is deficient in calcium or phosphorus, bone development is abnormal. Within 10 days after being placed on a rachitogenic diet, mink kits experience difficulty in walking. Lordosis, bending of leg bones and enlargements of the costochondral junctions are seen. Ash content of the dry fat-free femurs may decrease to 22–30% compared with 60–64% for normal animals.

2. Tetany

Tetany is a symptom complex characterized by increased neuromuscular excitability. After a variable period of latency, neuromuscular excitability increases to the point where spontaneous manifestations appear. One of the most important biochemical findings during tetany is diminished serum calcium concentration. This is usually between 7 and 8 mg/100 ml in latent and between 4 and 6 mg/100 ml in manifest tetany. However, this close parallelism between the severity of symptoms and the degree of hypocalcemia is not constant. Latent tetany may be present at low calcium levels, and manifest tetany may occur at concentrations as high as 8 mg/100 ml. Accordingly, other factors must participate in the pathogenesis of neuromuscular hyperirritability. The most important of these is probably the decreased Ca:P ratio.

Alkalosis, known as one cause of tetany, is usually thought to act by diminishing the effective calcium ion concentration at the neuromuscular junction.

3. Osteomalacia

The adult counterpart to rickets is osteomalacia. In the adult animal the growth of the bones has terminated and therefore the typical lesion of rickets—defective endochondral mineralization of the "zone of provisional calcification" of long bones—cannot occur. Inadequate supply of calcium and/or phosphorus and/or vitamin D in the adult animal is manifested by a resorption of bone already laid down. An excessive mobilization of minerals may be caused by an overfunctioning of the parathyroid, and/or a continued body demand for calcium and/or phosphorus. Most acute cases occur during pregnancy and lactation when excessive demands are made upon bones already depleted. Often the depletion occurs to a point where the bones break. A characteristic feature of the disease is a negative calcium and phosphorus balance. The blood serum may be low in one or both minerals, and tetany may be seen in cases with a low serum calcium.

Although the pathology of osteomalacia is similar in all domestic animals, its etiology varies according to the different types of diet used for different species of animals. Thus in the bovine and ovine animal it occurs generally as an aphosphorosis, in pigs as an acalcicosis, in dogs as an avitaminosis, and in horses as an hyperphosphorosis.

4. Aphosphorosis

The chronic form of aphosphorosis is best known through the classic work of Theiler and his co-workers on "styfziekte" in relation to botulism in South Africa (Theiler *et al.*, 1924, 1927). Since then aphosphorosis has been described in the bovine under various names as "mjölkhälta" (Svanberg, 1932), "peg-leg" (A. W. Turner *et al.*, 1935; Barnes and Jephcott, 1955), "bog-crook," or "bog-lame" (Curran, 1949; O'Donovan and Sheery, 1950; O'Moore, 1950), "cruban" (Carmichael, 1958), "stiffs" or "creeps" (A. L. Rose, 1954). A detailed review concerning the chronic form of aphosphorosis in ruminants has been given by Theiler and Green (1932). Recently McTaggart (1959) has described the syndrome of acute hypophosphatemia in heavy-milking cows.

The chief signs of aphosphorosis are bone-chewing (allotriophagia) and sudden onset of lameness. Enlargements around the lower end of the metacarpus and metatarsus and a peculiar stiff gait are frequently observed. Loss of body weight and decreased production are usually the first signs to be observed.

Generally it is found that affected animals have very low serum inorganic phosphate levels, whereas calcium and magnesium values are within normal range. The conditions can be reproduced experimentally by feeding animals diets low in phosphorus but otherwise adequate. The pastures contain very little phosphorus, especially during periods of drought. A high incidence of the disease is frequently associated with such periods. Symptoms may also develop during winter, when animals are being fed a diet low in phosphorus (Hutten and Uhlenbruck, 1952). A relative excess of calcium in the diet increases the severity of the disease.

Sheep and horses are not as susceptible to phosphorus deficiency as cattle. In New Zealand, osteomalacia in grazing sheep has been described as being associated with an antivitamin D effect of high carotene levels in green oats, while calcium and phosphorus intakes were adequate (Grant, 1955). In the United States low phosphorus levels have been reported in lame horses (Craige and Gadd, 1941).

5. Osteodystrophia Fibrosa or Osteitis Fibrosa

The nutritional origin of these diseases has gradually been established. It is now generally agreed that osteodystrophia fibrosa or osteitis fibrosa is a result of a secondary hyperparathyroidism.* In animals the nutritional secondary hyper-parathyroidism is typically caused by a diet imbalanced in favor of phosphorus. The clinical picture of secondary nutritional hyperparathyroidism appears, however, in different animal species so dissimilar, that diseases of quite different etiology could easily be expected.

a. HERBIVOROUS ANIMALS.   The disease is best known in horses. In the past it was prevalent among army horses fed roughages low in calcium and concentrates high in phosphorus. The disease usually manifests itself by a softening of the bones. In the literature it has been recorded under such various names as osteoporosis, osteomalacia, osteitis fibrosa, big head, or "bran" disease (H. Schmidt, 1940). An identical disease can be produced by feeding an excess of phosphorus over calcium. Any ratio of Ca:P lower than 0.8 may produce it. The development is rather slow, several months to a year. The disease can be stopped by furnishing an adequate calcium supply, thereby adjusting the Ca:P ratio to 1 or a little above. The development of the disease may be considerably faster, if the absolute amount of calcium given is low (Niimi and Kato, 1928; Niimi and Aoki, 1927; Scheunert, 1923).

Affected animals move with a stiff stilted gait, and often an examination of the head reveals slight bilateral enlargements of the bones of the face or rami of the mandibles. Frequent fractures of the head of the femur have been reported (Hellmich, 1938). Bone analyses reveal a significant decrease in ash content. No change in the Ca:P ratio is found, but marked decrease in magnesium content has been reported. Bardwell (1959) has drawn attention to the clinical aspects of the disease, especially pointing out that such diseases as navicular disease, ring bones, and spavins could well be local clinical manifestations of a general disease of the skeletal system. So-called mucoid degeneration of the nasal conchae has recently been classified as an expression of nutritional secondary hyperparathyroidism (Rubarth and Krook, 1968).

In an experiment reported by Krook and Lowe (1964) horses were fed a diet with a Ca:P ratio 1:3.6 for 23 weeks with calcium at an optimal level of 15.8 gm/day. The diet immediately caused hyperphosphatemia and weekly determinations showed that hyperphosphatemia reached maximum after 12–20 weeks. Serum calcium dropped to a minimum after 10 weeks and was partly or almost completely compensated after 23 weeks. Clinical symptoms were observed after 12 weeks.

Osteodystrophia fibrosa has been described in goats (Groenewald et al., 1940; Deckwer, 1950; Hansen et al., 1966). A similar condition with a striking depletion of the bones has been produced experimentally in dairy cows which had been continuously fed a diet low in calcium and relatively high in phosphorus (Becker et al., 1933).

b. OMNIVOROUS ANIMALS.   In swine the effect of imbalanced Ca:P rations was studied by Marek and Wellmann (1931). With low calcium and high phosphorus diets hyperostotic osteitis fibrosa was induced. After diets with Ca:P ratios from 1:5.5 to 1:11.6 Liégeois and Derivaux (1951) produced hyperphosphatemia followed by

---

*Two types of hyperparathyroidism are known: the primary form, caused by parathyroid neoplasia, and the secondary form, which has two subtypes, renal and nutritional. In both the compensatory hypertrophy is initiated by hypocalcemia. Quite often the hypocalcemia is found to be secondary to hyperphosphatemia.

hypocalcemia in pigs. At necropsy the parathyroids were found diffusely hyperplastic. Finally Brown *et al.* (1966) experimentally induced nutritional secondary hyperparathyroidism in pigs and identified the morphological and nutritional changes with those found in spontaneous cases of atrophic rhinitis.

The position of atrophic rhinitis in pigs as an infectious disease, a nutritional disease or a combination of both, has, however, not yet been clarified (Baustad *et al.*, 1967).

c. CARNIVOROUS ANIMALS.   In carnivorous animals the source of imbalanced dietary calcium and phosphorous is unsupplemented meat without access to the bones (Riser, 1961). This causes a disease in young animals known as "osteogenesis imperfecta," "juvenile osteoporosis," or "paper bone disease." The disease is characterized by extreme fragility of the whole skeleton. Fractures occur for no apparent reason and seem to cause little pain. The disease, nutritional secondary hyperparathyroidism, is more fulminating in carnivorous animals than in herbivores. It is a disease of young animals and usually found superimposed on rickets. Enlargements of facial bones are less apparent than in other animals.

The disease has been reproduced in young kittens placed on a minced heart diet. Roentgenologic signs of generalized osteitis fibrosa developed within 3 weeks, folding fractures of the long bones a few weeks later. Due to the extreme rapid resorption of bone there is apparently no time for fibrous replacement of the resorbed, and hence a hypostotic osteitis fibrosa is the result (Krook *et al.*, 1963). Continuous blood analysis during experimentally induced nutritional secondary hyperparathyroidism has not been reported (Krook, 1965). Single determinations have shown mild hypocalcemia and hyperphosphatemia. Single determinations of calcium and phosphorus, however, are not conclusive in nutritional secondary hyperparathyroidism.

V. MAGNESIUM METABOLISM

Sheep and cattle are the only domestic animals known to be subject to clinical disorders apparently due to magnesium deficiency. Magnesium metabolism therefore has been studied most extensively in these species.

A. DISTRIBUTION OF MAGNESIUM IN THE BODY

In terms of the amounts of each cation present in the body, magnesium is fourth, being surpassed only by calcium, sodium, and potassium. In cattle the magnesium content of the body in relation to body weight is given by the following equation (Blaxter and McGill, 1956):

$$Mg(gm) = 0.655 \text{ wt (kg)} - 3.5$$

Magnesium is present in all tissues. About 70% of the total body magnesium is in the skeleton, and approximately one-third of this is available for mobilization to soft tissues when dietary intake is inadequate. Taylor (1959) has demonstrated that magnesium present in bone exists in at least two different forms. About 70% of the bone magnesium could be removed relatively easily with dilute acid, while the remaining 30% was in more intimate association with the bone. Taylor, therefore, suggested that the easily removable magnesium was bound to the surface of the bone crystal, probably to the phosphate grouping of the apatite crystal, whereas the more firmly bound magnesium may be an integral part of the bone crystal lattice.

The magnesium of the skeleton acts as a labile source of magnesium, but there is a striking difference between the reactions of the young as compared with the adult bovine animal (Blaxter and McGill, 1956). In the immature animal the entire skeleton may lose 30–60% of its magnesium content in exchange reactions, whereas adults, due to the inability of the animal to mobilize magnesium from the skeleton, die in tetany with little or no depletion of their bone magnesium (Cunningham, 1936a,b). The existence of this difference between the young and the adult animal has been confirmed in ^{28}Mg disappearance studies in the bovine (Simesen et al., 1965). In cows the total exchangeable magnesium was found to amount to 20–24% of the total body magnesium compared to 30–45% in calves.

In sheep total exchangeable magnesium has been estimated by Field (1960), Care et al. (1965), and Hjerpe (1968a).

Apart from bone, magnesium occurs principally intracellularly. The concentration of magnesium in cells is about 36 mg/100 ml (30 mEq/liter) compared with a plasma concentration of about 2.4 mg/100 ml (2 mEq/liter). The mechanism maintaining this concentration gradient of about 1:15 across the cell membrane has been subject to much study (Rogers and Mahan, 1959; MacIntyre, 1959; Rogers et al., 1964). It is now thought that tissue magnesium exists in at least two different forms, one of which is free, ionic, and readily exchangeable, while the other is bound, and probably can be regarded as chelated, typically with adenosine triphosphate and the apoenzyme proteins to which Mg^{2+} is attached (Rogers, 1964).

The labile, exchangeable form exists in concentrations which are practically the same as Mg^{2+} in the extracellular water, and a simple diffusion equilibrium between these two and a more complex relation between the two intracellular forms has been suggested (Stevenson and Wilson, 1963).

The physiological function of magnesium may conveniently be divided into two parts: intracellular and extracellular.

1. Intracellular Function of Magnesium

Magnesium is an activator of numerous enzymes such as phosphatases and the enzymes catalyzing reactions involving adenosine triphosphate (ATP). Since ATP is required in such diverse functions as muscle contraction, protein, fat, nucleic acid, and coenzyme synthesis, glucose synthesis and utilization, methyl group transfer, sulfate, acetate and formate activation, and oxidative phosphorylation, it may be inferred that the action of magnesium extends to all the major anabolic and catabolic processes involving the main metabolites. Magnesium is an activator for enzymes that require thiamine pyrophosphate as a cofactor. One of them is the conversion of pyruvic acid to acetyl coenzyme A (acetyl CoA), an example of oxidative decarboxylation.

Excellent reviews giving detailed descriptions of the role of magnesium in biochemical processes (Aikawa, 1963) and in human magnesium metabolism (Wacker and Parisi, 1968) have appeared.

2. Extracellular Function of Magnesium

In the extracellular fluid magnesium has an important role to play in the production and the destruction of acetylcholine, the substance necessary for the transmission of impulses at the neuromuscular junction (Del Castillo and Engbäk, 1953). A low concentration of magnesium or more particularly a low $Mg^{2+}:Ca^{2+}$ ratio potentiates the release of acetylcholine. It therefore appears possible that a low concentration of magnesium in the extracellular fluid surrounding the muscle end plates may produce tetany through this mechanism (Blaxter et al., 1954). It is known that the activity of choline esterase is not affected during magnesium deficiency (Seekles and Van Asperen, 1949; Todd and Rankin, 1959).

During hibernation the serum magnesium has been found to increase from a normal of 3 mg/100 ml to about 6 mg/100 ml (Suomalainen, 1944). Serum calcium remained constant.

B. ABSORPTION AND EXCRETION

The availability of dietary magnesium is low compared with that of dietary calcium. The apparent digestibility of magnesium (the percentage of dietary magnesium which is not excreted in the feces) is 20–25% in ruminants compared with an average of 39% in monogastric animals (Gröning, 1959). R. H. Smith (1959a) found that calves fed a diet consisting basically of whole milk retained 39–54% of their dietary magnesium at ages less than 5 weeks. From about 3 weeks to about 16 weeks of age the mean fecal excretion of magnesium increased from 32 to 86% of the dietary magnesium (R. H. Smith, 1959b). For cattle on a variety of typical winter stall rations Rook et al. (1958) found 62–92% of the magnesium fed to be excreted in the feces compared with 82–83% when fed freshly cut herbage at stall. In pigs, 3–5 weeks of age, the average magnesium excreted in the feces has been found to be 65–84% of the dietary magnesium (Bartley et al., 1961).

1. Endogenous Magnesium

The magnesium in the feces is not solely dietary in origin. The large volumes of digestive secretions produced during digestion contain a considerable amount of endogenous magnesium. Knowledge of the amount of this endogenous fecal magnesium is important for determination of the "true" digestibility or availability of dietary magnesium. The apparent digestibility is a valid basis for estimating the "true"

$$\frac{\text{food Mg} - \text{fecal Mg}}{\text{food Mg}}$$

digestibility only when the endogenous magnesium in the feces is a small part of the total fecal magnesium. An increased fecal excretion of magnesium may be due either to a decreased absorption or to an increased production of endogenous magnesium.

Attempts to determine the endogenous magnesium in sheep using ^{28}Mg and methods originally developed for ^{32}P (Visek et al., 1953a) and ^{45}Ca (Hansard et al., 1954) have been made (Field, 1959; MacDonald et al., 1959), but Field (1961) has since questioned the validity of these methods, as he found both the comparative balance technique and the isotope dilution technique to overestimate the endogenous fecal magnesium.

Blaxter and Rook (1954) calculated the total endogenous loss of magnesium in milk-fed calves from the relationship between magnesium retention and intake. Since the loss via the urine is negligible, this value may be taken as the endogenous fecal magnesium (3–4 mg/kg body weight-day). R. H. Smith (1959a) estimated the endogenous fecal magnesium to be about 0.5 mg/kg body weight-day in milk-fed calves 2 to 5 weeks of age. This value increased to 2.2 mg/kg body weight-day in calves 26 to 32 weeks of age. For cows Blaxter and McGill (1956) have reported a figure of 3–5 mg/kg body weight-day. Simesen et al. (1962) measured the endogenous magnesium in milk-fed calves and in cows fed hay and cereals using intravenous injection of ^{28}Mg. Mean values of 3.5 and 1.5 mg/kg body weight were found for calves and cows, respectively. This result was in agreement with that reported by Blaxter and McGill (1956) for the calves, but considerably lower for the cows.

In sheep endogenous fecal magnesium has been estimated by Field et al. (1958), MacDonald et al. (1959), Care (1960), and Hjerpe (1968a). Values from 0.7 to 5.1 mg/kg body weight have been reported.

The size of the endogenous fecal magnesium may be increased by a greater flow of saliva stimulated by bulky diets such as roughages and grass (Rook and Storry, 1962). As pointed out by Care (1967), the endogenous fecal excretion of magnesium has in ruminants a very substantial magnitude.

2. Absorption

Up to about 1 month of age calves absorb magnesium in the large as well as in the small intestine (R. H. Smith, 1959c, 1962). With increasing age this ability is lost. From about 3 to 4 months of age the principal site of absorption appears to be the middle third of the small intestine (Field, 1961; Care and Van'T Klooster, 1965). The absorptive efficiency of magnesium has been found to decrease with increasing magnesium concentrations when concomitant plasma magnesium is normal. It has been shown that magnesium and calcium are absorbed as freely diffusing ions (Van'T Klooster, 1967). Normally, net absorption of magnesium does not take place from the rumen (Phillipson and Storry, 1965), but such absorption can occur when diets are liberally supplemented with magnesium salts (Care, 1967).

Ruminants have a particularly low efficiency of magnesium absorption. In these animals a large loss of magnesium takes place via the feces (70–95% of intake). However, a low efficiency of magnesium absorption and an increase in amounts absorbed with increasing intake has been shown in a number of animals. This seems to suggest that magnesium is absorbed by passive diffusion. Scott (1965) calculated that magnesium concentrations in the digesta of above 1.4 to 2.1 mmole/liter were necessary to overcome the fairly small electrical potential across the wall of the small intestine (7–15 mV, blood positive) before passive diffusion could occur. Van'T

Klooster (1967) measured the actual electrical potential difference and found it to vary between $+10$ and $+20$ mV (blood positive), and Care and Van'T Klooster (1965) found that magnesium absorption occurred only above the concentration given by Scott. Normally digesta from ruminants as well as from nonruminants contain appreciably higher total magnesium concentrations than 1.4 to 2.1 m mole/liter, but all the magnesium is not necessarily in the available ionic form.

If magnesium moves passively across the wall of the small intestine, the concentration of available magnesium in the digesta and the time of contact between the digesta and the absorbing surface is the major factors responsible for differences in the efficiency of magnesium absorption. In ruminants the concentration of magnesium ions in the digesta in the small intestine tends to be particularly low because of (1) the presence of materials in the digesta able to bind Mg^{2+} at the intestinal pH (Storry, 1961b; R. H. Smith and McAllan, 1966) and (2) the large amounts of water which is retained in the ileum (R. H. Smith, 1969).

Unlike calcium the absorption of magnesium is not influenced by vitamin D (R. H. Smith, 1957, 1958). Despite the disparity between the effects of vitamin D on calcium and magnesium absorption, a common transport system for absorption of calcium and magnesium has been postulated (Alcock and MacIntyre, 1960). Smith failed to find evidence for such a common mechanism for absorption of calcium and magnesium in milk-fed calves, but R. Allcroft and Ivins (1964) found that further addition of calcium to the diet of milk-fed calves caused a significant depression of serum and bone magnesium. Care and Van'T Klooster (1965) showed that calcium and magnesium interfered with absorption of each other and suggested that magnesium and calcium may be absorbed from ileum by a process of facilitated diffusion, whereas the calcium absorption from the duodenum was thought to be an active process sensitive to vitamin D (Care, 1967).

It has been shown that the chelating agent EDTA, which is known to bind calcium in prevalence of magnesium, inhibits the absorption of calcium from the small intestine of sheep, but promotes the absorption of magnesium from the proximal third of this region (Van'T Klooster and Care, 1966).

The estimates of availability of dietary magnesium for cattle of different ages have been given as 70% up to 5 weeks, 40% from 5 weeks to 5 months, and 20% for animals over 5 months of age (Agricultural Research Council, 1965). It has, however, been shown that the availability of magnesium varies considerably and may be very low in some types of feed given to cattle under normal farm conditions (Rook and Campling, 1962).

3.   Excretion

Magnesium is excreted mainly via three routes: the gastrointestinal tract, the kidney, and the mammary gland during lactation.

a. THE GASTROINTESTINAL TRACT.   As already mentioned, the main part of magnesium leaving the body appears in the feces. The fecal magnesium includes endogenous fecal magnesium, which is relatively higher for ruminants than for monogastric animals. After parenteral injection of ^{28}Mg in man, less than 1% of the injected dose was recovered in feces compared with about 20% in the sheep

(Field, 1959; MacDonald *et al.*, 1959). Field (1960) compiled data showing that the daily excretion of magnesium into the gastrointestinal tract of sheep is of the order of 60–200 mg magnesium or about the value found for endogenous magnesium (Field *et al.*, 1958; MacDonald *et al.*, 1959; Field, 1960).

Estimation of the availability of dietary magnesium by use of the relationship between urinary and dietary magnesium has been suggested (Field *et al.*, 1958). Such estimations, however, assume constant endogenous fecal magnesium, and even so, the figures obtained are of low accuracy.

b. THE KIDNEY.   Magnesium absorbed in excess of the body's requirements is excreted by the kidney. A. A. Wilson (1960) has critically reviewed existing knowledge of renal magnesium excretion and concludes "that excretion of magnesium is by a filter reabsorption mechanism in which the tubular reabsorption process is acting at or near its maximum rate, and that the excretion of magnesium is partly or wholly independent of other ions." Maximum tubular reabsorption rate is usually taken to be a physiological constant and in conjunction with the filtration rate fixes the threshold concentration in the plasma.

Rook *et al.* (1958) proved this correlation between serum concentration and urine output of magnesium and estimated the renal threshold for plasma magnesium to be less than 2.15 mg/100 ml. Later estimates (Storry and Rook, 1962; Rook and Storry, 1962; Meyer, 1963) have shown the renal threshold to be about 1.80–1.90 mg/100 ml in the bovine. In two sheep L'Estrange and Axford (1964b) have obtained threshold values of 1.37 and 1.90 mg/100 ml. From a practical point of view this means: if urine magnesium is present, no hypomagnesemia exists. [A special indicator test taking advantage of this fact has recently been developed (de Groot and Marttin, 1967)]. From a theoretical point it shows that the kidney plays a significant role in the magnesium homeostasis.

TABLE VI   REPRESENTATIVE VALUES FOR THE CALCIUM, MAGNESIUM, AND TOTAL PHOSPHORUS CONTENT OF MILK

Species	Calcium (gm/liter)	Magnesium (gm/liter)	Total P (gm/liter)
Cow[a]	1.25[b]	0.12[b]	0.96[b]
Sheep	1.93[c]	—	1.00[f]
Goat	1.30[b]	0.16[b]	1.06[b]
Horse	1.02[d]	0.09[d]	0.63[d]
Pig	2.10[e]	—	1.50[e]

[a]Colostrum-milk is usually not considered normal until about the fifth day after calving (C. W. Turner, 1930). The content of calcium, magnesium, and phosphorus are all high in colostrum, but as the milk becomes normal, a rapid decline toward a fairly constant level soon sets in (Garrett and Overman, 1940).
[b]Macy *et al.* (1953).
[c]Barnicoat *et al.* (1949).
[d]Holmes *et al.* (1947).
[e]Gregory *et al.* (1952).
[f]Basu and Mukherjee (1943).

TABLE VII   CONCENTRATION OF MAGNESIUM IN BLOOD OF VARIOUS ANIMALS

Species	Blood fraction[a]	Value (mg/100 ml)			Reference
		No. of animals sample	Mean	Standard deviation	
Shetlands pony	S	8	1.54	±0.16	Eriksen and Simesen (1970)
Horse	B	10	4.0	±0.62[b]	Eveleth (1937)
	S	30	2.5	±0.31	Jennings and Mulligan (1953)
	P	10	2.4	±0.32[b]	Eveleth (1937)
	C	10	6.8	±1.27[b]	Eveleth (1937)
Cattle	S	185	2.05	±0.25[b]	Crookshank and Sims (1955)
	S	90	2.3	±0.17	Mylrea and Bayfield (1968)
	B	833	2.3	±0.23	Lane et al. (1968)
	B	10	2.4	±0.32[b]	Eveleth (1937)
	P	10	2.8	±0.32[b]	Eveleth (1937)
	C	10	1.8	±0.78[b]	Eveleth (1937)
Sheep	B	10	3.3	±0.13[b]	Eveleth (1937)
	S	12	2.5	±0.3	White et al. (1957)
	P	10	2.9	±0.13[b]	Eveleth (1937)
	C	10	3.8	±0.29[b]	Eveleth (1937)
Pig	B	10	6.4	±0.78[b]	Eveleth (1937)
	P	10	3.2	±0.49[b]	Eveleth (1937)
	C	10	10.5	±1.46[b]	Eveleth (1937)
Rabbit	B	7	5.4	±0.74[b]	Eveleth (1937)
	P	7	3.2	±0.59[b]	Eveleth (1937)
	C	7	9.4	±2.63[b]	Eveleth (1937)
Dog	S[c]	10	2.1	±0.3	Eichelberger and McLean (1942)
Goat	B	3	3.7	±0.65[b]	Eveleth (1937)
	P	3	3.2	±0.35[b]	Eveleth (1937)
	C	3	4.5	±1.18[b]	Eveleth (1937)

[a]B = whole blood; P = plasma; S = serum; C = cells.
[b]Indicates that standard deviation was estimated from range and number of observations.
[c]Fat-free serum.

c. THE MAMMARY GLAND. The mineral constituents of milk are given in Table VI. As it appears from the table a heavily lactating cow may lose about 3 gm Mg/day by this route. This represents a large proportion of the dietary magnesium absorbed from the gut; therefore, any factor affecting either the rate of secretion or the concentration of magnesium in the milk will modify the requirement of magnesium. Robertson et al. (1960) and Rook and Storry (1962) provided evidence indicating that no significant fall in the magnesium content of milk occurs when intake of feed or of magnesium is reduced, or if hypomagnesemia develops.

About 20% of the magnesium in cow's milk is in the ionic form (Van Kreveld and Van Minnen, 1955), 30% is associated with the colloid, and the remaining 50% exists in unknown forms (Alexander and Ford, 1957).

VI. SERUM MAGNESIUM

Depending on the species blood serum normally contains 2–5 mg Mg/ 100 ml (see Table VII). In animals other than the ox, magnesium occurs at a higher concentration in erythrocytes than in plasma (Salt, 1950). There is apparently no exchange of magnesium between plasma and the red cells in the peripheral circulation (Aikawa, 1963). About 79% of the serum magnesium has been found to be ultrafiltrable independent of the total amount present (R. H. Smith, 1957).

REGULATION OF SERUM MAGNESIUM

Little is known regarding the factors involved in the regulation of the serum magnesium content of the blood. There is in some respects a reciprocal relationship between magnesium and calcium in the serum, e.g., in oxalate poisoning the decrease in serum calcium is accompanied by an increase in serum magnesium (Hallgren et al., 1959). During hypomagnesemia it has clearly been demonstrated that the regulation of serum magnesium is critically dependent on the daily magnesium intake. In contradiction to calcium no endocrine gland has been shown to exert a primary regulatory effect over plasma magnesium concentration. Three endocrine glands, the adrenals, the thyroids, and the parathyroids, appear to be involved.

Almost fifteen years ago Blaxter and McGill (1956) pointed out that there was no evidence from critical experimentation indicating that the endocrine glands had any specific effect on magnesium metabolism. They therefore suggested that the magnesium metabolism was regulated by a dynamic equilibrium in which the skeleton acted as a labile source of magnesium. Soft tissue magnesium was accepted of vital importance and therefore not available for magnesium homeostasis. As a first approximation the magnesium homeostasis was considered a result of a balance between intake from intestine and renal excretion. In an immature animal the entire skeleton acted as a labile source of surface minerals, whereas in the adult a very large part of the skeleton was inert.

1. The Adrenals

In man, hyperaldosteronism is associated with a negative magnesium balance and hypomagnesemia (Mader and Iseri, 1955). Studies in rats subsequently demonstrated that as a function of the dose, aldosterone caused increased excretion of magnesium in urine and feces (Hanna and MacIntyre, 1960). Somewhat similar findings were obtained with sheep (Oyaert, 1962; Care and Ross, 1963; Scott and Dobson, 1965).

In adrenal insufficiency, the opposite effect on magnesium metabolism occurs. Both in adrenalectomized laboratory animals and in patients with Addison's disease, serum magnesium concentration is increased (Wacker and Vallee, 1958). The effects of mineralocorticoids on magnesium homeostasis, however, appear to be secondary to their more important influences on potassium and sodium homeostasis. In contrast to these two ions, no influence of magnesium concentration on aldosterone secretion could be detected (Care and McDonald, 1963). Keynes and Care (1967) concluded after a reinvestigation of the possible role of mineralocorticoids in calcium and magnesium homeostasis in sheep from which the parathyroids, thyroids, and adrenals had all been removed that adrenal steroids may contribute to calcium and magnesium homeostasis in sheep, but their role in the intact animal is subordinate to that of the thyroid and parathyroid hormones.

2.   The Thyroid Glands

In man, thyrotoxicosis is associated with hypomagnesemia and negative magnesium balance, whereas in myxedema the serum concentration tends to be elevated and the balance is positive (Wacker and Parisi, 1968).

W. M. Allcroft (1947a) suspected some association between the level of serum magnesium and the degree of activity of the thyroid gland. Swan and Jamieson (1956) demonstrated that feeding of thyroprotein to lactating cows led to a decrease in serum magnesium. In growing rats Vitale et al. (1957) found that the depression of growth rate and the hypomagnesemia, which result from thyroxine feeding, could be partly overcome by supplementing the diet with large amounts of magnesium. In balance experiments with calves Meyer and Schmidt (1958) found that parenteral administration of thyroxine caused a transient hypomagnesemia brought about by an increased excretion of magnesium in both urine and feces. Thus most evidence suggests that increased thyroid activity tends to depress plasma magnesium concentration. Hypersecretion of thyroxine does, however, not appear to be one of the primary etiological factors in hypomagnesemic tetany (Todd and Thompson, 1962).

Thyrocalcitonin, the hormone secreted by the thyroid light cells, has only very little or no effect on plasma magnesium concentration (Care, 1967).

3.   The Parathyroid Glands

In 1963 MacIntyre et al. suggested a homeostasis mechanism for magnesium centered around the parathyroid glands. This hypothesis proposes, favored of a substantial amount of evidence, that elevation of plasma magnesium leads to inhibition of parathyroid secretion, whereas hypomagnesemia stimulates its release. From observations of parathyroidea-dependent hypercalcemia it was inferred that hypomagnesemia in magnesium-deficient rats stimulated the PTH secretion (Heaton, 1965; Gitelman et al., 1968). The proposal has finally been examined and confirmed in experiments in which parathyroid hormone concentration in plasma was measured directly by radioimmunoassay (Buckle et al., 1968).

The inverse relationship demonstrated between the magnesium concentration and the parathyroid gland activity is similar to that between the plasma concentration of calcium and that of PTH in peripheral plasma of cows (Sherwood et al., 1966). Since PTH exerts a prominent effect on the concentration of calcium in plasma relative to that on magnesium, it seems likely that the concentration of calcium in plasma exerts the major physiological control on parathyroid gland function. The PTH release, however, can be specifically influenced by the concentration of magnesium in plasma.

VII.   DISTURBANCES IN MAGNESIUM METABOLISM

Only cattle and sheep are known to be subject to clinical disorders, apparently due to magnesium deficiency. According to Green (1948) the disease can be grossly classified into two types, a rapidly developing and a slowly developing type. In calves and beef cattle the disease is generally of the slow type, whereas in milking cattle and sheep the onset in the majority of cases is rapid. Usually, but not invariably, the occurrence coincides with the first flush grass in the spring.

The fall in the blood level of serum magnesium may accordingly take place in a day or two as seen in the acute type, or the decline may be more gradual as seen in "out-wintered" cattle and stal -fed cattle on magnesium-poor diets.

The depletion of the magnesium ion concentration in the extracellular fluid, the fluid bathing neuromuscular junctions and synapses, apparently is responsible for the tetanic syndrome. The main symptoms are restlessness, twitching of the muscles, excitement, staggering gait, increased sensitivity to strange noises, and, finally, convulsions and death. The onset of symptoms, however, cannot be correlated directly with the concentration of magnesium in serum.

Since the very first report assigning this clinical picture to hypomagnesemia, the role of calcium has been discussed (Huffman and Robinson, 1926; C. W. Duncan et al., 1935). Thus Duckworth (1939) stated that a "principal effect of magnesium deficiency appears to be disturbance of normal calcium metabolism," and W. M. Allcroft (1947a) reported that 75% of 406 cows with hypomagnesemia also showed hypocalcemia.

A. Hypomagnesemia in Calves

This syndrome has been intimately associated with the feeding of whole milk for an abnormal length of time. The subject has been reviewed by Russell (1944), Blaxter and McGill (1956), and R. H. Smith (1964).

In 1923 McCandlish suggested that the nutritive failure of calves given whole milk for very long periods was related to their metabolism of magnesium. C. W. Duncan et al. (1935) subsequently demonstrated that the magnesium content of the blood serum of calves declined when they were given rations of whole milk supplemented with iron, copper manganese, and cod-liver oil. Blood calcium and phosphorus levels were reported to be within the normal range. The hypo-magnesemic nature of some naturally occurring tetanies, though, was not fully recognized until the work of Blaxter and his associates in the early 1950's.

In a series of studies it was pointed out that the hypomagnesemia in calves is a simple dietary deficiency of magnesium (Blaxter and Rook, 1954), and it was furthermore demonstrated that the pathological calcification of the endocardium and total vascular system observed in the so-called "milk syndrome" (L. A. Moore et al., 1936, 1938) was not associated with uncomplicated magnesium deficiency in calves. The calves were fed an artificial milk-substitute diet containing 0.5 mg Mg or less/100 ml. To this diet was added magnesium, so that different animals received from 0.5 to 19.0 mg Mg/100 ml. After 6–7 weeks on the experimental diet, three calves showed clinical symptoms of magnesium deficiency and died in convulsions. Two of the calves that died had received only the basal diet and the third received 1.64 mg Mg/100 ml. The concentration of serum magnesium had fallen to about 0.7 mg/100 ml when tetany appeared and to 0.5 mg/100 ml at death. One calf received 5.8 mg Mg/100 ml of diet for about 10 weeks and showed no clinical sign of deficiency, but serum magnesium steadily declined to 1.0 mg/100 ml. Calves which received 12.5

or 19.0 mg Mg/100 ml of diet were clinically normal and serum magnesium remained between 2.0 and 2.5 mg/100 ml.

No effect was noted on serum calcium and inorganic phosphate content during tetany, and no depletion of soft tissue magnesium was found either. During the 6 or 7 weeks on the low magnesium diet before death occurred, each calf lost about 2 gm of magnesium, whereas normal animals gained about 7 gm during the same time. Calves which grow the fastest usually show the greatest depression of serum magnesium (Blaxter and Sharman, 1955). One of the most characteristic symptoms observed was constant movement and flapping of the ears (Blaxter and Sharman, 1955; Parr, 1957).

The magnesium requirement for a growing calf was estimated to be 16–18 mg Mg/100 ml of diet, a much lower requirement than suggested by Huffman et al. (1941), but still considerably above the content of magnesium present in cow's milk (see Table V). Although applicable to some calves between 8 and 14 weeks, the figures of Blaxter and Rook are usually too high for younger calves and usually too low for older calves, which may develop hypomagnesemia on diets containing these and higher levels of magnesium (R. H. Smith, 1957).

1. Bone:Plasma Relationship

As mentioned, bone magnesium represents a store which can be called upon under conditions of deficiency. A study of the magnesium status of the skeleton during deficiency was made by R. H. Smith (1959b). In normal calves the magnesium content of the bone ash was about 0.80%. When plasma magnesium falls to about 1.6 mg/100 ml the bone ash contains about 0.60 to 0.67%, and at plasma levels of 0.7 the bone ash contains 0.40 to 0.48% of magnesium. During a depletion, plasma magnesium decreases only slowly after it has reached 0.7 mg/100 ml and further depletion of bone magnesium occurs with only a slight decrease of the plasma concentration.

The bone ash content of magnesium decreases with increasing age (Meyer, 1963). In adult cattle bone ash contains 0.55–0.70% of magnesium.

When hypomagnesemia is evident, it may take several weeks of oral magnesium supplementation to bring the level back to normal. Repeated subcutaneous injections of 1 gm Mg/day (given as the sulfate) can restore blood as well as bone ash magnesium at least in moderately deficient calves (R. H. Smith, 1959b).

2. Bone Sample and Its Diagnostic Value

During the final stages of convulsive attacks the serum magnesium is often increased, presumably due to the release of magnesium into the blood by rapidly contracting muscles (British Veterinary Association, 1957). Therefore a method to assess bone magnesium in the living animal as well as postmortem became desirable (Blaxter and Sharman, 1955). For this purpose rib biopsy has been used (Thomas and Okamoto, 1958). Later, R. H. Smith (1959b) suggested the use of vertebrae taken from the tail of the living animal. This method provides a satisfactory way of assessing bone composition, and the method offers obvious advantages over rib biopsy. In comparing ash analysis from different bones, Smith's findings are not in agreement with those of Blaxter and McGill (1956). However, the conclusions were based on findings in different bones. There might exist differences between bones at a stage of moderate depletion and the possibility still exists that bones losing magnesium more slowly will catch up with the bones losing magnesium more rapidly during more severe magnesium depletion.

The process of magnesium depletion of the bone apparently takes place as an exchange process in which magnesium is replaced by calcium on the bone crystal surface (Blaxter, 1955). Therefore, a diagnostic procedure estimating the Ca:Mg ratio as suggested by Blaxter and Sharman (1955) is clearly preferable under practical field conditions.

3.   Balance Experiments

R. H. Smith (1958) reported the mean fecal excretion of magnesium to be about 32% of the dietary intake at 3 weeks of age compared with about 86% at about 16 weeks of age. Thus with increasing age the ability to absorb magnesium decreases significantly. However, considerable variations between different calves were found. In general, the decrease reflects the onset of hypomagnesemia and might thus explain the inexplicable differences in susceptibility to hypomagnesemia found between groups of calves. Thus, for example, despite closely similar treatment the calves of Knoop et al. (1939) did not show hypomagnesemia until about 4 months of age, whereas those of Parr and Allcroft (1957) showed hypomagnesemia in 3–4 weeks.

It is not known whether the decreasing ability to utilize dietary magnesium is due to a decrease in absorption or an increase in endogenous fecal excretion or a combination of both. Neither vitamin D nor irradiation with ultraviolet light has any effect on this decrease. On the other hand, a marked decrease in calcium retention was also shown. However, this decrease could be prevented by vitamin D, provided the vitamin D intake was increased beyond that known to be adequate for calves (5–10 IU/kg body weight-day).

4.   Vitamin D and Serum Calcium and Magnesium

The convulsions reported in magnesium-deficient calves resemble convulsions due to low calcium, and in fact the reports of Parr (1957) and R. H. Smith (1958) seem to indicate a constant relationship between convulsions and hypocalcemia.

It has been shown that the addition of vitamin D (5–10 IU/kg body weight-day) to the milk does not prevent hypomagnesemia (C. W. Duncan et al., 1935; Huffman et al., 1941; Parr and Allcroft, 1957). R. H. Smith (1957), on the other hand, found that in calves not given vitamin D the development of hypomagnesemia was followed by a decrease in plasma calcium. The declines began about the same time and developed at about the same rate. If vitamin D (7,000–70,000 IU) or ultraviolet irradiation was given, the blood calcium values were rapidly brought back to normal. R. H. Smith (1957) reported a very interesting difference in the clinical picture in hypo-magnesemic-normocalcemic calves versus calves being hypocalcemic as well as hypomagnesemic. During the period in which the calves were hypocalcemic and moderately hypomagnesemic (1.4–1.5 mg/100 ml) they would suddenly collapse and remain almost motionless with their neck and legs stiff for periods varying from a few minutes to half an hour. On the other hand, calves having "pure" hypomagnesemia (the calves given ample vitamin D supplement) never started showing clinical signs before plasma magnesium had dropped to below 1 mg/100 ml. The initial signs then were nervousness, twitching ears, and staring eyes. Later they could be found staggering and unable to stand, but convulsions were never observed.

Recently, it has been shown that plasma creatine phosphokinase (CPK) levels are considerably elevated for about 24 hours after an acute phase of hypomagnesemic tetany in calves (Todd et al., 1969). After commencement of magnesium therapy the CPK levels decreased rapidly. The CPK activity was found closely related to the tetanic syndrome and not to hypomagnesemia per se. The diagnostic value of serum CPK is not yet known. Elevation of CPK activity has also been recorded in calves with muscular dystrophy (Todd and Thompson, 1968).

B. Hypomagnesemia in Adult Cattle

1. The Slow Type

Quite a number of reports have appeared concerning the type of hypomagnesemia in which animals exhibit low serum magnesium levels for some time, often for months. When serum magnesium levels approach critical low values, they are generally accompanied by mild clinical symptoms such as nervousness and increased excitability. In such cases certain conditions as fasting or reduced feed intake may precipitate the tetany–paresis syndrome. Often a combination of several adverse factors is found, but in most cases low dietary magnesium together with a low plane of nutrition are essential. Owing to underfeeding slight ketonemia is often seen. The incidence of the disease seems to increase with age and there is a tendency to recurrence in some animals. In the following section a short review will be given, dealing with some of the more important communications on this type of hypomagnesemia.

a. SEASONAL HYPOMAGNESEMIA. The first recorded study of seasonal hypomagnesemia in the bovine without clinical symptoms was made by W. M. Allcroft and Green (1938), when attention was drawn to the winter fall in serum magnesium in a herd of Hereford cows at pasture all year round without shelter or additional feeding. From August the serum magnesium fell to minimum levels in December with a return to normal levels in February. Values as low as 0.5 mg/100 ml were found for serum magnesium, but no changes occurred in the serum calcium levels. The pasture contained 0.20% magnesium (dry matter). It was noted that the additional feeding of 45 gm MgO/head per day in a mineral mixture alleviated the seasonal fall of serum magnesium, but did not maintain a normal level. W. M. Allcroft (1947b) extended these findings and showed that the low serum magnesium values were associated with adverse weather, especially with combined cold, wet, and windy periods. The lowest level of serum magnesium might occur any time between December and April. The conditions under which minimum serum magnesium was found were such that the heat loss from the body would be at the highest. When hay and cabbages were fed, the magnesium level rose to normal, only to fall again when supplementary feeding ceased. The clinical cases of hypomagnesemia, all of which showed very low serum magnesium and varying degree of hypocalcemia, coincided with the time when minimum serum magnesium values appeared, i.e. during periods with little or no growth of grass.

b. THE NORWEGIAN TETANY-PARESIS SYNDROME (Ender *et al.*, 1948; Breirem *et al.*, 1949). Special conditions during World War II forced the Norwegian farmers to feed rations containing herring meal and fodder cellulose, both very low in magnesium. Concentrates and grain were entirely suspended. The rations may be characterized as deficient in energy with an abundant supply of protein. This fodder caused a marked increase in metabolic diseases such as ketosis and tetany. Subnormal values of serum calcium and magnesium were found in paretic cows as well as in cows suffering from tetany. Both sets of symptoms often appeared simultaneously in the same herd.

This stimulated feeding experiments in which cows were given an ample supply of protein, calcium, and phosphorus, but a supply of energy 10–50% below theoretical requirements and deficient in magnesium. In these experiments it was shown that the tetany–paresis syndrome could be reproduced under strictly controlled conditions.

Some cows would show pronounced hypomagnesemia without showing clinical symptoms at all. In others the hypomagnesemia was accompanied by muscular irritability, twitchings, or tremor. A marked individual variation between different cows was seen. Fasting periods of 36 hours' duration or abrupt change in the diet brought about a drop in serum magnesium as well as in serum calcium in such cows. In eight cows, tetany or paresis was induced. Serum analysis revealed a picture similar to that described by Sjollema (1930) for grass tetany as shown in Table VIII. The daily intake of magnesium ranged from 4 to 11 gm. Supplements of magnesium (28 gm a day given as carbonate) could prevent the hypomagnesemia as well as the nervous symptoms and the tetany.

c. WINTER TETANY.   This type of disorder, mainly seen in beef cattle, may occur in stall-fed cattle (Mershon and Custer, 1958; Mershon, 1959) or in cattle during winter after the pasture growth has stopped (Udall, 1947). Generally the cows appear to be on fairly poor rations during development of the disease; in fact,

TABLE VIII   SERUM CALCIUM, MAGNESIUM, AND INORGANIC PHOSPHORUS CONCENTRATIONS IN GRASS TETANY[a]

	Calcium (mg/100 ml)	Inorganic phosphorus (mg/100 ml)	Magnesium (mg/100 ml)
Grass tetany according to Sjollema	6.5	4.5	0.5
Eight cows suffering from experimental tetany or paresis	6.7	3.4	0.7
The same 8 cows 2–5 days before onset of tetany or paresis	9.9	5.8	0.7

[a]Modified from Ender *et al* (1949a).

Marshak (1959) stated that the simplest means of controlling winter tetany was through improving the nutritional status of the herds. When pasture reappears, the disease disappears.

During winter months persistent low levels of magnesium may be found, but this hypomagnesemia is accompanied by few or no clinical symptoms. Certain cows, especially those with recent parturition, may suddenly come down with clinical symptoms ranging from moderate incoordination to paresis or tetany. In the syndrome hyperirritability has a dominant place whereas coma most often is absent. During the clinical stage, it is generally agreed that the hypomagnesemia is associated with a varying degree of hypocalcemia (Marshak, 1959). As an explanation for the variance in the clinical behavior, Mershon and Custer (1958) have suggested the Ca:Mg ratio.

Leffel and Mason (1959) fed cows hay obtained from two farms which had experienced a high incidence of winter tetany. The hay was given as the sole ration for 4–6 months before calving and in early lactation. The daily intake of magnesium ranged from 7 to 12 gm. Both in dairy cows and in the beef cows, severe hypomagnesemia was observed; but only beef cows developed tetany. Plasma sodium and potassium values were reported to be normal.

d. EFFECT OF UNDERFEEDING.   The pregnant or recently calved ruminant appears to be especially susceptible to an upset of this nature. Underfeeding (Swan and Jamieson, 1956; Pehrson, 1963) or fasting (Halse, 1958a, 1960; Robertson et al., 1960; Herd, 1966) has been found to be effective methods lowering the serum magnesium.

Swan and Jamieson (1956) thus obtained evidence that the following conditions may cause a lowering of the serum magnesium in milking cows: (1) feeding thyroprotein alone or in conjunction with underfeeding; (2) a sudden change in quality and quantity of the ration; (3) a sudden increase in the quantity of the ration; (4) calving, especially if accompanied by a reduction in grazing time; (5) estrus, if accompanied by marked homosexual activity and a disturbance of grazing behavior; and (6) strong winds, where there is a reduction of grazing time or, if not, a marked reduction in rumination time.

From Sweden Pehrson (1963) reported that a number of tetanic conditions in stable-fed cows occurred following the very wet summer of 1960. In all cases the tetany was found to be associated with hypomagnesemia and appeared more than 6 days after calving. Provision of 45 gm MgO daily prevented the hypomagnesemia as well as the tetanic conditions. Careful investigation showed that hypomagnesemia was also present in many symptom-free cows. It was shown that the energy requirements of the milking cows were not satisfied. The supply of magnesium was, however, a good deal higher than minimum requirements. The author states that the minimum requirements for dietary magnesium apparently become greater in combination with underfeeding.

The effect of fasting on the mineral metabolism of the lactating cow has been studied (Halse, 1958a, 1960; Robertson et al., 1960; Herd, 1966). These experiments extended and confirmed the experience of J. A. B. Smith et al. (1938), that starved cows may develop a clinical syndrome very similar to milk fever. A significant decrease in serum calcium and magnesium was found. In the cows showing symptoms similar to milk fever, the minimum calcium levels were not lower than in the cows which remained apparently normal. The magnesium levels, on the other hand, were decidedly lower just prior to the onset of "milk fever" than they were in other cows at any time during the experiment. In all cows the serum magnesium level had a tendency to remain low during the early stages of refeeding (see Fig. 2). A similar effect of fasting has been observed in sheep (Christian and Williams, 1960; Herd, 1966).

e. EFFECT OF ARTIFICIALLY LOW MAGNESIUM INTAKES.   Rook (1961, 1963) designed a diet extremely low in magnesium and fed it to cows. With this diet he showed that the critical low intake of magnesium was about 2 gm Mg daily. The ration, which was otherwise nutritionally adequate, produced hypomagnesemia in four lactating, housed cows in less than 8 days. In two of the cows the fall in magnesium was relatively slow and no symptoms appeared. In the other two the fall in serum magnesium was more rapid. Both developed tetany, one died. The day before the final tetanic attack the serum calcium and magnesium values were 9.5 and 0.28 mg%, respectively. At that time the cow was hyperexcitable and had mild tetany. The final attack, with collapse, violent tonic-clonic convulsions, opisthotonus with eyeballs suddenly withdrawn almost completely into the socket, took only 5–10 minutes.

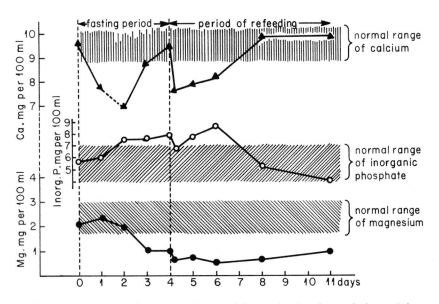

Fig. 2.   Change in serum calcium, magnesium, and inorganic phosphorus during a 4-day period of fasting.

2.   The Rapid Type: Grass Tetany

In the late 1920's a metabolic disturbance, now known as hypomagnesemic tetany, appeared in the veterinary literature. It affected cattle only, and was referred to under a variety of synonyms such as grass staggers (Sjollema, 1930; Sjollema and Seekles, 1930), Hereford disease, or lactation tetany (Lothian, 1931). The disease was probably not a new one, for unexplained sporadic, sudden death of cattle at pasture had previously been reported and given such labels as eclampsia, brain-fever, bovine hysteria, and the like (Robertson, 1960). However, the problem became prominent and work was started to elucidate the etiology of this syndrome.

The form of the disease first recognized occurred in cows in the spring within a few weeks after they were turned out to pasture following the winter feeding period (Sjollema, 1928; Sjollema and Seekles, 1929). The cases described by Lothian (1931) occurred mainly in "outwintered" cattle, and the clinical syndrome was similar to that described by Sjollema. The clinical–chemical findings confirmed this shortly after (Dryerre, 1932).

In nearly all descriptions of hypomagnesemic tetany, young rapidly growing grass is emphasized as being especially dangerous. Clover and herbs seem to be less dangerous. The disease occurs most frequently during the first weeks of the grazing season. In some years, however, it is also rather frequent in autumn, especially under wet conditions with relatively low temperature levels. Thus in Holland 95% of the cases reported occurred when the mean temperature was between 5 and 15° C ('tHart and Kemp, 1956). The same seems to be true for "wheat poisoning," tetany on winter grazing of oats in Argentina, and grass staggers in New Zealand. When frost occurs the number of cases declines rapidly (Inglis, 1960).

a. CLINICAL BIOCHEMICAL FINDINGS.   Sjollema first pointed out that a decline in the magnesium concentration of the blood was always present during hypo-magnesemic tetany, and he also noted that the pronounced hypomagnesemia in most cases was combined with a moderate hypocalcemia.

Blakemore and Stewart (1934) confirmed these findings and demonstrated that subnormal magnesium levels may be found in clinically normal herds where hypo-magnesemic tetany is present. This finding has been repeatedly confirmed. Recently Kemp (1958) demonstrated that the serum magnesium levels of 90 milking cows, grazing on pastures where hypomagnesemic tetany occurred, were reduced in nearly all cows. Of the 90 cows, only one had a serum magnesium level higher than 2.0 mg/100 ml, 38 showed levels between 1.1 and 2.0 mg/100 ml, whereas 51 cows, almost 60%, had serum magnesium levels below 1.1 mg/100 ml.

Todd and Thompson (1960) investigated most of the major blood electrolytes during hypomagnesemia without clinical symptoms. No consistent alterations were found in serum calcium, sodium, potassium, or chloride, or in carbon dioxide combining power. Similar results have been reported previously (Sjollema, 1930; Dryerre, 1932; Bartlett et al., 1957).

W. M. Allcroft (1947a) noted that hypocalcemia was present in 76% of 406 clinical cases of hypomagnesemia. Serum inorganic phosphate levels have been reported normal or low (Sjollema, 1930). Values below 2.0 mg/100 ml have been found (Hvidsten et al., 1959; Simesen, 1959). Van Koetsveld (1955) has demonstrated increased SO_4^{2+} values in serum from tetanic cows. During the tetanic stage a metabolic acidosis and moderate accumulation of lactate in the blood have been shown (Hendriks, 1962, 1964a). In sheep serious reductions in plasma magnesium have been found without effect on the proportions of bound magnesium and calcium present in plasma (Suttle and Field, 1969).

As a differential diagnostic method between milk fever and grass tetany, the proteinuria usually present during grass tetany has been recommended (Sjollema, 1930; Hopkirk et al., 1933; Metzger, 1936). The magnesium content of the urine, however, offers a much more reliable possibility for a differential diagnostic test. During milk fever the magnesium content in urine is about 50 mg % (Sjollema, 1930), whereas during hypomagnesemia the urine is devoid of magnesium (i.e., 2–3 mg %) (Ender et al., 1957; Kemp et al., 1961; Simesen, 1963b). An indicator paper which enables a semiquantitative determination of magnesium as a "bedside" test has been developed (de Groot and Marttin, 1967) and critically tested* (Simesen, 1968).

If a suspicion of hypomagnesemia exists before treatment of a paretic cow, the indicator paper makes it easy to confirm or invalidate such suspicion right on the spot. If the suspicion is confirmed, i.e., hypomagnesemia is a reality in the herd, preventive measures can be taken right away for the whole herd. Postmortem blood samples are of little value for diagnostic purposes as the magnesium level rises rapidly after death (Burns and Allcroft, 1967). In such cases a urine sample carefully removed from the bladder, preferably in connection with the taking of several blood samples from susceptible animals in the herd may supply the diagnosis (Simesen, 1964).

b. ETIOLOGICAL CONSIDERATIONS. In one of his earlier reports, Sjollema (1932a) suggested that hypomagnesemic tetany must have some connection with alteration in the methods of feeding and manuring. This point became evident in the early 1950's when a definite implication of such relationships was demonstrated in well-controlled experiments (Bartlett et al., 1954).

At that time it was known that (1) serum magnesium might fall very rapidly within a few days (R. Allcroft, 1954); (2) bones of adult animals with hypomagnesemic tetany did not exhibit depletion of magnesium (Cunningham, 1936a,b); (3) the condition occurred in cattle given grass with normal magnesium content (Sjollema, 1928, 1930); and (4) feeding magnesium oxide had a preventive effect (Blakemore and Stewart, 1934). Attempts to correlate the disease with a toxic factor or any special quality of the lush spring grass such as high intake of protein, potassium, nitrate (Sjollema, 1932a), or manganese (Blakemore et al., 1937) had been unsuccessful (Green, 1939), and the disease was thought to be of metabolic rather than nutritional origin (W. M. Allcroft, 1947b).

c. THE CHEMICAL AND BOTANICAL COMPOSITION OF SPRING PASTURE. Compared with hay, young grass has a strikingly high content of phosphorus. The calcium content is in the low range, whereas the magnesium appears to be adequate. The content of potassium is usually abundant, while the level of sodium is very low.

Mineral requirements of a cow milking 20 kg of milk daily compared with the amount of minerals contained in 18 kg of young grass (dry matter) or about 90 kg of fresh grass are shown in Table IX (modified from Werner, 1960).

Lush spring grass is rich in water (often more than 85%), soluble carbohydrates, and crude protein; whereas the content of crude fiber is low. During the growing season the content of crude fiber increases, while that of crude protein decreases. In autumn, especially during wet and rather cold weather, a second maximum in crude protein content may be reached (Brandsma, 1954). In spring grass a crude protein content of about 25% (dry matter) may be found. On the other hand, clover-rich pastures may produce herbage with protein contents between 25 and 30%.

---

*It is very important to avoid fecal contamination of the urine sample because of the magnesium content in feces.

TABLE IX   THEORETICAL MINERAL REQUIREMENTS COMPARED TO ACTUAL MINERAL CONTENTS OF A
DAY'S RATION OF GRASS

	Phos-phorus	Cal-cium	Magne-sium	Potas-sium	Sodium
Theoretical requirement (gm)	55	87	10	130	24
Young grass (gm)	88	84	29	300–500	12

Because hypomagnesemia rarely occurs on clover-rich pastures, the crude protein content has sometimes been considered of less importance in relation to hypomagnesemia. This may, however, more likely be due to the high calcium and magnesium content of clover. Usually clover and herbs contain at least twice as much calcium and magnesium as grasses.

While the content of phosphorus and crude protein decreases during the growing season, the content of magnesium and crude fiber slowly increases. The minimum magnesium level in pastures thus occurs in early spring and late autumn.

d. INFLUENCE OF DIFFERENT FERTILIZER TREATMENTS. Fertilizer treatment influences mineral composition of pasture as well as the botanical composition of the sward. Nitrogen fertilizers often reduce the proportion of clover, whereas application of phosphorus and potassium may quickly produce a clover-dominant sward.

Changes in the mineral composition of herbage after different fertilizing are shown in Table X (modified from Kemp, 1960).

'tHart and Kemp (1956) demonstrated that herbage from "tetany pastures" had a higher mean potassium and phosphorus content and a lower sodium, calcium, and magnesium content than herbage from pastures without tetany. The magnesium content of "tetany pastures" was about 10% below that of "nontetany pastures". Larvor and Guéguen (1963) followed the relations between grass composition and hypomagnesemia and found that tetany-prone grasses were significantly lower in magnesium and crude fiber content and higher in nonelaborated nitrogen. Wolton (1963) reviewed the various factors affecting herbage chemical composition and concluded: Nitrogen applications are essential to produce early bite and the bulk

TABLE X   INFLUENCE OF DIFFERENT FERTILIZER TREATMENTS

Dressing	Potas-sium	Magne-sium	Cal-cium	Sodium	Phos-phorus	Crude protein
Potash (K)	+[a]	−[b]	−	−	0[c]	0
Nitrogen (N)	[d]	+	+	+	0	+
K + N	+	−	−	−	0	+

[a] = increase.
[b] = decrease.
[c] = no change.
[d]Nitrogen applied to a sward high in potassium (more than 2%) will increase the percentage of potassium in the pasture. Applied to swards with a potassium content below 2%, on the other hand, it results in a decrease in the potassium content.

of spring growth. She therefore recommended that no more nitrogen is used than is required for immediate herbage production. Potassium applications should be deferred until the danger period has passed.

e. GRAZING EXPERIMENTS. The investigations of Bartlett *et al.* (1954) included a series of grazing experiments in which the influence of different fertilizer treatments on the incidence of hypomagnesemia was studied.

Dutch workers ('tHart and Kemp, 1956; Kemp, 1958) demonstrated that a high potassium content of grass promotes the incidence of hypomagnesemia. The incidence was further increased by a simultaneously high nitrogen content of the grass as shown in Table XI.

TABLE XI   DRESSING INFLUENCE ON SERUM MAGNESIUM

Dressing	Average serum Mg (mg/100 ml)	Dressing	Average serum Mg (mg/100 ml)
Low N, low K	2.43	High N, low K	2.15
Low N, high K	1.74	High N, high K	1.41

Plant magnesium uptake is powerfully influenced by the competition of potassium. This is absorbed preferentially from the soil by most plants. Therefore a decrease in the plant magnesium content may well be an indirect effect of potassium application.

Some workers do not agree on the importance of potassium in the development of hypomagnesemia (Ender *et al.*, 1957; Alten *et al.*, 1958; Smyth *et al.*, 1958). On the basis of potassium-feeding experiments Brouwer (1951), Kunkel *et al.* (1953), Sjollema *et al.* (1955a), and Van Koetsveld (1964) are of the opinion that potassium contributes to lower serum magnesium, whereas Green and Allcroft (1951), Eaton and Avampato (1952), and Daniel *et al.* (1952) have been unable to support such findings. Ender *et al.* (1957) have suggested the "tetanigen" effect observed to be more dependent on the simultaneously raised dietary level of phosphorus than on the high intake of potassium. Smyth *et al.* (1958) found that treatment of a sward with nitrogen alone or potassium alone did not render it more prone to a lowering of serum magnesium levels, whereas treatment with a combined dressing of nitrogen plus potassium resulted in a highly significant rapid decline in serum magnesium values followed by the onset of tetany. Application of magnesium in addition to nitrogen plus potassium resulted in maintenance of serum magnesium values within normal range. Blaxter *et al.* (1960) concluded that if potassium had anything to do with hypomagnesemia in cattle, it must be an indirect effect, i.e., by decreasing the magnesium content of the sward. High potassium content of the food neither had an influence on serum magnesium levels nor had it any influence on the potassium content of the blood cells. Recently, however, Suttle and Field (1969) have shown that an increase in potassium intake can reduce plasma magnesium and induce hypomagnesemic tetany in sheep, if the daily intake of magnesium is so low that the minimum magnesium requirements are barely met.

Sjollema (1932b) stated that the sulfur content of grass parallels the protein content. Since then, the importance of the high sulfur content of spring grass has been stressed by Van Koetsveld (1955), who demonstrated increased values of sulfate in serum from tetanic cows. Ender *et al.* (1957) reported that various inorganic substances, e.g., sulfates and phosphates, induce marked falls in the level of serum magnesium in sheep. In fertilizing experiments, they found sulfate of ammonia treated pasture, which contained about four times as much sulfur as calcium ammonium nitrate treated pasture, to be more tetanigen (Havre and Dishington, 1962). Tetany on pastures moderate in sulfate content were also reported. By means of balance experiments Gröning (1959) studied the influence of sulfate on the metabolism of magnesium in cattle. High sulfate content of the feed had no effect on the serum magnesium levels, whereas the excretion of magnesium in the urine decreased. Gröning concludes that even if sulfate should prove to possess a slight inhibitory effect upon magnesium absorption, a possibility which could not be excluded by his studies, this inhibition would not be of such magnitude as to explain the etiology of hypomagnesemic tetany.

A high content of nitrate in the grass has been suggested as a cause of grass tetany (Rathje, 1958), but a subsequent study of samples from pastures causing tetany did not support this hypothesis. Neither did Seekles and Sjollema (1932) nor Ender *et al.* (1957) in their above-mentioned studies find any indication of such relationship.

f. MINERAL INDICES. Several ratios such as K/(Ca + Mg) (Kemp and 'tHart, 1957), (Na × 100)/(K + Na + Ca + Mg) ('tHart and Kemp, 1957), (K × 100)/(K + Ca + Mg) (Verdeyen, 1953) and alkaline alkalinity* (Brouwer, 1957) have been suggested as indices for the relationship between a given sward and the degree of hypomagnesemia induced, when fed to cows. Rook and Wood (1960) have since demonstrated that no such relationship could be expected between the degree of hypomagnesemia in grazing cattle and the concentration of any particular mineral constituent or the magnitude of any mineral index. Ratios including potassium and sodium are clearly almost entirely dependent on the potassium and the sodium content of the sward and are likely to be most markedly influenced by an application of potash fertilizer, which increases the potassium and decreases the sodium content of herbage. For a particular sward and under any given sets of grazing conditions, however, an increased severity of hypomagnesemia, brought about by the application of nitrogenous or potash fertilizers, was generally associated with a lowering of the alkaline-earth alkalinity of the grazed herbage. But an attempt to use a single sward characteristic as a general diagnostic test for a pasture that is likely to produce a high incidence of hypomagnesemia and tetany in the grazing cow must inevitably fail (Rook and Wood, 1960). Butler (1963), on the other hand, finds that although the K/(Ca + Mg) ratio has not yet been shown to have any physiological or nutritional basis it does appear to be of particular significance in relation to the occurrence of grass tetany.

Seekles (1964) pointed out that, although the hypothesis of a relationship between the K/(Ca + Mg) ratio in the pasture and the occurrence of hypomagnesemic tetany may be supported by statistical data obtained from farms in certain areas and in

---

*Alkaline alkalinity: the sum of K + Na − Cl − S, when expressed in mEq/100 gm herbage, dry matter. Alkaline-earth alkalinity: the sum of Ca + Mg − P, when expressed in mEq/100 gm herbage, dry matter.

particular years, it is not well supported by data obtained over many years from samples collected throughout the whole area of the Netherlands.

In the spring a level of 0.20% of magnesium has been found to give protection even on "tetany-prone" pastures (R. Allcroft and Burns, 1968). In the autumn herbage magnesium levels of 0.25% seem closer to the critical level (Todd, 1967).

Increase in the magnesium content of the herbage brought about by a magnesium-containing fertilizer results in higher serum magnesium levels in grazing animals (Stewart, 1954; Reith, 1954; Bartlett et al., 1954; Parr and Allcroft, 1957; Smyth et al., 1958), and therefore Stewart and Reith (1956) concluded that grass tetany occurring on pasture must be regarded as a conditioned hypomagnesemic disorder, resulting either from an inadequate intestinal absorption of magnesium in the grass or from substances antagonizing the magnesium metabolism. Kemp (1960) subjected the relationship which might exist between the magnesium content of the herbage and the serum magnesium to a close valuation and demonstrated that the low serum magnesium levels only occur with magnesium contents of the herbage below 0.20% (dry matter). Furthermore, it was shown that in pasture with magnesium content below this value the low serum levels were associated with a higher percentage of crude protein.

g. RUMEN AMMONIA.   Head and Rook (1955) have drawn attention to the high ammonia concentration in the rumen of cows during the first days of grass feeding. The level rises from a general level of 10 to 20 mg/100 ml during winter stall-feeding conditions to a continuously high level of 40 to 60 mg/100 ml following the transfer to grass feeding. Simultaneously the urinary excretion fell to negligible amounts and the serum magnesium dropped from normal values to values of about 1 mg/100 ml. This decrease in urinary excretion of magnesium was suggested to reflect a reduced intestinal absorption of magnesium. Subsequently, addition of ammonium acetate or ammonium carbonate to the rumen (via a fistula) of cows fed a diet of hay and concentrates produced ruminal ammonia levels comparable with those observed on grass. The urinary magnesium excretion was reduced and a moderate reduction in serum magnesium levels seen.

h. BALANCE EXPERIMENTS.*   The above-mentioned findings induced a series of magnesium balance trials (Rook and Balch, 1958; Field et al., 1958; Kemp et al., 1960; Van der Horst, 1960; Meyer and Steinbeck, 1960). From the experiments it was learned that the change from winter stall feeds to herbage generally involves a decrease in the dietary magnesium intake. Head and Rook (1955) in their experiments reported a magnesium intake of about 21–25 gm/day on common winter rations compared with about 12.5 gm/day on rations of cut herbage. However, supposing unaltered "availability" (percentage of ingested magnesium not excreted in the feces) of the dietary magnesium, even such a daily magnesium intake should be sufficient (Ender et al., 1949b). The percentages of ingested magnesium excreted in the feces, however, were found to average 71.5–74.8% in cattle fed winter rations compared with 82–83% during grass feeding, i.e., the "availability" of magnesium in grass was lowered. This reduction in "availability" might be brought about by a lowering of the "true availability" or by an enlarged endogenous fecal magnesium,

---

*A transient hypomagnesemic effect on blood magnesium has been reported in connection with the application of a metabolic harness (Hendriks, 1964b).

as pointed out by Field (1960). Under normal dietary conditions the site of maximal magnesium absorption is in the midileum (Care and Van'T Klooster, 1965), i.e., below those parts of the intestinal tract into which the bulk of endogenous magnesium is secreted. If the process by which magnesium absorption takes place loses efficiency, not only does the ruminant fail to absorb dietary magnesium, but it also fails to absorb the magnesium secreted into the upper part of the digestive tract. A failure of the system by which magnesium is absorbed would thus lead to a reduction of the true absorption rate as well as to an increase in the endogenous fecal magnesium excretion (Care, 1967).

The decrease in magnesium absorption was at one time considered to be a result of an increased ruminal production of ammonia with subsequent elevation of pH in the upper part of the small intestine and precipitation of magnesium as magnesium ammonium phosphate (Simesen, 1959; Kemp et al., 1961). No significant changes in pH of ruminal, abomasal, or small intestinal contents have been observed in association with diets of spring grass, however (Simesen, 1963b; Van'T Klooster, 1967). Moreover, it is not usual to find a significant alteration in the ultrafiltrable magnesium concentration of digesta obtained from either duodenum or midileum of sheep when the diet is changed from hay to spring grass, despite a hypomagnesemic reaction to this dietary change (Care, 1967).

Feces of cows receiving a grass ration, on the other hand, has been found to contain less ultrafiltrable calcium and magnesium than the feces of cows fed winter rations (Van'T Klooster, 1967), whereas the percentage of water-extractable calcium and magnesium in samples of feces from a normal and a hypomagnesemic cow has been found without gross differences (Parr, 1961).

In the balance trials the change from winter rations to cut young grass was inevitably followed by an immediate fall in urinary magnesium excretion. Since this decrease in the urinary magnesium excretion preceded the fall in serum magnesium, it has been stated that urine magnesium is a better measure of the magnesium status of an animal than serum magnesium (Kemp, 1960).

Since calcium and magnesium are absorbed in the ionic state, and since the electrochemical potentials for the absorption from the ileum are comparatively small, a relatively small decrease in the concentration of ionized magnesium within the ileum would be sufficient to convert a net absorption of magnesium into a net secretion. The way in which the absorptive mechanism is impaired is still unknown. A common transport system for absorption of calcium and magnesium from the ileum has been postulated (Alcock and MacIntyre, 1960), and Care and Van'T Klooster (1965) suggested this system to be a process of facilitated diffusion. A calcium–magnesium interference at the absorption site in the ileum may therefore be a possible explanation. Another possibility is the binding of calcium and magnesium to suspended materials of the digesta as suggested by Storry (1961a,b). A third explanation would be a binding by some component derived from the diet, for example, a form of chelation favored by the high nonprotein nitrogen content of the spring grass (Larvor and Guéguen, 1963).

i. THE TRIGGER EFFECT.   The final insult that precipitates clinical symptoms of hypomagnesemic tetany in an already susceptible animal may be (1) a suddenly reduced feed intake (Halse, 1958b; Herd, 1966); (2) adverse weather (W. M. Allcroft, 1947b); (3) estrus (Swan and Jamieson, 1956); (4) oral application of relatively high doses of Na_2HPO_4 or Na_2SO_4 or both (Dishington, 1965); or (5) sudden reductions in dietary supplies of magnesium (Dishington and Tollersrud, 1967). Even the mere handling of a susceptible cow, pricking of a needle, unexpected noise, or the like may sometimes provoke an acute state of tetany.

As in man, tetany, the most distinctive symptom in the course of magnesium depletion, can occur when hypomagnesemia exists in the absence of other measurable serum electrolyte or acid-base abnormalities (Wacker and Parisi, 1968).

3. Methods of Prevention

In spite of the variety of different opinions on the exact etiology of hypomagnesemia there is a uniform agreement about the essential aim of the prevention: to increase the daily intake of magnesium. The provision of extra dietary magnesium may be given by means of drenching (Cunningham, 1934; Blakemore and Stewart, 1934; W. M. Allcroft and Green, 1938; R. Allcroft, 1954; Breirem et al., 1954; Jevnaker, 1955; Sjollema et al., 1955b), mixed in cattle cake (Seekles and Boogaert, 1955, 1956; Line et al., 1958), as magnesia–molasses mixtures (Todd et al., 1966; D. J. Horvath et al., 1967; Ross and Gibson, 1969), as foliar dusting of calcined magnesite on to pasture (Todd and Morrison, 1964; Poole, 1967; Kemp and Geurink, 1967), or via magnesium fertilization of the sward (Parr and Allcroft, 1957; Smyth et al., 1958; Bosch and Harmsen, 1958; Walsh and Conway, 1960), all effective means of prevention. In beef cattle it has been shown that effective control can be obtained by giving 4 oz calcined magnesite in a suspension of water sprayed on hay every second day (Herd et al., 1965).

Absorption of magnesium from the oxide has been shown to be better than from sulfate or carbonate (Storry and Rook, 1963; Meyer and Grund, 1963) and much better than from dolomite. For topdressing purposes it has been shown that magnesium sulfate as Epsom salt or kieserite is less suitable than calcined magnesite (R. Allcroft and Burns, 1968).

An extensive discussion on suitable methods to ensure an adequate intake under various types of management has been given (Burns and Allcroft, 1967).

A preventive effect of vitamin D has been suggested. Since the clinical syndrome usually is preceded by a fall in serum calcium (Bartlett et al., 1954) such an effect might be possible. It is well established, however, that such treatment does not prevent or reduce the degree of hypomagnesemia per se.

C. Miscellaneous Conditions

1. Hypomagnesemia in Sheep

The clinical symptoms of hypomagnesemia (grass staggers) in sheep were recognized fairly recently (Blumer et al., 1939; Barrentine, 1948; Stewart, 1954; Pook, 1955; Penny and Arnold, 1955; Inglis et al., 1959). The factors involved in hypomagnesemia in sheep are very similar to those in the development of hypomagnesemia in the cow (Hjerpe, 1968b) and have recently been reviewed (Hemingway et al., 1960). In sheep a striking variation between animals on similar treatment has been observed (L'Estrange and Axford, 1964a), and ewes with twins have been found more prone to hypomagnesemia than sheep with single lambs (Hvidsten, 1967). Oral supplementation of lactating ewes at pasture with magnesium, but no calcium, has been found effective in raising the concentration in serum of both calcium and magnesium to normal levels (L'Estrange and Axford, 1964b; Herd, 1966).

2. Wheat Pasture Poisoning

"Wheat pasture poisoning" is now usually regarded as a special feature of hypomagnesemic tetany (Sims and Crookshank, 1956). The combined effect of high potassium and high protein intake, known to be characteristic of lush wheat pasture grazing, was studied by means of balance trials (Fontenot et al., 1960). The findings of this study were consistent with the view that such rations may induce tetany by interfering with the absorption or retention of magnesium.

The effect of orally, intravenously, or subcutaneously administered calcium and magnesium has been studied by W. M. Allcroft (1947c). The anesthetic level of serum magnesium in the ruminant was found to be about 14 mg/100 ml and the lethal level about 20 mg/100 ml. Similar results have been reported in dogs (R. M. Moore and Wingo, 1942). When calcium is injected concurrently with magnesium, the level of magnesium necessary to cause death is considerably higher. It has recently been challenged (Somjen et al., 1966) if parenteral administration of magnesium salts could cause narcosis.

Hypermagnesemia is seen in advanced renal disease associated with uremia (Terkildsen, 1950).

REFERENCES

Aalund, O., and Nielsen, K. (1960). Nord. Veterinärmed. 12, 605.
Åkerblom, E. (1952). Nord Veterinärmed. 4, 471.
Agricultural Research Council (1965) "The Nutrient Requirement of Farm Livestock," No. 2. Ruminants: Technical Reviews and Summaries. Agr. Res. Council, London.
Aikawa, J. K. (1963). "The Measurement of Magnesium in Biologic Materials," Chapter 6, p. 42. Thomas, Springfield, Illinois.
Albright, F., and Reifenstein, E. C. (1948). "The Parathyroid Glands and Metabolic Bone Disease," p. 393. Williams & Wilkins, Baltimore, Maryland.
Albright, F., Bauer, W., Ropes, M. W., and Aub, J. C. (1929). J. Clin. Invest. 7, 139.
Alcock, N., and MacIntyre, I. (1960). Biochem. J. 76, 19.
Alexander, T. G., and Ford, T. F. (1957). J. Dairy Sci. 40, 1273.
Aliapoulios, M. A., Savery, A., and Munson, P. L. (1965). Federation Proc. 24, 322.
Allcroft, R. (1954). Vet. Record 66, 517.
Allcroft, R., and Burns, K. N. (1968). New Zealand Vet. J. 16, 109.
Allcroft, R., and Ivins, L. N. (1964). Rept. 3rd Intern. Meeting Diseases Cattle, Copenhagen, Nord. Veterinärmed, 1964, 16, Suppl. 1, p. 217.
Allcroft, W. M. (1947a). Vet. J. 103, 2 and 30.
Allcroft, W. M. (1947b). Vet. J. 103, 75.
Allcroft, W. M. (1947c). Vet. J. 103, 157.
Allcroft, W. M., and Folley, S. J. (1941). Biochem. J. 35, 254.
Allcroft, W. M., and Godden, W. (1934). Biochem. J. 28, 1004.
Allcroft, W. M., and Green, H. H. (1934). Biochem. J. 28, 2220.
Allcroft, W. M., and Green, H. H. (1938). J. Comp. Pathol. Therap. 51, 176.
Alten, F., Rosenberger, G., and Welte, E. (1958). Zentr. Veterinärmed. 5, 201.

Asbury, A. C. (1962). *J. Am. Vet. Med. Assoc.* **141**, 703.

Auger, M. L. (1926). *Compt. Rend.* **182**, 348.

Auger, M. L. (1927). *Rev. Gen. Med. Vet.* **36**, 625 and 689 (Transl. by C. J. Marshall); *J. Am. Vet. Med. Assoc.* **70**, 421 (1927).

Baer, J. E., Peck, H. M., and McKinney, S. E. (1957). *Proc. Soc. Exptl. Biol. Med.* **95**, 80.

Bardwell, R. E. (1959). *J. Am. Vet. Med. Assoc.* **135**, 72.

Barker, J. R. (1939). *Vet. Record* **51**, 575.

Barnes, J. E., and Jephcott, B. R. (1955). *Australian Vet. J.* **31**, 302.

Barnicoat, C. R., Logan, A. G., and Grant, A. I. (1949). *J. Agr. Sci.* **39**, 237.

Barrentine, B. F. (1948). *J. Animal Sci.* **7**, 535.

Bartlett, S., Brown, B. B., Foot, A. S., Rowland, S. J., Allcroft, R., and Parr, W. H. (1954). *Brit. Vet. J.* **110**, 3.

Bartlett, S., Brown, B. B., Foot, A. S., Head, M. J., Line, C., Rook, J. A. F., Rowland, S. J. and Zundel, G. (1957). *J. Agr. Sci.* **49**, 291.

Bartley, J. C., Reber, E. F., Yusken, J. W., and Norton, H. W. (1961). *J. Animal Sci.* **20**, 137.

Barto, L. R. (1932). *J. Am. Vet. Med. Assoc.* **80**, 251.

Bassett, C. F., Harris, L. E., and Wilke, C. F. (1951). *J. Nutr.* **44**, 433.

Basu, K. P., and Mukherjee, K. P. (1943). *Indian J. Vet. Sci.* **13**, 231.

Baustad, B., Teige, J., Jr., and Tollersrud, S. (1967). *Acta Vet. Scand.* **8**, 369.

Becker, R. B., Neal, W. M., and Shealy, A. L. (1933). *Florida. Univ., Agr. Expt. Sta. (Gainesville), Tech. Bull.* **262**.

Benzie, D., Boyne, A. W., Dalgarno, A. C., Duckworth, J., Hill, R., and Walker, D. M. (1959). *J. Agr. Sci.* **54**, 202.

Blakemore, F., and Stewart, J. (1934). *4th Rept. Director Inst. Animal Pathol., Cambridge Univ.* p. 103.

Blakemore, F., Nicholson, J. A., and Stewart, J. (1937), *Vet. Record* **49**, 415.

Blaxter, K. L. (1955). *Ciba Found. Symp. Bone Struct. Metab*, London 1956, p. 117.

Blaxter, K. L., and McGill, R. F. (1956). *Vet. Rev. Annotations* **2**, 35.

Blaxter, K. L., and Rook, J. A. F. (1954). *J. Comp. Pathol. Therap.* **64**, 176.

Blaxter, K. L., and Sharman, G. A. M. (1955). *Vet. Record* **67**, 108.

Blaxter, K. L., Rook, J. A. F., and MacDonald, A. M. (1954). *J. Comp. Pathol. Therap.* **64**, 157.

Blaxter, K. L., Cowlishaw, B., and Rook, J. A. F. (1960). *Animal Prod.* **2**, 1.

Bloom, F. (1957). *North Am. Vet.* **38**, 114.

Bloom, F. (1960). "The Blood Chemistry of the Dog and Cat." Gamma Publ. Inc., New York.

Blosser, T. H., and Albright, J. L. (1956). *Ann. N.Y. Acad. Sci.* **64**, 386.

Blosser, T. H., and Smith, V. R. (1950a). *J. Dairy Sci.* **33**, 81.

Blosser, T. H., and Smith, V. R. (1950b). *J. Dairy Sci.* **33**, 329.

Blumer, C. C., Madden, F. J., and Walker, D. J. (1939). *Australian Vet. J.* **15**, 24.

Boda, J. M., and Cole, H. H. (1954). *J. Dairy Sci.* **37**, 360.

Boda, J. M., and Cole, H. H. (1956). *J. Dairy Sci.* **39**, 1027.

Boogaerdt, J. (1954). Thesis, Utrecht.

Bosch, S., and Harmsen, H. E. (1958). *Mededel. Proefst. Akker-en Weidebouw. Wageningen* **10**, 9.

Brandsma, S. (1954). *Mededel. Landbouwhogeschool Wageningen* **54**, 245.

Breirem, K., Ender, G., Halse, K., and Slagsvold, P. (1949). *Acta Agr. Suecana* **3**, 89.

Breirem, K., Ender, F., Halse, K., and Slagsvold, P. (1954). *Meldinger Norg. Landbrukshøgskole* **34**, 373.

British Veterinary Association (1957). "The Husbandry and Diseases of Calves," p. 20. Brit. Vet. Assoc., London.

Brouwer, E. (1951). *Mededel. Landbouwhogeschool Wageningen* **51**, 91.

Brouwer, E. (1957). *E. P. A. Proj. Utrecht* No. 204, p. 161 (European Productivity Agency).

Brown, W. R., Krook, L., and Pond, W. G. (1966). *Cornell Vet.* **56**, Suppl. 1.

Buckle, R. M., Care, A. D., Cooper, C. W., and Gitelman, H. J. (1968). *J. Endocrinol.* **42**, 529.

Burns, K. N., and Allcroft, R. (1967). *Brit. Vet. J.* **123**, 340 and 383.

Bussolati, G., and Pearse, A. G. E. (1967). *J. Endocrinol.* **37**, 205.

Butler, E. J., (1963). *J. Agr. Sci.* **60**, 329.

Campbell, J. R. (1960). *Vet. Record* **72**, 1153.

Campbell, J. R., and Douglas, T. A. (1965). *Brit. J. Nutr.* **19**, 339.

Capen, C. C., Cole, C. R., and Hibbs, J. W. (1966a). *Pathol. Vet.* **3**, 350; see *Vet. Bull. (Commonwealth Bur. Animal Health)* **36**, Abstr. 4873 (1966).
Capen, C. C., Cole, C. R., Hibbs, J. W., and Wagner, A. R. (1966b). *Am. J. Vet. Res.* **27**, 1177.
Care, A. D. (1960). *Brit. Vet. Assoc. Conf. Hypomagnesaemia, London, 1960* p. 8 (discussion).
Care, A. D. (1967). *World Rev. Nutr. Dietet.* **8**, 127.
Care, A. D., and Duncan, T. (1967). *J. Endocrinol.* **37**, 107.
Care, A. D., and McDonald, I. R. (1963). *Biochem. J.* **87**, 2P.
Care, A. D., and Ross, D. B. (1963). *Res. Vet. Sci.* **4**, 24.
Care, A. D., Van'T Klooster, A. T. (1965). *J. Physiol. (London)* **177**, 174.
Care, A. D., Ross, D. B., and Wilson, A. A. (1965). *J. Physiol. (London)* **176**, 284.
Care, A. D., Sherwood, L. M., Potts, J. T., and Aurback, G. D. (1966). *Nature* **209**, 55.
Care, A. D., Duncan, T., and Webster, D. (1967). *J. Endocrinol.* **37**, 155.
Carlström, B. (1933). *Skand. Veterinärtidskr.* **23**, 229.
Carlström, G. (1969). Thesis, Skara, Sweden.
Carmichael, M. A. (1958). Quoted by McTaggart (1959).
Chang, K. Y., and Carr, C. W. (1968). *Biochim. Biophys. Acta* **157**, 127.
Christian, K. R., and Williams, V. J. (1960). *New Zealand J. Agr. Res.* **3**, 389.
Clark, G. W. (1925). *Univ. Calif. (Berkeley) Publ. Physiol.* **5**, 195.
Cole, C. R., Chamberlain, D. M., Hibbs, J. W., Pounden, W. D., and Smith, C. R. (1957). *J. Am. Vet. Med. Assoc.* **130**, 298.
Colovos, N. F., Keener, H. A., Teeri, A. E., and Davis, H. A. (1951). *J. Dairy Sci.* **34**, 735.
Comar, C. L., Monroe, R. A., Visek, W. J., and Hansard, S. L. (1953). *J. Nutr.* **50**, 459.
Conrad, H. R., Hansard, S. L., and Hibbs, J. W. (1956). *J. Dairy Sci.* **39**, 1697.
Copp, D. H., and Kuczerpa, A. V. (1967). *Resumé Commun. 5th Symp. Europ. Tissus Calcifié, 1967.* p. 11.
Copp, D. H., Cameron, E. C., Cheney, B. A., Davidson, A. G. F., and Henze, K. G. (1962). *Endocrinology* **70**, 638.
Craige, A. H., and Beck, J. D. (1941). *J. Am. Vet. Med. Assoc.* **98**, 315.
Craige, A. H., and Gadd, J. D. (1941). *Am. J. Vet. Res.* **2**, 227.
Cramer, C. F., Parkes, C. O., and Copp, D. H. (1969). *Can. J. Physiol. Pharmacol.* **47**, 181.
Crookshank, H. R., and Sims, F. H. (1955). *J. Animal Sci.* **14**, 964.
Crosfield, P. (1941). *Vet. Record* **53**, 593.
Cumming (1853). Quoted by Hutyra *et al.* (1946, p. 130).
Cunningham, I. J. (1934). *New Zealand J. Sci. Technol.* **15**, 414.
Cunningham, I. J. (1936a). *New Zealand J. Sci. Technol.* **17**, 775.
Cunningham, I. J. (1936b). *New Zealand J. Sci. Technol.* **18**, 419.
Curran, S. (1949). *Eire Dept. Agr., J.* **46**, 60.
Daniel, O., Hatfield, E. E., Shrewsberry, W. C., Gibson, M. E., and MacVicar, R. (1952). *J. Animal Sci.* **11**, 790.
Deckwer, N. (1950). *Berlin. Münch. Tierärztl. Wochschr.* **63**, 85.
de Groot, T., and Marttin, M. A. (1967). *Tijdschr. Diergeneesk.* **92**, 452.
Del Castillo, J., and Engbäk, L. (1953). *J. Physiol. (London)* **120**, 54P.
Dell, J. C., and Poulton, B. R. (1958). *J. Dairy Sci.* **41**, 1706.
Detweiler, D. K., and Martin, J. E. (1949). *Am. J. Vet. Res.* **10**, 201.
Dishington, I. W. (1965). *Acta Vet. Scand.* **6**, 150.
Dishington, I. W., and Tollersrud, S. (1967). *Acta Vet. Scand.* **8**, 14.
Dryerre, H. (1932). *Vet. Record* **12**, 1163.
Dryerre, H., and Greig, J. R. (1925). *Vet. Record* **5**, 225.
Dryerre, H., and Greig, J. R. (1928). *Vet. Record* **8**, 721.
Duckworth, J. (1939). *Nutr. Abstr. Rev.* **8**, 841.
Duckworth, J., Godden, W., and Thomson, W. (1943). *J. Agr. Sci.* **33**, 190.
Duncan, C. W., Huffman, C. F., and Robinson, C. S. (1935). *J. Biol. Chem.* **108**, 35.
Duncan, D. L. (1958). *Nutr. Abstr. Rev.* **28**, 695.
Earle, I. P., and Cabell, C. A. (1952). *Am. J. Vet. Res.* **13**, 330.
Eaton, H. D., and Avampato, J. E. (1952). *J. Animal Sci.* **11**, 761.
Eichelberger, L., and McLean, F. C. (1942). *J. Biol. Chem.* **142**, 467.
Eichelberger, L., Eisele, C. W., and Wertzler, D. (1948). *J. Biol. Chem.* **151**, 177.

Ender, F., Halse, K., and Slagsvold, P. (1948). *Norsk. Vet.-Tidsskr.* **60**, 1 and 41.

Ender, F., Halse, K., and Slagsvold, P. (1949a). *Rept. 14th Intern. Vet. Congr., London, 1949* Vol. 3, p. 14.

Ender, F., Helgebostad, A., and Bøhler, N. (1949b). *Nord. Veterinärmed.* **1**, 827.

Ender, F., Dishington, I. W., and Helgebostad, A. (1956). *Nord Veterinärmed.* **8**, 507.

Ender, F., Dishington, I. W., and Helgebostad, A. (1957). *Nord Veterinärmed.* **9**, 881.

Ender, F., Dishington, I. W., and Helgebostad, A. (1962). *Acta Vet. Scand.* **3**, Suppl. 1.

Erdtman, H. (1928). *Z. Physiol. Chem.* **177**, 211 and 231.

Eriksen, L. and Simesen, M. G. (1970). *Nord. Veterinärmed.* **22** (in press).

Eveleth, D. F. (1937). *J. Biol. Chem.* **119**, 289.

Field, A. C. (1959). *Nature* **183**, 983.

Field, A. C. (1960). *Brit. Vet. Assoc. Conf. Hypomagnesaemia, London, 1960, Brit. Vet. Ass.* p. 13.

Field, A. C. (1961). *Brit. J. Nutr.* **15**, 349.

Field, A. C., McCallum, J. W., and Butler, E. J. (1958). *Brit. J. Nutr.* **12**, 433.

Fish, P. A. (1927). *Cornell Vet.* **17**, 99.

Fish, P. A. (1928). *J. Am. Vet. Med. Assoc.* **73**, 10.

Fish, P. A. (1929a). *Cornell Vet.* **19**, 147.

Fish, P. A. (1929b). *J. Am. Vet. Med. Assoc.* **75**, 695.

Folin, O., and Svedberg, A. (1926). *J. Biol. Chem.* **70**, 405.

Folley, S. J. (1936). *Nature* **137**, 741.

Fontenot, J. P., Miller, R. W., Whitehair, C. K., and MacVicar, R. (1960). *J. Animal Sci.* **19**, 127.

Ford, E. J. H. (1958). *Vet. Rev. Annotations* **4**, 119.

Franklin, M. C., Reid, R. L., and Johnstone, I. L. (1948). *Commonwealth Australia, Council Sci. Ind. Res., Bull.* **240**, Parts I–IV.

Freudenberg, F. (1955). *Deut. Tierärztl. Wochschr.* **62**, 422.

Friedman, J., and Raisz, L. G. (1965). *Science* **150**, 1465.

Garm, O. (1950). *Acta Endocrinol.* **9**, 413.

Garm, O. (1951). *Proc. 6th Nord. Vet. Congr., Stockholm, 1951* p. 288.

Garrett, O. F., and Overman, O. R. (1940). *J. Dairy Sci.* **23**, 13.

Gershoff, S. N., Legg, M. A., O'Connor, F. J., and Hegsted, D. M. (1957). *J. Nutr.* **63**, 79.

Gitelman, H. J., Kukolj, S., and Welt, L. G. (1968). *J. Clin. Invest.* **47**, 118.

Glawischnig, E. (1962). *2nd Intern. Tagung Rinderkrankh., Wien, 1962* pp. 19–20.

Granström, R. (1908). *Z. Physiol. Chem.* **58**, 195.

Grant, A. B. (1955). *Vet. Rev. Annotations* **1**, 115.

Green, H. H. (1939). *Vet. Record* **51**, 1179.

Green, H. H. (1948). Quoted by Allcroft (1954).

Green, H. H., and Allcroft, R. (1951). *Rept. Natl. Inst. Dairying, Reading* p. 35.

Greenberg, D. M. (1945). *J. Biol. Chem.* **157**, 99.

Gregory, M. E., Kon, K., and Thompson, S. Y. (1952). *Rept. Natl. Inst. Dairying. Reading* p. 63.

Greig, J. R. (1926). *Vet. Record* **6**, 625.

Greig, J. R. (1929). *Vet. Record* **9**, 509.

Greig, J. R. (1930). *Vet. Record* **10**, 301.

Groenewald, J. W. (1935). *Onderstepoort J. Vet. Sci. Animal Ind.* **4**, 93.

Groenewald, J. W. (1949). *Rept. 14th Intern. Vet. Congr., London, 1952* Vol. 3 p. 34.

Groenewald, J. W., Thomas, A. D., and Dutoit, B. A. (1940). *Onderstepoort J. Vet. Sci. Animal Ind.* **15**, 299.

Gröning, M. (1959). Thesis, Hannover.

Gudmundsson, T. V., MacIntyre, I., and Soliman, H. A. (1966). *Proc. Roy. Soc.* **B164**, 460.

Hackett, P. L., Gaylor, D. W., and Bustad, L. K. (1957). *Am. J. Vet. Res.* **18**, 338.

Hallgren, W. (1955). *Nord. Veterinärmed.* **7**, 433.

Hallgren, W., Carlström, G., and Jönsson, G. (1959). *Nord. Veterinärmed.* **11**, 217.

Halse, K. (1948). *Skand. Veterinärtidskr.* **38**, 567.

Halse, K. (1958a). *Nord. Veterinärmed.* **10**, 1.

Halse, K. (1958b). *Nord. Veterinärmed.* **10**, 9.

Halse, K. (1960). *Proc. 8th Intern. Grassland Congr., Reading Engl., 1960* p. 553. Grassland Res. Inst., Hentley, England.

Hanna, S., and MacIntyre, I. (1960). *Lancet* **II**, 348.

Hansard, S. L., Comar, C. L., and Plumlee, M. P. (1954). *J. Animal Sci.* **13**, 25.

Hansen, Aas, M., Flatla, J. L., and Mikkelsen. T. (1966). *Rept. 10th Nord. Vet. Congr., Stockholm, 1966* p. 935.

Hart, E. B., Steenbock, H., Kline, O. L., and Humphrey, G. C. (1931). *J. Dairy Sci.* **14**, 307.

Havre, G. N., and Dishington, I. W. (1962). *Acta Agr. Scand.* **12**, 298.

Hayden, C. E. (1924–1925). *Rept. N.Y. State Vet. Coll.* p. 200.

Hayden, C. E. (1927). *Cornell Vet.* **17**, 121.

Hayden, C. E. (1929). *Cornell Vet.* **19**, 285.

Head, M. J., and Rook, J. A. F. (1955) *Nature* **176**, 262.

Heaton, F. W. (1965). *Clin. Sci.* **28**, 543.

Hellmich, K. (1938). *Tierärztl. Rundschau* **44**, 533.

Hemingway, R. G., Inglis, J. S. S., and Ritchie, N. S. (1960). *Brit. Vet. Assoc. Conf. Hypomagnesaemia, London, 1960* p. 58.

Hendriks, H. J. (1962). Thesis, Amsterdam.

Hendriks, H. J. (1964a). *Tijdschr. Diergeneesk.* **89**, 487.

Hendriks, H. J. (1964b). *Nature* **203**, 1306.

Herd, R. P. (1966). *Australian Vet. J.* **42**, 269

Herd, R. P., Schuster, N., and Coltman, M. (1965). *Australian Vet. J.* **41**, 142.

Hess, A. F., Benjamin, H. R., and Gross, J. (1931). *J. Biol. Chem.* **94**, 1.

Hibbs, J. W. (1947). *Thesis, Ohio State Univ. 1947.*

Hibbs, J. W. (1950). *J. Dairy Sci.* **33**, 758.

Hibbs, J. W., and Conrad, H. R. (1960). *J. Dairy Sci.* **43**, 1124.

Hibbs, J. W., and Pounden, W. D. (1955). *J. Dairy Sci.* **38**, 65.

Hibbs, J. W., Krauss, W. E., Monroe, C. F., and Pounden, W. D. (1945). *J. Dairy Sci.* **28**, 525.

Hibbs, J. W., Krauss, W. E., Pounden, W. D., Monroe, C. F., and Sutton, T. S. (1946). *J. Dairy Sci.* **29**, 767.

Hirsch, P. F., Gauthier, G. F., and Munson, P. L. (1963). *Endocrinology* **73**, 244.

Hjärre, A. (1930). Thesis, Uppsala, Sweden; *Acta Pathol. Microbiol. Scand, 1930* Suppl. 7.

Hjerpe, C. A. (1968a). *Cornell Vet.* **58**, 193.

Hjerpe, C. A. (1968b). *Am. J. Vet. Res.* **29**, 143.

Hoff-Jørgensen, E. (1946). *Biochem. J.* **40**, 189.

Holcombe, R. B. (1953). *Brit. Vet. J.* **109**, 359.

Holmes, A. D., Spelman, A. F., Smith, C. T., and Kuzmeski, J. W. (1947). *J. Dairy Sci.* **30**, 385.

Hopkirk, C. S. M., Marshall, D., and Blake, T. A. (1933). *Vet. Record* **13**, 355.

Horvath, D. J., Dozsa, L., Kidder, H. E., Warren, J. E., Jr., Bhatt, B., and Croushore, W. (1967). *J. Animal Sci.* **26**, 875.

Horvath, G., and Kutas, F. (1959). *Acta Vet. Acad. Sci. Hung.* **9**, 183.

Huffman, C. F., and Robinson, C. S. (1926). *J. Biol. Chem.* **69**, 101.

Huffman, C. F., Conley, C. L., Lightfoot, C. C., and Duncan, C. W. (1941). *J. Nutr.* **22**, 609.

Hutten, H., and Uhlenbruck, K. (1952). *Deut. Tierärztl. Wochschr.* **59**, 5.

Hutyra, F., Marek, J., and Manninger, R. (1946), "Special Pathology and Therapeutics of the Diseases of Domestic Animals." Baillière, London.

Hvidsten, H. (1967). *Z. Tierphysiol., Tierernähr. Futtermittelk.* **22**, 210.

Hvidsten, H., Ødelien, M., Baerug, R., and Tollersrud, S. (1959). *Acta Agr. Scand.* **9**, 261.

Inglis, J. S. S. (1960). *Rept. 8th Intern. Grassland Congr., Reading, Engl., 1960* p. 558. Grassland Res. Inst., Henley, England.

Inglis, J. S. S., Weipers, M., and Pearce, P. J. (1959). *Vet. Record* **71**, 755.

Jackson, H. D., Pappenhagen, A. R., Goetsch, G. D., and Noller, C. H. (1962). *J. Dairy Sci.* **65**, 897.

Jennings, F. W., and Mulligan, W. (1953). *J. Comp. Pathol. Therap.* **63**, 286.

Jevnaker, I. (1955). *Medlemsblad Norsk Vet. For.* **7**, 118.

Jonsgård, K. (1963). *Nord. Veterinärmed.* **15**, 28.

Jonsgård, K. (1965). *Nord. Veterinärmed.* **17**, 386; see *Vet Bull.* **36**, 717 Abstr. (1966).

Jönsson, G. (1960). Thesis, Uppsala, Sweden.

Kemp, A. (1958). *Neth. J. Agr. Sci.* **6**, 281.

Kemp, A. (1960). *Neth. J. Agr. Sci.* **8**, 281.

Kemp, A., and Geurink, J. H. (1967). *Agr. Dig.* **12**, 23.

Kemp, A., and 'tHart, M. L. (1957). *Neth. J. Agr. Sci.* **5**, 4.

Kemp, A., Deijs, W. B., Hemkes, O. J., and Van Es, A. J. H. (1960). *Brit. Vet. Assoc. Conf. Hypo-magnesaemia, London, 1960* p. 23.

Kemp, A., Deijs, W. B., Hemkes, O. J., and Van Es, A. J. H. (1961). *Neth. J. Agr. Sci.* **9**, 134.

Kenny, A. D., and Heiskell, C. A. (1965). *Proc. Soc. Exptl. Biol. Med.* **120**, 269.

Keynes, W. M., and Care, A. D. (1967). *Proc. Roy. Soc. Med.* **60**, 1136.

Kjeldberg, J. (1940). *Beretn. 5th Nord. Vet.-Møde, Copenhagen, 1939* p. 670; see *Vet. Bull. (Commonwealth Bur. Animal Health)* **12**, 230 (1942).

Kleiber, M., Smith, A. H., Ralston, N. P., and Black, A. L. (1951). *J. Nutr.* **45**, 253.

Klein, D. C., and Talmage, R. V. (1968). *Endocrinology* **82**, 132.

Klobouk, A. (1932). *Zverolek. Obz.* **6**, 13 and 25; see *Vet. Bull. (Commonwealth Bur. Animal Health)* **2**, 567 (1932).

Knoop, C. E., Krauss, W. E., and Hayden, C. C. (1939). *J. Dairy Sci.* **22**, 283.

Kronfeld, D. S. (1970). *In* "Parturient Hypocalcemia in Dairy Animals" (J. J. B. Anderson, ed.). Academic Press, New York.

Krook, L. (1965). *Rev. Can. Biol.* **24**, 63.

Krook, L., and Lowe, J. E. (1964). *Pathol. Vet.* **1**, Suppl.

Krook, L., Barrett, R. B., Usui, K., and Wolke, R. E. (1963). *Cornell Vet.* **57**, 224.

Kunkel, H. O., Burns, K. H., and Camp, B. J. (1953). *J. Animal Sci.* **12**, 451.

Lane, A. G., Campbell, J. R., and Krause, G. F. (1968). *J. Animal Sci.* **27**, 766.

Larson, B. L., and Kendall, K. A. (1957). *J. Dairy Sci.* **40**, 659.

Larvor, P., and Guéguen, L. (1963). *Ann. Zootech.* **12**, 39.

Leffel, E. C., and Mason, K. R. (1959). *Proc. Symp. Magnesium Agr., West Virginia Univ. 1959* p. 182.

Leslie, A. (1931). *Vet. Record* **11**, 1148.

L'Estrange, J. L., and Axford, R. F. E. (1964a). *J. Agr. Sci.* **62**, 341.

L'Estrange, J. L., and Axford, R. F. E. (1964b). *J. Agr. Sci.* **62**, 353.

Lichtwitz, A., Hioco, D., Parlier, R., and De Seze, S. (1961). *Presse Med.* **69**, 5 and 51.

Liégeois, F., and Derivaux, J. (1951). *Ann. Med. Vet.* **95**, 201.

Line, C., Head, M. J., Rook, J. A. F., Foot, A. S., and Rowland, S. J. (1958). *J. Agr. Sci.* **51**, 353.

Little, W. L., and Mattick, E. C. V. (1933). *Vet. Record* **13**, 238.

Little, W. L., and Wright, N. C. (1925). *Brit. J. Exptl. Pathol.* **6**, 129.

Little, W. L., and Wright, N. C. (1926). *Vet. J.* **82**, 185.

Littlejohn, A. I., and Hebert, C. N. (1969). *Vet. Record* **84**, 130.

Lode, T., and Øverås, J. (1968). *Medlemsblad Norsk Vet. For.* **20**, 101.

Lofgreen, G. P., and Kleiber, M. (1953). *J. Animal Sci.* **12**, 366.

Lofgreen, G. P., Kleiber, M., and Smith, A. H. (1951). *J. Nutr.* **43**, 401.

Lofgreen, G. P., Kleiber, M., and Smith, A. H. (1952). *J. Nutr.* **47**, 571.

Logan, M. A., Christensen, W. R., and Kirklin, J. W. (1942). *Am. J. Physiol.* **135**, 419.

Lothian, W. (1931). *Vet. Record* **11**, 585.

Luecke, R. W., Schmidt, D. A., and Hoefer, J. A. (1958). *J. Animal Sci.* **17**, 1185.

Luick, J. R., and Lofgreen, G. P. (1957). *J. Animal Sci.* **16**, 201.

Luick, J. R., Boda, J. M., and Kleiber, M. (1957a). *J. Nutr.* **61**, 597.

Luick, J. R., Boda, J. M., and Kleiber, M. (1957b). *Am. J. Physiol.* **189**, 483.

McCandlish, A. C. (1923). *J. Dairy Sci.* **7**, 94.

McChesney, E. W., and Giacomino, N. J. (1945). *J. Clin. Invest.* **24**, 680.

McClymont, G. L. (1947). *N. S. Wales, Dept. Agr., Diseases Animal Leaflet* No. 52.

MacDonald, D. C., Care, A. D., and Nolan, B. (1959). *Nature* **184**, 736.

MacGregor, J., and Brown, W. E. (1965). *Nature* **205**, 359.

MacIntyre, I. (1959). *Proc. Roy. Soc. Med.* **52**, 212.

MacIntyre, I., Boss, S., and Troughton, V. A. (1963). *Nature* **198**, 1058.

MacIntyre, I., Parsons, J. A., and Robinson, C. J. (1967). *J. Physiol. (London)* **191**, 393.

McLean, F. C., and Urist, M. R. (1955). "Bone." Univ. of Chicago Press, Chicago, Illinois.

McRoberts, M. R., Hill, R., and Dalgarno, A. C. (1965a). *J. Agr. Sci.* **65**, 1.

McRoberts, M. R., Hill, R., and Dalgarno, A. C. (1965b). *J. Agr. Sci.* **65**, 11.

McTaggart, H. S. (1959). *Vet. Record* **71**, 709.

Macy, I. G., Kelly, H. J., and Sloan, R. E. (1953). *Natl. Acad. Sci.—Natl. Res. Council, Publ.* **254**.
Mader, I. J., and Iseri, L. T. (1955). *Am. J. Med.* **19**, 976.
Madsen, D. E., and Nielsen, H. M. (1940). *North Am. Vet.* **21**, 81.
Madsen, D. E., and Nielsen, H. M. (1944). *J. Am. Vet. Med. Assoc.* **105**, 22.
Manston, R., and Payne, J. M. (1964). *Brit. Vet. J.* **120**, 167.
Marek, J., and Wellmann, O. (1931). "Die Rachitis," Vol II. Fischer, Jena.
Marsh, H., and Swingle, K. F. (1955). *Am. J. Vet. Res.* **16**, 418
Marshak, R. R. (1956). *Am. Vet. Med. Assoc.* **128**, 423.
Marshak, R. R. (1957). *Vet. Ext. Quart. Univ. Pa.* No. 146, p. 104.
Marshak, R. R. (1959). *Proc. Symp. Magnesium Agr., West Virginia Univ. 1959* p. 169.
Martin, T. J., Robinson, C. J., and MacIntyre, I. (1966). *Lancet* **II**, 9.
Mayer, G. P., Raggi, F., and Ramberg, C. F. (1965). *J. Am. Vet. Med. Assoc.* **146**, 839.
Mayer, G. P., Ramberg, C. F., and Kronfeld, D. S. (1966). *J. Am. Vet. Med. Assoc.* **149**, 402.
Meigs, E. B., Edward, B., Blatherwick, N. R., and Carry, C. A. (1919). *J. Biol. Chem.* **37**, 1.
Mellanby, E. (1949). *J. Physiol. (London)* **109**, 488.
Merrild, W. G., and Smith, V. R. (1954). *J. Dairy Sci.* **37**, 546.
Mershon, M. M. (1959). *J. Am. Vet. Med. Assoc.* **135**, 435.
Mershon, M. M., and Custer, F. D. (1958). *J. Am. Vet. Med. Assoc.* **132**, 396.
Metzger, H. J. (1936). *Cornell Vet.* **26**, 353.
Meyer, H. (1963). Thesis, Hannover.
Meyer, H., and Grund, H. (1963). *Tierärztl. Umschau* **18**, 181.
Meyer, H., and Schmidt, P. (1958). *Deut Tierärztl. Wochschr.* **65**, 602.
Meyer, H., and Steinbeck, H. (1960). *Deut Tierärztl. Wochschr.* **67**, 315.
Milhaud, G., Perault, A.-M., and Moukhtar, M. S. (1965). *Compt. Rend.* **261**, 813.
Miller, C. D. (1946). *J. Am. Dietet. Assoc.* **22**, 312; see *Nutr. Abstr. Rev.* **16**, 329 (1946–1947).
Møller, T., and Simesen, M. G. (1959). *Nord Veterinärmed.* **11**, 719.
Møllgaard, H. (1943). *Biedermanns Zentr., Abt. B. Tierernähr.* **15**, 1.
Montgomery, R. G., Savage, W. H., and Dodds, E. C. (1929). *Vet. Record* **9**, 319.
Moodie, E. W. (1960). *Vet. Record* **72**, 1145.
Moodie, E. W., and Robertson, A. (1961). *Res. Vet. Sci.* **2**, 217.
Moodie, E. W., and Robertson, A. (1962). *Vet. Sci.* **3**, 470.
Moore, L. A., Sholl, L. B., and Hallman, E. T. (1936). *J. Dairy Sci.* **19**, 441.
Moore, L. A., Hallman, E. T., and Sholl, L. B. (1938). *A.M.A. Arch. Pathol.* **26**, 820.
Moore, R. M., and Wingo, W. J. (1942). *Am. J. Physiol.* **35**, 140.
Muir, L. A., Hibbs, J. W., and Conrad, H. R. (1968). *J. Dairy Sci.* **51**, 1046.
Mullins, J. C., and Ramsay, W. R. (1959). *Australian Vet. J.* **35**, 140.
Murty, V. N., and Kehar, N. D. (1951). *Indian J. Physiol. Allied Sci.* **5**, 71.
Mylrea, P. J., and Bayfield, R. F. (1968). *Australian Vet. J.* **44**, 565.
Nelson, G. S., Guggiberg, C. W. A., and Mukundi, J. (1963). *Ann. Trop. Med. Parasitol* **57**, 332; see *Vet. Bull.* **34**, Abstr. 1002 (1964).
Nicolaysen, R. (1937). *Biochem. J.* **31**, 107.
Niedermeier, R. P., and Smith, V. R. (1950). *J. Dairy Sci.* **33**, 38.
Niedermeier, R. P., Smith, V. R., and Whitehair, C. K. (1949). *J. Dairy Sci.* **32**, 927.
Nielsen, K. (1966). Thesis, Copenhagen, Denmark.
Niimi, K., and Aoki, M. (1927). *J. Japan. Soc. Vet. Sci.* **6**, 345.
Niimi, K., and Kato, K. (1928). *J. Japan. Soc. Vet. Sci.* **7**, 181.
Nisbet, D. I., Butler, E. J., Smith, B. S. W., Robertson, J. M., and Bannatyne, C. C. (1966). *J. Comp. Pathol. Therap.* **76**, 159.
Nisbet, D. I., Butler, E. J., Robertson, J. M., and Bannatyne, C. C. (1968). *J. Comp. Pathol. Therap.* **78**, 73.
Nocard, E. (1885). *Bull. Soc. Cent. Med. Vet.* **39**, 121.
O'Donovan, J., and Sheery, E. J. (1950). *Eire Dept. Agr., J.* **47**, 34.
O'Moore, L. B. (1950). *Irish Vet. J.* **4**, 198 and 218.
Oslage, H. J., Farries, F. E., Zorita, E., and Becker, M. (1960). *Arch. Tierernähr.* **10**, 190 and 200.
Ott, G. L., and Coombes, A. I. (1941). *Vet. Med.* **36**, 202.
Owen, E. C. (1948). *Biochem. J.* **43**, 243.

Owen, J. R. (1954). *Missouri, Univ., Agr. Expt. Sta., Inform. Sheet* No. 497.

Oyaert, W. (1962). *Berlin. Münch. Tierärztl. Wochschr.* **75**, 323.

Palmer, L. S., and Eckles, C. H. (1930). *J. Dairy Sci.* **13**, 351.

Palmer, L. S., Cunningham, W. S., and Eckles, C. H. (1930). *J. Dairy Sci.* **13**, 174.

Parkinson, B., and Sutherland, A. K. (1954). *Australian Vet. J.* **30**, 232.

Parr, W. H. (1957). *Vet. Record* **69**, 71.

Parr, W. H. (1961). *Res. Vet. Sci.* **2**, 320.

Parr, W. H., and Allcroft, R. (1957). *Vet. Record* **69**, 1041.

Patwardhan, V. N., Chitre, R. G., and Sukhatankar, D. R. (1945). *Indian J. Med. Res.* **33**, 195.

Payne, J. M. (1963). *Vet. Record* **75**, 848.

Payne, J. M. (1964). *Vet. Record* **76**, 77.

Payne, J. M., and Leech, F. B. (1964). *Brit. Vet. J.* **120**, 385.

Payne, J. M., and Manston, R. (1967). *Vet. Record* **81**, 215.

Payne, J. M., Sansom, B. F., and Manston, R. (1963). *Vet. Record* **75**, 588.

Pearse, A. G. E., and Calvalheira, A. F. (1967). *Nature* **214**, 929.

Pedersen, J. G. A. (1940). *Kbh. Forsøgslab. Beretn.* No. 193; see *Nutr. Abstr. Rev.* **17**, 694 (1947–1948).

Pedersen, J. G. A. (1945). *Acta Pharmacol.* **1**, 219.

Pehrson, B. (1963). *Nord. Veterinärmed.* **15**, 937.

Penny, R. H. C., and Arnold, J. H. S. (1955). *Vet. Record* **67**, 772.

Petersen, W. E., Hewitt, E. A., Boyd, W. L., and Brown, W. R. (1931). *J. Am. Vet. Med. Assoc.* **79**, 217.

Phillipson, A. T., and Storry, J. E. (1965). *J. Physiol. (London)* **181**, 130.

Pook, H. L. (1955). *Vet. Record* **67**, 281.

Poole, D. B. (1967). *Irish Vet. J.* **21**, 10.

Pribyl, E. (1933). *Zverolek. Obz.* **7**, Suppl., 61 and 73; see *Nutr. Abstr. Rev.* **4**, 88 (1934–1935).

Quaterman, J., Dalgarno, A. C., and Adam, A. (1964). *Brit. J. Nutr.* **18**, 79.

Raghavachari, K. (1943). *Indian J. Vet. Sci.* **13**, 137.

Ramberg, C. F., Mayer, G. P., Kronfeld, D. S., Aurback, G. D., Sherwood, L. M., and Potts, J. T. (1967). *Am. J. Physiol.* **213**, 878.

Rapoport, S., and Guest, G. M. (1941). *J. Biol. Chem.* **138**, 269.

Rathje, W. (1958). *Z. Tierphysiol., Tierernähr. Futtermittelk.* **13**, No. 3, 155.

Reid, R. L., Franklin, M. C., and Hallsworth, E. G. (1947). *Australian Vet. J.* **23**, 136.

Reith, J. W. S. (1954). *Empire J. Exptl. Agr.* **22**, 305.

Ringarp, N., Rydberg, C., Damberg, O., and Boström, B. (1967). *Zentr. Veterinärmed.* **14**, 242.

Riser, W. H. (1961). *J. Am. Vet. Med. Assoc.* **139**, 117.

Roberts, S. J., Richard, C. G., and Bentick-Smith, J. (1951). *J. Am. Vet. Med. Assoc.* **119**, 380.

Robertson, A. (1949). *Vet. Record* **61**, 333.

Robertson, A. (1960). *Brit. Vet. Assoc. Conf. Hypomagnesaemia, London, 1960, Brit. Vet. Ass. 1960* p. 1.

Robertson, A., Marr, A., and Moodie, E. W. (1956). *Vet. Record* **68**, 173.

Robertson, A., Paver, H., Barden, P., and Marr, T. G. (1960). *Res. Vet. Sci.* **1**, 117.

Robinson, C. J., Martin, T. J., and MacIntyre, I. (1966). *Lancet II*, 83.

Robison, R. (1923). *Biochem. J.* **17**, 286.

Rogers, T. A. (1964). *Proc. Symp. Radioisotopes Animal Nutr. Physiol. Prague, 1965* p. 285. I.A.E.A., Vienna.

Rogers, T. A., and Mahan, P. E. (1959). *Proc. Soc. Exptl. Biol. Med.* **100**, 235.

Rogers, T. A., Simesen, M. G., Lunaas, T., and Luick, J. R. (1964). *Acta Vet. Scand.* **5**, 209.

Rook, J. A. F. (1961). *Nature* **191**, 1019.

Rook, J. A. F. (1963). *J. Comp. Pathol. Therap.* **73**, 93.

Rook, J. A. F., and Balch, C. C. (1958). *J. Agr. Sci.* **51**, 199.

Rook, J. A. F., and Campling, R. C. (1962). *J. Agr. Sci.* **59**, 225.

Rook, J. A. F., and Storry, J. E. (1962). *Nutr. Abstr. Rev.* **32**, 1055.

Rook, J. A. F., and Wood, M. (1960). *J. Sci. Food Agr.* **11**, 137.

Rook, J. A. F., Balch, C. C., and Line, C. (1958). *J. Agr. Sci.* **51**, 189.

Rose, A. L. (1954). *Australian Vet. J.* **30**, 172.

Rose, E., and Sunderman, F. W. (1939). *A. M. A. Arch. Internal Med.* **64**, 217.

Ross, E. J., and Gibson, W. W. C. (1969). *Vet. Record* **84**, 520.

Rubarth, S., and Krook, L. (1968). *Acta Vet. Scand.* **9**, 253.
Russell, F. C. (1944). *Imp. Bur. Animal Nutr. (Rowett Res. Inst.), Tech. Commun.* No. 15, p. 69.
Saarinen, P. (1950). *Maataloustieteellinen Aikakauskirja* **22**, 122; see *Nutr. Abstr. Rev.* **20**, 1058 (1950).
Saarinen, P., Comar, C. L., Marshall, S. P., and Davis, G. K. (1950). *J. Dairy Sci.* **33**, 878.
Salt, F. J. (1950). *Lab. J. (Lond.)* **8**, 357.
Scheunert, A. (1923). *Landwirtsch. Ztg.* **43**, 351.
Schmidt, H. (1940). *J. Am. Vet. Med. Assoc.* **96**, 441.
Schmidt, J. (1897). *Maanedsskr. Dyrlæg.* **9**, 225.
Schulhof, A. (1933). *Klin. Spisy Skoly Zverolek., Brno* **10**, 23; see *Nutr. Abstr. Rev.* **4**, 699 (1934–1935).
Scott, D. (1965). *Quart. J. Exptl. Physiol.* **50**, 312.
Scott, D., and Dobson, A. (1965). *Quart. J. Exptl. Physiol.* **50**, 42.
Seekles, L. (1964). *Rept. 3rd Intern. Meeting Diseases Cattle, Copenhagen, 1964* p. 119.
Seekles, L., and Boogaerdt, J. (1955). *Tijdschr. Diergeneesk.* **80**, 331.
Seekles, L., and Boogaerdt, J. (1956). *Tijdschr. Diergeneesk.* **81**, 281.
Seekles, L., and Sjollema, B. (1932). *Arch. Wiss. Prakt. Tierheilk.* **65**, 331.
Seekles, L., and Van Asperen, K. (1949). *Tijdschr. Diergeneesk.* **74**, 191.
Seekles, L., Sjollema, B., and Van der Kaay, F. C. (1931). *Tijdschr. Diergeneesk.* **58**, 750.
Seekles, L., Reitsma, P., De Man, T. J., and Wilson, J. H. G. (1958). *Tijdschr. Diergeneesk.* **83**, 125.
Seekles, L., Wilson, J. H. G., and Philips-Duphar, N. V. (1964). *Vet. Record* **76**, 486.
Sherwood, L. M., Potts, J. T., Jr., Care, A. D., Mayer, G. P., and Aurback, G. D. (1966). *Nature* **209**, 52.
Simesen, M. G. (1958). *Rept. 8th Nord. Vet. Congr., Helsingfors, 1958* Sect. B, No. 9, p. 344.
Simesen, M. G. (1959). *Main Papers, 16th Intern. Vet. Congr., Madrid, 1959* Vol. II, p. 85.
Simesen, M. G. (1963a). *In* "Clinical Biochemistry of Domestic Animals" (C. E. Cornelius and J. J. Kaneko, eds.), p. 441. Academic Press, New York.
Simesen, M. G. (1963b). *Proc. 17th Intern. Vet. Congr., Hannover, 1963* Vol. 1, p. 117
Simesen, M. G. (1964). *Nord. Veterinärmed.* **16**, Suppl. 1, 167.
Simesen, M. G. (1968). *Medlemsblad Danske Dyrlægeforen.* **51**, 848.
Simesen, M. G., Lunaas, T., Rogers, T. A., and Luick, J. R. (1962). *Acta Vet. Scand.* **3**, 175.
Simesen, M. G., Rogers, T. A., Lunaas, T., and Luick, J. R. (1965). *Proc. Symp. Radioisotopes Animal Nutr. Physiol. Prague, 1965*, p. 721. I.A.E.A., Vienna.
Sims, F. H., and Crookshank, H. R. (1956). *Texas Agr. Exptl. Sta., Bull.* **842**.
Sjollema, B. (1928). *Tijdschr. Diergeneesk.* **55**, 1016, 1085, 1121, and 1187.
Sjollema, B. (1930). *Vet. Record* **10**, 425 and 450.
Sjollema, B. (1932a). *Nutr. Abstr. Rev.* **1**, 621.
Sjollema, B. (1932b). *Zentr. Tierernähr.* **3**, 507.
Sjollema, B., and Seekles, L. (1929). *Tijdschr. Diergeneesk.* **56**, 979.
Sjollema, B., and Seekles, L. (1930). *Biochem. Z.* **229**, 358.
Sjollema, B., and Seekles, L. (1932). *Klin. Wochschr.* **11**, 989.
Sjollema, B., Grashuis, J., Van Koetsveld, E. E., and Lehr, J. J. (1955a). *Tijdschr. Diergeneesk.* **80**, 579.
Sjollema, B., Van Koetsveld, E. E., Grashuis, J., and Lehr, J. J. (1955b). *Tijdschr. Diergeneesk.* **80**, 1111.
Smith, A. H., Kleiber, M., Black, A. L., and Luick, J. R. (1955a). *J. Nutr.* **57**, 497.
Smith, A. H., Kleiber, M., Black, A. L., and Baxter, C. F. (1955b). *J. Nutr.* **57**, 507.
Smith, A. H., Kleiber, M., Black, A. L., and Lofgreen, G. P. (1956). *J. Nutr.* **58**, 95.
Smith, J. A. B., Howat, G. R., and Ray, S. C. (1938). *J. Dairy Res.* **9**, 310.
Smith, R. H. (1957). *Biochem. J.* **67**, 472.
Smith, R. H. (1958). *Biochem. J.* **70**, 201.
Smith, R. H. (1959a). *Biochem. J.* **71**, 306.
Smith, R. H. (1959b). *Biochem. J.* **71**, 609.
Smith, R. H (1959c). *Nature* **184**, 821.
Smith, R. H. (1962). *Biochem. J.* **83**, 151.
Smith, R. H. (1964). *Nord. Veterinärmed.* **16**, Suppl. 1, 143.
Smith, R. H. (1969). *Proc. Nutr. Soc. (Engl. Scot.)* **28**, 151.
Smith, R. H., and McAllan, A. B. (1966). *Brit. J. Nutr.* **20**, 703.
Smith, R. H., McAllan, A. B., and Hill, W. B. (1968). *Proc. Nutr. Soc. (Engl. Scot.)* **27**, 48A.
Smith, S. E., and Barnes, L. L. (1941), unpublished data. Ref. in "Nutrition Requirements of Mink and

Foxes," 1968, p. 45 Natl. Acad. Sci., Washington, D.C.

Smith, V. R., and Blosser, T. H. (1947). *J. Dairy Sci.* **30**, 861.

Smith, V. R., and Brown, W. H. (1963). *J. Dairy Sci.* **46**, 223.

Smith, V. R., and Merrild, W. G. (1954). *J. Dairy Sci.* **37**, 967.

Smith, V. R., Niedermeier, R. P., and Hansen, R. G. (1948). *J. Dairy Sci.* **31**, 173.

Smyth, P. J., Conway, A., and Walsh, M. J. (1958). *Vet. Record* **70**, 846.

Somjen, G., Hilmy, M., and Stephen, C. R. (1966). *J. Pharmacol. Exptl. Therap.* **154**, 652.

Stahl, P. D., and Kenny, A. D. (1967). *Endocrinology* **81**, 661.

Stevenson, D. E., and Wilson, A. A. (1963). "Metabolic Disorders of Domestic Animals." p. 75 Blackwell, Oxford.

Stewart, J. (1954). *Scot. Agr.* **34**, 68.

Stewart, J., and Reith, J. W. S. (1956). *J. Comp. Pathol. Therap.* **66**, 1.

Storry, J. E. (1961a). *J. Agr. Sci.* **57**, 97.

Storry, J. E. (1961b). *J. Agr. Sci.* **57**, 103.

Storry, J. E., and Rook, J. A. F. (1962). *J. Sci. Food Agr.* **13**, 621.

Storry, J. E., and Rook, J. A. F. (1963). *J. Agr. Sci.* **61**, 167.

Stott, G. H., and Smith, V. R. (1957). *J. Dairy Sci.* **40**, 897.

Straub, O. C., Peoples, S. A., and Cornelius, C. E. (1959). *Cornell Vet.* **49**, 324.

Suomalainen, P. (1944). *Sitzber. Finn. Akad. Wiss.* p. 163; see *Biol. Abstr.* **20**, 12101 (1946).

Suttle, N. F., and Field, A. C. (1969). *Brit. J. Nutr.* **23**, 81.

Svanberg, O. (1932). *Kgl. Lantbruksakad. Handl. Tidskr.* **71**, 41.

Swan, J. B., and Jamieson, N. D. (1956). *New Zealand Sci. Technol.* **A38**, 137, 316, and 363.

Talapatra, S. K., Ray, S. C., and Sen, K. C. (1948). *J. Agr. Sci.* **38**, 163.

Taylor, T. G. (1959). *J. Agr. Sci.* **52**, 207

Tenenhouse, A., Arnaud, C., and Rasmussen, H. (1965). *Proc. Natl. Acad. Sci. U. S.* **53**, 818.

Terkildsen, T. C. (1950). Thesis, Copenhagen, Denmark.

'tHart, M. L., and Kemp, A. (1956). *Tijdschr. Diergeneesk.* **81**, 84.

'tHart, M. L., and Kemp, A. (1957). *E. P. A. Proj. Utrecht* No. 204, p. 193 (European Productivity Agency).

Theiler, A., and Green, H. H. (1932). *Nutr. Abstr. Rev.* **1**, 359.

Theiler, A., Green, H. H., and DuToit, P. J. (1924). *J. Dept. Agr. S. Africa* **8**, 460.

Theiler, A., Viljoen, P. R., Green, H. H., DuToit, P. J., Meier, H., and Robinson, E. M. (1927). *Director. Vet. Educ. Res. S. Africa 11th & 12th Repts.* p. 821.

Thomas, J. W., and Okamoto, M. (1958). *U. S. Dept. Agr., A. R. S.* **44**.

Thomson, D. L., and Collip, J. B. (1932). *Physiol. Rev.* **12**, 309.

Todd, J. R. (1967). *Vet. Record* **81**, Clin. Suppl. VI.

Todd, J. R., and Morrison, N. E. (1964). *J. Brit. Grassland Soc.* **19**, 179.

Todd, J. R., and Rankin, J. E. F. (1959). *Vet. Record* **71**, 256.

Todd, J. R., and Thompson, R. H. (1960). *Brit. Vet. J.* **116**, 437.

Todd, J. R., and Thompson, R. H. (1962). *Res. Vet. Sci.* **3**, 449.

Todd, J. R., and Thompson, R. H. (1968). Unpublished observations; see Todd *et al.* (1969).

Todd, J. R., Scally, W. C. P., and Ingram, J. M. (1966). *Vet. Record* **78**, 888.

Todd, J. R., Horvath, D. J., and Anido, V. (1969). *Vet. Record* **84**, 176.

Turner, A. W., Kelley, R. B., and Dann, A. T. (1935). *J. Council Sci. Ind. Res.* **8**, 120.

Turner, C. W. (1930). *Missouri, Univ., Agr. Expt. Sta., Bull.* **285**, 65.

Udall, R. H. (1947). *Cornell Vet.* **37**, 314.

Van der Horst, C. J. G. (1960). *Tijdschr. Diergeneesk.* **85**, 1060.

Van Koetsveld, E. E. (1955). *Tijdschr. Diergeneesk.* **80**, 525.

Van Koetsveld, E. E. (1964). *Tijdschr. Diergeneesk.* **89**, 590.

Van Kreveld, A., and Van Minnen, G. (1955). *Neth. Milk Dairy J.* **9**, 1.

Van Maltits, L. (1945). *J. S. African Vet. Med. Assoc.* **16**, 9.

Van Soest, P. J., and Blosser, T. H. (1954). *J. Dairy Sci.* **37**, 185.

Van'T Klooster, A. T. (1967). *Thesis, Mededel. Landbouwhogeschool Wageningen* no: **67–5**.

Van'T Klooster, A. T., and Care, A. D. (1966). *Biochem. J.* **99**, 2.

Verdeyen, J. (1953). *Compt. Rend. Rech. IRSIA* **9**, 87.

Vigue, R. F., (1952). *Vet. Med.* **47**, 215.

Visek, W. J., Barnes, L. L., and Loosli, J. K. (1952). *J. Dairy Sci.* **35**, 783.

Visek, W. J., Monroe, R. A., Swanson, E. W., and Comar, C. L. (1953a). *J. Nutr.* **50**, 23.

Visek, W. J., Monroe, R. A., Swanson, E. W., and Comar, C. L. (1953b). *J. Dairy Sci.* **36**, 373.

Vitale, J. J., Hegsted, D. M., Nakamura, M., and Connors, P. (1957). *J. Biol. Chem.* **226**, 597.

Wacker, W. E. C., and Parisi, A. F. (1968). *New Engl. J. Med.* **278**, 658, 712, 772.

Wacker, W. E. C., and Vallee, B. L. (1958). *New Engl. J. Med.* **259**, 431, 475.

Walsh, M. J., and Conway, A. (1960). *Proc. 8th Intern. Grassland Congr., Reading, Engl. 1960* p. 548. Grassland Res. Inst., Henley, England.

Ward, G. M. (1956). *Ann. N. Y. Acad. Sci.* **64**, 361.

Ward, G. M., Blosser, T. H., and Adams, M. F. (1952). *J. Dairy Sci.* **35**, 587.

Ward, G. M., Blosser, T. H., Adams, M. F., and Crilly, J. B. (1953). *J. Dairy Sci.* **36**, 39.

Watts, P. S. (1959). *J. Agr. Sci.* **52**, 244 and 250.

Wenger, R. D. (1945). *North Am. Vet.* **26**, 289.

Wentworth, R. A., and Smith, S. E. (1961). *Proc. Cornell Nutr. Conf., 1961* p. 53.

Werner, W. (1960). *Landwirtsch. Forsch.* **12**, 133.

White, R. R., Christian, K. R., and Williams, V. J. (1957). *New Zealand J. Sci. Technol.* **A38**, 440.

Widmark, E., and Carlens, O. (1925a). *Svensk Veterinärtidskr.* **30**, 1 (Transl. by C. A. Nelson); *North Am. Vet.* **6**, 28 (1925).

Widmark, E., and Carlens, O. (1925b). *Biochem. Z.* **158**, 81.

Widmark, E., and Carlens, O. (1925c). *Biochem. Z.* **156**, 454.

Wieland, W. (1940). *Teirärztl. Rundschau* **46**, 522.

Wilson, A. A. (1955). *Brit. Vet. J.* **110**, 233.

Wilson, A. A. (1960). *Vet. Rev. Annotations* **6**, 39.

Wilson, L. T., and Hart, E. B. (1932). *J. Dairy Sci.* **15**, 116.

Wise, M. B., Smith, S. E., and Barnes, L. L. (1958). *J. Animal Sci.* **17**, 89.

Wise, M. B., Ordoveza, A. L., and Barrick, E. R. (1963). *J. Nutr.* **79**, 79.

Wolton, K. M. (1963). *N. A. A. S. Quart. Rev.* **14**, No. 59, 122.

Young, V. R., Richards, W. P. C., Lofgreen, G. P., and Luick, J. R. (1966). *Brit. J. Nutr.* **20**, 783.

10 Iron Metabolism

J. J. Kaneko

I. INTRODUCTION

Iron is an element of fundamental importance in the vital respiratory processes of life. It is an integral constituent of the respiratory pigment hemoglobin, myoglobin, and the heme enzymes, catalase, peroxidase, and the cytochromes. Although it is one of the most abundant elements in the environment, it is also the most common cause of anemia in man. Iron deficiency per se is of less importance in the adult domestic animal than in man. It is, however, of equally great importance in the young of all species during the period of rapid growth and particularly in those dependent on a milk diet exclusively. Disorders of iron metabolism may also arise from a variety of other causes in domestic animals. Thus, an understanding of iron metabolism is required for the clarification and differentiation of the anemias.

II.   IRON BALANCE

A. Distribution

The results of extensive iron balance studies have been reviewed by Drabkin (1951) and Granick (1954), and their estimates of iron distribution in the body are in close agreement (Table I). Of a total of 4 gm iron in a 70 kg man, approximately 65% is in hemoglobin, 3% in myoglobin, and 30% in the iron-storage compounds, ferritin and hemosiderin. The remainder is distributed among the heme enzymes (cytochromes, catalase, and peroxidase), nonheme enzymes, and the iron transport protein, transferrin or siderophilin. It has been estimated (Lintzel and Radeff, 1931) that the body iron content of pups ranges as high as 79 mg/kg body weight. Hemoglobin iron (43 mg/kg)* would account for greater than one-half. Thus, the percent distribution of iron in the dog is essentially similar to that found in man. More recently, Kolb (1963) has reviewed and presented extensive data on iron balance in farm animals which indicate that in its qualitative aspects, iron balance is similar in all species.

B. Function

Iron combines with a variety of proteins in nature and, depending on the type of combination, various functions are carried out. The most important function of iron is to combine with protoporphyrin (see Chapter 4) to form heme and the heme combines with various proteins to form the heme proteins. If the protein is a globin, hemoglobin and myoglobin are formed. If the protein is an apoenzyme, the heme enzymes such as the cytochromes, catalase, and peroxidase are formed. The heme enzymes are of fundamental importance in the vital respiratory processes of life, namely, in the cytochrome system, the ultimate site of O_2 utilization.

Hemoglobin is a protein of 68,000 MW composed of two α and two β polypeptide chains, four protoporphyrin molecules, and 4 moles of ferrous (Fe^{2+}) iron. Hemoglobin contains 3.4 mg iron per gram. The iron of hemoglobin binds oxygen (O_2) reversibly and it functions to transport oxygen and CO_2 to and from the tissues. Myoglobin is smaller, a single polypeptide of 17,000 MW, and binds only one molecule of heme. Myoglobin also binds O_2 reversibly and functions as a reserve supply of O_2 in the muscles. The high content of myoglobin in marine mammals, such as the seal and whale, is thought to permit their extended underwater activities (Kendrew et al., 1954). Without adequate iron, insufficient hemoglobin is produced, O_2 supply to the tissues is reduced, and all the clinical manifestations of anemia ensue.

The major functions of the nonheme iron compounds is iron transport and storage.

---

* Estimated for 9% blood volume, 14 gm Hb/100 ml, 0.34% iron in hemoglobin.

TABLE I DISTRIBUTION OF IRON IN HEME AND NONHEME[a] COMPOUNDS

Species (wt)	Heme iron		Nonheme iron		Reference
	gm	%	gm	%	
Dog (10 kg)	0.43	55	0.36	45	Lintzel and Radeff (1931)
Horse (400 kg)	11.5	67	5.6	33	Obara and Nakajima (1961a)
Cow (386 kg)	9.2	55	7.7	45	Kaneko (1963)
Man (70 kg)	2.67	67	1.33	33	Drabkin (1951)

[a]Approximate nonheme iron distribution is: 12%, hemosiderin; 13%, ferritin; 3%, myoglobin; 1%, transferrin, cytochromes, peroxidase, catalase; 4%, unknown.

Iron is transported in the plasma in the ferric (Fe^{3+}) form bound to a specific iron-binding protein, transferrin (T_f or siderophilin), which migrates with β_1-globulin under electrophoresis. The storage form of iron is also the Fe^{3+} form and is present in either ferritin or hemosiderin. These nonheme compounds will be discussed more fully in Section IV.

There is little established of the iron requirements of animals. The nutritional iron deficiency of calves fed only milk has been known for some time (Knoop *et al.*, 1935; Hibbs *et al.*, 1963), but few balance studies have been conducted (Matrone *et al.*, 1957). More is known of the iron requirements of baby pigs which are highly susceptible to iron deficiency. If the baby pig on a milk diet is kept in clean floored pens without access to iron sources, anemia can develop within a few weeks. Dietary iron requirements for young pigs can be met with iron contents in the feedstuffs of 60 mg/kg to 125 mg/kg feed (Matrone *et al.*, 1960; Ullrey *et al.*, 1960). Kolb (1963) estimated the iron requirements of farm animals as shown in Table II. The requirement for the cat is only an estimate, taking its size into account, based on its more rapid iron turnover as compared to the dog.

TABLE II ESTIMATED DIETARY IRON REQUIREMENTS FOR DOMESTIC ANIMALS[a]

Species	Iron (mg/day)
Calves	25–30
Yearling cattle	40–50
Milking cows	50–60
Pregnant cows	60–80
Sheep	10–15
Horse	50–80
Feeder pigs	30–40
Sow	40–60
Laying hen	2–3
Dog	10–30
Cat[b]	5–15

[a]Modified after Kolb (1963).
[b]Estimated on the basis of its turnover data and body size.

III. DIETARY IRON

The recommended (National Research Council, 1962) minimum daily requirement (MDR) for iron for the dog is 1.3 mg/kg body weight. However, a large percentage of this food iron is tightly bound to phytates and phosphates and is unavailable for absorption. It has been estimated (National Research Council, 1962) that approximately one-half of the food iron is available for absorption. The actual amount absorbed is also known to vary with the composition of the diet. Table III gives the iron content and estimated percent absorption for some foods. Highest iron contents (5–18 mg/100 gm) are found among the organ meats, eggs, and legumes, while milk and milk products, starches, and fruits generally contain less than 1 mg iron per 100 gm. The amount of the iron absorbed from these foods varies

TABLE III   IRON CONTENT OF SOME FOODS AND THEIR INTESTINAL ABSORPTION

Food source[a]	mg/100 gm	% Absorbed	Reference for absorption
Liver	6.6–18.0		
Brain	3.6		
Heart	4.6		
Kidney	7.9		
Spleen	8.9		
Pancreas	6.0		
Red meats	2.2–5.1	10.4–38.3 (20.3)	Layrisse et al. (1969)
Poultry	1.5–3.8		
Hemoglobin (uncooked)	340 mg	6.7–30.8 (15.6)	Layrisse et al. (1969)
		1.0–21.0 (19)	Callender et al. (1957)
Hemoglobin (cooked)	340 mg	0–16 (7)	Callender et al. (1957)
Fish	0.4–1.1	1.9–42.4 (18.3)	Layrisse et al. (1969)
Fish (cnd)	0.9–2.7		
Egg yolk	7.2		
Eggs, whole	2.7	0.5–5.0 (1.4)	Chodos et al. (1957)
Nuts	1.9–5.0		
Dried fruits	1.4–6.9		
Wheat	3.0–4.3	1.1–7.4 (4.5)	Hussain et al. (1965)
		0.4–22.5 (7.9)	Layrisse et al. (1969)
Wheat germ	8.1		
Wheat bran	16.7		
Legumes	4.7–8.0	0.7–6.4 (3.2)	Layrisse et al. (1969)
Soybean flour	13	1.7–42.2 (17.9)	Layrisse et al. (1969)
Green vegetables	1.6–3.0	1.7–5.8	Layrisse et al. (1969)
		0.5–2.3	Chodos et al. (1957)
Root vegetables	0.5–1.0	0.5–2.3	Chodos et al. (1957)
Cornmeal	1.0–2.7	0.2–14.8 (5.9)	Layrisse et al. (1969)
Milk, whole	0.07		
Coarse hays[b]	14–22		
Grains[b]	3.0–14		
Blood meal[b]	311		
Fish meal[b]	21–80		

[a]Compiled from various nutritive and feed tables.

[b]mg/100 gm dry weight.

from less than 10% for egg and liver iron to as high as 30% for muscle and hemo-globin iron (Moore, 1961; Moore and Dubach, 1951). This would indicate that the actual absorption of iron would be considerably less than one-half of the MDR of 1.3 mg/kg. It has been estimated from radioiron feeding studies that normal dogs absorb 5–10% of ingested iron (Hahn *et al.*, 1939; Stewart and Gambino, 1961). In general, anemia increases iron absorption. Thus, iron absorption is increased in hemolytic anemia, iron-deficiency, pregnancy, and blood loss and is decreased in transfusional polycythemia, iron loading, and aplastic anemia. During early life and during periods of rapid growth, iron absorption also increases.

IV. IRON METABOLISM

A. ABSORPTION

The central role of the absorptive mechanism in iron metabolism has long been recognized but has not been clearly defined. There has recently been extensive and renewed interest in control of iron absorption as evidenced by the number of excellent reviews (Conrad, 1967; Callender, 1967; Bothwell, 1968). A critique of iron absorption studies has been published by Cook *et al.* (1969).

1. Lumenal Factors

Dietary iron is principally in the Fe^{3+} form and occurs either as organic or in-organically bound iron. A large percentage of food iron is bound to phytates and phosphates. These forms are unavailable for absorption and a number of lumenal factors affect this availability. Dietary iron must first enter the acid environment of the stomach. The acidity in the stomach is sufficient to release iron from proteins and also to maintain the available Fe^{3+} and Fe^{2+} in solution (Cook *et al.*, 1964). In this way, gastric HCl appears to potentiate Fe^{2+} absorption (Jacobs *et al.*, 1964).

The iron next passes into the alkaline environment of the small intestine. In the upper duodenum, the pH and the redox potential appear to be optimum and reducing substances such as ascorbic acid reduce Fe^{3+} to Fe^{2+} which is more soluble in the alkaline condition. These factors also help to maintain iron in the Fe^{2+} state that is available for absorption. Foods containing large amounts of oxalates, phytates, or phosphates which bind more of this iron in the duodenum may further decrease the availability of the iron. Thus, the composition of the diet as well as the amount of iron affects the availability of iron for absorption in the intestine. The pancreatic enzymes, however, do not appear to play a role (Balcerzak *et al.*, 1967).

2. Mucosal Factors

Iron in the Fe^{2+} from is known to be absorbed throughout the intestine but the transfer of iron to the plasma occurs mainly in the duodenum (Manis and Schacter, 1962). The control of body iron content is unique in that it appears to be controlled by the rate of absorption rather than by excretion. McCance and Widdowson (1937, 1938) in their well-known studies demonstrated the limited excretion of iron by animals. Later studies of Hahn *et al.* (1943) and Granick (1946) led to the "mucosal block" theory of control of iron absorption by the intestinal mucosal cell. This concept held that when all the apoferritin in the mucosal cell was saturated with iron to form ferritin, no further uptake could occur.

Therefore, the amount of apoferritin and its degree of saturation would control iron absorption (Granick, 1954). This concept did not receive experimental support (Brown et al., 1958; Chodos et al., 1957) but did provide impetus for seeking other control mechanisms for iron absorption. It has become clear from metabolic studies that iron absorption in general varies (1) inversely with the body iron stores and (2) directly with the rate of erythropoiesis. This would imply a mechanism of "feedback" control by which the absorptive process in the duodenum is governed by the body's need for iron. This concept also places the mucosal cell in a central role in the control of iron absorption and has caused renewed interest in its role.

Conrad et al. (1964) studied the incorporation of ^{59}Fe into intestinal lumen cells by autoradiography. Their studies suggested that iron is incorporated into the intestinal cells as they are being formed in the crypts of Lieberkühn. The iron stays in these cells as they migrate upward toward the top of the intestinal villus and is lost when the cell is exfoliated, if it was not transferred to the plasma. The total iron content of the cell appears to control iron uptake in an inverse manner. Since the intestinal cell turnover is about 2–3 days (Creamer, 1967), this also serves as a means of excretion of body iron. Thus, the mucosal cell once again appears to be the site of regulatory control of iron absorption and excretion, although not in the manner proposed by Granick (1954).

Iron in the mucosal cell is thought to occur in two forms: a storage or slowly turning-over pool of Fe^{3+} iron which is probably ferritin (Charlton et al., 1965), and a more rapidly turning-over "labile" pool of iron. The content of ferritin in the mucosal cell is thought to be about 8% of the total protein-bound Fe^{3+} (Pinkerton, 1969). The intake of iron occurs by two phases: phase I, absorption into the mucosal cell, and phase II, its transfer into the plasma (Wheby et al., 1964). The iron-transfer step appears to be rate-limiting because the cell increases iron absorption during periods of high lumenal content but the transfer to plasma remains constant (Manis and Schacter, 1962). The iron-transfer system is an active transport process which requires ATP and oxygen (Manis and Schacter, 1964; Jacobs et al., 1966).

Conrad and Crosby (1963) and Conrad (1967) have proposed that iron absorption is regulated primarily through the mucosal cell. According to this concept the iron deposits within the mucosal cells regulates, within limits, the amount of iron that enters the body. Mucosal cell iron may enter the body or remain in the cell to be lost when the cell is exfoliated. In iron deficiency, little iron is in the cell because of increased body requirements. Therefore, absorption is enhanced and little iron is excreted. In iron overload, iron from the body iron pool loads the mucosal cell and blocks further uptake from the intestine. When the cell is exfoliated, the excess iron is lost with it and excretion is thereby also enhanced. Pinkerton (1969) speculates that an unknown carrier substance and a hypothetical "iron transferase" enzyme participates in the transfer to the plasma at the cell membrane.

The absorption of intact heme by the mucosal cell appears to be a separate and distinct phenomena. Heme can be absorbed and transferred to the plasma intact or it can be broken down and its Fe^{2+} transported to the plasma (Conrad et al., 1966; Weintraub et al., 1968). Both mechanisms appear to operate in the dog.

3. Metabolic Factors

As previously mentioned, the rate of erythropoiesis and the state of the tissue iron stores are important stimuli for iron absorption. Accelerated erythropoiesis, whether caused by hemorrhage, hemolysis, or hypoxia, always seems to be associated with increased iron absorption. Conversely, decreased erythropoiesis diminishes absorption. Numerous studies, however, have failed to uncover a humoral or other messenger substance which links erythropoiesis or iron stores to the gut (Beutler and Buttenweiser, 1960).

B. TRANSPORT

After the movement of iron through the mucosal cell, it is rapidly and tightly bound to a specific iron-binding protein in the plasma. This protein has been called transferrin or siderophilin, has an electrophoretic mobility of β_1-globulin, and is found in Cohn's Fraction IV_7. The transferrins are actually a group of proteins distinguishable by their electrophoretic mobility on starch and are under genetic control (Smithies and Hiller, 1959). The various types of transferrins do not show differences in their iron transport functions and can therefore be considered in this discussion as a single entity with respect to iron transport.

Transferrin (T_f) is a colorless protein with a molecular weight of about 90,000 and an ability to tightly bind 2 moles of ferric iron. The Fe–transferrin (Fe–T_f) complex has a characteristic salmon-pink color which is the basis for a technique to measure the unbound transferrin in plasma (Cartwright and Wintrobe, 1949; Rath and Finch, 1949). This is usually referred to as the unbound iron-binding capacity (UIBC) and expressed as μg Fe/100 ml serum or plasma. Normally, approximately two-thirds of the T_f is unbound to iron. The other one-third is bound to Fe^{3+} and, therefore, serum iron concentration is a measure of the bound transferrin. The total iron-binding capacity (TIBC) is the sum of the serum iron concentration and the UIBC. Its major role in iron metabolism is the transport of iron to and from the various "compartments" or acceptor sites in the body. Thus, it occupies a central position in the body exchange mechanism which are shown in Fig. 1. Iron is given up by transfer at the surface of the cell membrane of receptor cells, principally those of the bone marrow for hemoglobin synthesis (see Chapter 4, Fig. 5).

C. TURNOVER

The scheme in Fig. 1 summarizes the internal iron exchange or turnover of iron in the animal body. It was evident early (McCance and Widdowson, 1937, 1938) that iron was uniquely confined or trapped in an essentially closed cycle within the body with little loss by the normal routes of excretion. It is generally accepted that about 1 mg/day is absorbed and excreted. A large percentage of the total body iron such as that contained in the intact erythrocytes, ferritin, or hemosiderin is not a readily available part of the metabolic pool. A smaller and more readily available pool of iron which is called the "labile iron pool" is also shown in Fig. 1. The concept of this "labile iron pool" has arisen largely as the result of study of intermediate iron metabolism. By analysis of radioiron turnover data, it was postulated that a small

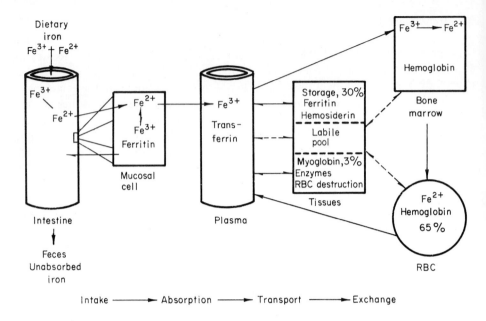

Fig. 1.   Pathways of iron metabolism. The single arrow shows a unidirectional flow of iron to emphasize the limited excretion of iron and its "closed" cycle in the body. (Kaneko, 1964, reprinted by permission.)

portion of the total body iron pool was in sufficient rapid flux with major iron metabolic sites in the body as to be considered a single pool. This pool was called the "labile iron pool" and recently Pollycove and Maqsood (1962) identified a pool of this type on the cell membranes of the immature erythrocytic bone marrow cells in the dog.

The flux of iron between the various compartments as shown in Fig. 1 is most readily studied by labeling the plasma transferrin, following the plasma disappearance and appearance of radioactivity in the various other compartments. Sophisticated analyses of these complex curves result in a description of erythropoiesis and iron metabolism in quantitative terms (Pollycove and Mortimer, 1961). The figures for the distribution of iron (Fig. 1, Table I) are in part a result of analysis of these curves. From these curves, the flux of iron in the plasma and between pools may also be calculated and some ferrokinetic data on iron turnover derived from the curves are given in Table IV.

D. STORAGE

In the tissues, iron that is not required for hemoglobin synthesis is transferred to the reticuloendothelial cells of the liver, spleen, and bone marrow for incorporation into the iron-storage compounds, ferritin and hemosiderin. Ferritin is a soluble ferric hydroxide–phosphoprotein complex consisting of apoferritin, a protein, and iron.

Ferritin is a large compound (MW 460,000) which contains about 23% Fe in the Fe^{3+} form. It is colorless, soluble, and cannot be detected by light microscope.

TABLE IV   PLASMA IRON TURNOVER (FERROKINETICS) IN DOMESTIC ANIMALS[a]

Animal	Half-time $T_{\frac{1}{2}}$ (min)	Fractional transfer rate, k (day^{-1})	Transfer rate (Tr) (mg/day)	Transfer rate (Tr) or plasma iron turnover rate (PITR)		Maximum erythrocyte ^{59}Fe uptake (% dose)	References
				Tr/kg BW (mg/kg/day)	Tr/100-ml plasma (mg/100 ml/day)		
Horse	75–103 (88.8)	(10.6)	111–153 (132)	0.45–0.65 (0.55)	0.77–1.48 (1.18)	74–77 (76)	Obara and Nakajima (1961b)
Cow	187	5.3	106	0.27	0.27	55	Kaneko (1963)
Calf	88–137 (117)	8.0–11.3 (8.7)	45–104 (74)	0.50–0.64 (0.57)	1.18–1.49 (1.30)	66–82 (73)	Kaneko and Mattheeuws (1966)
Sheep	85–110	9.9–11.7 (94)		0.42–0.65 (0.56)	1.91–2.26 (1.99)	74–87 (78)	Baker and Douglas (1957b)
Pig	43–100 (71.4)	2.3–10.0 (14.0)	(10.3)	0.40–1.66 (1.11)	1.30–4.13 (1.57)	72–100 (92)	Bush et al. (1956b)
Dog	39–63 (56)	16–40 (18.2)			1.71–2.22 (1.96)	58–93 (75)	Kaneko (1964)
Cat	(40)	(24.8)			1.75–1.86 (1.80)	19–21 (20)	Kaneko (1969)

[a]Values from the various sources have been recalculated where necessary to be consistent.

Ferritin is one of the main storage forms of iron in the body. Hemosiderin is the other major storage form. The chemical nature of hemosiderin is unclear although there is evidence that it contains ferritin (Richter, 1958). Hemosiderin differs from ferritin in that it is insoluble, contains more Fe^{3+} (25–33%), and the granules are coarse enough to be seen with the light microscope. The iron of hemosiderin is visible microscopically as blue granules after staining with Prüssian blue. The iron of ferritin and hemosiderin appears to be readily available when need occurs. The repletion of stores, however, occurs slowly.

E. EXCRETION

As previously mentioned, actual excretion of iron in the normal body amounts to no more than 1 mg/day. The large amounts of iron in the feces are almost entirely unabsorbed dietary iron. The normal routes for excretion of body iron are through the major excretory routes in the body. The very small amounts lost in exfoliated skin cells, hair, nails, milk, and urine remain relatively constant. As mentioned in Section IV, A, control of excretion may be exercised by the amount of iron contained in the mucosal cells when they are sloughed at the end of their life span. In times of need, little iron is contained in the mucosal cell and therefore little iron is lost by this route. In iron-overload, body iron moves into the mucosal cell to block further uptake and when the mucosal cell is sloughed, its iron load is also lost (Conrad and Crosby, 1963). Thus, the mucosal cell participates in iron metabolism as a major controlling mechanism of iron excretion as well as absorption.

V.   TESTS OF IRON METABOLISM

The number of laboratory tests of iron metabolism is not extensive and the most useful of these are (1) hematology, (2) serum iron, (3) iron-binding capacity, and (4) stainable iron in the bone marrow. Ferrokinetic studies utilizing ^{59}Fe permit the quantitation of iron absorption, turnover, and excretion but the technique continues to be most useful in its research applications. It will become apparent that a combination of these techniques should be employed to evaluate suspected disorders of iron metabolism.

A.   HEMATOLOGY

The hematological techniques employed for the examination of animal bloods have been described in detail by Schalm (1965). Evidence of anemia should be sought in the hemoglobin (Hb) determination, packed cell volume (PCV), and in the erythrocyte (RBC) count. The stained blood film should always be examined in particular for cell size (anisocytosis, macrocytosis, microcytosis), shape (poikilocytosis, leptocytosis), and Hb pigmentation (polychromasia, hypochromasia). From the Hb, PCV, and RBC, useful erythrocyte indices may be empirically calculated:

$$\text{Mean corpuscular volume (MCV)} = \frac{\text{PCV (\%)}}{\text{RBC (millions)}} \times 10 = \mu^3$$

Mean corpuscular hemoglobin concentration (MCHC) $= \dfrac{\text{Hb (gm/ 100 } \mu)}{\text{PCV (\%)e}} = \%$

On the basis of cell size (MCV) and hemoglobin concentration (MCHC), a morphological classification of the anemias has been devised:

MCV	MCHC
High = macrocytic	—
Normal = monocytic	Normal = normochromic
Low = microcytic	Low = hypochromic

Any combination of the above can occur and the finding of a microcytic hypochromic anemia is most commonly associated with iron deficiency and more rarely as a result of a block in heme synthesis. Thus, it can also occur in pyridoxine-responsive anemia or in copper deficiency.

B. SERUM IRON

The abundance of iron in the environment and the microgram quantities of iron in the serum require that extra care be taken in the serum iron determination. An accurate measure of iron is dependent on freedom from contamination from time of sampling to its final determination. Specially cleaned iron-free glassware should be used throughout, with extra care taken during sampling, and the use of disposable sampling equipment is to be recommended.

Most procedures for the determination of serum or plasma iron are based on the separation of the Fe^{3+} from transferrin, its reduction to Fe^{2+}, and the colorimetric determination of Fe^{2+} using such reagents as thiocyanate, o-phenanthroline, or 2, 2'-dipyridyl. The method of Peters et al. (1956) has proved to be satisfactory in our laboratories and some representative data are given in Table V.

C. UNBOUND IRON-BINDING CAPACITY

The iron-binding capacity of the serum is most often referred to as the unbound iron-binding capacity (UIBC) or the latent iron-binding capacity (LIBC). As the name implies, this represents that portion of the plasma transferrin which is not bound to Fe^{3+}, hence unbound or latent. UIBC is measured by the amount of iron that the plasma can bind and is, therefore, expressed as μg Fe/ 100 ml. Since the serum iron (SI) determination represents the portion of the transferrin which was bound to Fe^{3+}, the total iron-binding capacity (TIBC) is the sum of the SI and the UIBC.

The Fe-transferrin (Fe-T_f) complex has a characteristic salmon-pink color (Schade and Caroline, 1946) and its colorimetric determination is the basis of several methods of determination (Cartwright and Wintrobe, 1949; Rath and Finch, 1949). A more recent method (Ressler and Zak, 1958), based on iron determination, is more readily employed. The UIBC in some domestic animals is also given in Table V.

TABLE V   SERUM IRON AND UNBOUND IRON-BINDING CAPACITY IN DOMESTIC ANIMALS[a]

	Horse	Cow	Calves	Sheep	Pig	Dog	Cat
Serum iron (SI)[b]	73–140	57–162	114–170	166–222	91–199	94–122	68–215
	(111 ±11)	(97 ±29)	(148)	(193 ±7)	(121 ±33)	(108)	(140)
Unbound iron-binding capacity (UIBC)[b]	200–262	63–186	139–264		100–262	170–222	105–205
	(218 ±21)	(131 ±36)	(218)	(141 ±10)	(196 ±39)	(200)	(150)

[a]Compiled from: horse, cow, pig: Kolb (1963), Planas and De Castro (1960), Obara et al. (1957); calves (4–13 months): Kaneko and Mattheeuws (1966); sheep: Baker and Douglas (1957a,b); dog and cat: Kaneko (1964, 1969).
[b]μg/100 ml.

D. Bone Marrow Stain for Iron

The amount of hemosiderin in the body is about one-half of the storage iron. It contains more iron than ferritin (30% vs 23%) and it forms granules large enough to be seen with the light microscope. Hemosiderin appears as a dark yellowish-brown pigment. After staining with Prussian Blue, these granules are blue. The amount of hemosiderin is graded qualitatively from 0 to 4+ on a bone marrow smear with the normal amount being 2+.

The stain consists of (Davidsohn and Nelson, 1969) 4 gm potassium ferrocyanide and 20 ml distilled water. Concentrated HCl is added until a white precipitate is formed and then filtered. A marrow smear is fixed in formalin vapor for 10 minutes in a Coplin jar. The smear is flooded with the filtered stain for 30 minutes. The iron of ferritin and hemosiderin are stained blue and the amount is graded 0 to 4+.

E. Ferrokinetics

The ferrokinetic technique originally introduced by Huff *et al.* (1950) is now widely employed to study iron metabolism. In this method, the recipient's own transferrin is labeled with ^{59}Fe *in vitro* by incubating its plasma with ^{59}Fe and then reinjecting the labeled plasma intravenously. The serum iron and iron-binding capacity are determined before addition of isotope and the dosage of ^{59}Fe which does not exceed the binding capacity is added and incubated. At intervals after injection, blood

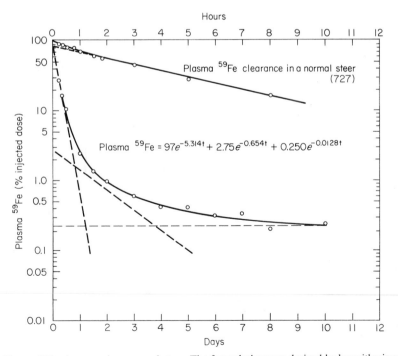

$$\text{Plasma } ^{59}\text{Fe} = 97e^{-5.314t} + 2.75e^{-0.654t} + 0.250e^{-0.0128t}$$

Fig. 2.   Plasma ^{59}Fe clearance in a normal steer. The formulation was derived by logarithmic analysis. (Kaneko, 1963, by permission.)

samples in heparin for plasma radioactivity are obtained. The time course of the plasma radioactivity is then plotted on semilogarithmic coordinates using appropriate scales (Fig. 2).

The disappearance rate during the first few minutes or hours can be used to determine the plasma volume by isotope dilution after extrapolation to time zero:

$$\text{Plasma volume (PV)} = \frac{\text{total activity injected}}{\text{activity at time zero (ml plasma)}} = \text{ml}$$

In actuality, the rate of plasma disappearance is an extremely complex curve. This curve can be resolved by logarithmic analysis as in the example in Fig. 2 where the formula of the curve is given by a 3-component polynomial expression. Each component presumably represents the relative rate of change of all ^{59}Fe atoms which are in sufficiently rapid equilibrium so as to represent a single pool of these atoms. Recently, Pollycove and Mortimer (1961) have proposed an anatomical compartmentation of these iron pools in man based on theoretical and experimental information of this type. Their mathematical formulations of the curves were of even greater complexity.

A more simplified approach to ferrokinetics has been to use only the initial rapid component of the plasma iron disappearance curve which follows the mixing period. From the half-time ($T_{\frac{1}{2}}$), the slope of the line, (k) is calculated:

$$k = \frac{0.693}{T_{\frac{1}{2}}}$$

The slope, k, represents the relative rate of change or the fraction (or number of times if greater than 1), of a pool which is transferred or replaced per unit time. This is termed the fractional transfer rate, k. The reciprocal of k, $1/k$, is then the turnover time, T_t, the time required for a complete replacement or turnover of the iron pool. The slope k, is also proportional to the transfer rate, Tr, divided by the pool size:

$$k \text{ (day}^{-1}) = \frac{\text{Tr}}{\text{pool size (mg Fe)}}$$

The plasma iron pool size is given by the product of the plasma iron concentration times the plasma volume. From the slope, k, the Tr into or out of the plasma can then be calculated and is given in mg Fe/day. If the body weight is known, it can be standardized by division:

$$\text{Tr/kg} = \frac{k \text{ (day}^{-1}) \times \text{pool size (mg Fe)}}{\text{BW (kg)}} = \text{mg Fe/kg/day}$$

This is the plasma iron turnover rate or PITR as used by Huff et al. (1950).

A more convenient standardization is to express Tr in mg Fe/100 ml plasma/day. This standardization has the advantage that the plasma volume is not required and the calculation reduces to:

$$\text{Tr/100 ml} = k \text{ (day}^{-1}) \times \frac{\text{mg Fe}}{100 \text{ ml plasma}} = \text{mg Fe/100 ml/day}$$

It should be apparent also that its accuracy is largely dependent on an accurate determination of SI. Table IV gives the plasma iron turnover data in a number of domestic animals. These turnover data are probably the most useful quantitative indices of erythropoiesis.

2. Red Blood Cell Iron Incorporation

Together with the plasma ferrokinetic studies, the rate of iron incorporation into the erythrocyte (RBCII) can also be measured by following the time course of radioactivity in the erythrocytes (Fig. 3). Pollycove and Mortimer (1961) have evaluated RBCII rate curve in their extensive mathematical treatment of these data. Under usual conditions, however, a measure of the percent incorporation into the RBC suffices for most purposes. These values are also shown in Table IV.

VI. DISORDERS OF IRON METABOLISM

Disorders of iron metabolism are a worldwide problem and the most common causes of anemia in man. In animals, dietary disorders of a similar nature are of great importance in the young, especially those on a milk-only diet. There are no indications that an animal's need for iron are grossly dissimilar to man's and the variety of disorders listed in Table VI provides some indication of the clinical biochemical significance of iron metabolism. Iron deficiency, whether from a milk-only diet in the young or induced by other causes, e.g., chronic hemorrhage, is by far the most common iron metabolic disorder. Rarely does iron overload occur.

TABLE VI   IRON METABOLISM IN VARIOUS DISEASE STATES[a]

Disease	Serum iron	Unbound iron-binding capacity	BM iron stores	Transfer rate	RBC iron incorporation
Microcytic hypochromic anemias					
Iron deficiency (chronic blood loss, dietary, etc.)	Decr	Incr	Decr	Incr	Incr
Chronic inflammation	Decr	Decr	Normal	Decr	Decr
Pyridoxine-responsive	Incr	Normal	Incr	Decr	Decr
Macrocytic anemia					
Nutritional, malabsorptive	Incr	Normal	Incr	Decr	Decr
Hemolytic anemia	Incr	Decr	Incr	Incr	Incr
Refractory anemia	Incr	Decr	Incr	Decr	Decr
Iron overload	Incr	Decr	Incr	Decr	Decr
Acute liver disease	Incr	Decr	Incr	Incr	Incr
Hypoproteinemia	Decr	Decr			
Late pregnancy	Decr	Incr	Decr	Normal	Normal
Endocrinopathy hypothyroid	Decr			Decr	Decr

[a]Compiled from Pollycove (1966) and Conrad (1967).

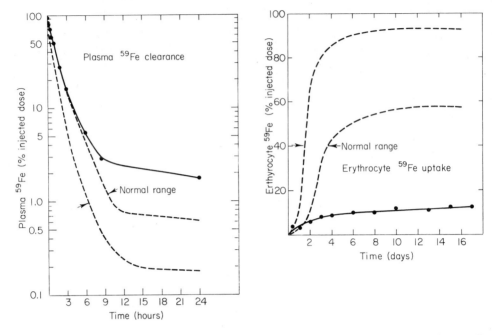

Fig. 3. Iron metabolism in dogs. The dotted lines show the normal range in dogs for plasma ^{59}Fe clearance and RBC ^{59}Fe uptake. The delayed clearance and low incorporation are evident in refractory anemia. (Kaneko, 1964, by permission.)

A. IRON DEFICIENCY

Iron deficiency is defined as a reduction in total body iron stores and depending on the degree of reduction, can be mild, moderate, or severe. Iron deficiency can be differentiated from other nutritional anemias by the finding of small, pale RBC in the blood smear or a microcytic hypochromic anemia based on the RBC indices. The extent of the morphological change depends on the degree and severity of the deficiency. In mild iron deficiency, the iron stores may be depleted and the serum iron low but morphological and hemoglobin changes have not yet occurred. In the moderate and severe deficiences, iron stores have been depleted and, with insufficient iron to meet the replacement needs for hemoglobin, anemia occurs. Thus, differentiation from other causes of anemia can be made by the finding of a decreased SI, increased UIBC, and decreased iron stores together with the microcytic hypochromic anemia.

The mechanism for iron incorporation into hemoglobin has already been described in Chapter 4. Hemoglobin synthesis has a high priority for tissue iron stores and these will be depleted to maintain normal hemoglobin.

Since iron is absorbed in only limited amounts, causes which induce excessive loss of iron also readily induce iron deficiency. In fact, in most cases, iron-deficiency anemia must be considered to be evidence of bleeding until another cause is demonstrated. Since hemoglobin contains 3.4 mg Fe/gm, the loss of 1 ml of blood (15 gm Hb/100 ml) represents the loss of about 0.5 mg Fe from the body:

$$3.4 \text{ mg Fe/gm} \times \frac{0.15 \text{ gm}}{\text{ml}} = 0.51 \text{ mg/ml}$$

This 0.5 mg/day represents about one-half or more of the normal daily iron absorption and thus chronic losses of a few milliliters per day can easily lead to iron deficiency. Bleeding can be caused by a wide variety of intestinal and external causes. Intestinal hemorrhage or loss can occur with lesions of the wall, intestinal parasites, or coagulation defects. Hookworm infestation can cause severe anemia. Conversely, failure of absorption, such as in the rare malabsorption syndromes (Kaneko *et al.*, 1965), induce iron deficiency in addition to all the other manifestations of absorptive failure.

Microcytic hypochromic anemias may also be caused by factors which block the heme synthetic pathway. Thus, in addition to iron deficiency, the anemia of chronic infection and pyridoxine-responsive anemia are usually microcytic hypochromic. A number of conditions associated with iron deficiency are given in Table VII.

Lastly, the ferrokinetic studies permit a quantitation of iron turnover. In general, increased iron turnover is associated with iron deficiency or increased erythropoiesis or both. Decreases are observed in depression of erythropoiesis (Table VI).

B. Iron Overload

Frank iron overload is a relative rarity among animals. Idiopathic hemochromatosis with hereditary implications as seen in man has not been reported to occur in animals. Iron overload, may, however, result from excessive iron therapy or as a transfusion hemosiderosis.

C. Other Disorders

Iron metabolic studies have been carried out in a number of naturally occurring and experimental disease conditions in animals, particularly in those associated with anemia. Rapid iron turnover with a degree of ineffective erythropoiesis, i.e., bone marrow hemolysis, has been observed in equine infectious anemia (Obara and

TABLE VII CONDITIONS ASSOCIATED WITH IRON DEFICIENCY

1. Excess iron loss—chronic hemorrhage
   a. Tumors associated with hemorrhage
   b. Intestinal parasites
   c. Coagulation defects
2. Deficient iron intake
   a. Dietary iron deficiency
   b. Protein deficiency
   c. Copper deficiency?
   d. Malabsorptive syndromes
3. Increased iron requirements
   a. Growth
   b. Pregnancy
4. Chronic inflammation and infection

Nakajima, 1961b). In cattle, increased iron turnover has been observed in experimental anaplasmosis (Hansard and Foote, 1959), erythropoietic porphyria (Kaneko, 1963; Kaneko and Mattheeuws, 1966), polycythemia vera (Fowler *et al.*, 1964), and familial polycythemia (Kaneko *et al.*, 1968). In studies with copper deficient Swine, Bush *et al.* (1956a) demonstrated an increased iron turnover which was in keeping with their conclusion that iron and copper metabolism were closely related in erythropoiesis. They (Bush *et al.*, 1956a) also studied iron metabolism in experimental hemolytic anemia, pyridoxine anemia, and pteroylgutamic acid deficient anemia in pigs. Iron turnover was increased in all these conditions and the rate of erythropoiesis, as might be expected, was markedly increased in hemolytic anemia, slightly increased in pteroylglutamic acid deficiency, and decreased in pyridoxine deficiency. Many iron metabolism studies have been carried out on an experimental basis but relatively few have been conducted in naturally occurring disease states in dogs. Ferrokinetic studies demonstrated increased iron turnover in hemolytic anemia and a decreased iron turnover in depression anemia (Kaneko, 1964). In a polycythemic cat, it was recently shown that iron turnover was increased (Kaneko, 1969). As pointed out earlier, the ferrokinetic studies are likely to remain as research tools in the laboratory but their use in experimental and naturally occurring disease has provided a sounder basis for evaluation of the other more readily utilized parameters of iron metabolism.

REFERENCES

Baker, N. F., and Douglas, J. R. (1957a). *Am. J. Vet. Res.* **18**, 295.
Baker, N. F., and Douglas, J. R. (1957b). *Am. J. Vet. Res.* **18**, 142.
Balcerzak, S. P., Peternel, W. W., and Heinle, E. W. (1967). *Gastroenterology* **53**, 257.
Beutler, E., and Buttenweiser, E. (1960). *J. Lab. Clin. Med.* **55**, 274.
Bothwell, T. H. (1968). *Brit. J. Haematol.* **14**, 453.
Brown, E. B., Jr., Dubach, R., and Moore, C. V. (1958). *J. Lab. Clin. Med.* **52**, 335.
Bush, J. A., Jensen, W. N., Athens, J. W., Ashenbrucker, H., Cartwright, G. E., and Wintrobe, M. M. (1956a). *J. Exptl. Med.* **103**, 701.
Bush, J. A., Jensen, W. N., Ashenbrucker, H., Cartwright, G. E., and Wintrobe, M. M. (1956b). *J. Exptl. Med.* **103**, 161.
Callender, S. T. (1967). *Brit. Med. Bull.* **23**, 263.
Callender, S. T., Mallett, B. J., and Smith, M. O, (1957). *Brit. J. Haematol.* **3**, 186.
Cartwright, G. E. and Wintrobe, M. M. (1949). *J. Clin. Invest.* **28**, 86.
Charlton, R. W., Jacobs, P., Torrance, J. D., and Bothwell, T. H. (1965). *J. Clin. Invest.* **44**, 543.
Chodos, R. B., Ross, J. F., Apt, L., Pollycove, M., and Halkett, J. A. (1957). *J. Clin. Invest.* **36**, 314
Conrad, M. E. (1967). *Borden's Rev. Nutr. Res.* **28**, 49.
Conrad, M. E., and Crosby, W. H. (1963). *Blood* **22**, 406.
Conrad, M. E., Weintraub, L. R., and Crosby, W. H. (1964). *J. Clin. Invest.* **43**, 963.
Conrad, M. E., Weintraub, L. R., Sears, D. A., and Crosby, W. H. (1966). *Am. J. Physiol.* **211**, 1123.
Cook, J. D., Brown, G. M., and Valberg, L. S. (1964). *J. Clin. Invest.* **43**, 1185.
Cook, J. D., Layrisse, M., and Finch, C. A. (1969). *Blood* **33**, 421.
Creamer, B. (1967). *Brit. Med. Bull.* **23**, 226.
Davidsohn, I., and Nelson, D. A. (1969). *In* "Todd-Sanford Clinical Diagnosis by Laboratory Methods" (I. Davidsohn and J. B. Henry, eds.), 14th ed. p, 203. Saunders, Philadelphia.
Drabkin, D. L. (1951). *Physiol. Rev.* **31**, 345.
Fowler, M. E., Cornelius, C. E., and Baker, N. F. (1964). *Cornell Vet.* **54**, 154.
Granick, S. (1946). *Science* **103**, 107.
Granick, S. (1954). *Bull. N.Y. Acad. Med.* [2] **30**, 81.

Hahn, P. F., Bale, W. F., Lawrence, E. O., and Whipple, G. H. (1939). *J. Exptl. Med.* **69**, 739.

Hahn, P. F., Bale, W. F., Ross, J. F., Balfour, W. M., and Whipple, G. H. (1943). *J. Exptl. Med.* **78**, 169.

Hansard, S. L., and Foote, L. E. (1959). *Am. J. Physiol.* **197**, 711.

Hibbs, J. W., Conrad, H. R., Vandersall, T. H., and Gale, C. (1963). *J. Dairy Sci.* **46**, 1118.

Huff, R. L., Hennessy, T. G., Austin, R. E., Garcia, J. F., Roberts, B. M., and Lawrence, J. H. (1950). *J. Clin. Invest.* **29**, 1041.

Hussain, R., Walker, R. B., Layrisse, M., Clark, P., and Finch, C. A. (1965). *Am. J. Clin. Nutr.* **16**, 464.

Jacobs, P., Bothwell, T. H., and Charlton, R. R. (1964). *J. Appl. Physiol.* **19**, 187.

Jacobs, P., Bothwell, T. H., and Charlton, R. W. (1966). *Am. J. Physiol.* **210**, 694.

Kaneko, J. J. (1963). *Ann. N.Y. Acad. Sci.* **104**, 689.

Kaneko, J. J. (1964). *13th Gaines Vet. Symp. Athens, Ga.* p. 2.

Kaneko, J. J. (1969). Unpublished data.

Kaneko, J. J., and Mattheeuws, D. R. G. (1966). *Am. J. Vet. Res.* **27**, 923.

Kaneko, J. J., Moulton, J. E., Brodey, R. S., and Perryman, V. D. (1965). *J. Am. Vet. Med. Assoc.* **146**, 463.

Kaneko, J. J., Zinkl, J., Tennant, B. C., and Mattheeuws, D. R. G. (1968). *Am. J. Vet. Res.* **29**, 949.

Kendrew, J. C., Parrish, R. G., Marrack, J. R., and Orlans, E. S. (1954). *Nature* **174**, 946.

Knoop, C. E., Krauss, W. E., and Washburn, K. G. (1935). *J. Dairy Sci.* **18**, 337.

Kolb, E. (1963). *Advan. Vet. Sci.* **8**, 49.

Layrisse, M., Cook, J. D., Martinez, C., Roche, M., Kuhn, I. N., Walker, R. B., and Finch, C. A. (1969). *Blood* **33**, 430.

Lintzel, W., and Radeff, T. (1931). *Arch. Tierernaehr. Tierzucht* **6**, 313.

McCance, R. A., and Widdowson, E. M. (1937). *Lancet* **II**, 680.

McCance, R. A., and Widdowson, E. M. (1938). *J. Physiol. (London)* **94**, 148.

Manis, J. G., and Schacter, D. (1962). *Am. J. Physiol.* **203**, 73.

Manis, J. G., and Schacter, D. (1964). *Am. J. Physiol.* **207**, 893.

Matrone, G., Conley, C., Wise, G. H., and Waugh, L. K. (1957). *J. Dairy Sci.* **40**, 1437.

Matrone, G., Thomason, E. L., and Bunn, C. R. (1960). *J. Nutr.* **72**, 459.

Moore, C. V. (1961). *Harvey Lectures* **55**, 67.

Moore, C. V., and Dubach, R. (1951). *Trans. Assoc. Am. Physicians* **64**, 245.

National Research Council (1962) *Natl. Acad. Sci.—Natl. Res. Council, Publ.* **989**.

Obara, J., and Nakajima, H. (1961a). *Bull. Natl. Instr. Animal Health (Japan)* **42**, 45.

Obara, J., and Nakajima, H. (1961b). *Japan. J. Vet. Sci.* **23**, 247.

Obara, J., Yamamoto, H., and Nakajima, H. (1957). *Bull. Natl. Inst. Animal Health (Japan)* **33**, 103.

Peters, T., Giovanniello, T. J., Apt, L., and Ross, J. F. (1956). *J. Lab. Clin. Med.* **48**, 280.

Pinkerton, P. H. (1969). *Ann. Internal Med.* [N. S.] **70**, 401.

Planas, J., and De Castro, S. (1960). *Nature* **187**, 1126.

Pollycove, M. (1966). *In* "The Metabolic Basis of Inherited Disease" (J. B. Stanbury, J. B. Wyngaarden, and D. S. Fredrickson, eds.), p. 780. McGraw-Hill, New York.

Pollycove, M., and Maqsood, M. (1962). *Nature* **194**, 152.

Pollycove, M., and Mortimer, R. (1961). *J. Clin. Invest.* **40**, 753.

Rath, C. E., and Finch, C. A. (1949). *J. Clin. Invest.* **28**, 79.

Ressler, M., and Zak, B. (1958). *Am. J. Clin. Pathol.* **30**, 87.

Richter, G. W. (1958). *J. Biophys. Biochem. Cytol.* **4**, 55.

Schade, A. L., and Caroline, L. (1946). *Science* **104**, 340.

Schalm, O. W. (1965). "Veterinary Hematology" Lea & Febiger, Philadelphia, Pennsylvania.

Smithies, O., and Hiller, O. (1959). *Biochem. J.* **72**, 121.

Stewart, W. B., and Gambino, S. R. (1961). *Am. J. Physiol.* **201**, 67.

Ullrey, D. E., Miller, E. R., Thompson, O. A., Ackerman, I. M., Schmidt, D. A., Hoefer, J. A., and Leucke, R. W. (1960). *J. Nutr.* **70**, 187.

Weintraub, L. R., Weinstein, M. B., Huser, H. J., and Rafal, S. (1968). *J. Clin. Invest.* **47**, 531.

Wheby, M. S., Jones, L. G., and Crosby, W. H. (1964). *J. Clin. Invest.* **43**, 1433.

Author Index

Numbers in italics refer to the pages on which the complete references are listed.

Challis, T. W., 238, *244*
Chamberlain, D. M., 331, *367*
Chance, R. E., 22, *49*
Chandrasekharan, K. P., 222, *225*
Chang, K. Y., 316, *367*
Channick, B. J., 277, 286, *287*
Chanutin, A., 109, *125*
Chao, K., 4, 40, *51*
Chao, P. Y., 273, *288*
Chapman, R. G., 141, *157*
Chapman, W. L., 222, *224*
Charlton, R. R., 381, *395*
Charlton, R. W., 382, *394, 395*
Chase, W. E., 109, *125*
Chen, Y. P., 211, *226*
Cheney, B. A., 321, *367*
Chernick, S. S., 25, *49*
Cherny, P. J., 61, *96*
Chernyak, N. Z., 177, *225*
Cherrick, G. R., 199, *225*
Chevallier, F., 79, *94*
Chevreul, M. E., 54, *93*
Chiaravalle, A., 166, *229*
Childs, W. A., 113, 116, *127*
Chitre, R. G., 338, *372*
Chodos, R. B., 380, 382, *394*
Chow, B. F., 109, *125*
Chrétien, M., 248, *288*
Christensen, W. R., 322, *370*
Christian, K. R., 347, 356, *367, 375*
Chute, H. L., 102, *126*
Clare, H. T., 153, *157*
Clark, A. R., 275, 277, *288*
Clark, B., 64, *93*
Clark, C. H., 102, *125*, 196, 205, 215, *224*
Clark, G. W., 318, *367*
Clark, J. D., 102, 113, 117, *125*
Clark, P., 380, *395*
Clark, S. T., 308, 309, *309, 310*
Clark, T. J., 276, 278, 285, *291*
Clarkson, M. J., 195, 196, *225*
Clegg, R. E., 100, 106, 107, 110, *125*
Clements, J. A., 55, *93*
Cline, J. J., 135, *157*
Cline, M. J., 270, 271, *288*, 299, *309*
Cochrane, D., 100, *125*
Cochrane, W. A., 39, *49*
Coffey, R. J., 241, *244*
Coffin, D. L., 243, *244, 245*, 255, 256, *288*
Cohly, M. A., 103, *128*
Coghlan, J. P., 268, 275, 277, *288*
Cohen, E., 233, *245*
Cohen, E. S., 196, *225*
Cohn, C., 189, 190, 214, *225, 230*
Cohn, M., 111, 113, 117, *126*
Cole, R., 331, *367*

Cole, H. H., 321, 330, 331, *366, 367*
Cole, P. G., 165, *225*
Cole, W. H., 109, *125*
Coleman, D. L., 137, *158*
Coleman, R., 64, *93*
Collip, J. B., 321, *374*
Colovos, N. F., 336, *367*
Colowick, S. P., 8, 23, *49*
Coltman, M., 364, *369*
Comar, C. L., 306, 307, *310*, 315, 316, 317, 344, *367, 369, 373, 375*
Comer, E. O'B., 103, *125*
Comfort, J. E., 307, *310*
Common, R. H., 107, *125*
Conley, C. L., 351, 352, *369*, 379, *395*
Conn, E. F., 83, *93*
Conn, J. W., 248, *289*
Conner, G. H., 255, 284, *291*
Conney, A. H., 14, *49*
Connors, P., 349, *375*
Conrad, H. R., 331, *367, 369, 371*, 379, *395*
Conrad, M. E., 381, 382, 386, 391, *394*
Conway, A., 360, 362, 364, *374, 375*
Cook, J. D., 380, 381, *394, 395*
Cookson, G. H., 136, *157*
Coombes, A. I., 338, *371*
Copp, D. H., 283, *290*, 321, 322, *367*
Cooper, C. W., 349, *366*
Cooper, R. W., 168, 204, 211, *229*
Cori, G. T., 4, 6, 8, 9, 23, *49*
Cornblath, M., 4, 40, *51*
Cornelius, C. E., 17, *49*, 88, *93*, 104, 112, 123, *125*, 135, 145, 149, *157, 158*, 163, 168, 169, 170, 171, 176, 179, 180, 182, 184, 186, 187, 189, 191, 192, 193, 194, 195, 196, 197, 200, 201, 202, 203, 204, 205, 206, 207, 208, 209, 210, 212, 215, 218, 220, *225, 226, 227, 228*, 303, 306, 308, *310*, 325, *374*, 394, *394*
Corner, A. H., 109, *125*
Cornwall, H. J. C., 203, 205, *227*
Correl, J. W., 72, *93*
Cos, J. J., 273, *288*
Cottereau, P., 219, 221, *225, 226*
Cotui, F. W., 29, *49*
Coupland, R. E., 273, *288*
Courtice, F. C., 301, *310*
Courtois, G., 168, 196, 197, 203, 205, 212, 217, *225*
Cowgill, G. R., 106, *125*
Cowlishaw, B., 360, *366*
Cragle, R. G., 295, *309*
Craig, P., 255, 267, 278, 279, 280, *288, 291*
Craige, A. H., 332, 339, *367*
Cream, J. J., 272, *288*
Creamer, B., 382, *394*
Cramer, C. F., 322, *367*
Cranston, W. I., 199, *230*

Subject Index